Walter F Mance

OXFORD MEDICAL PUBLICATIONS

The Genetics of
Renal Tract Disorders

OXFORD MONOGRAPHS ON MEDICAL GENETICS

General Editors:

ARNO G. MOTULSKY   MARTIN BOBROW
PETER S. HARPER   CHARLES SCRIVER

Former Editors:

J. A. FRASER ROBERTS   C. O. CARTER

OXFORD MONOGRAPHS ON MEDICAL GENETICS No 14

The Genetics of Renal Tract Disorders

M. D'A. CRAWFURD

Senior Clinical Scientific Officer,
Division of Inherited Metabolic Disease,
Clinical Research Centre, Harrow, Middlesex

Consultant Clinical Geneticist,
Kennedy Galton Centre, Northwick Park Hospital,
Harrow, Middlesex

OXFORD   NEW YORK   TOKYO
OXFORD UNIVERSITY PRESS
1988

Oxford University Press, Walton Street, Oxford OX2 6DP
Oxford New York Toronto
Delhi Bombay Calcutta Madras Karachi
Petaling Jaya Singapore Hong Kong Tokyo
Nairobi Dar es Salaam Cape Town
Melbourne Auckland
and associated companies in
Beirut Berlin Ibadan Nicosia

Oxford is a trade mark of Oxford University Press

British Library Cataloguing in Publication Data
Crawfurd, M. d'A.
The genetics of renal tract disorders. —
(Oxford monographs on medical genetics;
N. 14).
1. Kidneys — Diseases — Genetic aspects
I. Title
616.6' 1042   RC903
ISBN 0–19–261147–X

Library of Congress Cataloging in Publication Data
Crawfurd, M. d'A. (Martin d'A.)
The genetics of renal tract disorders.
(Oxford monographs on medical genetics; no. 14)
(Oxford medical publications)
Bibliography: p.
Includes index.
1. Urinary organs—Diseases—Genetic aspects.
2. Urinary organs—Abnormalities. I. Title. II. Series.
III. Series: Oxford medical publications. [DNLM:
1. Metabolism, Inborn Errors—familial &genetics.
2. Urologic Diseases—familial &genetics. WJ 101 C899g]
RC900.5.C73   1988   616.6'.042   87–15280
ISBN 0–19–261147–X

Set by Cotswold Typesetting Ltd, Cheltenham
Printed in Great Britain by St Edmundsbury Press,
Bury St Edmunds, Suffolk

Dedicated to
the memory of Lionel Penrose
who stimulated and fostered my
early interest in human genetics.

Preface

This book has been written with two groups of readers in mind. Firstly it is hoped it will prove of value to clinicians and pathologists working with renal disease whose experience of at least some forms of renal disease is inevitably limited by the nature of their specialty. The paediatrician for example will only occasionally see the early onset of adult polycystic kidney whereas the adult renal physician will seldom, if ever, meet the infantile form; likewise many severe congenital renal defects, regularly seen by the neonatal pathologist, may seldom reach the renal pathologist. By covering the diagnosis and genetics, including counselling aspects, of the whole field the book should have something to contribute to each of these groups. Secondly it attempts to provide a reference source for medical geneticists, bringing together material that is widely scattered in the literature and inadequately covered in most textbooks of renal disease. As with any monograph it will inevitably be outdated by the time it is published but this is an inescapable limitation.

An attempt has been made to cover the whole field of renal tract disorders but the exact lines of demarcation with other fields have to be arbitrary. Brief selective accounts have been included of the genetics of hypertension and of diabetes mellitus; the former remains a controversial topic and the latter is a currently developing field. Any attempt to deal fully with either would have imbalanced the book and the reader with particular interest in these subjects will find adequate accounts included in the references. The lower urinary tract malformations overlap with those of the reproductive tract. No attempt has been made to cover the various intersex states, the account being confined to those malformations involving the renal tract itself only. It is hoped that all the more important general metabolic and other systemic disorders involving the renal tract have been included but some which only do so to a minor degree have been omitted and doubtless a few will have been overlooked.

There are numerous multiple congenital anomaly, or dysmorphic, syndromes in which renal tract abnormality is either a common or only an occasional feature. These have been dealt with at relevant points in the book rather than create a 'catalogue' chapter on its own. Here too there will doubtless be disorders that have been overlooked.

A recurring problem in renal tract disorder is that of classification and the related question of genetic heterogeneity. Whenever there is controversy on these questions the differing views are presented and the reader left to form his own judgement, rather than take the dogmatic stance that would be more appropriate to an introductory or under-graduate text. Likewise alternative terms are presented where they are in current use. Fortunately, although there is some confusion over terms used in classification, and to label specific disorders, the terms used in describing pathological appearances and function are reasonably consistent.

The brief outline of human inheritance in the first chapter is included as an aide memoire for the non-geneticist and can of course be omitted by readers who do not need it. Further accounts are to be found in the chapter on genetics by R. M. Winter in the 5th edition of *Clinical physiology* by C. S. Wilcox, published by Blackwell, and more fully in J. A. Fraser Roberts' *An introduction to medical genetics*, published by Oxford University Press as a companion volume to this *Monographs in Medical Genetics* series, and in other texts included among the refer-ences at the end of the book. The clinical geneticist or scientifically qualified medical geneticist may find it helpful to read the very brief outline of renal structure and function. Fuller accounts are to be found in several standard works such as Chapter 5 of *Clinical physiology*, mentioned above, Sir Douglas Black and N. F. Jones' *Renal disease* 4th edn, published by Blackwell (1979), Seldin and Giebisch's *The kidney: physiology and pathophysiology* (1985), and de Wardener's *The kidney: an outline of normal and abnormal function*, 5th edition (1985).

In the main body of the work each disorder is briefly described with an outline of the main clinical and biochemical features and a note of the methodology used for establishing a precise diagnosis, together with appropriate histological or other illustrations. This is followed by a statement on population incidence when this has been estimated and a discussion of the genetics of the condition. The references are given at the end of each such section for ease of consultation. For details of genetic methodology the reader is referred to Professor A. E. H. Emery's book *Methodology in medical genetics,* and to Murphy and Chase's *Principles of genetic counselling.* These and further sources are listed among the references at the end of the book.

On the vexed question of the use of possessive or non-possessive forms of eponyms compromise has been adopted, retaining the older form for long established names, for example Wilson's disease, but adopting the modern American usage for more recently described disorders, for example Ivemark syndrome.

I have drawn on reviews in several early texts on renal or genetic disease, in particular Osman (1934), Gates (1946), Kemp (1951), Sorsby (1953), Touraine (1955) and Lynch and Egan (1973); and also Professor Harry Harris' review in the 3rd edition of Sir Douglas Black's book

(1976), the 4th edition of the same book, edited by Black and Jones (1979), the 2nd edition of Suki and Eknoyan (1981) and 4th and 5th editions of Stanbury *et al.* (1978, 1983) and Rubin and Barratt (1975).

London and Hertfordshire   M. d'A. C.
1987

Acknowledgements

I am grateful to: Dr R. W. E. Watts and Dr M. A. C. Ridler for their helpful comments on parts of the manuscript, and to the former for Figs 1.6 and 9.3; to Dr Ann Chandley for Fig. 1.1; and to Dr A. Price for the microscope slide for Fig. 12.1. Mr Keith Bullock kindly did the drawings for Figs 1.3–1.5, 1.7–2.6, 3.2–6.3, and 10.1; and Mrs Sheila Kingsley and Cathy Headhouse-Benson typed the manuscript. Miss Janet MacKenzie kindly undertook the photomicrography for Figs 9.2–9.5 and 12.1. I would also like to thank the Medical Research Council's Clinical Research Centre for their assistance over the typing and Oxford University Press for their patience. The author would be grateful for comments from readers on his sins of commission or omission, which are of course entirely his own responsibility.

Contents

1. Mechanism of human inheritance

1.1. HUMAN CHROMOSOME CONSTITUTION

Man is an eukaryotic organism with nucleated cells and a *diploid* chromosomal constitution. The germ cells are *haploid* with a single set of 23 chromosomes made up of 22 autosomes and an X chromosome in ova, and 22 autosomes plus an X or a Y chromosome in spermatozoa (Fig. 1.1). At fertilization the diploid state is restored with 46 chromosomes, designated 46,XY or 46,XX, one chromosome of each pair being maternally derived and the other paternally.

The development in recent years of several techniques of differential staining or banding (Fig. 1.2) has enabled the precise identification of each chromosome pair. As a result the recognition of common variants sometimes makes it possible to distinguish the maternal and paternal chromosome of a pair.

Abnormalities of chromosomal number or morphology constitute one major group of genetic disorders. Several of these include renal abnormalities as a minor part of the spectrum of abnormalities they produce and this aspect of their effects is discussed in the text. Chromosomal disorders can be diagnosed in the fetus early in pregnancy by culture and cytogenetic analysis of cells obtained by amniocentesis at about 16 weeks of pregnancy, or by chorionic villus biopsy at 8–12 weeks.

1.2. THE CHEMICAL BASIS OF INHERITANCE

Each chromosome is composed of nucleochromatin, which is itself a single long molecule of *deoxyribonucleic acid* (DNA) with associated histone and non-histone proteins. The DNA of each chromosome carries the code for the synthesis of a number of polypeptide chains by the cell and can be considered as a string of *genes*, each gene along its length being the segment of the DNA that codes for one polypeptide chain. The role of the histone and non-histone proteins is only just beginning to be understood but it is likely that they are involved in the regulation of gene action, the switching on and off of genes, both in short term regulation and in permanent differentiation during development.

1

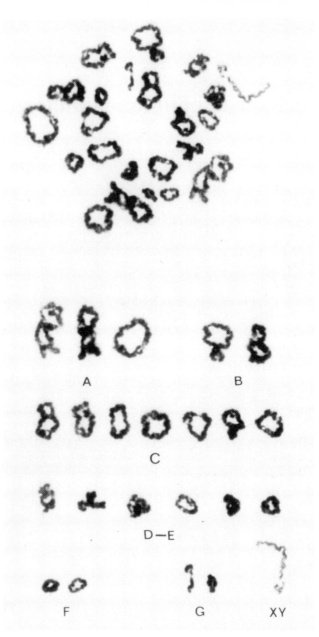

Fig. 1.1. The 22 autosomal bivalents and the XY bivalent from a cell at the diakinesis stage of meiosis from a normal male. Kindly provided by Dr Ann Chandley.

Group	Chromsome pairs	Group	Chromosome pairs
A	1–3	E	16–18
B	4 and 5	F	19 and 20
C	6–12	G	21 and 22
D	13–15		

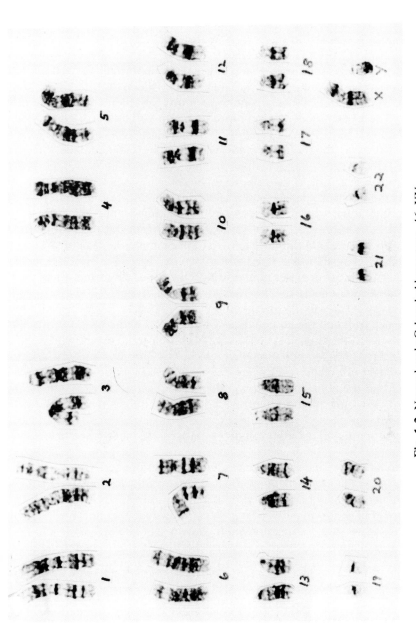

Fig. 1.2. Normal male G-banded karyotype, 46, XY.

1.3. MENDELIAN INHERITANCE IN MAN

Since the chromosomes are paired the genes must also be paired, the analogous genes at the same *locus* on the two chromosomes of a pair being termed *alleles*. These alleles frequently exist in alternative forms, which may be common or rare, normal or abnormal. A well-known example of common, normal variants are the alleles of the ABO blood group system, and one of a common abnormal variant is the sickle cell gene. The existence of two or more common variants at a given locus constitutes a *polymorphic system* or polymorphism, which, at least where one of these is functionally abnormal, can only be maintained through some selective advantage, such as the increased resistance of individuals with sickle cell trait to malaria. Rare variants are largely maintained by fresh mutation, such, for example, as that for adult polycystic kidneys.

An individual who possesses two identical alleles at a given locus is said to be *homozygous*, as for example two O genes at the ABO locus; one who possesses different alleles, as for example the A and B alleles for the ABO system, is termed *heterozygous*. The two alleles at a locus, whether identical or different, constitute the *genotype* at that locus, and their observed effects the *phenotype*. The genotype OO results in the phenotype 'O'; similarly the genotype β^A/β^S results in the phenotype sickle cell trait and the homozygous β^S/β^S results in the phenotype sickle cell disease. For a gene carried on the X chromosome males, who do not have a second corresponding allele on their Y chromosome, are said to be *hemizygous*. Genes producing disease may do so in both the hetero-zygote and the abnormal homozygote and are then termed *dominant*, or may do so only in the abnormal homozygote when they are termed *recessive*.

Fully dominant disorders show a pattern of inheritance from one generation to another with transmission of the gene by affected individuals only and with both sexes equally affected (Fig. 1.3). On average half the offspring of an affected person will also be affected. This classic pattern may be modified by a number of factors. Some dominant diseases fail to be manifested in every individual carrying the gene in heterozygous state, a phenomenon known as *incomplete penetrance*. Such non-manifesting heterozygotes nevertheless still transmit the gene and can give rise to the apparent 'skipping' of a generation. Diseases in which this may occur include retinoblastoma and myotonic dystrophy. Many dominant disorders become manifest at some stage of life after birth, for example adult polycystic kidney usually appears in late childhood or early adult life, and Huntington's chorea usually in early middle age. With such disorders one cannot be sure that a patient at risk of developing the disease will not do so until he or she is past the

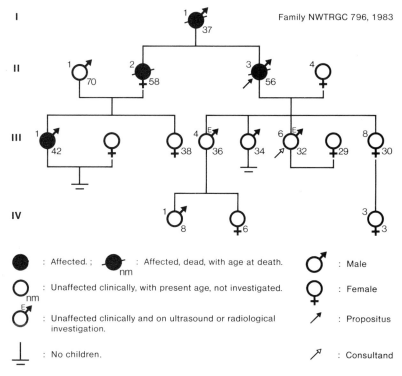

Fig. 1.3. Pedigree illustrating autosomal dominant inheritance of adult polycystic kidney disease.

maximum age of onset. There are frequently also significant correlations in age of onset between close relatives. These considerations affect genetic advice for such diseases. It must also be remembered that for many severe dominant disorders a high proportion of cases are sporadic, due to fresh mutation. In apparently sporadic cases it is important to examine, and if necessary investigate, the parents very carefully before giving genetic advice in case an affected parent has not been diagnosed, as for example in tuberose sclerosis. Very rarely when a couple who both have the same dominant disorder have children an affected homozygote is produced in whom the disease is almost invariably far more severe than in the heterozygote.

A quite different pattern of inheritance is seen with autosomal recessive diseases. In this situation the heterozygote is a clinically normal carrier of the gene and only the homozygote is affected. This results in the appearance of the disease in one or more children of a single sibship whose parents are normal (Fig. 1.4). Most such diseases are rare but

Pedigree

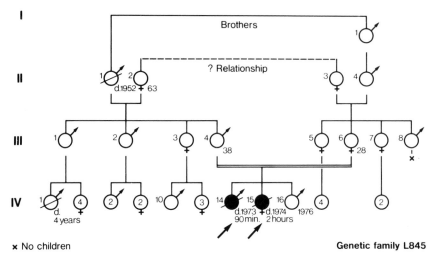

x No children   Genetic family L845

Fig. 1.4. Pedigree illustrating autosomal recessive inheritance of Meckel's syndrome. Symbols: ♂=male, ♀=female, ●=affected, ○=unaffected clinically, with present age, ∅=dead. From Crawfurd *et al.* (1978) *J. Med. Genet.* **15**, 242, with permission from the *Journal of Medical Genetics.*

there are a great many of them, nearly 1300 being listed in McKusick's catalogue (McKusick 1983). The two sexes are equally affected and, on average, one child in four of two heterozygous parents is affected. When the disease is rare there is an increased incidence of parental consanguinity, most often a first-cousin relationship. This increased parental consanguinity is not seen with common recessive disorders, such as cystic fibrosis of the pancreas, which affects about 1 in 2000 live-born children in the United Kingdom with a heterozygote frequency of 1 in 22. Instead an increased incidence of affected first cousins is observed.

The question as to why certain mutations result in a phenotype with dominant inheritance and others result in a recessive pattern has not been fully answered. To some extent the distinction is an artifact of the method of observation. For example if the occurrence of sickle cell disease in a community is observed clinically then the expression of the sickle gene is seen to follow a recessive pattern, only affected homozygotes being observed, but if all individuals are screened by a red-cell sickling test or by haemoglobin electrophoresis then heterozygotes as well as homozygotes are seen and by these criteria the expression of the gene is dominant. In another sense there is a real difference which probably reflects the function of the protein encoded by the gene. Apart from the porphyrias and some lipoprotein disorders virtually all inborn errors of metabolism are recessive, either autosomal or X-linked recessive. In this group of diseases the basic defect is a failure to synthesize an active enzyme through non-synthesis or more often synthesis of an altered inactive enzyme. Studies by Kacser and Burns (1973) and by Rapoport *et al.* (1976) have shown that for most metabolic steps the reduction of the normal level of enzyme activity by a half has little, if any, effect on flux of the metabolite catalysed, hence the recessive pattern. The defective protein in dominant disorders has with few exceptions not been identified. However, from the observed phenotype of dominant disorders, we can conjecture that some of them will involve structural proteins of the membrane or other cellular organelles and that some others will involve proteins involved in the direction of differentiation. In both of these situations it is likely that a significant reduction in the amount of normal protein synthesized would have clinically observable effects.

A third type of inheritance is that associated with genes on the X chromosome. As with autosomal genes, the expression of X-linked genes may be dominant or recessive. X-linked dominant diseases, which are comparatively few, show a pattern of inheritance in which affected women transmit the disease to half of their children of both sexes but affected males transmit it to all their daughters but none of their sons (Fig. 1.5). An apparent exception to this rule is seen in diseases that appear to affect only females. This arises from lethality of the gene in hemizygous males resulting in their early spontaneous abortion. In X-linked recessive diseases (Fig. 1.6), typified by haemophilia, only the hemizygous male and the exceedingly rare homozygous female are affected. Heterozygous females are symptomless carriers of the gene who transmit the gene to, on average, half their sons and half their daughters. The former are affected and the latter are again carriers. In those diseases in which the affected males survive to have children all their daughters are carriers but their sons are unaffected. With X-linked recessive diseases it is often possible to investigate female relatives on the maternal side to determine whether or not they are heterozygous and, therefore, at risk of having affected sons. The degree of expression of the gene in such female heterozygotes shows considerable variation as a result of chance variation in different tissues in the proportion of cells in which the X-chromosome bearing the normal or the abnormal gene is inactivated (Lyon 1961). In those families with a sporadic case of an affected male, investigation of the mother and other female relatives on her side of the family will sometimes indicate whether or not the single case is due to a fresh mutation or inheritance.

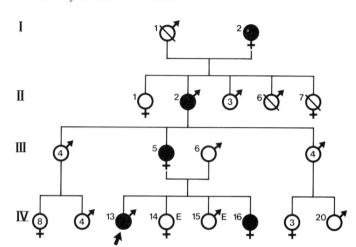

● Affected (I 2: reliably reported; II 2: skeletal disease observed; III 5,
  IV 13 and 16: skeletal disease and hypophosphataemia observed.)

Fig. 1.5. Pedigree illustrating X-linked dominant inheritance of familial hypo-phosphataemia (vitamin-D-resistant rickets). Symbols: ♂=male, ♀=female, Ø=dead, E=normal on examination. From Burnett *et al.* (1964) *Am. J. Med.* **36,** 222, with permission from the *American Journal of Medicine.*

1.4. EARLY PRENATAL DIAGNOSIS

With an increasing number of metabolic disorders, whether autosomal or X linked, it is becoming possible to determine at about 16–18 weeks of pregnancy whether or not a fetus carried by a mother at risk is affected or not. In most cases this requires culture of amniotic cells followed by specific enzyme assay but in a few the diagnosis can be made by chemical analysis of the supernatant amniotic fluid.

In the last few years it has become possible to diagnose haemoglobin disorders using recombinant DNA techniques from samples of fetal blood taken by the technique of fetoscopic aspiration. Recombinant DNA techniques are now being extended to inborn errors of metabolism generally and to other single gene, and perhaps eventually even polygenic, defects (Emery 1981, 1984; Weatherall 1982). Many inborn errors of metabolism can also be diagnosed prenatally by chorionic villus biopsy in the first trimester, either by recombinant DNA methods on the uncultured villus sample or by enzyme assay on the cultured or uncultured tissue.

Other techniques that can be used in early antenatal diagnosis include direct viewing of the fetus through a fetoscope to detect external

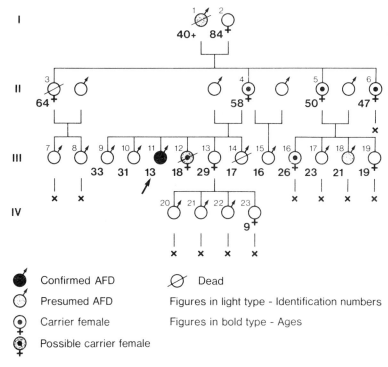

Fig. 1.6. Pedigree illustrating X-linked recessive inheritance of Anderson–Fabry disease (AFD) (Angiokeratoma corporis diffusum). Symbols: X=no children. Kindly provided by Dr R. W. E. Watts.

morphological abnormalities, and ultrasound that will detect a variety of external or internal morphological defects such as neural tube defects or polycystic kidneys. In all these cases the aim is to terminate the pregnancy if severely handicapping fetal abnormality is established but otherwise to allow it to continue. In the case of severe X-linked recessive disorders that cannot be diagnosed prenatally, a possible alternative is to determine fetal sex and terminate if it is male.

1.5. RECOMBINANT DNA GENETICS

The last few years have seen the rapid development of a range of new genetic techniques that involve working with DNA itself. Many of these techniques make use of DNA probes in which a sequence of DNA of interest is incorporated into a viral genome or plasmid to form a recombinant DNA genome that can be propagated in a bacterium.

Weatherall (1982) has used the term 'New Genetics' in an excellent review of the subject. When used to study the molecular basis of human disease, or simply for pre- or postnatal diagnosis of homozygotes or heterozygotes for inherited diseases, the usual approach is fairly straightforward. Because the DNA is being analysed, rather than the gene product, any cell line and not just those expressing the gene concerned may be used. Moreover, although it is an advantage in developing DNA methods for the study of a particular disease to know and be able to isolate the gene product, this is not essential. Indeed, in a disease for which the search for the basic protein defect has been very elusive, such as cystic fibrosis, it may prove easier to isolate the gene first and work back from that to the gene product. This may well be the case for many inherited renal diseases such as adult and infantile polycystic kidney, Alport's disease, and congenital nephrosis.

The key to studying any disease at the molecular level is to obtain a specific DNA probe or probes. These may be derived from genomic DNA or made from complementary DNA (cDNA), the latter being the most frequently used. If the gene product can be isolated and purified specific DNA probes can be prepared in several ways. One is to prepare an antibody to the gene product and use this to isolate polysomes on which the nascent protein is being synthesized. These will carry the specific mRNA, which in turn can be used as the substrate for a viral reverse transcriptase that will make a cDNA complementary to the mRNA. Another method is to undertake an amino acid sequence of the protein gene product and then synthesize short oligonucleotides that would code for a short part of the sequence obtained. The most efficient of these can then be used as the final probe. Alternatively, cloned fragments of total nuclear, genomic DNA can be screened for variant forms that segregate in families in linkage with the disease, or if the specific mRNA is available hybridize to it. One refinement of this procedure, if the gene has been assigned to a specific chromosome, is to first sort that chromosome on a fluorescence-activated cell sorter and then use the DNA of the sorted chromosomes. Theoretically, specific mRNA itself could be used as a probe, but this cannot be so readily propagated as can DNA.

Once a suitable probe has been obtained the steps in its use for diagnostic purposes are illustrated in Fig. 1.7. Firstly DNA is extracted from cells obtained from patients or their relatives, along with normal subjects as controls. The cells used may be peripheral blood lymphocytes or cultured lymphoblastoid or fibroblast cell lines postnatally, or cultured amniotic fluid cells or uncultured trophoblast obtained by chorionic villus biopsy prenatally. Secondly the extracted DNA is fragmented into relatively short segments. The usual method of doing

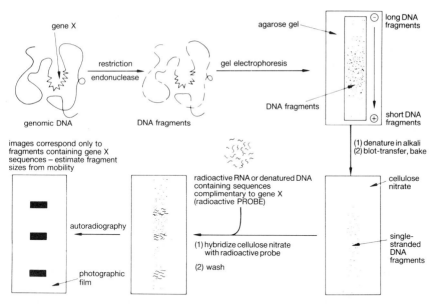

Fig. 1.7. Diagram to illustrate restriction enzyme digestion, agarose electrophoresis, Southern blotting and autoradiography of genomic DNA sequences. From *Principles of gene manipulation*, 2nd edn. by R. W. Old and S. B. Primrose, (1981), with permission from Blackwell Scientific Publications and Professor Old.

this is to use bacterial endonucleases that cleave DNA only at specific nucleotide sequences. Such enzymes are often referred to as restriction enzymes and digestion of aliquots of DNA from the same sample with them will yield identical fragments. The third step is to separate these fragments according to their length by electrophoresis in agarose gels. The next step is the well-known Southern blot, named after Dr Ed Southern who described it. This consists in transferring the DNA in the gel to a nitrocellulose filter by drawing it in buffer from the gel to the filter laid on top by means of many layers of absorbent paper laid on top of the gel and filter. The DNA binds to the filter and is subsequently permanently fixed to it by heat treatment. The fifth step is incubation of the DNA or cDNA probe, usually labelled with a high activity radioactive isotope, with the filter. During this procedure the single stranded probe will hybridize to any complimentary sequence in the single-stranded denatured DNA on the filter. In the sixth and final step any such hybridization is revealed by autoradiography.

More sophisticated procedures may involve isolation of a DNA sequence of interest and the determination of its nucleotide sequence.

Once this is done the amino acid sequence of the protein product can be predicted, and indeed synthesized in a cell-free system.

The advent of recombinant DNA techniques has given new clinical relevance to the phenomenon of genetic linkage. A few of the DNA probes in use hybridize to the coding sequences (exons) of a specific gene within the cellular DNA, or to intervening sequences within the gene between the coding sequences (introns). Where a mutational site involves a recognition sequence for a restriction enzyme, or a whole gene is deleted, such probes will detect mutations associated with inherited disease. A good example is a probe used in conjunction with the restriction enzyme MstII (Chang *et al.* 1982) which normally cuts the DNA at the site of the nucleotide involved in the β^S mutation in sickle cell disease. In the presence of β^S DNA the enzyme fails to cut the DNA at this point, giving rise to a fragment larger than that normally recognized by the probe. A type of mutation recognized in some forms of thalassaemia occurs within an intron and may result in a defect in the splicing together of the transcribed exons to form the messenger RNA. However, the majority of DNA probes currently being used to detect mutant forms of human DNA associated with inherited disease recognize normal DNA variants or polymorphisms (restriction fragment length polymorphisms) within the non-coding sequences flanking the gene of interest. If such a polymorphism is sufficiently close to the gene to be unlikely to be separated from it by crossing over (or *recombination*) during gametogenesis it may be useful as a diagnostic marker of the disease. Better still two DNA polymorphisms, one either side of the gene concerned, will greatly reduce the chance of unrecognized recombination.

It is important to appreciate that although these methods provide potentially powerful and precise tools their clinical application is at present limited. A probe for the mutant gene itself will only distinguish a mutant form causing disease from other variants, normal or disease producing, if there is a restriction enzyme which will cleave at the site of the mutation, or a deletion causing loss of a restriction site or large enough to interfere with hybridization. Such situations prevail for sickle cell disease and some of the common forms of thalassaemia. Less common inherited diseases are likely to be highly heterogeneous, with many different mutations of their genes being found in different families so that in only a few instances would such favourable situations prevail. One possible future answer to this problem may be the production of a range of synthetic oligonucleotide probes for each disease, each probe being specific for a known mutation.

With the more widely used approach of probes recognizing normal DNA polymorphisms linked to the disease gene, the problem of the heterogeneity of the mutations responsible is avoided but a new problem is introduced. This is that the probe will only provide useful information in a particular family if the potentially informative relatives are heterozygous so that segregation of the polymorphism, and of the disease gene with it, may be observed. The value of a particular polymorphism will depend on its closeness to the disease gene and the frequencies of its variant forms when analysed with particular restriction enzymes. In consequence it will often be the case that when a recombinant DNA method of diagnosis is available it cannot be applied to a particular family. The proportion of families who can be helped will increase as more polymorphisms are discovered, and these are located closer to the disease gene, especially if they lie either side of it. When eventually such polymorphisms have been detected at close intervals all along each human chromosome then mapping of inherited diseases will be relatively easy, and it may become feasible to analyse genetic predisposition to the multifactorially determined disorders discussed below.

1.6. LINKAGE, ASSIGNMENT, AND SYNTENY

Genes, or specific DNA sequences, shown to be on the same chromosome are said to be *syntenic*. Assignments of genes to specific chromosomes may be made in several ways. The demonstration of X- or Y-linked inheritance of course assigns a gene to the X or Y chromosome, as for example X-linked inheritance of haemophilia or Y-linked inheritance of variation in the length of the heterochromatic region of the Y chromosome. The demonstration of linkage of a gene to another gene already assigned to a specific chromosome is a second method. Direct assignment, to a whole chromosome or regional assignments to part of a chromosome, may be made by a variety of techniques including somatic cell hybridization, *in situ* DNA hybridization, assignment using chromosomal translocations, deletion mapping, and other methods. There are now regional assignments of genes and DNA sequences for each of the human chromosomes (Human Gene Mapping 7 1984) for a total of over 500 separate loci.

The demonstration that two or more genes are syntenic does not imply that they are genetically linked. Indeed most syntenic genes will be sufficiently far apart that they are as likely to be separated by crossing over at meiosis as not. That is, their inheritance together from a parent carrying both genes is no more likely than if they were on different chromosomes.

At the opposite extreme two genes may be so close together on the same chromosome as virtually never to be separated at meiosis, that is never to show recombination. They are said to show complete linkage and to have a recombinant frequency of zero. In between there are varying degrees of linkage from the maximum at recombinant frequency of 0 to no linkage at 50 per cent (0.5) recombination. In family studies account has to be taken of the fact that the two genes under study, present in the same individual, may if linked be on the same chromosome (linkage in coupling), or on opposite chromosomes of a pair (linkage in repulsion). A study of the two, or better three or more, generation distribution of the gene within a family will establish the phase. By scoring the number of recombinants for the two genes in a large number of families the probability of linkage at a range of recombinant frequencies (lod score) can be calculated. If such a study shows a DNA polymorphism to be closely linked to a disease gene then that polymorphism can be used for diagnosis. For example a study of two families with Huntington's chorea found close linkage to a DNA polymorphism on chromosome 4 (Gusella *et al.* 1983). If further studies with this probe, currently under way, confirm close linkage then the probe will not only have assigned the Huntington's chorea gene to chromosome 4, but will provide a means of diagnosing presymptomatic carriers and of prenatal diagnosis. In due course comparable probes should become available for the diagnosis of at least some of the more common inherited renal diseases such as Alport's disease, and indeed has already been reported for adult polycystic kidney disease. In some diseases the use of DNA probes for diagnosis may be simplified if there is linkage disequilibrium between the disease gene and the DNA marker. This is the case when the abnormal allele occurs with greater frequency than would be expected in association with just one of the alternative alleles of the polymorphic marker locus, as for example was found in sickle cell disease.

1.7. GENETICS OF COMMON DISEASES

In the very large group of common diseases and congenital malformations not showing Mendelian inheritance there is nevertheless often an increased incidence of the disorder among close relatives. Evidence from family and twin studies often indicates that at least part of this familial occurrence is genetically determined. Usually the aetiology is complex, with the genetic component due to the action of several mostly unidentified genes, each playing a small part in predisposing to the disease rather than directly determining it. The importance of genetic factors may be high, as with idiopathic severe mental subnormality and maturity onset diabetes mellitus, or low, as in most forms of congenital heart disease.

It is likely that little progress will be made in understanding these diseases until at least some of the specific genes and environmental factors involved are identified. An important step in this direction is the discovery that certain diseases show an association with specific HLA antigens, as for example that of juvenile ketotic diabetes with HLA-B8, DW3 and DW4 (see Chapter 8 and leading article, BMJ 1980). Another is the separation of disorders with a specific aetiology from a large heterogeneous group of disorders. Examples include the recognition of mental retardation due to maternal phenylketonuria or to the fragile X syndrome, and the more recent recognition of familial hypercholesterol-aemia and hyperlipidaemia type III as causes of early onset ischaemic heart disease. These latter examples are potentially of great clinical importance as the recognition of individuals with a high degree of genetic predisposition enables preventive measures to be concentrated on those individuals for whom they will be most effective.

1.8. GENETIC COUNSELLING

Genetic counselling (Harper 1984), that is, giving families advice on the risks of developing or transmitting specific disorders and on prenatal diagnosis or other options, is based on a three-step process. The first, and most important, step is that of diagnosis of the disorder present in the family. This may be purely clinical, as in the recognition and diag-nosis of dysmorphic syndromes (see Smith 1982), or may involve radio-logical, histological, biochemical, cytogenetic, or other investigations. Such investigations may involve symptomless relatives, for diagnosis of the carrier state, as well as affected family members. Because of the over-riding importance of accurate diagnosis genetic counselling should always be undertaken by medically qualified persons in the first instance. The second step is that of obtaining a full family history. When the diag-nosis and family history together indicate a simply inherited disorder then the third step, that of assessing recurrence risk, can be based on straightforward deduction on the basis of mendelian inheritance.

In the case of an autosomal dominant disorder, the prima facie risk of inheriting the gene and developing the disease for a child of an affected individual will be 1 in 2, because the affected individual carries one disease allele and one normal allele with equal chances of transmission. This *a priori* 1 in 2 risk may have to be modified where there is known to be incomplete penetrance, that is, carriers who never manifest the disease, sex influence on expression, or late onset. In this last case the older the at-risk subject becomes without developing signs of the disease the less likely it becomes that he or she will eventually do so. This is well exemplified by Huntington's chorea with onset typically in the fourth to fifth decade. In dominant diseases with incomplete penetrance or late onset there may be specific tests, ranging from clinical methods like the use of audiometry to recognize deafness in Alport's disease, through ultrasound to detect cystic kidneys or enzyme assays for inborn errors of metabolism, to the use of DNA probes for the gene itself or a linked flanking marker, that will diagnose the asymptomatic or presymptomatic carrier.

In autosomal recessive disorders both parents are heterozygotes, each with an equal chance of transmitting the normal or abnormal allele. Hence for any future child of such a couple, usually detected through the previous birth of an affected child, the risk of inheriting the disease determining gene from both parents and of being an affected homozygote is 1 in 4. Carrier detection tests may identify heterozygous relatives, including phenotypically normal children, other than the parents.

The position for X-linked diseases is more complex. Where a woman is known to be a heterozygous carrier, from pedigree evidence such as having had two affected sons, or one affected son and one or more affected male relatives on her maternal side, or from the evidence of biochemical or other investigations, then the risk that any future son will be affected, or daughter be a carrier, is 1 in 2. When a woman has had one affected son and has had no other affected relative she may be a carrier or her son may have a fresh mutation. Since one-third of sporadic cases of lethal X-linked diseases are fresh mutations the *a priori* risk that the mother is a carrier is two-thirds. However, various independent sources of information may modify this risk, for example pedigree evidence, such as unaffected brothers of the affected boy or other unaffected male relatives on the maternal side, or quantitative results of carrier detection tests. Using Bayesian probability methods a final probability of heterozygosity, allowing for all conditional information, can be calculated for the mother or any other female relative, such as a sister or an aunt. A detailed exposition of Bayesian methods, which is beyond the scope of this book, is given by Murphy and Chase (1975).

Where the disorder does not appear to be so inherited then risks are determined empirically. By this is meant estimation of risks from the observation of the frequency of recurrence in a sufficiently large number of relevant families in like circumstances. Such risks are to be found in published papers and monographs (for example see Harper 1984), but judgement has to be exercised in interpreting these in individual con-sultations, both in deciding on the proper figures to quote and in interpreting their significance to the family. Finally, as discussed above, the position regarding prenatal diagnosis or other possible measures such as adoption or artificial insemination has to be explained. The essential point is that the counsellor is helping the family to take decisions in the light of the best available information rather than directing them as to what they should do.

References

British Medical Journal (leading article) (1980). HLA and disease. *Br. Med. J.* **2**, 1485–6.

Chang, J. C., Golbus, M. S. and Kan, Y. W. (1982). Antenatal diagnosis of sickle cell anaemia by sensitive DNA assay. *Lancet* **1**, 1463.

Emery, A. E. H. (1981). Recombinant DNA technology. *Lancet* **2**, 1406–9.

—— (1984). *An introduction to recombinant DNA*. John Wiley, Chichester.

Gusella, J. F., Wexler, N. S., Conneally, P. M., Naylor, S. L., Anderson, M. A., Tanzi, R. E., Watkins, P. C., Ottinak, K., Wallace, M. R., Sakogachi, A. Y., Young, A. B., Shoulson, L., Bonilla, E. and Martin, J. B. (1983). A polymorphic DNA marker genetically linked to Huntington's disease. *Nature* **306**, 234–8.

Harper, P. S. (1984). *Practical genetic counselling*, 2nd edn. John Wright Bristol.

Human Gene Mapping 7 (1984). Seventh International Workshop on Human Gene Mapping. *Cytogenet. Cell Genet.* **37**, Nos. 1–4.

Kacser, H. and Burns, J. A. (1973). The control of flux. *Symp. Soc. Exp. Biol.* **27**, 65–104.

Lyon, M. (1961). Gene action in the X-chromosome of the mouse (*Mus musculus* L.). *Nature* **190**, 372–3.

McKusick, V. A. (1983). *Mendelian inheritance in man*, 6th edn. The Johns Hopkins University Press, Baltimore.

Murphy, E. A. and Chase, G. A. (1975). *Priciples of genetic counselling*. Year Book Medical Publishers, Chicago.

Rapoport, T. A., Heinrich, R. and Rapoport, S. M. (1976). The regulatory principles of glycolysis in erythrocytes *in vivo* and *in vitro*. A minimal comprehensive model describing steady states, quasi-steady states and time dependent processes. *Biochem. J.* **154**, 449–69.

Smith, D. W. (1982). *Recognizable patterns of human malformation*, 3rd edn. W. B. Saunders, Philadelphia, London and Toronto.

Weatherall, D. J. (1982). *The new genetics and clinical medicine*, Nuffield Provincial Hospitals Trust, London.

2. Normal renal structure and function

2.1. EMBRYOLOGY

The renal tract is of largely mesodermal origin, the kidney itself developing from the mesoderm of the nephrogenic portion of the inner cell mass which gives rise to the nephrogenic cord. This in turn evolves cranially into the rudimentary tubules of the pronephros and mesonephros and caudally into the metanephros or permanent kidney. The nephric or Wolffian duct develops from local mesoderm between the ninth and fourteenth somites in relation to the pronephric nephrons, which in fact fail to canalize and subsequently degenerate.

In the 3 mm embryo the thoracic region of the inner cell mass gives rise to the mesonephros. At the same time cord-like condensations form, and later canalize and fuse with the Wolffian duct laterally, and are invaginated medially by glomerular tufts of capillaries to form Malphigian corpuscles. Mesonephic tubules elongate and become convoluted in a manner similar to that of the proximal convoluted tubule of the adult kidney. By the 7 mm embryo stage there are 32 mesonephric tubules apparent, which extend caudally as far as the third lumbar segment. These, like their pronephric precursors, also degenerate. This takes place in a caudal direction and is complete by the time the embryo reaches 21 mm in length, apart from those tubules that become associated with gonads.

The metanephros comprises that part of the developing kidney caudal to the third lumbar segment. It is formed from two main components: the ureteric bud and the nephrons. The ureteric bud develops from a primitive nephric duct. It grows dorsally and caudally to enter the lower end of the nephrogenic cord where it expands to form the renal pelvis. In its vicinity a mesodermal condensation, the metanephric blastema, forms through induction by the ureteric bud. In turn the blastema induces terminal branching of the bud from which primary tubules grow out into the metanephric tissue. From the primary tubules successive generations of tubules (ureteric trees) develop eventually into a lobulated organ composed of a series of pyramids. Each pyramid contains collecting tubules opening into the papillary ducts, which in turn open into minor calyces and finally major calyces. The nephrons are induced in metanephrogenic tissue by mesodermal condensation in relation to terminal tubules of the ureteric bud. They start as small vesicles that elongate to form metanephric tubules. Further elongation and convolution lead to distal contact with ureteric tubules and eventual fusion. At the same time the proximal end of the nephron thins, its epithelium becoming columnar to squamous. Adjacent to this proximal development a mesodermal condensation appears in which vascular spaces develop, which unite to form the capillaries of the glomerulus and join extraglomerular cortical capillaries, which in turn link up with afferent and efferent arterioles. The squamous epithelium of the tubule envelopes the glomerular capillary tuft to form Bowman's capsule. The rest of the tubule evolves further into the proximal and distal tubules and the loop of Henle.

A short, readable account of renal embryology is given by Winick and McCrory (1968), and Stephens (1983) also describes the normal embryology of the kidney, ureter, bladder, and cloaca in the relevant chapters of his book.

2.2. ANATOMY

The gross anatomy of the kidney is illustrated in Fig. 2.1. The renal columns of cortical tissue dip down between the pyramids. The ratio of pyramids to papillae to minor calyces is approximately 3:2:1. The calyceal-lining epithelium is continuous with that of the collecting tubules, that is to say that the papillae invaginate the calyces. The external layer of each minor calyx fuses with the renal capsule, and the

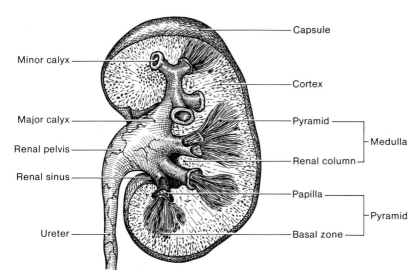

Fig. 2.1. The gross anatomy of the kidney.

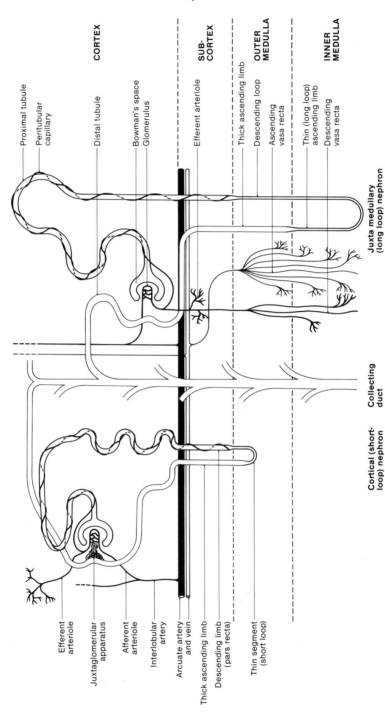

Fig. 2.2. The relation of nephrons and their collecting ducts to their vascular supply and to the zones of the kidney. Adapted from Figures 6 and 15 in *The mammalian kidney*, by D. B. Moffat (1975), with the permission of Cambridge University Press and Professor Moffat.

spaces between the minor calyces, the renal sinuses, are covered by renal capsule.

The dissected histological structure of a single collecting duct and two of its associated nephrons, one cortical and the other juxtamedullary, is illustrated in Fig. 2.2. In both types of nephron there is a Malpighian corpuscle composed of a glomerulus, that is, a tuft of 20 to 40 capillary loops supplied by a single afferent arteriole and rejoining to form a single efferent arteriole, and its enveloping Bowman's capsule. In both types the capsule is continued as a proximal tubule, a loop of Henle, and a distal tubule that drains into a collecting duct. There are, however, important distinctions between the two types.

Cortical nephrons have a glomerulus, situated in the outer two-thirds of the cortex, with a muscular afferent arteriole and a juxtaglomerular apparatus involving a specialized region of their distal tubule. The afferent arteriole and apparatus receive sympathetic innervation. Their efferent arteriole gives off peritubular capillary and cortical branches. Some glomeruli contain granular peripolar cells. Although they do not themselves contain renin they are found in close anatomical relationship to the renin-containing cells of the juxtaglomerular apparatus (Gardiner and Lindop 1985) and hence may play some part in the regulation of renin secretion. The loops of Henle of the cortical nephrons dip only a short distance into the medulla. The structure of the juxtaglomerular apparatus is shown in Fig. 2.3. It consists of the afferent and efferent arterioles of the glomerulus, lacis cells filling the space between the two

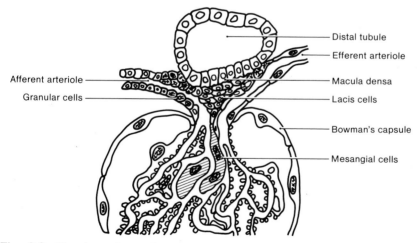

Fig. 2.3. The juxtaglomerular apparatus. Adapted from Figure 74 in *The mammalian kidney* by D. B. Moffat (1975), with the permission of Cambridge University Press and Professor Moffat.

arterioles and the adjacent portion of the distal tubule, a modification of
the wall of the distal tubule at this point to form columnar cells known as
the *macula densa,* and the granular epithelioid cells which synthesize
renin and lie in the angle between the afferent arteriole and the distal
tubule. It is thought that the macula densa is a receptor through which
changes in electrolyte concentration of the distal tubular fluid influence
the activity of the juxtaglomerular apparatus. The lacis cells resemble
and are continuous with the glomerular mesangial cells.

The juxtamedullary nephrons lack a juxtaglomerular apparatus. Their
glomeruli are situated in the inner third of the cortex, or subcortex, close
to the medulla. Their afferent arterioles do not have a muscular wall or
sympathetic supply. Their efferent arterioles have a wider lumen than
those of the cortical nephrons but unlike them do have a muscular coat
and sympathetic innervation. The efferent arterioles branch to form
peritubular capillaries and descending vasa recta. The latter are long
capillaries dipping down into the medulla along side the corresponding
loop of Henle. They loop back up as the ascending vasa recta, which
have about twice as many branches as their descending counterparts.
The ascending vasa recta drain to the arcuate veins. The loops of Henle
of the juxtamedullary nephrons have much longer thin loops than the
cortical nephrons and dip much deeper into the medulla. Their loops and
vasa recta lie in close proximity to the collecting ducts of their own
nephrons and their associated cortical nephrons. This anatomical
propinquity is important in relation to water reabsorption within the
medulla.

2.2.1. Ultrastructure

The glomerulus, in addition to the glomerular capillary tuft already
described, contains at its centre mesangial cells embedded in a spongy
mesangial matrix filling the spaces between the capillary loops. These
mesangial cells are irregularly shaped with long processes extending
between the capillaries. They contain bundles of filaments and are joined
to one another by gap junctions to form a syncytium, and in the cortical
nephrons are in continuity with the lacis cells of the juxtaglomerular
apparatus. These features suggest that the mesangial and lacis cells may
be able to contract together to control blood flow through the glomerular
capillaries. Further functions are phagocytosis of particulate matter that
passes through the filtration membrane, and probably synthesis of
erythropoietin (Kurtz *et al.* 1983).

The visceral layer of Bowman's capsule consists of epithelial cells, or
podocytes, which are closely applied to the basement membrane of the
capillary loops of the glomerulus and which may in fact synthesize the

basement membrane, which has a very rapid turnover. The podocytes have a central cell body, containing the nucleus and the main cytoplasmic organelles, and thick processes called trabeculae that radiate out from the body and envelop the capillaries to which the cell is applied, rather like an octopus. Contact between the podocyte and the capillary is via pedicels or foot processes of the trabeculae, which interdigitate with the trabeculae of neighbouring podocytes. The podocytes, and also mesangial cell processes and endothelial tubes of the glomerular capillaries, have been beautifully demonstrated by scanning electron microscopy following sequential digestion of renal tissue with trypsin, pepsin, and pronase E (Jones 1985).

The filtration membrane comprises the capillary endothelium and the basement membrane. The endothelium consists of very thin endothelial cells and oval or circular fenestrations, 50–100 nm in diameter, that allow direct contact between the blood in the lumen and the basement membrane. The membrane in humans has been variously estimated as being between 100 and 400 nm thick. It has a filamentous structure and contains collagen and other protein constituents.

On electron microscopy three layers can be identified: a central *lamina densa*, bounded by a *lamina rara externa* on the epithelial side and a *lamina rara intima* on the endothelial side. At the level of fine ultrastructure, using negative staining, a three-dimensional meshwork has been demonstrated. The strands of this meshwork have a mean diameter of 1.25 nm in humans and are interwoven to enclose fine pores of about 2 to 5 nm diameter (Ota *et al.* 1979). An essentially similar ultrastructure has been demonstrated for tubular basement membrane (Makino *et al.* 1981). The foot processes of the podocytes are embedded in the outer surface of the membrane. At the outer edge of the basement membrane the foot processes are connected by a thin membrane or diaphragm covering a space of about 20–45 nm width between the foot processes. This cleft is termed the slit pore, but because of its diaphragm it is not an open pore. It is through these slit pores that the glomerular filtrate has to pass to reach the lumen of Bowman's capsule. The cleft diaphragm has a central longitudinal filament from which cross-bridges pass alternatively to either side. About three-quarters of the slit area lies opposite fenestrations in the capillary endothelium. The foot processes on their free surface are covered by a layer of polyanionic glycoprotein (Kunz *et al.* 1985) through which the glomerular filtrate has to percolate. The main features of the structure of the filtration membrane, as outlined above, are illustrated in Fig. 2.4.

The glomerular basement membrane in the rat is made up of collagen type IV, localized to the lamina interna, to which a glycoprotein, laminin, found in the laminae rarae is covalently linked (Courtoy *et al.* 1982).

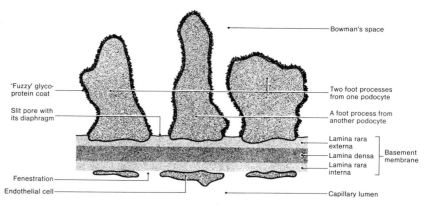

Fig. 2.4. The ultrastructure of the glomerular filtration membrane. Adapted from Moffat in *Renal disease*, 4th edn. by Sir Douglas Black and F. F. Jones (1979), with the permission of Blackwell Scientific Publications and Professor Moffat.

Laminin is thought to be involved in the attachment of the epithelial and endothelial cells to the basement membrane (Terranova *et al.* 1980). The localization of laminin, and other constituents, within the basement membrane has been demonstrated by immunochemical methods (Abrahamson 1986; Mohan and Spiro 1986). A proteoglycan, comprising a peptide core with a heparan sulphate like glycosaminoglycan moiety, is also covalently linked to the collagen type IV scaffold of the glomerular basement membrane (Parthasarathy and Spiro 1981). As discussed below these heparan sulphate side chains of the proteoglycans are strongly anionic and create a charge barrier which regulates permeability. A further component, of unknown function, also covalently linked to the collagen is the amyloid P (Dyck *et al.* 1980). The presence of type IV collagen in human glomerular basement membrane and mesangium has been confirmed using a monoclonal antibody (Scheinman and Tsai 1984). Ultrastructural alterations in the basement membrane have been described in several inherited renal diseases but it is not yet clear whether any of these is a direct result of the mutation in the disease concerned.

The ultrastructure of the tubules and collecting ducts varies. The proximal convoluted tubule is lined by columnar epithelium with a brush border on its luminal surface, and an external basement membrane on its serosal surface. There are channels between the cells, intercellular spaces, which are closed at the luminal end by 'tight junctions'. The serosal surface is folded into microvilli. The thin segment has elongated epithelial cells, and the distal tubule a lining similar to that of the thin segment but with many more mitochondria in the cytoplasm of the epithelial cells. An exceptional area is the macula densa already described. The collecting ducts have columnar epithelial cells whose height increases towards the inner medulla.

2.3. PHYSIOLOGY

The kidney has six main functions. These are: the elimination of waste products of metabolism and of foreign substances from the body; the maintenance of normal body fluid volume and of the concentrations of solutes in the fluid; the maintenance of normal plasma pH; the synthesis of hormones such as renin by the juxtaglomerular apparatus (see Barajas and Salido 1986), which is involved in the regulation of extracellular fluid volume and systematic arterial blood pressure, and whose gene structure has been determined (Hardman *et al.* 1984; Miyazaki *et al.* 1984); the synthesis of erythropoietin, which regulates the rate of proliferation of red-cell precursors, and whose gene has recently been cloned (Lin *et al.* 1985), and of certain prostaglandins and kallikrein (see Peart 1977; Epstein 1986); and finally the modification of body metabolites, as for example the hydroxylation of 25-hydroxycholecalciferol to the 1,25-dihydroxy form (Fraser and Kodicek 1970; Mawer *et al.* 1973). The first three of these functions, excretion of waste substances and the maintenance of solute concentration and pH of the milieu interieur, are performed by filtration through the glomerulus followed by selective reabsorption and secretion in the tubules and collecting ducts.

2.3.1. Glomerular filtration

Glomerular filtration is a physical rather than an active biological process. The glomerular capillary membrane is about 50 times as permeable as that of other peripheral capillaries, allowing a filtrate of plasma to pass essentially unaltered, apart from the retention of protein molecules above a molecular weight of about 40 000 to 70 000. The exact size above which particles do not pass the membrane is dependent on ionic charge.

Experimental studies with charged particles of varying size, such as cationic ferritin molecules (Rennke *et al.* 1975) or dextrans (Chang *et al.* 1975), suggest that anionic particles are electrostatically repelled by the anionic glycoproteins of the pedical coat so that they permeate less readily than similar-sized neutral or cationic particles. Corroborative evidence for a charge effect comes from experimentally induced proteinuria using puromycin in which there is a partial loss of negatively charged sialic acid rich glycoprotein sites on the surface of glomerular epithelial cells (Michael *et al.* 1970; Charest and Roth 1985). There is a further charge barrier within the basement membrane itself consisting of the heparan sulphate rich anionic polysaccharide side chains of the membrane proteoglycans referred to above. These are arranged in orderly rows within the lamina rara externa and interna (Kanwar and Farquhar 1979a and b). That these heparan sulphate rich sites are an important component of the charge barrier is demonstrated by the increased permeability to ferritin (Kanwar *et al.* 1980) and albumin (Rosenzweig and Kanwar 1982) that follows their removal.

Filtration is dependent on the high hydrostatic pressure in the glomerular capillaries relative to that in Bowman's capsule. This pressure gradient is higher than the opposing colloid osmotic pressure of the plasma in the capillary lumen. Since filtration itself raises plasma protein concentration the net filtration pressure falls from the afferent to efferent poles of the capillary bed.

Whether or not under normal physiological conditions this fall is sufficient to reach equilibrium between net hydrostatic and oncotic pressures before the end of the capillary bed is not clear. Under conditions of filtration equilibrium there would be a reserve filtration area in the glomerular capillary bed that could be recruited by increased renal plasma flow. Under filtration disequilibrium, the more traditional view based on direct studies of mammalian glomeruli (Brenner *et al.* 1972; Maddox *et al.* 1974), there is a reserve of filtration pressure and filtration can be increased by increasing capillary hydrostatic pressure. That equilibrium may, at least in some circumstances, be reached is supported by evidence of variation in filtration fraction, the proportion of the total renal plasma flow filtered, and, in glomerular filtration coefficient, the product of the total glomerular capillary surface area and hydraulic permeability. The calculated estimate of the latter, for example, has been shown to vary strikingly in response to angiotensin (Blantz *et al.* 1976), to plasma protein concentration (Baylis *et al.* 1976), and to plasma flow (Gertz *et al.* 1969; Daugharty *et al.* 1971).

Since there is no evidence for any change in intrinsic permeability of the filtration membrane in the absence of renal disease, it seems more likely that these observations reflect changes in the area of membrane available for filtration, as a result of filtration equilibrium being reached. In addition vascular shunts within the glomerular plexus, or juxta-glomerular apparatus, may regulate the proportion of plasma flowing through the capillary bed. An anatomical basis for a shunt in cortical nephrons has been demonstrated in the form of a continuous arteriole traversing the juxtaglomerular apparatus (Ljungqvist 1975).

Regulation of intraglomerular plasma flow may be even more complex as there is evidence of capillary constriction, in response to angiotensin, mediated by mesangial cells (Becker 1971; Hornych *et al.* 1972; Osborne *et al.* 1975; Blantz *et al.* 1976), as well as variation in tone of the muscular wall of the afferent arteriole of cortical nephrons, under the control of the juxtaglomerular apparatus, in response to changes in perfusion pressure.

The autoregulation which this mechanism provides can be overridden only by sympathetic stimulation. The juxtamedullary nephrons, lacking a juxtaglomerular apparatus, do not show autoregulation. Hence increased tone of cortical afferent arterioles leads to a relative redistribution of blood to the juxtamedullary nephrons. The muscular efferent arterioles of the juxtamedullary nephrons increase their tone in response to sympathetic stimulation or antidiuretic hormone (ADH) and relax in response to prostaglandins.

The glomerular filtration rate in the healthy adult human male of average body surface area (1.73 m^2) is about 120 millilitres per minute. However, there is diurnal variation, and the rate is reduced by exercise, postural hypotension, dehydration, and even pain.

Renal clearance of specific solutes depends on the glomerular filtration rate, which itself is the product of the filtration coefficient and the mean effective pressure, and plasma concentration of the solute. In clinical practice the clearance is estimated by multiplying the urine concentration (Umg/ml) by the rate of urine excretion (Vml/min) and dividing by the plasma concentration of (Pmg/ml). UV will be the rate of urine excretion of the solute in mg/min and UV/P, the renal clearance, will represent the volume of plasma cleared in millilitres.

Unfortunately such estimates although widely used are liable to substantial inaccuracy, mainly because of difficulties in the accurate measurement of 24-hour urine volumes as a measure of rate of urine excretion. The method is not an assessment of glomerular clearance alone as the final clearance is also influenced by tubular function. However, substances that are fully cleared from plasma by glomerular filtration and are neither secreted nor reabsorbed by the tubules can be used to estimate glomerular filtration rate. Inulin, creatinine, and mannitol have all been used for this purpose. The problems inherent in 24-hour urine collection can be avoided by using the newer radioactive chelate methods in which a single injection is administered, followed by the taking of blood samples only. These methods use [51Cr]EDTA (ethylenediaminetetra-acetic acid) (Chantler *et al.* 1966; Granerus and Aurell 1981), or the more recently introduced technectium-labelled chelate [99mTc] Diethylenetriamine pentacetate (DTPA) (Veall and Gibbs 1982; Watts *et al.* 1983), and give an estimate of glomerular filtration rate comparable to that obtained with inulin.

2.3.2. Tubular reabsorption

The most important function of the tubules is reabsorption of water and solutes from the glomerular filtrate. For example, despite the filtration of 120 ml/min, only 1 ml/min is excreted in the urine so that over 99 per cent of water is reabsorbed. Similarly, about 99 per cent of sodium, 94 per cent of potassium, 98 per cent of calcium, 100 per cent of glucose, 97 per cent of amino acids, but only 42 per cent of urea are reabsorbed. In practice net reabsorption of a solute is measured by comparing its renal clearance to that of inulin or a radioactive chelate.

The traditional view that reabsorption is mainly active by means of specific transport systems in the tubule cells, or for a few substances such as urea by passive diffusion, is now recognized to be an oversimplification. In particular, studies in recent years have shown that the peritubular vascular circulation and the vasa recta play an important role in reabsorption throughout the tubular and collecting duct system.

The bulk of reabsorption takes place in the proximal tubule, some 80–85 per cent of the glomerular filtrate being absorbed. This has been referred to as fixed reabsorption as it is a roughly constant proportion (Haberle and Shiigai 1978). Sodium and water are absorbed together, and as 90 per cent of the osmolality of the filtrate is due to sodium salts, there is no appreciable change in osmolality of the filtrate remaining. The mechanism is primary reabsorption of sodium, which takes water with it. That this mechanism is active, and is the main energy requiring activity of the kidney, is shown by the fact that the rate of sodium reabsorption of the kidney is proportional to renal oxygen consumption.

Active transport implies transport against either a chemical concentration gradient or an electrochemical gradient. In the proximal tubule it is primarily the latter, with a 2–4 mV potential across the tubule cell in the initial part of the tubule. The principle transport system is probably Na^+, K^+-dependent ATPase of the sodium pump, which is involved in extrusion of sodium from the tubule cell into the interspaces and peritubular space. Sodium cotransport during absorption of other solutes plays a part in initial uptake into the tubule cell and may indeed be rate limiting.

It is also known that the peritubular capillary differs in two important aspects from other peripheral capillaries. Firstly, in marked contrast to the glomerular capillary, it has a low hydrostatic pressure, only about 6.5 mmHg (865 Pa) in the rat, which is a fifth to a quarter of that in systemic capillaries (Wunderlich and Schnermann 1969; Falchuk and Berliner 1971). Secondly, because the peritubular capillaries derive from glomerular efferent arterioles, they have a high colloid osmotic pressure. Windhanger (1974) has reviewed experiments which have shown that capillary oncotic pressure influences proximal tubular reabsorption. This probably occurs via the intercellular spaces of the tubule wall.

High interstital protein concentration may also facilitate fluid flux from the tubular cellular space (O'Connor 1984). Beyond the first portions of the proximal tubule a high luminal concentration of chloride created by preferential absorption of bicarbonate in the initial portion of the tubule, along with the high peritubular bicarbonate thus created, provides a further driving force for passive reabsorption of sodium, which is, however, dependent on the primary active initial transport.

It has been generally assumed that the peritubular capillary is the continuation of the efferent arteriole of the glomerulus of its own nephron. However, the situation is more complex as individual nephrons, especially medullary nephrons, may derive an efferent blood supply from glomeruli of other nephrons or even from other zones of the kidney (Beeuwkes 1971; Beeuwkes and Bonventre 1975).

Substances that are actively reabsorbed, being dependent on a specific transport mechanism, have a maximal reabsorptive capacity (T_m). This is typified by glucose, which is normally fully reabsorbed. At a plasma level of 10.6 mmol/l and a normal glomerular filtration rate the transport system is saturated and all excess in the filtrate is excreted. Phosphate has a lower T_m than glucose, which is normally below the filtered load so that some is excreted.

Phosphate reabsorption in the proximal nephron involves two independent transport mechanisms; one is of high capacity but insensitive to parathyroid hormone (parathormone), and the other is of lesser capacity but very responsive to inhibition by this hormone (Dennis *et al.* 1977). Sulphate reabsorption also takes place in the proximal tubule but is independent of phosphate reabsorption (Cole and Scriver 1984). Chloride is reabsorbed along with sodium and water. Potassium has its own transport system and like sodium is about 80 per cent reabsorbed in the proximal tubule.

Urate reabsorption is probably complete, but it is also secreted giving a net clearance of about 8 ml/min.

Most amino acids are reabsorbed by means of group specific systems for (i) cystine, lysine, arginine, and ornithine; (ii) proline, hydroxproline, and glycine and (iii) glutamic and aspartic acids, threonine, and most other amino acids. Proximal tubular reabsorption is summarized in Fig. 2.5.

The loop of Henle provides the mechanism for regulating water and salt reabsorption. The loops of cortical nephrons have virtually no thin ascending segment. Within such loops some 25 per cent of filtered sodium is reabsorbed, but less than 15 per cent of filtered water. The rate of salt reabsorption is directly proportional to the sodium load leaving

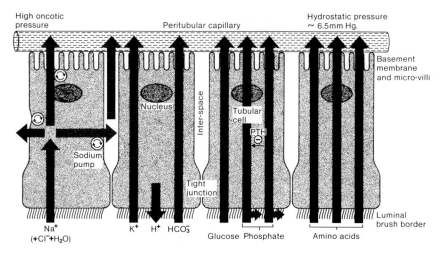

Fig. 2.5. The pathways of reabsorption in the proximal renal tubule. (PTH = parathormone.)

the proximal tubule (Giebisch and Windhager 1973), as is that in the proximal tubule itself. Absorption is active and takes place in the pars recta or descending limb at about half the rate of that in the proximal convoluted tubule. Reabsorption in the thick ascending limb is generally regarded as being due to active transport of chloride ions, inhibited by frusemide, establishing an electrochemical gradient for passive outward diffusion of sodium. However, Westenfelder and Kurtzman (1981) have produced evidence that it is sodium which is actively reabsorbed in the thick ascending limb. The ascending limb as a whole is virtually impermeable to water (Burg and Green 1973; Rocha and Kokko 1973). As a result of reabsorption in the loop a relatively dilute fluid is delivered to the distal tubule.

The primary function of the juxtamedullary nephrons is the conservation or rejection of water. Their loops of Henle are the active components of a complex medullary system comprising the long loops of the juxtamedullary nephrons themselves, their associated vasa recta, and the collecting ducts. This system involves contrary direction of flow in the ascending and descending limbs of the loops, and in the ascending and descending vasa recta, the effect of which is to set up a gradient of osmolality in the medulla from cortex to papillary tip (Wirz 1956), which is largely due to increasing concentrations of sodium and chloride ions and urea (Ullrich and Jarausch 1956).

The primary mechanism that initiates this gradient is the transport of chloride ions by the ascending limb in a similar manner to that in the loops of cortical nephrons. Sodium diffuses passively out with the chloride, or perhaps vice versa, but not water as the ascending limb is impermeable, resulting in a rise in salt concentration in the adjacent medullary interstital fluid. As a consequence water is drawn out of the nearby permeable descending limb, setting up an osmotic gradient between a more concentrated fluid in the descending limb and a relatively dilute one in the ascending limb.

The creation of this gradient led Hargitay and Kuhn (1951) to postulate their counter-current hypothesis of the mechanism of urine concentration. Earlier views of this mechanism assumed active transport of chloride out of the thin and thick ascending limbs and limited permeability of the descending limb to sodium diffusion. More recent views assign active chloride transport to the thick ascending limb in the outer medulla only and complete solute impermeability to the descending limb (Kokko and Rector 1972; Stephenson 1972, 1973a and b).

These two slightly differing views lead to what have been termed the 'active' and 'passive' models respectively. The latter hypothesis lays stress on the osmotic stratification, within the inner medulla, created by passive diffusion of water, salt, and urea arising from the differing permeabilities of the membrane structure involved. Hargitay and Kuhn (1951) referred to the active transport of salt by cells of the ascending limb, and the resultant loss of water and fluid concentration in the adjacent descending limb, as a 'single effect'. This slightly concentrated fluid in the descending limb moves further down the limb in its progression along the nephron and is subjected to the same process of concentration by loss of water to the surrounding hypertonic interstitium. This process continues at each level until the fluid turns the hairpin bend at the bottom of the loop to enter the ascending limb.

Hence at any level of the medulla the single effect is concentrating the fluid in the descending limb by passive diffusion of water into a relatively hypertonic environment, while that in the ascending limb is diluted, according to both hypotheses, by salt loss into a relatively hypotonic environment. This small single effect is multiplied at each level to achieve the final concentration at the bend of the loop. This mechanism is termed a counter-current multiplier. Under the 'active' hypothesis the concentration is assisted by some diffusion of salt into the descending limb and its active transport out of the thin as well as the thick, ascending limb. Whereas according to the 'passive' hypothesis this is achieved, apart from active salt transport in the thick ascending limb, purely by passive diffusion of water out of the ascending limb and a net excess of salt loss over urea gain by diffusion in the thin ascending limb. According to this view fluid entering the ascending limb contains salt at a higher concentration than surrounding interstitial fluid despite osmotic equilibrium which is maintained by a higher urea concentration in the interstitium.

Marsh and Azen (1975) have shown that the difference in urea concentration is confined to the lower fifth of the thin ascending limb and that subsequent dilution is due to sodium chloride reabsorption. However, their observations do not finally settle the question as to whether this transport is active or passive although they do favour active transport of sodium by the thin ascending segment. These two variants of the counter-current multiplier effect are illustrated in the diagrams in Fig. 2.6 taken from Kokko and Rector (1972).

The distal tubules, and the collecting ducts, are permeable to water only in the presence of ADH (vasopressin). ADH is secreted in response to high plasma osmolality and in its presence the distal tubule reabsorbs water independently of sodium so that when dilute urine is formed sodium is reabsorbed in excess of water and vice versa. Sodium is reabsorbed actively under the influence of aldosterone and exchanged for potassium and hydrogen ions, which are secreted into the lumen. The distal tubules also actively reabsorb chloride and bicarbonate and secrete ammonia. They are impermable to urea.

The collecting ducts run in close proximity to the loops of Henle. The amount of water in the duct fluid depends on the rate of sodium and water reabsorbed by the cortical nephrons. In the presence of ADH water diffuses out passively into the hypertonic interstitial fluid of the medulla rendering the urine in the duct more concentrated. A urine osmolality up to 1200 mosmol/1 is formed, that is, up to four times the osmolality of plasma. Most of the water entering the medullary interstitium in this way is removed via the venous vasa recta. When plasma osmolality is low less ADH is secreted and the walls of collecting ducts and distal tubules become relatively impermeable to water, resulting in the excretion of a dilute urine with an osmolality down to one-tenth that of plasma.

The vasa recta, like the loop of Henle, are also exposed to the medullary osmolar gradient. Since fluid leaves the descending vasa recta and enters the ascending vasa, owing to the excess of oncotic pressure over opposing hydrostatic pressure (Sanjana *et al.* 1975), rapid blood flow through the vasa will tend to wash out the gradient. This tendency is countered in two ways. Firstly the medullary blood flow is low owing to the resistance created by the length of the vasa recta and by the greater resistance of juxtamedullary efferent arterioles to plasma flow. Secondly the vasa recta themselves act as a counter-current exchange system. At any level their osmolality is intermediate between that of the fluid in the adjacent ascending and descending limbs.

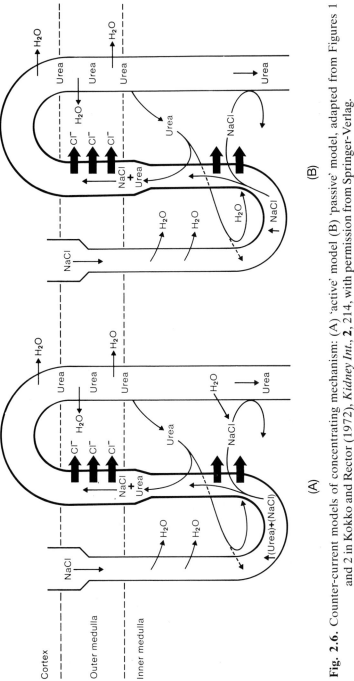

Fig. 2.6. Counter-current models of concentrating mechanism: (A) 'active' model (B) 'passive' model, adapted from Figures 1 and 2 in Kokko and Rector (1972), *Kidney Int.*, **2**, 214, with permission from Springer-Verlag.

The presence of ADH slows plasma flow in the vasa by acting directly on the juxtamedullary efferent arterioles. This slowing increases the concentration gradient in the medulla. A further effect of the increased efferent arteriolar resistance is an increase in filtration fraction and hence of the sodium load on which the single effect can act. The 2:1 ratio of the venous to arterial vasa recta facilitates the removal of water transported across the collecting ducts by the former. During diuresis these effects are reversed, and plasma flow is increased as the concentration gradient is lessened.

2.3.3. Urea excretion

Urea excretion depends on the amounts filtered and reabsorbed; in humans it is not secreted. Transport of urea is passive, being greatest when urine concentration is high and minute volume low. When urine is copious and dilute only about one third of the filtered urea is reabsorbed compared with half on average. However, the ratio of urea clearance to filtration rate is variable and the urea concentration in the outer medulla may be up to 10 times that in the urine. About 40 per cent of filtered urea is reabsorbed in the proximal tubule by diffusion from the relatively high concentration in the tubular lumen to the lower concentration in the peritubular interstitial fluid and capillary. This depends indirectly on active sodium reabsorption as the greater the reabsorption of sodium and water the higher is the luminal concentration of urea and the fraction reabsorbed. Conversely if the blood urea level rises urea reabsorption is diminished.

Permeability to urea varies along the nephron. The descending limb of the loop and the distal tube are impermeable to urea, whereas the thin ascending limb is moderately permeable, and the permeability of the collecting duct increases towards the distal end.

Reabsorption of urea is dependent on the functioning of the counter-current system. The local gradients of concentration result in diffusion of urea out of the collecting duct into the medullary interstitium and from there into the thin ascending limb and thence via the lumen it passes back to the collecting duct (see Fig. 2.6). A consequence of this recycling of urea is that the increase in urea excretion with increasing urine flow is not linear, falling off sharply above a flow of 2 ml/min. With diuresis water permeability of the collecting duct is reduced and the urea concentration in the duct lumen falls. This reduces the concentration difference between the duct fluid and the interstitium with less reabsorption of urea and increased excretion in relation to the amount filtered.

Urea reabsorption is not only dependent on the counter-current system, but plays an important part in it. It has long been recognized that a more concentrated urine is formed when urea is the principle solute present. The urea concentration in the medullary interstitium increases the outflow of water from the descending limb of Henle's loop thereby concentrating salt in the loop and promoting its passive diffusion from the thin ascending limb. This augmentation of the 'single effect' in turn increases water reabsorption from the collecting ducts and concentrates both urea and non-urea solutes in the urine.

2.3.4. Tubular secretion

Tubular secretion is an important mechanism of renal clearance in amphibia but much less so in mammals. Net tubular excretion, that secretion greater than reabsorption, is indicated by a clearance greater than that of inulin. Substances that are secreted include hippuric acid and its derivatives such as *p*-amino-hippuric acid, aromatic sulphates and glucuronides, potassium in the distal tubule, and in humans creatinine, urate, and urobilinogen. Hydrogen ions and ammonia are generated in the distal tubular epithelium and then secreted, which does not of course constitute clearance.

Substances such as *p*-amino-hippurate, phenol red, diodone, and some penicillins have a maximal tubular secretory capacity. Their excretion within this capacity can be used as a measure of renal plasma flow. For example, *p*-amino-hippurate has a secretory clearance approximately 90 per cent of renal plasma flow (RPF). Hence a clearance of 600 ml/min indicates an RPF of about 700 ml/min and a renal blood flow of about 1250 ml/min.

Both glomerular and tubular function may be disturbed in renal disease. As far as genetically determined disease is concerned developmental defects of the kidney as a whole, or of parts of the nephron, and other structures of the genito-urinary tract are well recognized in the various types of cystic disease and in malformations. Genetic factors are also involved in certain types of neoplastic change in the renal tract. Specific defects of several tubular transport systems are inherited in a mendelian manner. Specific primary defects of the glomerular basement membrane may be involved in several inherited renal disorders such as Alport's disease and congenital nephrosis.

Accounts of the anatomy and physiology of the kidney are to be found in Moffat (1975) and Black and Jones (1979).

References

Abrahamson, D. R. (1986). Post-embedding colloidal gold immunolocalization of laminin to the lamina rara interna, lamina densa and lamina rara externa of renal glomerular basement membranes. *J. Histochem. Cytochem.* **34**, 847–53.

Barajas, L. and Salido, E. (1986). Editorial: juxtaglomerular apparatus and the renin–angiotensin system. *Lab. Invest.* **54**, 361–4.

Baylis, C., Shinagawa, L., Wilson, C. B. and Brenner, B. M. (1976). A relationship between systemic protein concentration and glomerular capillary ultrafiltration coefficient (Kf). *Fed. Proc.* **35**, 542.

Becker, C. G. (1971). Demonstration of actomyosin in mesangial cells of the renal glomerulas. *Circulation* **43** and **44**, Suppl. II: 66.

Beeuwkes, R. (1971). Efferent vascular patterns and early vascular–tubular relations in the dog kidney. *Am. J. Physiol.* **221**, 1361–74.

—— and Bonventre, J. V. (1975). Tubular organization and vascular–tubule relations in the dog kidney. *Am. J. Physiol.* **229**, 695–713.

Black, Sir Douglas and Jones N. F. (eds.) (1979). *Renal disease*, 4th edn. Blackwell, Oxford, London, and Edinburgh.

Blantz, R. C., Konnen, K. S. and Tucker, B. J. (1976). Angiotensin II effects upon the glomerular microcirculation and ultrafiltration coefficient of the rat. *J. Clin. Invest.* **57**, 419–34.

Brenner, B. M., Troy, J. L., Daugharty, T. M., Deen, W. M. and Robertson, C. R. (1972). Dynamics of glomerular ultrafiltration in the rat. II. Plasma-flow dependence of GFR. *Am. J. Physiol.* **223**, 1184–90.

Burg, M. B. and Green, N. (1973). Function of the thick ascending limb of Henle's loop. *Am. J. Physiol.* **224**, 659–68.

Chang, R. L. S., Deen, W. M., Robertson, C. R. and Brenner, B. M. (1975). Permselectivity of the glomerular capillary wall. III. Restricted transport of polyanions. *Kidney Int.* **8**, 212–18.

Chantler, C., Garnett, E. S., Parsons, V. and Veall, N. (1966). GFR measurements in man by the single injection method using ^{51}Cr-EDTA. *Clin. Sci.* **37**, 169–80.

Charest, P. M. and Roth, J. (1985). Localization of sialic acid in kidney glomeruli: regionalization in the podocyte plasma membrane and loss in experimental nephrosis. *Proc. Nat. Acad. Sci.* **82**, 8508–12.

Cole, D. E. C. and Scriver, C. R. (1984). The effects of mendelian mutation on renal sulphate and phosphate transport in man and mouse. *Pediatr. Res.* **18**, 25–9.

Courtoy, P. J., Timpl, R. and Farquhar, M. G. (1982). Comparative distribution of laminin, type IV collagen and fibronectin in the rat glomerulus. *J. Histochem. Cytochem.* **30**, 874–86.

Daugharty, T. M., Troy, J. and Brenner, B. M. (1971). Glomerular dynamics and the concept of filtration pressure equilibrium (FPE). *Am. Soc. Nephrol.* **5**, 17.

Dennis, V. W., Bello-Reuss, E. and Robsinson, R. R. (1977). Response of phosphate transport to parathyroid hormone in segments of rabbit nephron. *Am. J. Physiol.* **233**, F29–F38.

Dyck, R. F., Lockwood, C. M., Kershaw, M., McHugh, N., Duance, V. C., Baltz, M. L. and Pepys, M. B. (1980). Amyloid P-component is a constituent of normal human glomerular basement membrane. *J. Exp. Med.* **152**, 1162–74.

Epstein, M. (ed.) (1986). Prostaglandins and the kidney. Proceedings of a symposium. *Am. J. Med.* **80**(1A), 1–84.

Falchuk, K. H. and Berliner, R. W. (1971). Hydrostatic pressures in peritubular capillaries and tubules in the rat kidney. *Am. J. Physiol.* **220**, 1422–6.

Fraser, D. R. and Kodicek, E. (1970). Unique biosynthesis by kidney of a biologically active vitamin D metabolite. *Nature* **228**, 764–6.

Gardiner, D. S. and Lindop, G. B. M. (1985). The granular peripolar cell of the human glomerulus: a new component of the juxtaglomerular apparatus? *Histopath.* **9**, 675–85.

Gertz, K. H., Brandis, M., Braun-Schubert, G. and Boylan, J. W. (1969). The effect of saline infusion and hemorrhage on glomerular filtration pressure and single nephron filtration rate. *Pflügers Arch.* **310**, 193–205.

Giebisch, G. and Windhager, E. E. (1973). Electrolyte transport across renal tubular membranes. In *Handbook of physiology* eds. Orloff, J. and Berliner, R. W. Sect. 8, 'Renal physiology', pp. 315–76. American Physiological Society, Washington DC.

Granerus, G. and Aurell, M. (1981). Reference values for ^{51}Cr-EDTA clearance as a measure of glomerular filtration rate. *Scan. J. Clin. Lab. Invest.* **41**, 611–16.

Haberle, D. A. and Shiigai, T. (1978). Flow-dependent volume reabsorption in the proximal convolution of the rat kidney—the role of glomerular-borne tubular fluid for the maintenance of glomerulotubular balance. In *New aspects of renal function* (workshop conference Hoechst), Vol. 6, eds. Vogel and Ulrich. Excerpta Medica, Amsterdam, Oxford.

Hardman, J. A., Hort, Y. J., Catanzaro, D. F., Tellam, J. T., Baxter, J. D., Morris, B. J. and Shine, J. (1984). Primary structure of the human renin gene. *DNA* **3**, 457–68.

Hargitay, B, and Kuhn, W. (1951). Das Multiplikationsprinzip als Grundlage der Harnkonzentrierung in der Niere. *Z. Elektrochem.* **55**, 539–58.

Hornych, H., Beaufils, M. and Richet, G. (1972). The effect of exogenous angiotensin on superficial and deep glomeruli in the rat kidney. *Kidney Int.* **2**, 336–43.

Jones, D. B. (1985). Methods in laboratory investigation: enzymatic dissection of the glomerulus. *Lab. Invest.* **52**, 453–61.

Kanwar, Y. S. and Farquhar, M. G. (1979a). Presence of heparan sulfate in the glomerular basement membrane. *Proc. Nat. Acad. Sci.* **76**, 1303–7.

—— and Farquhar, M. G. (1979b). Anionic sites in the glomerular basement membrane: *in vivo* and *in vitro* localization to the laminae rarae by cationic probes. *J. Cell Biol.* **81**, 137–53.

——, Linker, A. and Farquhar, M. G. (1980). Increased permeability of the glomerular basement membrane to ferritin after removal of glycosaminoglycans (heparan sulphate) by enzyme digestion. *J. Cell Biol.* **86**, 688–93.

Kokko, J. P. and Rector, F. C. (1972). Countercurrent multiplication system without active transport in inner medulla. *Kidney Int.* **2**, 214–23.

Kunz, A., Brown, D., Vassalli, J.-D., Kontturi, M., Kumpulainen, T. and Orci, L. (1985). Ultrastructural localization of glycocalyx domains in human kidney podocytes using the lectin–gold technique. *Lab. Invest.* **53**, 413–20.

Kurtz, A., Jelkmann, W., Sinowatz, F. and Bauer, C. (1983). Renal mesangial cell cultures as a model for study of erythropoietin production. *Proc. Nat. Acad. Sci.* **80**, 4008–11.

Lin, F. K., Suggs, S., Lin, C.-H., Browne, J. K., Smalling, R., Egrie, J. C., Chen, K. K., Fox, G. M., Martin, F., Stabinsky, Z., Badrawi, S. M., Lai, P.-H. and Goldwasser, E. (1985). Cloning and expression of the human erythropoietin gene. *Proc. Nat. Acad. Sci.* **82**, 7580–4.

Ljungqvist, A. (1975). Ultrastructural demonstration of a connection between afferent and efferent juxtamedullary glomerular arterioles. *Kidney Int.* **8**, 239–44.

Maddox, D. A., Deen, W. M., Brenner, B. M., Troy, J. L. and Surface, R. W. (1974). Dynamics of glomerular ultrafiltration. VI. Studies in the primate. *Kidney Int.* **5**, 271–8.

Makino, H., Ota, Z., Takaya, Y., Miyoshi, A. and Ofuji, T. (1981). Molecular sieve in rat tubular basement membrane as measured by negative staining. *Renal Physiol., Basel* **4**, 180–90.

Marsh, D. J. and Azen, S. P. (1975). Mechanism of NaCl reabsorption by hamster thin ascending limbs of Henle's loop. *Am. J. Physiol.* **228**, 71–9.

Mawer, E. B., Backhouse, J., Taylor, C. M., Lumb, G. A. and Stanbury, S. W. (1973). Failure of formation of 1,25-dihydroxycholecalciferol in chronic renal insufficiency. *Lancet* **1**, 626–8.

Michael, A. F., Blau, E. and Vernier, R. L. (1970). Glomerular polyanion: alteration in amino-nucleoside nephrosis. *Lab. Invest.* **23**, 649–57.

Miyazaki, H., Fukamizu, A., Hirose, S., Hayashi, T., Hori, H., Ohkubo, H., Nakanishi, S. and Murakami, K. (1984). Structure of the human renin gene. *Proc. Nat. Acad. Sci.* **81**, 5999–6003.

Moffat, D. B. (1975). *The mammalian kidney.* Cambridge University Press.

Mohan, P. S. and Spiro, R. G. (1986). Macromolecular organization of basement membranes. Characterization and comparison of glomerular basement membrane and lens capsule components by immunochemical and lectin affinity procedures. *J. Biol. Chem.* **261**, 4328–36.

O'Connor, W. J. (1984). Tubular reabsorption in normal renal function. *Renal Physiol., Basel* **7**, 193–204.

Osborne, M. J., Drox, B., Meyer, P. and Morel, F. (1975). Angiotensin II: renal localization in glomerular mesengial cells by auto-radiography. *Kidney Int.* **8**, 245–54.

Ota, Z., Makino, H., Miyoshi, A., Hiramatsu, M., Takahashi, K. and Ofuji, T. (1979). Molecular sieve in glomerular basement membrane as revealed by electron microscopy. *J. Electron Microsc.* **28**, 20–8.

Parthasarathy, N. and Spiro, R. G. (1981). Characterization of the glycosamino-glycan portion of the glomerular basement membrane and its relationship to the peptide portion. *J. Biol. Chem.* **256**, 507–13.

Peart, W. S. (1977). The kidney as an endocrine organ. *Lancet* **2**, 543–8.

Rennke, H. G., Cotran, R.S. and Venkatachalam, M. A. (1975). Role of molecular charge in glomerular permeability. *J. Cell Biol.* **67**, 638–46.

Rocha, A. S. and Kokko, J. P. (1973). Sodium chloride and water transport in the medullary thick ascending limb of Henle. *J. Clin. Invest.* **52**, 612–23.

Rosenzweig, L. J. and Kanwar, Y. S. (1982). Removal of sulfated (heparan sulfate) or non-sulfated (hyaluronic acid) glycosaminoglycans results in increased permeability of the glomerular basement membrane to ^{125}I bovine serum albumin. *Lab. Invest.* **47**, 177–84.

Sanjana, V. M., Johnston, P. A., Deen, W. M., Robertson, C. R., Brenner, B. M. and Jamison, R. L. (1975). Hydraulic and oncotic pressure measurements in inner medulla of mammalian kidney. *Am. J. Physiol.* **288**, 1921–6.

Scheinman, J. I. and Tsai, C. (1984). Monoclonal antibody to type IV collagen with selective basement membrane localization. *Lab. Invest.* **50**, 101–12.

Stephens, F. D. (1983). *Congenital malformations of the urinary tract,* pp. 3–14, 162–3, 186–7, and 381–90. Praeger, New York.

Stephenson, J. L. (1972). Central core model of the renal counterflow system. *Kidney Int.* **2**, 85.

—— (1973a and b). Concentrating engines and the kidney. I. Central core model of the renal medulla. *Biophys. J.* **13**, 512–45. II. Multisolute central core systems. *ibid.* 546–67.

Terranova, V. P., Rohrbach, D. H. and Martin, G. R. (1980). Role of laminin in the attachment of PAM 212 (epithelial) cells to basement membrane collagen. *Cell* **22**, 719–26.

Ullrich, K. J. and Jarausch, K. H. (1956). Untersuchungen zum Problem der Harnkonzentrierung und Verdunnung. Uber die Verteilung der Elektrolyten (Na, K, Ca, Mg, Cl, anorg, phosphat). Harnstoff, Aminosauren und exogenem Kreatinin in Rinde und Mark der Jundeniere bei verschiedenen Diuresezustanden. *Pflügers Arch.* **62**, 537–50.

Veall, N. and Gibbs, G. P. (1982). The accurate determination of tracer clearance rates and equlibrium distribution of tracer clearance volumes from single injection plasma measurements using numerical analysis. In *Radionuclides in nephrology,* eds. Joekes, A. M., Constable, A. R., Brown, N. J. G. and Tauxe, W. N. pp. 125–30. Academic Press/Grune and Stratton, New York.

Watts, R. W. E., Veall, N. and Purkiss, P. (1983). Sequential studies of oxalate dynamics in primary hyperoxaluria. *Clin. Sci.* **65**, 627–33.

Westenfelder, C. and Kurtzman, N. A. (1981). Bartter's syndrome: a disorder of active sodium and/or passive chloride transport in the ascending limb of Henle's loop. *Mineral and Electrolyte Metabolism* **5**, 135–42.

Windhager, E. E. (1974). Some aspects of proximal tubular salt reabsorption. *Fed. Proc.* **33**, 21–4.

Winick, M. and McCrory, W. W. (1968). Renal differentiation: a model for the study of development. *Birth Defects Orig. Art. Series* **4**, (5), 1–14.

Wirz, H. (1956). Der osmotische Druck in den corticalen Tubuli der Rattenniere. *Helv. Physiol. Pharmacol. Acta* **14**, 354–62.

Wunderlich, P. and Schnermann, J. (1969). Continuous recording of hydrostatic pressure in renal tubules and blood capillaries by use of a new pressure transducer. *Pflügers Arch.* **313**, 89–94.

3. Urinary tract anomalies in chromosomal disorders

Renal and lower urinary tract abnormalities, mainly malformations such as horseshoe or unilateral fused kidney, duplication defects, agenesis or hypoplasia, hydronephrosis and hydroureter, renal dysplasia or cystic disease, and hypospadias, small penis, hypoplastic or bifid scrotum, and cryptorchidism are commonly found in chromosomal disorders. Although certain renal anomalies are typical of specific chromosome disorders the general picture is one of a remarkable lack of specificity. Indeed no one renal malformation is unique to any specific chromosomal disorder. Another striking observation, in those chromosome disorders in which renal malformation does occur, is that, despite apparently identical loss or gain of either whole chromosomes, or of specific chromosome regions carrying presumably identical genes and chromatin, the phenotypic effects from case to case are remarkably variable, both as regards renal malformation and other defects. This is true even for monozygotic twins concordant for a chromosome disorder (Lemli and Smith 1963).

An overview of renal anomalies in chromosomal disorders suggests that two main processes are involved. The first and primary process is developmental error or growth failure during embryogenesis of the renal tract. This is clearly the case in horseshoe kidney, duplication defects, and lower urinary tract malformation. It is probably also the case in renal agenesis and renal hypoplasia with normal renal histology and in simple hypogenitalism. The second process is that of the effects of urinary tract obstruction, secondary to developmental error, on subsequent development proximal to the site of obstruction. This is obvious in hydronephrosis and hydroureter. The description of multiple, largely subcapsular cortical microcysts in many chromosomal disorders, such as trisomy 13, strongly resembles the type of cystic disorder seen in incomplete ureteric or urethral obstruction in the fetus, classified by Osathanondh and Potter (1964) as type 4 despite their description of a kidney from trisomy 13 under their type 3. Other descriptions of cystic kidney and dysplasia with or without renal hypoplasia in chromosomal disorders strongly resemble the dysplastic or dysgenic kidney that largely occur as sporadic defects. This picture may follow complete early lower urinary tract obstruction or result from gross developmental error.

40

In the accounts of urinary tract anomaly in specific chromosomal disorders to follow in this chapter no attempt is made to provide comprehensive reference lists of every mention in the literature of such abnormalities in chromosomal disorder. Rather a selection of papers that illustrate the types of defects that have been described is quoted for each chromosomal disorder for which urinary tract anomaly has been reported. Most of the chromosome anomalies not mentioned are rare. The omission of any specific anomaly merely indicates that no mention of urinary tract disorder in that anomaly has been found in the literature, not that its occurrence is excluded.

Of the major human aneuploid chromosomal disorders both trisomy 13 and 18 are frequently associated with renal abnormality, and the former with hypospadias. Hypoplasia of the genitalia is occasionally seen in the XYY male (Carakushansky *et al.* 1968), and more commonly in Klinefelter's syndrome. Deletion of the long arm of the Y chromosome has been reported in association with various abnormalities including, in one family, hypospadias (Muldal and Ockey 1962), and a long Y chromosome with a stag-horn calculus in a boy showing extremely bizarre behaviour (Harvey *et al.* 1970). Renal malformation is also common in Turner's syndrome (45,X). Urinary tract developmental anomaly occurs with only slightly increased frequency in Down's syndrome. Fabia and Drolette (1970) in a study of 2421 cases of Down's syndrome found the incidences quoted in Table 3.1.

Stern and Lewis (1958) in discussing equivocal evidence for a slightly low plasma calcium and high phosphate in children with Down's syndrome specifically excluded impaired renal function as a possible cause. On the other hand Deaton (1973) in a survey of 1018 Down's children, nine of whom died, found renal failure to be the cause of death

Table 3.1 *Incidence of urinary tract malformation in patients with Down's syndrome (Fabia and Drolette 1970).*

Malformation	Affected males	Affected females	Incidence per 1000 LB Down's patients
Hydroureter or hydronephrosis	2	2	1.7
Cystic kidney	2	0	0.8
Agenesis or hypoplasia of kidney	2	2	1.7
Congenital bladder obstruction	1	1	0.8
Miscellaneous	0	2	0.8
Total	7	7	5.8
	14		

in three, but does not comment further on this category. One may speculate that the known susceptibility of Down's patients to infection might increase the frequency of pyelonephritis. As early as 1966 Warkany *et al.* reviewed congenital malformations, including those of the urogenital system, in the autosomal trisomies. They noted cystic kidneys in 10 out of 32 autopsied cases of trisomy 13–15 as well as duplication defects and cryptorchidism. Among 84 autopsies reported in trisomy 18 they noted 18 instances of horseshoe kidney and 22 of duplication defects. Cystic kidney was present in only nine cases and unilateral renal agenesis or hypoplasia in only six. Cryptorchidism was reported only twice. They confirm the paucity of reports of renal anomaly in Down's syndrome, but quote early figures of 50 per cent cryptorchidism at birth (Benda 1960) and 27 per cent for all ages (Oster 1953).

Apart from these well known chromosomal disorders many of the partial monosomies and trisomies are associated, either frequently or only occasionally, with genito-urinary abnormalities.

In the selection of patients with renal anomalies for chromosomal analysis only limited guidelines can be provided because of the lack of specificity and variable expression of renal malformations in chromosomal disorders mentioned earlier. In general, isolated renal malformations in an otherwise normal child are most unlikely to be chromosomal in origin. Renal malformation forming part of a recognized clinical syndrome will require cytogenetic analysis only if chromosomal disorder is a known cause. Such analysis should be performed on any patient in whom renal anomaly is part of a cluster of malformations or dysmorphic features of unknown origin.

3.1. THE MAJOR CHROMOSOMAL DISORDERS

3.1.1. Trisomy 13 (47,XX or XY, +13)

The first report of renal anomaly in trisomy 13 was in a child with D trisomy who had large retroperitoneal masses suggestive of polycystic kidney and on an intravenous pyelogram showed enlargement of the right kidney with dilatation of the calyces (Lubs *et al.* 1961). Unfortunately no autopsy was obtained when she died at 7 weeks. Smith and his colleagues (1963) surveying 14 cases published up to that time recorded a renal anomaly in at least six out of nine with autopsy findings. These included most of the main types of anomaly that have since been described in trisomy 13, namely hydroureter and hydronephrosis (cases 163 and 408 of Smith *et al.* 1963), double renal pelvis and ureter (case 288 of Smith *et al.* 1963), and polycystic kidney (Northcutt 1962).

The earliest report of histologically studied polycystic kidney in trisomy 13 showed the cysts to be cortical microcysts (Sergovich *et al.* 1963). A fuller account is given by Marin-Padilla *et al.* (1964) who confirmed that the cysts are predominantly small. They observed abnormal atrophic fetal lobulations containing cysts, with normal lobulations in between. The cysts were formed by dilated Bowman's capsules. The associated glomerular tufts were frequently morphologically abnormal, commonly showing multiple vascular tufts (Fig. 3.1). Taylor *et al.* (1970) observed renal anomaly in all three of their cases, which were confirmed as polycystic kidney at autopsy in two of the three.

Several authors have attempted to estimate the frequency of the different clinico-pathological abnormalities in trisomy 13, including renal anomalies. Apart from Smith and his colleagues (1963) similar observations were made by Koenig *et al.* (1962) and Rosenfield *et al.* (1962). Taylor (1967) reviewed 55 cases mainly from the literature and also studied 27 cases herself, seen at the Paediatric Research Unit, Guy's Hospital Medical School (1968). She found polycystic kidney in a third of her own autopsy cases and a half of those from the literature. Duplication anomalies were present in a seventh of her own cases. These features in particular were helpful in distinguishing trisomy 13 from trisomy 18. She found just under a tenth of her own and a third of published cases of trisomy 13 had hydronephrosis or hydroureter, compared with 23 per cent of her own cases of trisomy 18. Horseshoe kidney did not occur in Taylor's own series of trisomy 13 but did so in 23 per cent of her cases of trisomy 18. Two of her male trisomy 13 cases had hypospadias, and other authors have reported micropenis and cryptorchidism (Powars *et al.* 1964; Smith 1964). Just under a half of Taylor's cases had a normal renal tract. Nevertheless renal anomaly may be seen in cases of partial trisomy 13, as instanced by the finding of hydronephrosis in a patient with a duplication of the long arm of chromosome 13 (Delhanty and Shapiro 1962) and of renal agenesis in the case of Ishmael and Laurence (1965). Neibuhr (1977), reviewing partial trisomy 13, found renal anomaly in three out of eight mosiac cases and in six out of 10 translocation cases with trisomy of the distal one- to two-thirds of the chromosome. A curious observation is that of a thickened renal tubular membrane in an infant with a double aneuploid mosaicism trisomy 13 and XXY (47,XY,+13/48,XXY,+13) (Ebbin *et al.* 1972). Recently Cowen *et al.* (1979) reported apparent absence of the right kidney on intravenous pyelography in a patient, without evidence of mosaicism, still alive at 9 years of age.

3.1.2. Trisomy 18 (47,XX or YX,+18)

Horseshoe kidney was a feature of the second reported case of trisomy 18 (Smith *et al.* 1960, case 8), and indeed horseshoe kidney or unilateral

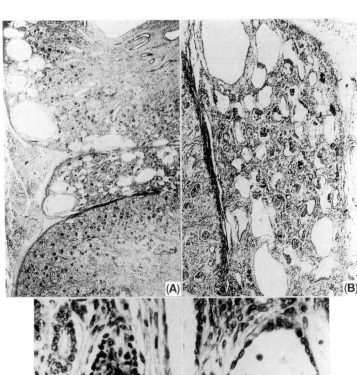

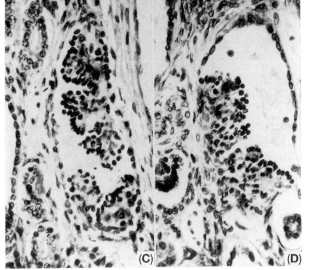

Fig. 3.1. Renal cortical cysts in trisomy 13, from Marin-Padilla *et al.* (1964) *Cytogenetics and cell genetics*, **3**, 258, with permission from S. Karger, AG, Basel. (A) Low power view to show normal and abnormal fetal lobulations; (B) Detail of atrophic fetal lobulation from A, showing numerous cysts, the smaller of which are dilated glomerular spaces; (C) Detail of single dilated glomerulus with several vascular poles; (D) Detail of single dilated glomerulus with broad vascular pole.

fused kidney is the most common renal malformation in this chromosomal disorder. Horseshoe kidney occurred in two of the seven cases reviewed by Smith *et al.* (1962), unilateral fused kidney in two and horseshoe kidney in one of three cases of Townes *et al.* (1963), and horseshoe kidney in three out of 19 of Taylor's (1968) cases. A detailed autopsy anatomical study, including description of a J-shaped unilateral fused kidney, in a case of trisomy 18 is presented by Barash *et al.* (1970). Other renal anomalies reported include duplication anomalies, unilateral renal agenesis, hydronephrosis, and renal cortical cysts. Townes *et al.* (1963) described histological cysts involving both Bowman's capsules and proximal tubules.

The overall incidence of renal anomaly in different studies is remarkably consistent. Lejeune (1964) found 58 per cent of cases had renal anomaly, Hamerton (1971) reviewing 150 published cases found 57 per cent and Taylor (1968) found 10 out of 16 (63 per cent) among her own cases. Urinary tract anomalies were observed in two out of three spontaneously aborted fetuses with trisomy 18 reported by Byrne and Blanc (1985). Like partial trisomy 13, partial trisomy 18 may still be associated with renal anomaly, as in the case reported by the author (Crawfurd 1961) in which an apparent extra E-group chromosome had a deletion of part of the long arm and the patient had left-sided hydronephrosis and hydroureter, as well as the clinical picture of trisomy 18. Hsu *et al.* (1971) in a review of cases of trisomy 22 have reinterpreted the extra chromosome in this case as a 22 instead of a deleted 18. However, neither the morphology of the extra chromosome nor the clinical picture support this contention.

In addition to renal malformation, cryptorchidism is a constant finding in the male (Taylor 1968), and the kidney may show the comparatively benign condition of nodular renal blastema, or diffuse nephroblastomatosis, in association with malformations (Bove *et al.* 1969). Wilm's tumour may arise in kidneys with nodular blastema and this combination has been reported in trisomy 18 (Geiser and Schindler 1969).

3.1.3. Turner's syndrome (45,X)

Turner's syndrome, ovarian dysgenesis, was well recognized as being frequently associated with renal malformation, especially horseshoe kidney, long before its karyotype became established (Meyer 1925; Hortling 1955; Bishop *et al.* 1960). The association of the 45,X karyotype with these renal anomalies, in both live-born births and spontaneously aborted fetuses, was later confirmed (Lemli and Smith 1963; Hung and LoPresti 1965; Byrne and Blanc 1985). Other renal abnormalities that are seen include double kidney or ureter, unilateral renal agenesis, cystic kidney or hydronephrosis, as are indeed seen in other chromosomal disorders thus underlining the non-specificity of these defects. The overall incidence of renal anomaly in 45,X Turner's syndrome is variously quoted as 60 to 70 per cent, but in one study (Gordon and O'Neill 1969) renal anomaly was not observed in any of 10 infantile cases.

3.1.4. Sex chromosome polyploid syndromes

The external genitalia; penis, testes, and sometimes scrotum are often small in childhood patients with Klinefelter's syndrome. In adult life the testes are of course atrophic. Cryptorchidism and hypospadias are reported to occur as occasional abnormalities. One of 17 cases reviewed by Hamerton (1971) had hypospadias but follow-up studies on 47,XXY infants detected in neonatal surveys have not detected hypospadias (Eller *et al.* 1971; Puck *et al.* 1975; Ratcliffe 1976). It may be that reports of malformation of the genitalia, as distinct from hypoplasia, are chance associations biasing ascertainment. Although early reports of males with the 47,XXY karyotype frequently mention cryptorchidism and penal or scrotal hypoplasia, it would appear that hypospadias and other lower urinary tract malformations are rare. Higher degrees of X and Y ploidy in the male (48,XXXY or XXYY, 49,XXXXY, and 49,XXXYY) all show a greater tendency to hypogonadism and hypogenitalism (Zollinger 1969; McGann *et al.* 1970; Simpson *et al.* 1974), intellectual impairment, behavioural disturbance, congenital heart disease and minor skeletal defects such as radio-ulnar synostosis especially in the 49,XXXXY syndrome (Zaleski *et al.* 1966). None of these further male sex chromosomal anomalies, nor females with 47,XXX or higher degrees of X ploidy, show any increased incidence of renal malformation, although renal malformation is mentioned in a boy with a 49,XXXX karyotype (Fraccaro *et al.* 1960a and b). Hypospadias is again rare in these syndromes and also in the syndrome of the XX male (Yunis *et al.* 1975). Wilms' tumour has been described in a male pseudohermaphrodite with XX/XY mosaicism (Denys *et al.* 1967).

3.2. OTHER CHROMOSOMAL DISORDERS

3.2.1. Chromosome 1

A family with segregation of a translocation between chromsomes 1 and 7 has been reported in which two offspring had an unbalanced form of the translocation with effective trisomy for the 1q32 → qter segment of chromosome 1 and deletion of the chromosome 7q34 → qter segment.

The infants had cyclopia or cebocephaly and urethral stenosis with hydronephrosis or horseshoe kidneys with hydroureters, respectively (Schinzel 1984).

In another recent report an infant is described with an interstitial deletion in the long arm of chromosome 1, del(q23→q25). There were facial and limb defects comparable to those previously reported in similar deletion cases, a congenital heart defect and hypoplastic kidneys (Silengo *et al.* 1984).

3.2.2. Chromosome 3

Boué *et al.* (1974) described an infant with a duplication 3q21qter and deletion 3p25ter as an aneuploid derivative of a parental inversion. The child had amongst other abnormalities hyperplastic, polycystic kidneys, double ureter, hydronephrosis, and cryptorchidism. An identical inversion was reported with similar duplication deletion anomaly in three children by Allderdice *et al.* (1975). Renal malformations included: (1) duplicated right ureter, (2) large kidneys with thin cortical surface cysts, and (3) large kidneys with left hydronephrosis and hydroureter. Similar renal malformations have been described in more recently reported cases (see De Grouchy and Turleau 1984). A recent literature review noted renal or urinary tract anomalies in 11 out of 23 reported cases of 3q duplication (Wilson *et al.* 1985).

Deletion of the short arm of chromosome 3 is typically associated with microcephaly and dolicocephaly, micrognathia, epicanthus, ptosis, low set or malformed ears, postaxial polydactyly and growth or mental retardation. Microcysts of the kidney due to dilated glomeruli in the cortex and dilated tubules in the cortex and medulla, with increased interstitial connective tissue, have been described in a single case (Beneck *et al.* 1984).

3.2.3. Chromosome 4

Deletion of the short arm of this chromosome (Wolf-Hirschhorn or 4p− syndrome) appears to be almost constantly associated in males with hypospadias and frequently with cryptorchidism (Leao *et al.* 1966; Arias *et al.* 1970; Miller *et al.* 1970; Fryns *et al.* 1973; Centerwall *et al.* 1975; Neu *et al.* 1975). This was so in 13 out of 14 cases reviewed by Rethore (1977b). Guthrie *et al.* (1971) noted the presence of small kidneys in one out of four cases of short arm chromosome 4 deletions. Arias *et al.* (1970) noted bilateral ureteric reflux in their case 1, and Wilcock *et al.* (1970) observed dilated renal pelvis and calyces due to fibrous obstruction of the ureters. Mikelsaar *et al.* (1973) reported bilateral renal agenesis in a stillborn 4p— fetus. Similar genital abnormalities, along with short penis, are seen in trisomy for the short arm of chromosome 4 (Rethore *et al.* 1974, Rethore 1977a). Hydronephrosis has been reported twice (Gustavson *et al.* 1964; Hustinx *et al.* 1975) and prolapsed bladder once (Giovanelli *et al.* 1974, case 1). Cryptorchidism is invariable in males with partial trisomy for the long arm and renal abnormalities have been found in most autopsied cases (Rethore 1977a), but not all cases of partial 4q trisomy (Baccichetti *et al.* 1975). The renal malformations described have included hydronephrosis and hydroureter with vesico-ureteral reflux (Surana and Conen 1972; Schrott *et al.* 1974), horseshoe kidney (Shaw *et al.* 1965), unilateral renal agenesis or bilateral renal hypoplasia (Francke 1972; Dutrillaux *et al.* 1975, case 3; Vogel *et al.* 1975, cases 2 and 3). Partial long arm deletion for chromosome 4 (partial 4q monosomy) is recorded as being associated with renal hypoplasia with dysplasia (Carter *et al.* 1969), calyceal dilatation (Ockey *et al.* 1967), and with renal duplication (Carnevale and de los Cobos 1973; Golbus *et al.* 1973) and hypospadias with genital hypoplasia (Van Kempen 1975).

3.2.4. Chromosome 5

Monosomy for the short arm ('Cri-du-chat' or 5p— syndrome) is one of the better-known chromosomal anomalies. Hypospadias, cryptorchidism, and renal malformations are all exceptional defects. In her review of cri-du-chat syndrome Rethore (1977b) mentions nine reports of renal malformations including horseshoe kidney (Lejeune *et al.* 1964, case 5; Bach *et al.* 1968; Hoehn and Engel 1969), renal hypoplasia (Giorgi *et al.* 1965), renal agenesis or radiologically non-functioning kidney (Sidbury *et al.* 1964; Capotorti and Ferrante 1966; McGavin *et al.* 1967), and precalyceal ectasia (Lejeune *et al.* 1964, case 2).

3.2.5. Chromosome 6

Therkelsen *et al.* (1971) reported a family in which partial trisomy for the short arm of chromosome 6 was present in two brothers. The picture included small kidneys with urinary infections and proteinuria. Thorburn *et al.* (1969) described an infant with a partial B-group long arm trisomy. This infant died at 5 weeks of age. At autopsy the kidneys, sited at the pelvic brim, showed extensive 'congenital' glomerulosclerosis with eosinophilic cell infiltration and scattered cortical nephrocalcinosis. Unfortunately both these reports were from the prebanding days and the precise identification of chromosomes 6 as being the one involved is not confirmed.

3.2.6. Chromosome 7

Complete trisomy 7 has only rarely been reported in spontaneous abortuses (Byrne and Bland 1985), and in only two near-term fetuses. Both of the latter fetuses showed Potter's syndrome. In one this was associated with unilateral renal agenesis and contralateral polycystic kidney with hydronephrosis (Yunis *et al.* 1980). In the other there was bilateral renal agenesis (Pflueger *et al.* 1984). Partial trisomy for the short arm, especially the 7p2 region, was reported as being associated with cryptorchidism and a small penis in a boy (Carnevale *et al.* 1978), and with renal cysts in a girl (Berry *et al.* 1979).

Urinary tract abnormalities do not appear to have been reported in partial trisomy for the long arm of this chromosome. Normal findings on intravenous pyelography have been reported for deletions of both the short arm (Friedrich *et al.* 1975) and the long arm (Harris *et al.* 1977; Kousseff *et al.* 1977). On the other hand Shokeir *et al.* (1973) found parenchymal renal atrophy with calyceal and ureteric dilatation associated with vesico-ureteral reflux in a 22-year-old woman with long arm chromosome 7 deletion, and Crawfurd *et al.* (1979) found hypospadias and hypogenitalism in an infant with a short arm 7 deletion.

3.2.7. Chromosome 8

Renal malformations, apart from hydronephrosis (Caspersson *et al.* 1972, case 10; Malpuech *et al.* 1972; Kakati *et al.* 1973; Aller *et al.* 1975; Kondo *et al.* 1975), are rare in the relatively frequent anomaly of trisomy 8, although cryptorchidism is common even in mosaic cases (Bijlsma *et al.* 1972; Crandall *et al.* 1974). However, in several presumed cases of 8 trisomy, from prebanding-technique days, renal cysts, agenesis, and other anomalies have been described (Wolf and Reinwein 1965; van Eys *et al.* 1970; Juberg *et al.* 1970; Riccardi *et al.* 1970; Cassidy *et al.* 1975; Gorlin *et al.* 1975). Wilms' tumour has been reported in a case of trisomy 8 in which the chromosomal anomaly could be detected only in fibroblasts (Niss and Passarge 1976).

Trisomy for the distal portion of the long arm of 8 has been described as a separate syndrome from the complete trisomy. Renal anomalies have not been reported (Fryns *et al.* 1974), nor have they been described in trisomy for the short arm (Rosenthal *et al.* 1973).

3.2.8. Chromosome 9

Trisomy of the whole chromosome 9, either pure or mosaic, is associated with cryptorchidism in some and scrotal hypoplasia and micropenis in most affected males (Feingold and Atkins 1973; Bowen *et al.* 1974). Microcysts of Bowman's capsule have also been reported (Bowen *et al.* 1974; Francke *et al.* 1975).

Tetrasomy of the short arm of chromosome 9 has been described in three cases, all mosaic. The facial abnormalities are similar to those of trisomy for the short arm but in addition there are multiple severe malformations which include the kidney. The renal malformation in one case consisted of hypoplasia of the right kidney (Ghymers *et al.* 1973).

Monosomy of the short arm is associated with hypospadias in about two-thirds of male cases (Alfi *et al.* 1973, 1976; Rethore 1977a).

A new syndrome has recently been reported in which the phenotype included bilateral hydroureter and a unilateral small dysplastic kidney. The karyotype showed an interstitial deletion within the long arm of chromosome 9 with breaks at 9q22 and 9q32 (Ying *et al.* 1982).

3.2.9. Chromosome 10

Renal malformation may be present in partial trisomy of the long arm of this chromosome, and when present may contribute to early death. Both hydronephrosis and renal dysplasia (Mulcahy *et al.* 1974), and renal cysts (Talvik *et al.* 1973; Moreno-Fuenmayor *et al.* 1975, case 2), have been described. Unilateral renal hypoplasia has also been reported (Yunis and Sanchez 1974) and also decreased renal function (Bühler *et al.* 1967).

In five out of 12 reported cases of deletion of the short arm of chromosome 10 there were urinary tract anomalies, and in a further three of these cases cryptorchidism or hypoplastic scrotum (Elstner *et al.* 1984). In the first such case renal dysplasia, with on the left hypoplasia and acute pyelonephritis, and in both kidneys scattered foci of cartilage were reported (Shokeir *et al.* 1975).

In trisomy for the short arm the genitalia in the male may be hypoplastic (Schleiermacher *et al.* 1974, case 1; Yunis *et al.* 1976). In an autopsied case bilateral cystic kidneys and one blind-ending ureter were found (Hustinx *et al.* 1974). Renal agenesis (Cantu *et al.* 1975, case 2) and renal dysplasia (Yunis *et al.* 1976) have also been described.

3.2.10. Chromosome 11

Severe malformation is common in trisomy for the long arm of chromosome 11, including urogenital malformations, and in males invariable micropenis (Rott *et al.* 1972; Laurent *et al.* 1975; Francke 1977). The renal malformations reported include renal agenesis and renal artery anomalies (Francke 1972; Rott *et al.* 1972; Giraud *et al.* 1975). The majority of cases result from a 3:1 segregation of a parental t(11;22) translocation (Schinzel *et al.* 1981).

Long arm 11 deletions were associated with hypospadias and ectopic testes in one of two males reported (Jacobsen *et al.* 1973). Severe renal malformations, including duplication defects and hydronephrosis, were present in two patients from Jacobsen *et al.* (1973) family, and in the single case of Sirota *et al.* (1984), but are certainly not present in all cases (Taillemite *et al.* 1975; Turleau *et al.* 1975).

Because of the marked prepronderance of females among such deletions, and of XY sex chromosomal constitution and ambiguous genitalia in chromosome 11 short arm deletions, Franck and Riccardi (1977) suggested that in the presence of an XY sex chromosome constitution intact 11 long arms are necessary for survival, and intact 11 short arms for normal genito-urinary development.

The association of an 11p13 deletion with Wilms' tumour and the aniridia, genito-urinary malformation, mental retardation triad is fully discussed in Chapter 10.

3.2.11. Chromosome 12

In partial monosomy for the short arm of chromosome 12 cryptorchidism is common, and micropenis is an occasional feature (Magnelli and Therman 1975; Orye and Craen 1975; Tenconi *et al.* 1975).

3.2.12. Chromosome 13

Apart from trisomy 13 discussed earlier many cases of partial chromosome 13 deletions have been described. Niebuhr (1977) has reviewed 72 such cases and on the basis of whether they have simple or complex deletions or ring chromosomes and of their phenotype has defined four categories. There are ring chromosome cases with normal thumbs: category 1, rings or deletions with thumb aplasia or hypoplasia: categories 2a and 2b, deletions with retinoblastoma: category 3, and deletions with neither thumb abnormality nor retinoblastoma: category 4. The precise localization of the deletion is not clear in all cases but the cumulated evidence suggests that category 1 is associated with deletion of the 13q telomere and distal band (13q34−), category 2 with various proximal to mid long arm deletions involving loss of at least the band 13q31, category 3 with an interstitial deletion of the proximal part of the long arm involving loss of a segment in the region of bands q14–q22, and category 4 with an interstitial deletion of the long arm between bands 13q21 and 13q31. Examples of the deletions associated with the different categories are illustrated in Fig. 3.2.

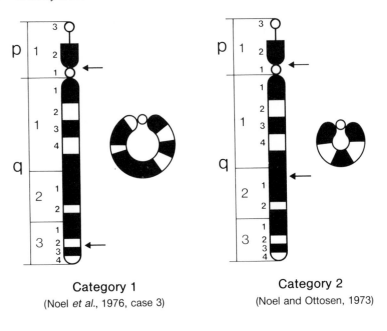

Category 1
(Noel *et al.*, 1976, case 3)

Category 2
(Noel and Ottosen, 1973)

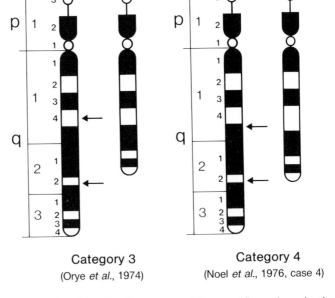

Category 3
(Orye *et al.*, 1974)

Category 4
(Noel *et al.*, 1976, case 4)

Fig. 3.2. Diagnosis of breakpoints reported by specific authors in the different types of chromosome 13 long arm deletion, as defined by Niebuhr (1977).

The frequency of urinary tract malformations in these different categories is shown in Table 3.2. However, the absolute numbers in each category are small, mostly 10 or less.

Table 3.2 *Urinary tract malformation in 13q deletion*

Malformation	Category of deletion and cases affected (%)				
	1	2a	2b	3	4
Hypospadias	33	100	66	33	0
Bifid scrotum	28	100	66	0	0
Renal anomaly	57	50	100	0	66

Bifid scrotum is seen with or without perineal fistula, and in some patients epispadias replaces hypospadias. Cryptorchidism is also seen, especially in the cases with distal long arm deletions (category 2b) (Allderdice *et al.* 1969) or ring 13 (categories 1 and 2a) (Reisman *et al.* 1965; Tolksdorf *et al.* 1969; Lehrke *et al.* 1971). Whilst several phenotype abnormalities, such as abnormal nuclear projections, elevated HbF, retinoblastoma, polydactyly, and absent thumbs, appear to be associated with trisomy or monosomy for specific regions of the long arm this is not the case for renal malformations, except that they do not seem to be associated with deletions with the retinoblastoma phenotype (Wilson *et al.* 1969, 1973). The renal malformations seen include renal hypoplasia in a patient with a ring chromosome (Bain and Gauld 1963), and hydronephrosis in an unusual case with del 13(q14) without retinoblastoma or thumb defect but with intestinal atresia (Nishikawa *et al.* 1985). A recent report of partial 13q monosomy and partial 18p trisomy in a stillborn infant describes hypoplastic kidneys and a bicornuate uterus (Beneck *et al.* 1986). Ring chromosomes involving a D-group chromosome have been described, such as the three cases reported by Lejeune *et al.* (1968), without significant urogenital anomaly. However, as these cases were reported before banding techniques had become available the ring D may have involved a chromosome 14 or 15 rather than a 13.

3.2.13. Chromosome 14

Syndromes with partial trisomy of the long arm of chromosome 14 have been described involving either the proximal or the distal part of the long arm. The more common proximal trisomy, although associated with severe malformation, has not usually been reported as showing urinary tract anomaly. An exception is a case in which there was unilateral renal agenesis with contralateral renal hypoplasia and cystic change (Cottrall *et al.* 1981).

Partial trisomy for the distal long arm may be associated with cryptorchidism, micropenis, or hypospadias but not renal anomaly (Atkin and Patil 1983).

3.2.14. Chromosome 15

Trisomy for the distal part of the long arm of chromosome 15 was associated with cryptorchidism in each of six male patients in one family (Schnatterly *et al.* 1984).

3.2.15. Chromosome 16

Trisomy for the short arm of this chromosome may be associated with cryptorchidism (Roberts and Duckett 1978), and partial trisomy for the long arm with micropenis and cryptorchidism (Hatanaka *et al.* 1984).

3.2.16. Chromosome 17

'Deformed kidney' has been described in trisomy of the short arm of this chromosome in a single case (Docherty *et al.* 1983), renal abnormalities in two cases, and cryptorchidism in one case of duplication of the short arm (Feldman *et al.* 1982). Consistent cryptorchidism in male patients, and renal malformations in autopsied cases, have also been described in the reported cases of duplication of the distal part of the long arm of chromosome 17 (Naccache *et al.* 1984).

The Miller–Dieker syndrome of lissencephaly with growth retardation and dysmorphic features has in the past been regarded as probably an autosomal recessive disorder. Recently Dobyns and colleagues have reported effective monosomy for the 17p 13.3 band on the short arm of chromosome 17 in several cases. In one of these this was due to an unbalanced translocation inherited from a balanced parent (Dobyns *et al.* 1983; Dobyns *et al.* 1984; Stratton *et al.* 1984), and in another to the recombinant product of a parental pericentric inversion (Greenberg *et al.* 1986). In reviewing the earlier literature they suggest that some previous cases were also associated with this deletion. They mention cystic renal dysplasia or polycystic kidneys in two patients, and renal agenesis or cryptorchidism in others.

Smith and colleagues (1986) have described a slightly more proximal deletion (17) (p 11.2) in nine patients. In two of these there were abnormalities of the ureterovesical junction.

3.2.17. Chromosome 18

Abnormalities of male genitalia have been reported in deletions involving both the short and long arms of chromosome 18. Genital anomalies are unusual, being present in only six out of 22 male patients reviewed by Rethore (1977b), in the comparatively common short arm deletion.

Micropenis has been reported twice (Jacobsen and Mikkelsen 1968, case 1; McDermott *et al.* 1968), hydronephrosis once (Giraud *et al.* 1971), and testicular ectopy three times (De Grouchy *et al.* 1963; Lejeune *et al.* 1966; Vaillaud *et al.* 1970).

In contrast, the same anomalies along with hypoplastic scrotum are all common in long arm deletions or 'carp-mouth' syndrome (Parker *et al.* 1972; Schinzel *et al.* 1975). Rethore (1977b) on reviewing the 18q– syndrome noted ectopic testes in 10 out of 22 males. Furthermore horseshoe kidney (De Grouchy *et al.* 1964; Wertelecki *et al.* 1966, case 6) and unilateral renal agenesis (Law and Masterton 1966) have also been reported in long arm deletion. Lurie and Lazjuk (1972) in a review of the literature estimated that 3 per cent of 18p– cases and 7 per cent of 18q– cases have renal abnormalities, and 18 and 44 per cent respectively have genital anomalies with values for ring 18 intermediate between the 18p– and 18q– cases.

3.2.18. Chromosome 19

Lange and Alfi (1976) reported two sibs who inherited trisomy for the long arm of chromosome 19 from their mother who carried a balanced translocation t(19;22) (q13;p13). Their clinical abnormalities included hypospadias and hypoplasia of the testes in the male sib and multicystic kidneys in both. In the male there was a right hydronephrosis and hydroureter and in the female an ectopic malrotated left kidney and left hydroureter.

3.2.19. Chromosome 20

Trisomy 20 mosaicism is a comparatively common finding in amniotic fluid cell cultures. Although it does not appear to be an *in vitro* artefact it has never been confirmed in neonatal tissues and cannot be regarded as being indicative of fetal maldevelopment (Nisani *et al.* 1984). There is evidence that the mosaicism may originate, or at least be reflected, in fetal urinary tract tissues including renal fibroblast cultures (Boué *et al.* 1979).

3.2.20. Chromosome 21

Reports of a ring chromosome or of proximal deletion of chromosome 21 include hypospadias and cryptorchidism as almost constant clinical features (Warren and Rimoin 1970; Armendares *et al.* 1971) in male patients. Renal agenesis (Reisman *et al.* 1966) has also been reported in ring 21, and in a case studied by Rethore *et al.* (1976), with proximal 21 deletion horseshoe and bifid kidneys were found.

3.2.21. Chromosome 22

Reported cases of apparent trisomy for chromosome 22 are now generally regarded as instances of effective trisomy 11q derived from an 11;22 translocation (De Grouchy and Turleau 1984). They show the clinical features, including micropenis and renal malformations seen in 11q trisomy. True trisomy 22 is seen only in early spontaneous abortuses. Partial trisomy for the proximal long arm has been termed 'cat-eye syndrome' and is characterized by coloboma and imperforate anus. It has been reported in association with a variety of renal malformations including unilateral renal agenesis or renal hypoplasia, horseshoe kidneys, duplication defects, ectopia, and obstruction with or without hydronephrosis (Gerald *et al.* 1968, 1972; Thomas *et al.* 1969; Noël and Quack 1970; Weber *et al.* 1970; Cory and Jamison 1974; Kunze *et al.* 1975; Pierson *et al.* 1975). They have also been reported in several patients with incomplete cat-eye syndrome (Zellweger *et al.* 1962; Ishmael and Laurence 1965; Schachenmann *et al.* 1965; Beyer *et al.* 1968; Gerald *et al.* 1968). Nevertheless typical cat-eye syndrome can occur without renal anomaly (Pfeiffer *et al.* 1970). This syndrome overlaps phenotypically with the full trisomy 22 syndrome and also with the VATER anomaly (Quan and Smith 1972) and the Holt–Oram syndrome (Silver *et al.* 1972) as pointed out by Lindenbaum (1978). Renal malformation has not been reported in ring chromosome 22 cases (Lindenbaum *et al.* 1973; Rethore 1977b). Complete or partial trisomy 22 should not be confused with the syndrome of imperforate anus, and digital and vertebral anomaly described by Say *et al.* (1971) in which no chromosomal anomaly has been reported, but which can include renal agenesis. Two sisters with apparently normal karyotypes but phenotypically characteristic cat-eye syndrome have been reported (Franklin and Parslow 1972). Renal anomaly was detected in neither. Intravenous pyelography was normal in the second sister and autopsy revealed no renal anomaly in the first.

In comparison with partial trisomy for the proximal long arm, that for the distal long arm is rare. The trisomic segment has varied from a 22q11 to 22q13 breakpoint to 22qter. It is characterized by severe mental and motor retardation, failure to thrive and growth retardation, hypotonia, congenital hydrocephalus, cleft palate, congenital heart defect, sacral pits, and a facial dysmorphology with micrognathia, broad nasal bridge, low set ears, and long philtrum. Four out of five reported cases have also shown renal aplasia or dysplasia (Jotterand-Bellomo 1976/77; Schinzel 1981, case 2 but not the cytogenetically identical case 1; Bendel *et al.* 1982 (first case); Annerén *et al.* 1984).

3.2.22. Triploidy

The great majority of triploid fetuses are aborted. In the rare cases with birth after 28 weeks gestation hypospadias, cryptorchidism, and Leydig cell hyperplasia are commonly seen and micropenis and bifid scrotum occasionally seen in the male. Cystic renal dysplasia and occasionally hydronephrosis are seen in both sexes (Walker *et al.* 1973; Al Saadi *et al.* 1976; Gosden *et al.* 1976).

References

Al Saadi, A., Juliar, J. F., Harm, J., Brough, A. J., Perrin, E. V. and Chen, H. (1976). Triploidy syndrome. A report on tiny live-born (69,XXY) and one still-born (69,XXX) infants. *Clin. Genet.* **9**, 43–50.

Alfi, I., Donnell, G. N., Crandall, B. F., Derencsenyi, A. and Menon, R. (1973). Deletion of the short arm of chromosome No. 9(46,9p−): a new deletion syndrome. *Ann. Génét.* **16**, 17–22.

——, Sanger, R. G. and Donnel, G. M. (1975). Trisomy 22: clinically identifiable syndrome. In *New chromosomal and malformation syndromes,* ed. Bergsma, D. *Birth Defects Orig. Art. Series.* **11** (5), 241–5.

——, Donnell, G. N., Allderdice, P. W. and Derencsenyi, A. (1976). The 9p− syndrome. *Ann. Génét.* **19**, 11–16.

Allderdice, P. W., Davis, J. G., Miller, O. J., Klinger, H. P., Warburton, D., Miller, D. A., Allen, F. N. Jr, Abrams, C. A. L. and McGilvray, E. (1969). The 13q− deletion syndrome. *Am. J. Hum. Genet.* **21**, 499–512.

——, Browne, N. and Murphy, D. P. (1975). Chromosome 3 duplication q21 →qter deletion p25 →pter syndrome in children of carriers of a pericentric inversion inv(3) (p25q21). *Am. J. Hum. Genet.* **27**, 699–718.

Aller, V., Abrisqueza, J. A., Perez, A., Martin, M. A., Goday, C. and Del Mazo, J. (1975). A case of trisomy 8 mosaicism 47,XX,+8/46,XX. *Clin. Genet.* **7**, 232–7.

Annerén, G., Gustavson, K.-H. and Jagell, S. (1984). Partial trisomy for the distal part of chromosome 22 (22q12 →qter) in a mentally retarded girl with congenital birth defects. *Hereditas* **100**, 115–19.

Arias, D., Passarge, E., Engle, M. A. and German, J. (1970). Human chromosomal deletion: two patients with the 4p− syndrome. *J. Pediatr.* **76**, 82–8.

Armendares, S., Buentello, L. and Cantu-Garza, J. M., (1971). Partial monosomy of a G group chromosome (45,XY,−G/46,XY,Gr): report of a new case. *Ann. Génét.* **14**, 7–12.

Atkin, J. F. and Patil, S. (1983). Duplication of the distal segment of 14q. *Am. J. Med. Genet.* **16**, 357–66.

Baccichetti, C., Tenconi, R., Anglani, F. and Zacchello, F. (1975). Trisomy 4q 32 → qter due to a maternal 4/21 translocation. *J. Med. Genet.* **12**, 425–7.

Bach, Ch., Gautier, M., Schaefer, P. and Moszer, M. (1968). La maladie du cri-du-chat. Une observation anatomoclinique *Sem. Hôp. Paris (Ann. Pédiatr.)* **44**, 339–43.

Bain, A. D. and Gauld, I. K. (1963). Multiple congenital abnormalities associated with ring chromosome. *Lancet* **2**, 304–5.

Barash, B. A., Freedman, L. and Opitz, J. M. (1970). Anatomic studies in the 18-trisomy syndrome. *Birth Defects Orig. Art. Series* **6** (4), 3–15.

Benda, C. A. (1960). *The child with mongolism (congenital acromicria)*. Grune & Stratton, New York.

Bendel, R. P., Baldinger, S., Millard, C. and Arthur, D. C. (1982). Two successive partial trisomies for opposite halves of chromosome 22 in a mother with a balanced translocation. *J. Med. Genet.* **19**, 313.

Beneck, D., Oreco, M. A., Wolman, S. R., McMorrow, L. E., Jansen, V. and Cason, J. (1986). Partial monosomy 13q and partial trisomy 18p: case report with necropsy findings. *J. Med. Genet.* **23**, 260–3.

——, Suhrland, M. J., Dicker, R., Greco, M. A. and Wolman, S. R. (1984). Deletion of the short arm of chromosome 3: a case report with necropsy findings. *J. Med. Genet.* **21**, 307–10.

Berry, A. C., Honeycombe, J. and Macoun, S. J. R. (1979). Two children with partial trisomy for 7p. *J. Med. Genet.* **16**, 320–1.

Beyer, P., Ruch, J.-V., Rumpler, Y. and Girard, J. (1968). Observation d'un enfant débile mental et polymalformé dont le caryotype montre la presence d'un petit extra-chromosome mediocentrique. *Pédiatrie* **23**, 439–42.

Bijlsma, J. B., Wijffels, J. C. H. M. and Tegelaers, W. H. H. (1972). C8 trisomy mosaicism syndrome. *Helv. Paediatr. Acta* **27**, 281–98.

Bishop, P. M. F., Lessof, M. H. and Polani, P. E. (1960). Turner's syndrome and allied conditions. *Mem. Soc. Endocrinol* No. **7**, 162–72.

Boué, J., Hirschhorn, K., Lucas, M., Moszier, M. and Bac, C. (1974). Aneusomies de recombinaison, consequences d'une inversion pericentrique d'un chromosome 3 paternal. *Ann. Pédiatr.* **21**, 567–73.

——, Nicolas, H., Barichard, F. and Boué, A. (1979). Le clonage des cellules du liquide amniotique, aide dans l'interpretation des mosaiques chromosomiques en diagnostic prenatal. *Ann. Génét.* **22**, 3–9.

Bove, K. E., Koffler, H. and McAdams, A. J. (1969). Nodular renal blastema: definition and possible significance. *Cancer* **24**, 323–32.

Bowen, P., Ying, K. L. and Chung, G. S. H. (1974). Trisomy 9 mosaicism in a newborn infant with multiple malformations. *J. Pediatr.* **85**, 95–7.

Bühler, U. K., Bühler, E. M., Sartorius, J. and Standler, G. R. (1967). Multiple Misbildungen bei partieller Trisomie C (12) als Manifestation einer erblichen E/C(18/12) Translokation. *Helv. Paediatr. Acta* **22**, 41–53.

Byrne, J. and Blanc, W. A. (1985). Malformations and chromosome anomalies in spontaneously aborted fetuses with a single umbilical artery. *Am. J. Obstet.*

Gynecol. **151**, 340–2.

Cantu, J.-M., Salamanca, F., Buentello, L., Carnevale, A. and Armendares, S. (1975). Trisomy 10p. A report of two cases due to a familial translocation rcp (10;21) (p11;p11). *Ann. Génét.* **18**, 5–11.

Capotorti, L. and Ferrante, E. (1966). D/B translocation in an infant with 45 chromosomes and with some phenotypic manifestations of the cri-du-chat syndrome. *Acta Paediatr. Lat. (Reggio Emilio)* **19**, 471–88.

Carakushansky, G., Neu, R. L. and Gardner, L. I. (1968). XYY with abnormal genitalia. *Lancet* **2**, 1144.

Carnevale, A. and de Los Cobos, L. (1973). A child with multiple congenital malformations and a 46,XX,t(13q+;Dq−)/45,XX,−B,−D,+ der (B), t(Bq+;Dq−) karyotype. *J. Med. Genet.* **10**, 376–9.

——, Frias, S. and Del Castillo, V. (1978). Partial trisomy of the short arm of chromosome 7 due to a familial translocation rcp (7;14) (p11;p11). *Clin. Genet.* **14**, 202–6.

Carter, R., Baker, E. and Hayman, D. (1969). Congenital malformations associated with a ring 4 chromosome *J. Med. Genet.* **6**, 224–7.

Caspersson, T., Lindsten, J., Zech, L., Buckton, K. E. and Price, W. H. (1972). Four patients with trisomy 8 identified by the fluorescence and giemsa banding technique. *J. Med. Genet.* **9**, 1–7.

Cassidy, S. B., McGee, B. J., van Eys, J., Nance, W. E. and Engel, E. (1975). Trisomy 8 syndrome. *Pediatrics* **56**, 826–31.

Centerwall, W. B., Thompson, W. P., Allen, I. E. and Fobes, C. D. (1975). Translocation 4p− syndrome. A general review. *Am. J. Dis. Child* **129**, 366–70.

Cory, C. C. and Jamison, D. L. (1974). The cat eye syndrome. *Arch. Ophthalmol.* **92**, 259–62.

Cottrall, K., Magrath, I., Bootes, J. A. H., Prouten, V., Brooker, C., Stewart, A. and Richards, B. W. (1981). A case of proximal 14 trisomy with pathological findings. *J. Ment. Defic. Res.* **25**, 1–6.

Cowen, J. M., Walker, S. and Harris, F. (1979). Trisomy 13 and extended survival. *J. Med. Genet.* **16**, 155–61.

Crandall, B. F., Bass, H. N., Marcy, S. M., Glovsky, M. and Fish, C. H. (1974). The trisomy 8 syndrome: two additional mosaic cases. *J. Med. Genet.* **11**, 393–8.

Crawfurd, M. d'A. (1961). Multiple congenital anomaly associated with an extra autosome. *Lancet* **2**, 22–4.

——, Kessell, I., Liberman, M., McKeown, J. A., Mandalia, P. Y. and Ridler, M. A. C. (1979). Partial monosomy 7 with interstitial deletions in two infants with different congenital abnormalities. *J. Med. Genet.* **16**, 453–60.

Deaton, J. G. (1973). The mortality rate and causes of death among institutionalized mongols in Texas. *J. Ment. Defic. Res.* **17**, 117–22.

De Grouchy, J. and Turleau, C. (1984). *Clinical atlas of human chromosomes,* 2nd edn. John Wiley, New York.

——, Lamy, M., Thieffry, S., Arthuis, M. and Salmon, C. (1963). Dysmorphie complexe avec oligophrenie: délétion des bras courts d'un chromosome 17–18. *C. R. Acad. Sci. (Paris)* **256**, 1028–9.

——, Royer, P., Salmon, Ch. and Lamy, M. (1964). Délétion partielle des bras longs du chromosome 18. *Pathol. Biol.* **12**, 579–82.

Delhanty, J. D. A. and Shapiro, A. (1962). An unusual acrocentric found in a case of idiocy with microphthalmia. *J. Ment. Defic. Res.* **6**, 38–40.

Denys, P., Malvaux, P., van den Berge, H., Tanghe, W. and Proesmans, W. (1967). Association d'un syndrome anatomopathologique de pseudohermaphrodisme masculin, d'une tumeur de Wilms, d'une nephropathie parenchymateuse et d'un mosaicisme XX/XY. *Arch. Fr. Pédiatr.* **24**, 729–39.

Dobyns, W. B., Stratton, R. F., Parke, J. T., Greenberg, F., Nussbaum, R. L. and Ledbetter, D. H. (1983). The Miller–Dieker syndrome: lissencephaly and monosomy 17p *J. Pediatr.* **102**, 552–8.

——, —— and Greenberg, F. (1984). Syndromes with lissencephaly. I: Miller–Diecker and Norman–Roberts syndromes and isolated lissencephaly. *Am. J. Med. Genet.* **18**, 509–26.

Docherty, Z., Hulten, M. A. and Honeyman, M. M. (1983). De novo tandem duplication of 17p11 → cen. *J. Med. Genet.* **20**, 138–42.

Dutrillaux, B., Laurent, C., Forabosco, A., Noel, B., Suerinc, E., Bemont, M.-C. and Cotton, J. B. (1975). La trisomie 4q partielle. Apropos de trois observations. *Ann. Génét.* **18**, 21–7.

Ebbin, A. J., Lim, R. C., Towner, J. W. and Wilson, M. G. (1972). A double aneuploid mosaic: trisomy 13 and XXY. *J. Med. Genet.* **9**, 365–7.

Eller, E., Frankenburg, W., Puck, M. and Robinson, A. (1971). Prognosis in newborn infants with X-chromosomal abnormalities. *Pediatrics*, **47**, 681–8.

Elstner, C. L., Carey, J. C., Livingston, G., Moeschler, J. and Lubinsky, M. (1984). Further delineation of the 10p deletion syndrome. *Pediatrics* **73**, 620–75.

Eys, J. van, Nance, W. E. and Engel, E. (1970). C autosomal trisomy with mosaicism: a new syndrome? *Pediatrics* **45**, 665–71.

Fabia, J. and Drolette, M. (1970). Malformations and leukaemia in children with Down's syndrome. *Pediatrics* **45**, 60–70.

Feingold, M. and Atkins, L. (1973). A case of trisomy 9. *J. Med. Genet.* **10**, 184–7.

Feldman, G. M., Baumer, J. G. and Sparkes, R. S. (1982). Brief clinical report: the dup (17p) syndrome. *Am. J. Med. Genet.* **11**, 299–304.

Ferrandez, A. and Schmid, W. (1971). Potter-Syndrom (Nierenagenesie) mit chromosomaler Aberration beim Patienten und Mosaik beim Vater. *Helv. Paediatr. Acta* **26**, 210–14.

Fraccaro, M., Kaijser, K. and Lindsten, J. (1960a and b). A child with 49 chromosomes. *Lancet* **2**, 899–902 and 1303.

Francke, U. (1972). Quinacrine mustard fluorescence of human chromosomes. Characterization of unusual translocations. *Am. J. Hum. Genet.* **24**, 189–213.

—— (1977). Abnormalities of chromosomes 11 and 20. Chapter 8 in *New chromosomal syndromes,* ed. Yunis, J. J. pp. 251–8. Academic Press, New York.

——, Benirschke, K. and Jones, O. W. (1975). Prenatal diagnosis of trisomy 9. *Humangenetik* **29**, 243–50.

Frank, J. and Riccardi, V. M. (1977). The 11q− syndrome. *Hum. Genet.* **35**, 241–6.

Franklin, R. C. and Parslow, M. I. (1972). The cat-eye syndrome. Review and two further cases occuring in female siblings with normal chromosomes. *Acta Paediatr. Scand.* **61**, 581–6.

Friedrick, U., Lyngbye, T. and Oster, J. (1975). A girl with karyotype

46,XX,del(7)(qter → p15:). *Humangenetik* **26**, 161–5.

Fryns, J. P., Eggermont, E., Verresen, H. and van Den Berghe, H. (1973). The 4p− syndrome with a report of two necropsy cases. *Humangenetik* **19**, 99–109.

——, Verresen, H., van Den Berghe, H., van Kerckvoorde, J. and Cassiman, J. J. (1974). Partial trisomy 8: trisomy of the distal part of the long arm of chromosome number 8+ (8q2) in a severely retarded and malformed girl. *Humangenetik* **24**, 241–6.

Geiser, C. F. and Shindler, A. M. (1969). Long survival in a male with 18 trisomy syndrome and Wilms' tumor. *Pediatrics* **44**, 111–16.

Gerald, P. S., Davis, C., Say, B. M. and Wilkins, J. L. (1968). A novel chromosomal basis for imperforate anus (the 'cat's-eye' syndrome). *Pediatr. Res.* **2**, 297.

——, ——, —— and —— (1972). Syndromal associations of imperforate anus: the cat eye syndrome. *Birth Defects Orig. Art. Series* **8** (2), 79–84.

Ghymers, D., Hermann, B., Distéche, C. and Frederic, J. (1973). Tétrasomie partielle du chromosome 9, à l'état de mosaique, chez un enfant porteur de malformations multiples. *Humangenetik* **20**, 273–82.

Giorgi, P. L., Ceccarelli, M. and Paci, A. (1965). Su un caso di sindrome del 'cri-du-chat' con peculiari anomalie fenotipiche. *Minerva Pediat.* **17**, 1972–5.

Giovanelli, G., Forabosco, A. and Dutrillaux, B. (1974). Translocation familiale t(4;22) (p11;p12) et trisomie 4p chez deux germains. *Ann. Génét.* **17**, 119–24.

Giraud, F., Hartung, M., Mattei, J. F., Passeron, P. and Coignet, J. (1971). Mosaic 46,XY/45,X and deletion 18p−. *Ann. Génét.* **14**, 59–62.

——, Mattei, J.-F., Mattei, M.-G. and Bernard, R. (1975). Trisomie partielle 11q et translocation familiale 11–22. *Humangenetik* **28**, 343–7.

Golbus, M. S., Conte, F. A. and Daentl, D. L. (1973). Deletion of the long arm of chromosome 4 (46,XX,4q−) associated with congenital anomalies. *J. Med. Genet.* **10**, 83–5.

Gordon, R. R. and O'Neill, E. M. (1969). Turner's infantile phenotype. *Br. Med. J.* **1**, 483–5.

Gorlin, R. J., Cervenka, J., Moller, K., Horrobin, M. and Witkop, C. J. (1975). A selected miscellany. Trisomy 8 mosaicism. *Birth Defects Orig. Art. Series* **11** (2), 48–50.

Gosden, M., Wright, M. O., Paterson, W. G. and Grant, K. A. (1976). Clinical details, cytogenic studies, and cellular physiology of a 69,XXX fetus, with comments on the biological effect of triploidy in man. *J. Med. Genet.* **13**, 371–80.

Greenberg, F., Stratton, R. F., Lockhart, L. H., Elder, F. F. B., Dobyns, W. B. and Ledbetter, D. H. (1986). Familial Miller–Diecker syndrome associated with pericentric inversion of chromosome 17. *Am. J. Med. Genet.* **23**, 853–9.

Gustavson, K.-H., Finley, S. C., Finley, W. H., and Jalling, B. (1964). A 4-5/21-22 chromosomal translocation associated with multiple congenital abnormalities. *Acta Paediatr. (Stockholm)* **53**, 172–81.

Guthrie, R. D., Aase, J. M., Asper, A. C. and Smith, D. W. (1971). The 4p− syndrome. A clinically recognizable chromosomal syndrome. *Am. J. Dis. Child.* **122**, 421–6.

Hamerton, J. L. (1971). *Human cytogenetics*, Vol. II *Clinical cytogenetics.* p. 32. Academic Press, New York and London.

Harris, E. L., Wappner, R. S., Palmer, C. G., Hall, B., Dinno, N., Seashore, M. R.

and Breg, W. R. (1977). 7q deletion syndrome (7q32 → 7qter). *Clin. Genet.* **12**, 233–8.

Harvey, P. W., Muldal, S. and Wauchob, D. (1970). Antisocial behaviour and a large Y chromosome. *Lancet* **1**, 887–9.

Hatanaka, K., Ozaki, M., Suzuki, M., Murata, R. and Fujita, H. (1984). Trisomy 16q13 → qter in an infant from a t(11;16) (q25;q13) translocation-carrier father. *Hum. Genet.* **65**, 311–15.

Hoehn, H. and Engel, W. (1969). Screening for minute deletions in patients with suspected cri-du-chat syndrome and apparently normal karyotype. *Humangenetik* **8**, 105–10.

Hortling, H. (1955). Congenital kidney anomalies in 'Turner's syndrome'. *Acta Endocrinol.* **18**, 548–52.

Hsu, L. Y. F., Shapiro, L. R., Gertner, M., Lieber, E. and Hirshhorn, K. (1971). Trisomy 22: a clinical entity. *J. Pediatr.* **79**, 12–19.

Hung, W. and LoPresti, J. M. (1965). Urinary tract anomalies in gonadal dysgenesis. *Am. J. Roentgenol., Rad. Therap. Nucl. Med. [N.S.]* **95**, 439–41.

Hustinx, Th. W. J., Ter Haar, B. G. A., Scheres, J. M. J. C. and Rutten, F. J. (1974). Trisomy for the short arm of chromosome No. 10. *Clin. Genet.* **6**, 408–15.

——, Gabriels, F. J. M., Kirkels, V. G. H. J., Korten, J. J., Scheres, J. M. J. C., Joosten, E. M. G. and Rutten, R. J. (1975). Trisomy 4p in a family with a t(4;15). *Ann. Génét.* **18**, 13–19.

Ishmael, J. and Laurence, K. M. (1965). A probable case of incomplete trisomy of a chromosome of the 13–15 group. *J. Med. Genet.* **2**, 136–41.

Jacobsen, P. and Mikkelsen, M. (1968). The 18p− syndrome. Report of two cases. *Ann. Génét.* **11**, 211–16.

——, Hauge, M., Henningsen, K., Hobolth, N., Mikkelsen, M. and Philip, J. (1973). An (11;21) translocation in four generations with chromosome 11 abnormalities in the offspring. *Hum. Hered.* **23**, 568–85.

Jotterand-Bellomo, M. (1976/77). Trisomie 22, *Arch. Genet.* **49/50** 134–66.

Juberg, R. C., Gilbert, E. F. and Salisbury, R. S. (1970). Trisomy C in an infant with polycystic kidneys and other malformations. *J. Pediatr.* **76**, 598–603.

Kakati, S., Nihill, M. and Sinha, A. K. (1973). An attempt to establish trisomy 8 syndrome. *Humangenetik* **19**, 293–300.

Kempen, C. Van (1975). A patient with congenital anomalies and a deletion of the long arm of chromosome 4 [46,XY, del(4)(q31)]. *J. Med. Genet.* **12**, 204–6.

Koenig, E. U., Lubs, H. A. and Brandt, I. K. (1962). The relationship between congenital anomalies and autosomal chromosome abnormalities. *Yale J. Biol. Med.* **35**, 189–205.

Kondo, I., Tomisawa, T., Matsura, A., Ibuki, Y., Yamashita, A. and Hara, Y. (1975). A case of trisomy 9 mosaicism. *Ann. Paediatr. Japan.* **21**, 48–50.

Kousseff, B. G., Hsu, L. Y. F., Paciuc, S. and Hirschhorn, K. (1977). A partial long arm deletion of chromosome 7: 46,XY, del (7) (q32). *J. Med. Genet.* **14**, 144–7.

Kunze, J., Tolksdorf, M. and Wiedermann, H.-R. (1975). Cat Eye-Syndrom. Klinische und cytogenetische Differentialdiagnose. *Humangenetik* **26**, 271–89.

Lange, M. and Alfi, O. S. (1976). Trisomy 19q. *Ann. Génét.* **19**, 17–21.

Laurent, C., Biemont, M.-Cl., Bethenod, M., Cret, L. and David, M. (1975). Deux observations de trisomie 11q (q 23.1 → qter) avec la meme anomalie des organes genetaux. *Ann. Génét.* **18**, 179–84.

Law, E. M. and Masterton, J. G. (1966). Partial deletion of chromosome 18.

(letter). *Lancet* **2**, 1137.

Leao, J. C., Neu, R. and Gardner, L. I. (1966). Hypospadias and other anomalies associated with partial deletion of short arms of chromosome No. 4. *Lancet* **1**, 493–4.

Lehrke, R., Thelen, T. and Lehrke, R. Jr. (1971). Syndrome associated with Group D chromosome deletions. *Lancet* **2**, 98–9.

Lejeune, J. (1964). *Chromosomes humains,* Vol. 1. Gauthier-Villars, Paris.

——, Gautier, M., Lafourcade, J., Berger, R. and Turpin, R. (1964). Délétion partielle du bras court du chromosome 5. Cinquieme cas de syndrome du cri du chat. *Ann. Génét.* **7**, 7–12.

——, Berger, R., Rethore, M. O., Paolini, P., Boisse, J. and Mozziconacci, P. (1966). Sur un cas de délétion partielle du bras court de chromosome 18, résultant d'une translocation familiale 18 c–17. *Ann. Génét.* **9**, 27–31.

——, Lafourcade, J., Berger, R., Cruveiller, J., Rethoré, M. O., Dutrillaux, B., Abonyi, D. and Jerome, H. (1968). Le phenotype [Dr] etude de trois cas de chromosomes D en anneau. *Ann. Génét.* **11**, 79–87.

Lemli, L. and Smith, D. W. (1963). The XO syndrome: a study of the differentiated phenotype in 25 patients. *J. Pediatr.* **63**, 577–88.

Lindenbaum, R. H. (1978). Chromosomal syndromes. In *Developmental defects and syndromes* by Salmon, M. A. p. 358. H. M. & M. Publishers, Aylesbury.

——, Bobrow, M. and Barber, L. (1973). Monozygotic twins with ring chromosome 22. *J. Med. Genet.* **10**, 85–9.

Lubs, H. A. Jr., Koenig, E. U. and Brandt, I. K. (1961). Trisomy 13–15: a clinical syndrome. *Lancet* **2**, 1001–2.

Lurie, I. W. and Lazjuk, G. I. (1972). Partial monosomies 18. Review of cytogenetical and phenotypical variants. *Humangenetik* **15**, 203–22.

McDermott, A., Insley, J., Barton, M. E., Rowe, P., Edwards, J. H. and Cameron, A. H. (1968). Arrhinencephaly associated with a deficiency involving chromosome 18. *J. Med. Genet.* **5**, 60–7.

McGann, B. R., Alexander, M. and Fox, F. A. (1970). XXXY chromosomal abnormality in a child. *Calif. Med.* **112**, 30–2.

McGavin, D. D. M., Cant, J. S., Ferguson-Smith, M. A. and Ellis, P. M. (1967). The cri-du-chat syndrome with an apparently normal karyotype. *Lancet* **2**, 326–30.

Magnelli, N. C. and Therman, E. (1975). Partial 12p deletion: a cause for a mental retardation, multiple congenital abnormality syndrome. *J. Med. Genet.* **12**, 105–8.

Malpuech, G., Dutrillaux, B., Fonck, Y., Gaulme, J. and Bouche, B. (1972). Trisomie 8 en mosaique. *Arch. Fr. Pédiatr.* **29**, 853–9.

Marin-Padilla, M., Hoefnagel, D. and Benirschke, K. (1964). Anatomic and histopathological study of two cases of D_1 (13–15) trisomy. *Cytogenetics* **3**, 258–84.

Meyer, R. (1925). Zum Mangel der Geschlechtsdrusen mit und ohne Zwittrige Erscheinungen. *Arch. Pathol. Anat. Physiol.* **255**, 33–46.

Mikelsaar, A.-V. N., Lazjuk, G. J., Lurie, J. W., Tüür, S., Käosaar, M. E., Mikelsaar, R. and Loolaid, V. E. (1973). A 4p-syndrome. A case report. *Humangenetik* **19**, 345–7.

Miller, O. J., Breg, W. R., Warburton, D., Miller, D. A., de Capoa, A., Allderdice, P. W., Davis, J., Klinger, H. P., McGilvray, E. and Allen, F. N. Jr. (1970). Partial deletion of the short arm of chromosome No. 4 (4p−): clinical studies in five unrelated patients. *J. Pediatr.* **77**, 792–801.

Moreno-Fuenmayor, H., Zachai, E. H., Mellman, W. J. and Aronson, M. (1975). Familial partial trisomy of the long arm of chromosome 10 (q24–26). *Pediatrics* **56**, 756–61.

Mulcahy, M. T., Jenkyn, J. and Masters, P. L. (1974). A familial 10/13 translocator: partial trisomy C in an infant associated with familial 10/13 translocation. *Clin. Genet.* **6**, 335–40.

Muldal, S. and Ockey, C. H. (1962). Deletion of Y chromosome in a family with muscular dystrophy and hypospadias. *Br. Med. J.* **1**, 291–4.

Naccache, N. F., Vianna-Morgante, A. M. and Richieri-Costa, A. (1984). Brief clinical report: duplication of distal 17q: report of an observation. *Am. J. Med. Genet.* **17**, 633–9.

Neu, R. L., Shott, R. J. and Gardner, L. I. (1975). 4p− phenotype in an infant with t(4p−; 19p or 19q+) mat translocation. *Am. J. Dis. Child.* **129**, 366–70.

Niebuhr, E. (1977). Partial trisomies and deletions of chromosome 13. Chapter 9 in *New chromosomal syndromes,* ed. Yunis, J. J. pp. 273–99. Academic Press, New York.

Nisani, R., Chemke, J., Rappaport, S. and Felsenburg, T. (1984). Genetic counselling for trisomy 20 mosaicism in amniotic fluid cell cultures. *Acta Obstet. Gynecol. Scand.* **63**, 273–5.

Nishikawa, A., Mitomori, T., Matsuura, A., Inoue, A., Mori, A. and Takahashi, M. (1985). A 13q− syndrome with extensive intestinal atresia. *Acta Paediatr. Scand.* **74**, 305–8.

Niss, R. and Passarge, E. (1976). Trisomy 8 restricted to cultured fibroblasts. *J. Med. Genet.* **13**, 229–34.

Noël, B. and Quack, B. (1970). Petit métacentrique surnuméraire chez un polymalformé. *J. Genet. Hum.* **18**, 45–55.

Northcutt, R. C. (1962). Multiple congenital anomalies in a negro infant with 13–15 trisomy. *S. Med. J.* **55**, 385–9.

Ockey, C. H., Feldman, G. V., Macaulay, M. E. and Delaney, M. J. (1967). A large deletion of the long arm of chromosome No. 4 in a child with limb abnormalities. *Arch. Dis. Child.* **42**, 428–34.

Orye, E. and Craen, M. (1975). Short arm deletion of chromosome 12. Report of two new cases. *Humangenetik* **28**, 335–42.

Osathanondh, V. and Potter, E. L. (1964). Pathogenesis of polycystic kidneys. *Arch. Pathol.* **77**, 459–512.

Oster, J. (1953). *Mongolism.* Danish Science Press, Copenhagen.

Parker, C. E., Mavalwala, J., Koch, R., Hatashita, A. and Derencsenyi, A. (1972). The syndrome associated with the partial deletion of the long arm of chromosome 18 (18q−). *Calif. Med.* **11** (4), 65–71.

Penchaszadeh, V. B. and Coco, R. (1975). Trisomy 22. Two new cases and delineation of the phenotype. *J. Med. Genet.* **12**, 193–9.

Perez-Castillo, A., Abrisqueta, J. A., Martin-Lucas, M. A., Goday, C., del Mazo, J. and Aller, V. (1975). A new contribution to the study of 22 trisomy. *Humangenetik* **30**, 265–71.

Pfeiffer, R. A., Heimann, K. and Heiming, E. (1970). Extra chromosome in 'cat-eye' syndrome. *Lancet* **2**, 97.

Pflueger, S. M. V., Scott, C. I. and Moore, C. M. (1984). Trisomy 7 and Potter syndrome. *Clin. Genet.* **25**, 543–8.

Pierson, M., Gilgenkrantz, S. and Saborio, M. (1975). Syndrome dit de l'oeil de chat avec nanisme hypophysaire et développement mental normal. *Arch. Fr. Pédiatr.* **32**, 835–48.

Powars, D., Rohde, R. and Graves, D. (1964). Foetal haemoglobin and neutrophil anomaly in the D_1-trisomy syndrome. *Lancet* **1**, 1363–4.

Puck, M., Tennes, K., Frankenburg, W., Bryant, K. and Robinson, A. (1975). Early childhood development of four boys with 47,XXY karyotype. *Clin. Genet.* **7**, 8–20.

Quan, L. and Smith, D. W. (1972). The VATER association: vertebral defects, anal atresia, tracheo-esophageal fistula with esophageal atresia, radial dysplasia. *Birth Defects Orig. Art. Series.* **8**, (2), 75.

Ratcliffe, S. G. (1976). The development of children with sex chromosome abnormalities. *Proc. R. Soc. Med.* **69**, 189–91.

Reisman, L. E., Darnell, A. and Murphy, J. W. (1965). Abnormalities with ring chromosome. *Lancet* **2**, 445.

——, Kasahara, S., Chung, C.-Y., Darnell, A. and Hall, B. (1966). Anti-mongolism. Studies in an infant with a partial monosomy of the 21 chromosome. *Lancet* **1**, 394–7.

Rethoré, M. O. (1977a). In *Chromosomes in biology and medicine.* Vol. II. *New chromosomal syndromes,* ed. Yunis, J. J. pp. 119–83. Academic Press, New York.

—— (1977b). Deletions and ring chromosomes. In *Handbook of clinical neurology* eds. Vinken, J. P. and Bruyn, G. W. Vol. 26–7. *Congenital malformations of the brain and skull.* pp. 549–620. North-Holland, Amsterdam.

——, Dutrillaux, B., Giovanelli, G., Forabosco, A., Dallapiccola, B. and Lejeune, J. (1974). La Trisomie 4p. *Ann. Génét.* **17**, 125–8.

——, Noel, B., Couturier, J., Prieur, M., Lafourcade, J. and Lejeune, J. (1976). Le syndrome r (22). A propos de 4 nouvelles observations. *Ann Génét.* **19**, 111–17.

Riccardi, V. M., Atkins, L. and Holmes, L. B. (1970). Absent patellae, mild mental retardation, skeletal and genitourinary anomalies and C group autosomal mosaicism. *J. Pediat.* **77**, 664–72.

Roberts, S. H. and Duckett, D. P. (1978). Trisomy 16p in a liveborn infant and a review of partial and full trisomy 16. *J. Med. Genet.* **15**, 375–81.

Rosenfield, R. L., Breibart, S., Isaacs, H. Jr., Klevit, H. D. and Millman, W. J. (1962). Trisomy of chromosomes 13–15 and 17–18: its association with infantile arteriosclerosis. *Am. J. Med. Sci.* **244**, 763–79.

Rosenthal, I. M., Krmpotic, E., Bocian, M. and Szego, K. (1973). Trisomy of the short arm of chromosome 8: association with translocation between chromosomes 8 and 22; 46,XY,22−,t(8p22q)+. *Clin. Genet.* **4**, 507–16.

Rott, H. D., Schwanitz, G., Grosse, K.-P. and Alexandrow, G. (1972). C 11/D 13-translocation in four generations. *Humangenetik* **14**, 300–5.

Say, B., Balchi, S., Pirnar, T. and Tuncbilek, E. (1971). A new syndrome of dysmorphogenesis: imperforate anus with polyoligodactyly and skeletal (mainly vertebral) anomalies. *Acta Paediatr. Scand.* **60**, 197–202.

Schachenmann, G., Schmid, W., Fraccaro, M., Mannini, A., Tiepolo, L., Perona, G. P. and Sartori, E. (1965). Chromosomes in coloboma and anal atresia. *Lancet* **2**, 290.

Schinzel, A. (1981). Incomplete trisomy 22. II. Familial trisomy of the distal segment of chromosome 22q in two brothers from a mother with a trans-location, t(6;22)(q27;q13). *Hum. Genet.* **56**, 263–8.

—— (1984). Cyclopia and cebocephaly in two newborn infants with unbalanced segregation of a familial translocation rcp (1;7)(q32;q34). *Am. J. Med. Genet.* **18**, 153–61.

——, Hayashi, K. and Schmid. W. (1975). Structural aberrations of chromosome 18. II. The 18q− syndrome. Report of three cases. *Humangenetik* **26**, 123–32.

——, Schmid, W., Auf Dermaur, P., Moser, H., Degenhardt, H. K., Geisler, M. and Grubisic, A. (1981). Incomplete trisomy 22. I. Familial 11/22 translocation with 3:1 meiotic disjunction. Delineation of a common clinical picture and report of nine new cases from six families. *Hum. Genet.* **56**, 249–62.

Schleiermacher, E., Schliebitz, U. and Steffens, C. (1974). Brother and sister with triosmy 10p: a new syndrome. *Humangenetik.* **23**, 163–72.

Schnatterly, P., Bono, K. L., Robinow, W., Wyandt, H. E., Kardon, N. and Kelly, T. E. (1984). Distal 15q trisomy: phenotypic comparison of nine cases in an extended family. *Am. J. Hum. Genet.* **36**, 444–51.

Schrott, H. G., Sakaguchi, S., Francke, U., Luzzatti, L. and Fialkow, P. J. (1974). Translocation t(4q−; 13q+) in three generations resulting in partial trisomy of the long arm of chromosome 4 in the fourth generation. *J. Med. Genet.* **11**, 201–5.

Sergovich, F., Madronich, J. S., Barr, M. L., Carr, D. H. and Langdon, W. A. (1963). The D trisomy syndrome: a case report with a description of ocular pathology. *Can. Med. Assoc. J.* **89**, 151–7.

Shaw, M. W., Cohen, M. M. and Hildebrandt, H. M. (1965). A familial 4/5 reciprocal translocation resulting in partial trisomy B. *Am. J. Hum. Genet.* **17**, 54–70.

Shokeir, M. H. K., Ying, K. L. and Pabello, P. (1973). Deletion of the long arm of chromosome No. 7: tentative assignment of the Kidd (Jk) locus. *Clin. Genet.* **4**, 360–8.

——, Ray, M., Hamerton, J. L., Bauder, F. and O'Brien, H. (1975). Deletion of the short arm of chromosome No. 10. *J. Med. Genet.* **12**, 99–113.

Sidbury, J. B. Jr., Schmickel, R. D. and Gray, M. (1964). Findings in a patient with apparent deletion of short arm in one of the B group chromosomes. (Abs.). *J. Pediatr.* **65**, 1098.

Silengo, M. C., Davi, G. F., Bianco, R., Biagioli, M., Guala, A., Franceschini, P. and Novelli, G. (1984). Interstitial deletion of chromosome 1 (q23–q25). Report of a case. *Clin. Genet.* **25**, 549–52.

Silver, W., Steier, M., Schwartz, O. and Zeichner, M. B. (1972). The Holt–Oram syndrome with previously undescribed associated anomalies. *Am. J. Dis. Child.* **124**, 911–14.

Simpson, J. L., Morillo-Cucci, G., Horwith, M., Stiefel, F. H., Feldman, F. and German, J. (1974). Abnormalities of human sex chromosomes. VI. Monozygotic twins with the complement 48,XXXY. *Humangenetik* **21**, 301–8.

Sirota, L., Shabtai, F., Landman, I., Halbrecht, I. and Dulitzsky, F. (1984). New anomalies in the 11q− syndrome. *Clin. Genet.* **26**, 569–73.

Smith, A. C. M., McGavran, L., Robinson, J., Waldstein, G., Macfarlane, J., Zonona, J., Reiss, J., Lahr, M., Allen, L. and Magenis, E. (1986). Interstitial deletion of (17) (p.11.2 p.11.2) in nine patients. *Am. J. Med. Genet.* **24**, 393–414.

Smith, D. W. (1964). Autosomal abnormalities. *Am. J. Obstet. Gynec.* **90**, 1055–77.

——, Patau, K., Therman, E. and Inhorn, S. L. (1960). A new autosomal trisomy syndrome: multiple congenital anomalies caused by an extra chromosome. *J. Pediatr.* **57**, 338–45.

——, ——, —— and —— (1962). The No. 18 trisomy syndrome. *J. Pediatr.* **60**, 513–27.

——, ——, ——, —— and De Mars, R. I. (1963). The D_1 trisomy syndrome. *J. Pediatr.* **62**, 326–41.

Stern, J. and Lewis, W. H. P. (1958). Calcium, phosphate and phosphatase in mongolism. *J. Ment. Sci.* **104**, 880–3.

Stratton, R. F., Bobyns, W. B., Airhart, S. D. and Ledbetter, D. H. (1984). New chromosomal syndrome: Miller–Dieker syndrome and monosomy 17p13. *Hum. Genet.* **67**, 193–200.

Surana, R. B. and Conen, P. E. (1972). Partial trisomy 4 resulting from a 14/18 reciprocal translocation. *Ann. Génét.* **15**, 191–4.

Taillemite, J.-L., Baheux-Morlier, G. and Roux, Ch. (1975). Délétion interstitielle du bras long d'un chromosome 11. *Ann Génét.* **18**, 61–3.

Talvik, T., Mikelsaar, A.-V., Mikelsaar, R., Käosaar, M. and Tüür, S. (1973). Inherited translocations in two families t(14q+; 10q−) and t(13q−;21q). *Humangenetik* **19**, 215–26.

Taylor, A. I. (1967). Patau's, Edwards' and Cri-du-chat syndromes: a tabulated summary of current findings. *Dev. Med. Child. Neurol.* **9**, 78–86.

—— (1968). Autosomal trisomy syndromes: a detailed study of 27 cases of Edwards' syndrome and 27 cases of Patau's syndrome. *J. Med. Genet.* **5**, 227–52.

Taylor, M. B., Juberg, R. C., Jones, B. and Johnson, W. A. (1970). Chromosomal variability in the D_1 trisomy syndrome. *Am. J. Dis. Child.* **120**, 374–81.

Tenconi, R., Baccichetti, C., Anglani, F., Pellegrino, P. A., Kaplan, J. C. and Junien, C. (1975). Partial deletion of the short arm of chromosome 12 (p11;p13). Report of a case. *Ann. Génét.* **18**, 95–8.

Therkelsen, A. J., Klingg, T., Henningsen, K., Mikkelsen, M. and Schmidt, G. (1971). A family with a presumptive C/F translocation in five generations. *Ann Génét.* **14**, 13–21.

Thomas, Ch., Cordier, J., Gilbenkrantz, S., Reny, A. and Raspiller, A. (1969). Un syndrome rare: atteinte colobomateux du globe oculaire, atresie anale, anomalies congenitales multiples et presence d'un chromosome surnumeraire. *Ann. Oculist (Paris)* **202**, 1021–31.

Thorburn, M. J., Smith-Read, E. H. McN. and Peck, J. E. (1969). A translocation t(Bq+;Cq−) in a West Indian family and a report of a second family showing a possible long arm group B translocation. *Arch. Dis. Child.* **44**, 106–12.

Tolksdorf, M., Wiedmann, H.-R. and Goll, U. (1969). Ring D_1 chromosome and multiple malformations. *Lancet* **2**, 1009.

Townes, P. L., Kreutner, K. A., Kreutner, A. and Manning J. (1963). Observations on the pathology of the trisomy 17–18 syndrome. *J. Pediatr.* **62**, 703–9.

Turleau, C., Chavin-Colin, F., Roubin, M., Thomas, D. and de Grouchy, J. (1975). Monosomie partielle 11q et trigonocephalie. Un nouveau syndrome. *Ann. Génét* **18**, 257–60.

Vaillaud, J. C., Martin, J. and Ayraud, N. (1970). A new case of partial deletion of the short arm of chromosome 18. *Ann. Génét.* **13**, 120–2.

Vogel, W., Siebers, J. W., Gunkel, J., Hass, B., Knörr-Gartner, H., Niethammer, D. G. and Noel, B. (1975). Un einheitlicher Phänotyp bei Partial Trisomie 4q. *Humangenetik* **28**, 103–12.

Walker, S., Andrews, J., Gregson, N. M. and Gault, W. (1973). Three further cases of triploidy in man surviving to birth. *J. Med. Genet.* **10**, 135–41.

Warkany, J., Passarge, E. and Smith, L. R. (1966). Congenital malformations in autosomal trisomy syndromes. *Am. J. Dis. Child.* **112**, 502–17.

Warren, R. J. and Rimoin, D. L. (1970). The G deletion syndromes. *J. Pediatr.* **27**, 658–63.

Weber, F. M., Dooley, R. R. and Sparkes, R. S. (1970). Anal atresia, eye anomalies, and an additionial small abnormal acrocentric chromosome (47,XX,mar+): report of a case. *J. Pediatr,* **26**, 594–7.

Wertelecki, W., Schindler, A. M. and Gerald, P. S. (1966). Partial deletion of chromosome 18. *Lancet* **2**, 641.

Wilcock, A. R., Adams, F. G., Cooke, P. and Gordon, R. R. (1970). Deletion of short arm of No. 4 (4p−)—a detailed case report. *J. Med. Genet.* **7**, 71–6.

Wilson, G. N., Dasouki, M. and Barr, M. (1985). Further delineation of the dup (3q) syndrome. *Am. J. Med. Genet.* **22**, 117–23.

Wilson, M. G., Melnyk, J. and Towner, J. W. (1969). Retinoblastoma and deletion D(14) syndrome. *J. Med. Genet.* **6**, 322–7.

——, Towner, J. W. and Fujimoto, R. (1973). Retinoblastoma and D-chromosome deletion. *Am. J. Hum. Genet.* **25**, 57–61.

Wolf, U. and Reinwein, H. (1965). Chromosomenmosaik, C-trisomie/normal. *Humangenetik* **1**, 686–7.

Ying, K. L., Curry, C. J. R., Rajani, K. B., Kassel, S. H. and Sparkes, R. S. (1982). De novo interstitial deletion in the long arm of chromosome 9: a new chromosome syndrome. *J. Med. Genet.* **19**, 68–70.

Yunis, E., de la Cruz, E., Nossa, M. A. and Guttierez, G. (1975). XX males: two new cases. *Clin. Genet.* **7**, 394–9.

——, Silva, R. and Giraldo, A. (1976). Total trisomy 10p. *Ann Génét.* **19**, 57–60.

——, Ramirez, E. and Uribe, J. G. (1980). Full trisomy 7 and Potter syndrome. *Hum. Genet.* **54**, 13–18.

Yunis, J. J. and Sanchez, O. (1974). A new syndrome resulting from partial trisomy for the distal third of the long arm of chromosome 10. *J. Pediatr.* **8**, 567–70.

Zaleski, W. A., Houston, C. S. and Pozsonyi, J. (1966). The XXXXY chromosome anomaly: report of three new cases and review of 30 cases from the literature. *Can. Med. Assoc. J.* **94**, 1143–54.

Zellweger, H., Mikamo, K., and Abbo, H. G. (1962). Two cases of nonmongoloid trisomy G. *Ann. Paediatr.* **199**, 613–24.

Zollinger, H. (1969). Das XXXY Syndrom. *Helv. Paediatr. Acta* **24**, 589–99.

4. Inherited metabolic diseases involving the kidney

The inherited metabolic diseases, or inborn errors of metabolism, were the first group of human diseases to be shown to be inherited in accordance with Mendel's laws. The physician Archibald Garrod, a friend of the geneticist Bateson, studied several rare metabolic diseases. He proposed the concept of a metabolic block in which a defect in the activity of a specific enzyme resulted in a failure of normal conversion of one metabolite to another, and first illustrated this idea in alkaptonuria (Garrod 1899). He demonstrated that the darkening of the urine of patients with alkaptonuria was due to excessive excretion of homo-gentisic acid, or alkaptone, which on exposure to light is oxidized to the dark pigment melanin. Garrod postulated that the excess of homogentisic acid was due to a block in its catabolism to acetoacetic acid and predicted that this block would be shown to be due to defective activity of a specific enzyme, homogentisic acid oxidase. This prediction was fulfilled over 50 years later by La Du and colleagues in 1958. In his studies on alkaptonuria, albinism, cystinuria, and pentosuria Garrod observed that sibs, but not parents, of his patients were often affected, and that the parents were often consanguineous (1902). This led him to propose, on the advice of Bateson, that these diseases were inherited in a mendelian autosomal recessive manner, and to formulate the 'one-gene–one-enzyme' hypothesis in his Croonian Lectures (1908), and in his seminal monograph *Inborn errors of metabolism* published in 1909 with a second edition in 1923. This concept, in its essentials, is still the accepted basis of inborn errors of metabolism. It has been more precisely defined by Beadle (1945, 1959) with his colleague Tatum (1941) in *Neurospora crassa*. We know now that many enzymes are polymers containing more than one type of polypeptide chain and, therefore, determined by more than one gene. On the other hand many proteins have non-enzymatic functions (Horowitz and Leupold 1951). Such non-enzymatic proteins include transport proteins such as haemoglobin and transferrin, structural proteins of cell membranes and the cytoskeletal system or secreted proteins such as collagen, membrane receptor proteins, antibodies, and developmental inducers. These ideas have led to a restatement of the one-gene–one-enzyme hypothesis as the one-cistron–one-polypeptide chain hypothesis. Furthermore not all inherited deficiencies in enzyme activity are due to mutations in a structural gene for a polypeptide chain in that enzyme. Instead of a defective enzyme being synthesized, due to a point or mis-sense mutation, there may be no enzymic protein synthesized at all, owing either to a deletion of the structural gene or to a mutation of a regulatory gene. An apparent failure of synthesis may be due to a point mutation in the structural gene leading to premature termination or to the formation of a highly unstable protein.

An understanding of the molecular changes in the protein gene product in inherited diseases came through three major technical advances. The first of these was the electrophoretic separation of different haemoglobins by Linus Pauling and his colleagues (1949). They demonstrated that patients with sickle cell disease were homozygous for a gene determining production of haemoglobin S, and that carriers, who gave a positive sickling test, were heterozygous with a mixture of haemoglobins A and S in their red cells. Since then it has proved possible by this simple method to diagnose the presence of any abnormal haemoglobin associated with an alteration in the electric charge on the molecule. The next innovation was Ingram's use of Sanger's technique of peptide fingerprinting and the development of amino acid composition analysis and sequencing. This enabled him to identify the precise amino acid substitution in the β-chain of haemoglobin S (Ingram 1956), the first occasion in which it was proved, for any organism, that a structural gene mutation could produce a single amino acid substitution in its gene product. Since then similar identifications have been made for most of the numerous known haemoglobinopathies. The third advance was Perutz's use of X-ray crystallography to elucidate the tertiary and quaternary structure of normal and abnormal haemoglobins. In an elegant series of studies he has related specific amino acid substitutions to observed changes in structure, and hence function, of the molecule and in this way has correlated molecular alteration with clinical phenotype. He reviewed this work in the *British Medical Bulletin* (Perutz 1976).

More recently attention has shifted from the product to the gene itself. Molecular genetic techniques have revealed much evidence on the precise structure and organization of the DNA of both normal and mutant genes in micro-organisms, and latterly eukaryotes, including humans. As far as the last is concerned most of the work has once again concentrated on haemoglobins. This work has, for example, revealed the existence of non-coding DNA sequences within genes, *introns*, as well as between genes; of evolutionary vestigeal genes, *pseudogenes*; and of polymorphic restriction fragment length variant regions of DNA, either point mutational or tandem reduplicational variants. These polymorphic variants may be in genetic linkage with structural genes, and a particular variant in linkage disequilibrium with a specific disease mutant of a structural gene acting as a signpost to it (see discussion in Chapter 2). Proudfoot and colleagues (1980) have recently reviewed the structure and transcription of human globin genes, while Wyman and White (1980) have described one highly polymorphic DNA site. Molecular genetic methods, along with those based on somatic cell hybrids and chromosomal structural variants, have greatly facilitated the mapping of human genes and their assignment to specific chromosomes or chromosomal regions (Malcolm *et al.* 1981). Clinically molecular genetic techniques have provided new methods for the prenatal diagnosis of both thalassaemias (Little *et al.* 1980) and haemoglobinopathies (Kan and Dozy 1978; Chang and Kan 1981). As mentioned in Chapter 1 an excellent review of the clinical applications of molecular biology is that of Weatherall (1982).

Studies on enzymatic human inborn errors of metabolism, comparable to those published on human haemoglobin and its disorders, are only just beginning to be undertaken, and not yet at all on transport or other non-enzymatic renal defects. It was not until 1952 that Cori first confirmed Garrod's hypothesis that inherited metabolic blocks are due to specific enzyme deficiencies when she showed that Von Gierke's disease is due to lack of activity of glucose 6-phosphatase. These inborn errors where the enzyme defect has been extensively studied have, like the haemoglobin disorders, revealed considerable genetic heterogeneity. The outstanding example has been glucose 6-phosphate dehydrogenase deficiency. McKusick (1983) lists 272 variants including the usual Gd^B gene. Yoshida (1967) demonstrated a single amino acid substitution in one variant. He has also shown (1973) that, whereas there was little correlation between the level of residual enzyme activity assayed under optimal conditions and clinical phenotype, there was excellent correlation when assays were performed at physiological pH and in the presence of physiological concentrations of metabolites. Amino acid sequencing of a series of mutant forms of a single enzyme has not been undertaken in humans but Fincham and coworkers did so for nicotinamide adenine dinucleotide phosphate (NADP)-dependent glutamate dehydrogenase in *Neurospora crassa* and were able in consequence not only to map the mutational sites within the gene but also to demonstrate the precise amino acid substitutions involved (Holder *et al.* 1975; Brett *et al.* 1976; Kinsey *et al.* 1980). Recently Fincham has reported the complete nucleotide sequence of the wild type gene (Kinneard and Fincham 1983).

Studies of most other human inborn errors in which a specific enzyme deficiency has been demonstrated have been limited to analysis of kinetics, pH optima, stability, and electrophoretic differences. These may indicate genetic heterogeneity but in some inborn errors the deficiency in enzyme activity is too profound for valid comparison between different patients at the enzyme level, as for example the mucopolysaccharidoses IH, IS and IHS (Hurler, Scheie and Hurler/Scheie variants of mucopolysaccharidoses type I). In other diseases the opportunity for detailed enzyme analysis is limited by lack of expression in readily available tissue, as in phenylketonuria where the defective enzyme is expressed only in liver (Crawfurd *et al.* 1981). In some inborn errors, without detectable enzyme activity, such as classical galactosaemia, the presence of a protein material cross-reacting with antisera to the normal enzyme has confirmed the synthesis of a defective enzyme molecule (Tedesco and Mellman 1971). Unfortunately the absence of such cross-reacting material does not indicate total lack of enzyme synthesis as a defective gene product may lack the antigenic sites of the normal enzyme.

A novel approach was that of Nadler and associates (1970) in galactosaemia. They produced somatic cell hybrids by fusing fibroblasts from seven different patients with galactosaemia and from normal subjects. They observed complementation, in the form of restored enzyme activity, in three of the hybrids derived from two deficient lines, and postulated interallelic complementation of point mutations. They recognized that intergenic complementation could have been involved but on either interpretation they clearly demonstrated genetic heterogeneity within classical galactosaemia.

Probably the greatest advances in future for the analysis of the molecular defect, and for improved diagnostic methods, will come from genetic manipulative techniques such as have already been applied in the haemoglogin disorders. As yet there have been only a few published reports of such studies on inborn errors and other inherited diseases. Savio Woo and his colleagues have isolated a cDNA probe for the prenatal diagnosis of phenylketonuria that is informative in at least some families (Woo *et al.* 1982, 1984). Caskey's group has used hypoxanthine-guanine phosphoribosyltransferase cDNA probes to study Lesch–Nyhan disease (Nussbaum *et al.* 1983; Wilson *et al.* 1983a and b).

The general principles of genetics in relation to the inborn errors has been discussed at some length as they provide the most clear-cut illustration of simply inherited disorders. The same general principles apply to other simply inherited disorders in which no metabolic defect has been demonstrated, whether renal or otherwise. Whilst the lack of knowledge of the gene product in most such diseases precludes work on the protein concerned it does not prevent direct study of the gene itself. Demonstration of a DNA restriction fragment length polymorphic variant segregating in close linkage with the clinical phenotype provides the possibility of isolating the gene, or more simply of direct diagnosis of

Disease	Enzyme deficient in kidney	Material deposited in kidney	Mode of inheritance
1. Von Gierke's disease (Glycogenosis I)	Glucose 6-phosphatase	Glycogen	AR
2. Fabry's disease	α-galactosidase A	Neutral glycosphingolipid	XR
3a. GM$_1$ gangliosidosis type 1 (infantile GM$_1$ gangliosidosis)	Acid-β-galactosidase (Not confirmed in kidney but deficient in leucocytes, brain, liver, and cultured fibroblasts)	GM$_1$ ganglioside	AR
3b. GM$_1$ gangliosidosis type 2 (juvenile GM$_1$ gangliosidosis)			
3c. GM$_2$ gangliosidosis type 2 (Sandhoff's disease)	Hexosaminidase A and B (deficient in all tissues examined but not confirmed in kidney)	Increased proportion of GM$_2$ ganglioside in visceral tissues; accumulation of GM$_{A2}$ and globoside, especially in kidney	AR
4. Cystinosis, infantile and juvenile forms	?	Accumulation of free cystine in lysosomes of kidney and other tissues with deposition of cystine crystals	AR
5. Wilson's disease	?	Copper	AR
6. Hereditary amyloidoses:			
(a) Nephropathic forms including familial Mediterranean fever	?	Amyloid	AR and AD
(b) Neuropathic types I and III	?	Amyloid	AD
7. Glutamylribose 5-phosphate storage disease	? An ADP ribose protein hydrolase	Glutamyl ribose 5-phosphate	XR
8. Hurler's disease (MPS IH)	α-iduronidase	Mucopolysaccharide material in renal epithelial cell lysosomes	AR

Abbreviations: AR=autosomal recessive, AD=autosomal dominant, XR=X-linked recessive

Table 4.2. *Inherited metabolic diseases with renal involvement: (B) diseases with secondary renal damage*

(i) Due to exercise-induced myoglobinuria:

Disease	Primary enzyme deficiency	Mode of inheritance
1. McArdle's disease (glycogenosis V)	Muscle phosphorylase	AR
2. Glycogenosis type VIII	Muscle phosphofructokinase	AR
3. Forbes' disease (glycogenosis III)	Amylo-1,6-glucosidase	AR
4. Pompe's disease (glycogenosis II)	α-1,4-glucosidase	AR
5. Phosphohexose isomerase deficiency	Phosphohexose isomerase	AR
6. Malignant hyperpyrexia	?	AD

(ii) Due to other metabolites:

Disease	Primary enzyme deficiency	Circulating toxic metabolite	Mode of inheritance
1. Hereditary fructose intolerance	Fructose 1-P-aldolase	Probably fructose 1-P-which accumulates in the kidney damaging tubules	AR
2. Galactosaemia	Galactose 1-P-uridyltransferase	Probably galactose 1-P which accumulates in the kidney, along with galactitol, damaging tubules	AR

Disease		Circulating metabolite	
3. Hereditary tyrosinaemia (hepatorenal type)	?	Excrete high levels of tyrosine and other amino acids along with P-hydroxy-phenolic acids. Which of these is toxic to the kidney is not known	AR
4. Familial lecithin: cholesterol acyltransferase deficiency	Lecithin: cholesterol acyltransferase	Low density lipoprotein	AR
5. Hypophosphatasia	? Alkaline phosphatase of liver and bone	Probably calcium, resulting in nephrocalcinosis	AR
(iii) Cause not known:			
Disease		*Circulating metabolite*	
1. Zellweger's disease (cerebro-hepato-renal syndrome)	Enzyme defect unknown	Pipecolic acid	AR
2. Nephrosialidosis	α-(2-6) neuraminidase	—	AR

Abbreviations: AR=autosomal recessive, AD=autosomal dominant, XR=X-linked recessive

Table 4.3. *Inherited metabolic diseases with renal involvement: (C) diseases with renal stone or crystal formation (Chapter 5)*

Disease	Primary enzyme defect	Type of renal stone or crystal	Mode of inheritance
1. Familial hyperparathyroidism	?	Mixed calcium stones	AD
2. Hyperoxaluria:			
(a) Type I: glycolic aciduria	Soluble α-ketoglutarate: glyoxylate carboligase is deficient in liver, spleen, and kidney	Calcium oxalate stones and nephrocalcinosis secondary to increased oxalate synthesis	AR
(b) Type II: L-glyceric aciduria	D-glyceric dehydrogenase is deficient in leucocytes		AR
3. Cystinuria (see Chapter 4)	Renal tubule amino acid transport defect	Cystine stones	AR
4. Lesch–Nyhan disease	Hypoxanthine–guanine phosphoribosyltransferase	Uric acid stones	XR
5. PRPP synthetase overactivity	PRPP synthetase	Uric acid stones	XR
6. Hereditary xanthinuria	Xanthine oxidase	Xanthine stones	AR
7. Hereditary orotic aciduria			
(a) Type 1	Deficiency of orotate phosphoribosyltransferase and of orotidine 5'-P-decarboxylase	Orotic acid crystals	AR
(b) Type 2	Deficiency or orotidine 5'-P-decarboxylase alone		AR
8. 2,8-dihydroxyadeninuria	Adenine phosphoribosyltransferase	2,8-dihydroxyadenine crystals and stones	AR

Abbreviations: AR = autosomal recessive, AD = autosomal dominant, XR = X-linked recessive heterozygotes or homozygotes pre- or postnatally. Such an approach has been used in different laboratories for Duchenne muscular dystrophy (Murray *et al.* 1982; Davies *et al.* 1983; Harper *et al.* 1983; O'Brien *et al.* 1983; Pembrey *et al.* 1984) and Huntington's chorea (Gusella *et al.* 1983) and is currently being pursued for cystic fibrosis, diabetes, and other diseases. It could equally readily be undertaken for some of the more common renal diseases.

The enzymatic inborn errors are not of course primarily renal diseases but several of them do have secondary renal damage of varying severity. The inborn errors with renal damage can be divided into three groups: firstly those in which the kidney is directly involved in the primary metabolic block with deposition of metabolic precursors in renal tissue and often with the enzyme defect demonstrable in the kidney, as in Von Gierke's disease; secondly those in which the kidney is damaged by a circulating substance, as in the tubular damage of galactosaemia, or the various disorders which may be complicated by myoglobinuria; and finally those in which the kidney is damaged by renal stone or crystal formation, as in hyperoxaluria (see Tables 4.1–4.3). The enzymic metabolic diseases will be discussed in this chapter, followed in the next chapter by diseases with renal stone formation or crystalluria, and in the following chapter by the renal transport defects, such as cystinuria. Treatment of inborn errors is not discussed. Apart from dietary management, of those disorders amenable to this approach, treatment of inborn errors of metabolism is largely experimental. The current state of practice and of experimental approaches is reviewed in the proceedings of the second CRC symposium, *Advances in the Treatment of Inborn Errors of Metabolism* (Crawfurd *et al.* 1982).

References

Beadle, G. W. (1945). Biochemical genetics. *Chem. Ren.* **37**, 15.

—— (1959). Genes and chemical reactions in *Neurospora. Science* **129**, 1715–19.

—— and Tatum, E. L. (1941). Genetic control of biochemical reactions in *Neurospora. Proc. Nat. Acad. Sci.* **27**, 499–506.

Brett, M. G. K., Chambers, A. A., Holder, A. A., Fincham, J. R. S. and Wooton, J. C. (1976). Mutational aminoacid replacements in *Neurospora crassa* NADP-specific glutamate dehydrogenase. *J. Mol. Biol.* **106**, 1–22.

Chang, J. C. and Kan, Y. W. (1981). Antenatal diagnosis of sickle cell anaemia by direct analysis of the sickle mutation. *Lancet* **2**, 1127–9.

Cori, G. T. and Cori, C. F. (1952). Glucose-6-phosphatase of the liver in glycogen storage disease. *J. Biol. Chem.* **199**, 661–7.

Crawfurd, M. d'A., Gibbs, D. A. and Sheppard, D. M. (1981). Studies on human phenyelalanine mono-oxygenase. I. Restricted expression. *J. Inher. Metab. Dis.* **4**, 191–5.

——, —— and Watts, R. W. E. (eds.) (1982). *Advances in the treatment of inborn errors of metabolism.* John Wiley, New York, Chichester, Brisbane and Toronto.

Davies, K. E., Pearson, P. L., Harper, P. S., Murray, J. M., O'Brien, T., Sarfarazi, M. and Williamson, R. (1983). Linkage analysis of two cloned DNA sequences flanking the Duchenne muscular dystrophy locus on the short arm of the human X chromosome. *Nucl. Acids Res.* **11**, 2303–12.

Garrod, A. E. (1899). A contribution to the study of alkaptonuria. *Proc. R. Med. Chir. Soc.* n.s. **2**, 130.

—— (1902). The incidence of alkaptonuria: a study in chemical individuality. *Lancet* **2**, 1616–20.

—— (1908). *Inborn errors of metabolism* (Croonian Lectures). *Lancet* **2**, 1, 73, 142, and 214.

—— (1923). *Inborn errors of metabolism,* Oxford University Press, London.

Gusella, J. F., Wexler, N. S., Conneally, P. M., Naylor, S. L., Anderson, M. A., Tanzi, R. E., Watkins, P. C., Ottina, K., Wallace, M. R., Sakaguchi, A. Y., Young, A. B., Shoulson, I., Bonilla, E. and Martin, J. B. (1983). A polymorphic DNA marker genetically linked to Huntington's disease. *Nature* **306**, 234–8.

Harper, P. S., O'Brien, T., Murray, J. M., Davies, K. E., Pearson, P. and Williamson, R. (1983). Use of linked DNA polymorphisms for genotype prediction in families with Duchenne muscular dystrophy. *J. Med. Genet.* **20**, 252–4.

Holder, A. A., Wooton, J. C., Baron, A. J., Chambers, G. K. and Fincham, J. R. S. (1975). The aminoacid sequence of *Neurospora* NADP-specific-glutamate dehydrogenase. Peptic and chymotryptic peptides and the complete sequence. *Biochem. J.* **149**, 757–73.

Horowitz, N. H. and Leupold, U. (1951). Some recent studies bearing on the one gene one enzyme hypothesis. *Symp. Quant. Biol.* **16**, 65.

Ingram, V. M. (1956). A specific chemical difference between the globins of normal human and sickle-cell anaemia haemoglobin. *Nature* **178**, 792–4.

Kan, W. Y. and Dozy, A. M. (1978). Antenatal diagnosis of sickle-cell anaemia by DNA analysis of amniotic fluid cells. *Lancet* **2**, 910–12.

Kinniard, J. H. and Fincham, J. R. S. (1983). The complete nucleotide sequence of the *Neurospora crassa am* (NADP-specific glutamate dehydrogenase) gene. *Gene* **26**, 253–60.

Kinsey, J. A., Fincham, J. R. S., Siddig, M. A. M. and Keighren, M. (1980). New mutational variants of Neurospora NADP-specific glutamate dehydrogenase. *Genetics* **95**, 305–16.

La Du, B. N., Zannoni, V. G., Laster, L. and Seegmiller, J. E. (1958). The nature of the defect in tyrosine metabolism in alcaptonuria. *J. Biol. Chem.* **230**, 251–60.

Little, P. F. R., Annison, G., Darling, S., Williamson, R., Camba, L. and Modell, B. (1980). Model for antenatal diagnosis of β-thalassaemia and other monogenic disorders by molecular analysis of linked DNA polymorphisms. *Nature* **285**, 144–7.

McKusick, V. A. (1983). *Mendelian inheritance in man,* 6th edn. pp. 1110–29. Johns Hopkins University Press, Baltimore and London.

Malcolm, S., Barton, P., Murphy, C. and Ferguson-Smith, M. A. (1981). Chromosomal localization of a single copy gene by *in situ* hybridization—human β-

globin genes on the short arm of chromosome 11. *Ann. Hum. Genet.* **45**, 135–41.

Murray, J. M., Davies, K. E., Harper, P. S., Meredith, L., Mueller, C. R. and Williamson, R. (1982). Linkage relationship of a cloned DNA sequence on the short arm of the X chromosome to Duchenne muscular dystrophy. *Nature* **300**, 69–71.

Nadler, H. L., Chacko, C. M. and Rachmeler, M. (1970). Interallelic complementation in hybrid cells derived from human diploid strains deficient in galactose-1-phosphate uridyl transferase activity. *Proc. Nat. Acad. Sci.* **67**, 976–82.

Nussbaum, R. L., Crowder, W. E., Nyhan, W. L. and Caskey, C. T. (1983). A three-allele restriction-fragment-length polymorphism at the hypoxanthine phosphoribosyltransferase locus in man. *Proc. Nat. Acad. Sci.* **80**, 4035–9.

O'Brien, T., Harper, P. S., Davies, K. E., Murray, J. M., Sarfarazi, M. and Williamson, R. (1983). Absence of genetic heterogeneity in Duchenne muscular dystrophy shown by a linkage study using two cloned DNA sequences. *J. Med. Genet.* **20**, 249–51.

Pauling, L., Itano, H. A., Singer, S. J. and Wells, I. C. (1949). Sickle cell anemia, a molecular disease. *Science* **110**, 543–8.

Pembrey, M. E., Davies, K. E., Winter, R. M., Elles, R. G., Williamson, R., Fazzone, T. A. and Walker, C. (1984). Clinical use of DNA markers linked to the gene for Duchenne muscular dystrophy. *Arch. Dis. Child.* **59**, 208–16.

Perutz, M. F. (1976). Structure and mechanism of haemoglobin. *Brit. Med. Bull.* **32**, 195–208.

Proudfoot, N. J., Shander, M. H. M., Manley, J. L., Gefter, M. L. and Maniatis, T. (1980). Structure and in vitro transcription of human globin genes. *Science* **209**, 1329–36.

Tedesco, T. A. and Mellman, W. J. (1971). Galactosemia: evidence for a structural gene mutation. *Science* **172**, 727–8.

Weatherall, D. J. (1982). *The new genetics and clinical practice.* Nuffield Provincial Hospitals Trust, London.

Wilson, J. M., Frossard, P., Nussbaum, R. L., Caskey, C. T. and Kelly, W. N. (1983a). Human hypoxanthine–guanine phosphoribosyltransferase: detection of a mutant allele by restriction endonuclease analysis. *J. Clin. Invest.* **72**, 767–72.

——, Young, A. B. and Kelley, W. N. (1983b). Hypoxanthine–guanine phosphoribosyltransferase deficiency: the molecular basis of the clinical syndromes. *New Engl. J. Med.* **309**, 900–10.

Woo, S. L. C., Lidsky, A. S., Guttler, F., Chandra, T. and Robson, K. J. H. (1983). Cloned human phenylalanine hydroxylase gene allows prenatal diagnosis and carrier detection of classical phenylketonuria. *Nature* **306**, 151–5.

——, ——, ——, Thirumalachary, C. and Robson, K. J. H. (1984). Prenatal diagnosis of classical phenylketonuria by gene mapping. *JAMA* **251**, 1998–2002.

Wyman, A. R. and White, R. (1980). A highly polymorphic locus in human DNA. *Proc. Nat. Acad. Sci.* **77**, 6754–58.

Yoshida, A. (1967). A single amino acid substitution (asparagine to aspartic acid) between normal (B plus) and the common Negro variant (A plus) of human glucose-6-phosphate dehydrogenase. *Proc. Nat. Acad. Sci.* **57**, 835–40.

—— (1973). Hemolytic anemia and G6PD deficiency. *Science* **179**, 532–7.

4.1. DISEASES WITH RENAL DEPOSITION OF METABOLITE OR OTHER MATERIAL

4.1.1. Von Gierke's disease (glycogenosis I or hepatorenal glycogen storage disease)

Glycogen storage disease with hepatic and renal enlargement was first described by von Gierke (1929). In 1932 Pompe drew attention to the existence of two types: one with predominant liver enlargement that has continued to carry von Gierke's name, and the other with a more generalized excess storage of glycogen in many tissues including the heart. Cori and Cori (1952) reported a deficiency of glucose 6-phosphatase in the liver in the hepatic form. This was the first recognition of a specific hepatic enzyme deficiency in an inherited metabolic disorder. Subsequently other enzyme deficiencies were recognized in glycogen storage diseases, which Cori and Cori numbered sequentially starting with von Gierke's disease as number I and currently up to glycogen synthetase deficiency as number IX.

The clinical picture is dominated by hepatic enlargement from birth which goes on to produce obvious abdominal protuberance. The kidneys also become enlarged, as seen on pyelography, but cannot be felt clinically owing to the enlarged liver. The children show a proportionate reduction in stature (Fine *et al.* 1969), and in later childhood tend to develop increased adiposity of soft tissues and poor flabby musculature (van Creveld 1961; Howell *et al.* 1962; Spencer-Peet *et al.* 1971; Howell 1978). A characteristic perimacular fundal lesion has been described (Fine *et al.* 1968). Bleeding, particularly associated with platelet dysfunction, can be a significant clinical problem (Corby *et al.* 1974), presumably due to the reduced glucose 6-phosphatase activity in the platelets (Negishi *et al.* 1974). The affected children are subject to attacks of fasting hypoglycaemia but are resistant to ketosis (Howell *et al.* 1962). Many patients develop hyperuricaemia which can lead in later childhood or early adult life to gouty arthritis and nephropathy or tophaceous gout (Howell 1965; Alepa *et al.* 1967), although uric acid stone formation is uncommon. Senior and Loridan (1968a and b) have developed a technique for differentiating glycogenoses types I–IV on the basis of the response of blood levels of glucose and lactate to oral glycerol loading, along with response to adrenaline and glucagon.

The renal disturbance in von Gierke's disease is a Fanconi-like syndrome with aminoaciduria, glucosuria, and phosphaturia (Lampert *et al.* 1967; Garty *et al.* 1974) and is associated with renal enlargement with glycogen accumulation due to deficiency of glucose 6-phosphatase in the kidney. The gouty nephropathy of older patients is a later complication.

Unfortunately renal transplantation does not improve glucose metabolism (Emmett and Narins 1978).

There have been reports of the disease in sibs from very early on (Ellis and Payne 1940; Sarmiento and Cortes Mendoza 1947; Van Creveld 1961; Alepa *et al.* 1967) and the disease has been described in all populations including Asians (Kapila *et al.* 1956). The autosomal recessive mode of inheritance has been amply confirmed (Illingworth 1964; Sidbury 1965) but as with so many well-studied inherited disorders there is evidence for genetic heterogeneity. Stamm and Webb (1975) reported a partial enzyme deficiency in an adult patient. Senior and Loridan (1968a and b) postulated the existence of a form with normal *in vitro* glucose 6-phosphatase activity but failure to liberate glucose from glucose 6-phosphate *in vivo*. Hsia and Kot (1959) claimed to be able to detect heterozygotes as well as patients on the basis of high levels of glucose 6-phosphate and fructose 6-phosphate in red blood cells. Sokal and colleagues (1961) were unable to confirm these findings and indeed obtained very much lower levels in all subjects. Hsia (1961) using improved methods largely agreed with Sokal and colleagues but did obtain levels in three out of five affected children and in one heterozygote above his normal range. The most extensive studies on heterozygotes have utilized assay of glucose 6-phosphatase, mainly in intestine. Field and his associates found reduced levels in all the parents of five affected children consistent with autosomal recessive inheritance (Field *et al.* 1965; Field and Drash 1967) and Williams and coworkers (1963) obtained similar results. Negishi and others (1974) found reduced activity in the platelets of patients and intermediate levels in their parents. Prenatal diagnosis has not been reported.

References

Alepa, F. P., Howell, R. R., Klinenberg, J. R. and Seegmiller, J. E. (1967). Relationships between glycogen storage disease and tophaceous gout. *Am. J. Med.* **42**, 58–66.

Cori, G. T. and Cori, C. F. (1952). Glucose-6-phosphatase of the liver in glycogen storage disease. *J. Biol. Chem.* **199**, 661–7.

Corby, D. G., Putnam, C. W. and Greene, H. L. (1974). Impaired platelet function in glucose-6-phosphatase deficiency. *J. Pediatr.* **85**, 71–6.

Van Creveld, S. (1961). The clinical progress of glycogenesis. *Triangle,* **5**, 137–44.

Ellis, R. W. B. and Payne, W. W. (1940). In *Biochemistry of diseases,* eds. Bodansky, M. and Bodansky, O. p. 247. Macmillan, New York.

Emmett, M. and Narins, R. G. (1978). Renal transplantation in type I glycogenosis: failure to improve glucose metabolism. *JAMA* **239**, 1642–4.

Field, J. B. and Drash, A. L. (1967). Studies in glycogen storage disease. II. Heterogeneity in the inheritance of glycogen storage diseases. *Trans. Assoc. Am. Physicians* **80**, 284–96.

82   *Inherited metabolic diseases involving the kidney*

——, Epstein, S. and Egan, T. (1965). Studies in glycogen storage diseases. I. Intestinal glucose-6-phosphatase in patients with von Gierke's disease and their parents. *J. Clin. Invest.* **44**, 1240–7.

Fine, R. N., Frasier, S. D. and Donnell, G. N. (1969). Growth in glycogen storage disease type I. Evaluation of endocrine function. *Am. J. Dis. Child.* **117**, 169–77.

——, Wilson, W. A. and Donnell, G. N. (1968). Retinal changes in glycogen storage disease type I. *Am. J. Dis. Child.* **115**, 328–31.

Garty, R., Cooper, M. and Tabachnik, E. (1974). The Fanconi syndrome associated with hepatic glycogenosis and abnormal metabolism of galactose. *J. Pediatr.* **85**, 821–3.

von Gierke, E. (1929). Hepato-nephromegalia Glykogenia (Glykogenspeicher-krankheit der Leber und Nieren). *Bietr. Pathol. Anat.* **82**, 497–513.

Howell, R. R. (1965). The inter-relationship of glycogen storage disease and gout. *Arthritis Rheum.* **8**, 780–5.

—— (1978). The glycogen storage diseases. In *The metabolic basis of inherited disease*, 4th edn. eds. Stanbury, J. B., Wyngaarden, J. B. and Fredrickson, D. S., pp. 137–59. McGraw-Hill, New York.

——, Ashton, D. M. and Wyngaarden, J. B. (1962). Glucose-6-phosphatase deficiency glycogen storage disease. Studies on the interrelationships of carbohydrate, lipid and purine abnormalities. *Pediatrics* **29**, 553–65.

Hsia, D. Y.-Y. (1961). Blood glucose-6-phosphate in heterozygous carriers and patients with liver glycogen disease (von Gierke's disease). *Nature* **192**, 266–7.

—— and Kot, E. G. (1959). Detection of heterozygous carriers in glycogen storage disease of the liver (von Gierke's disease). *Nature* **183**, 1331–2.

Illingworth, B. (1964). In: *Control of glycogen metabolism. Ciba Foundation Symposium,* eds. Whelan, W. J. and Cameron, M. P. p. 334. Churchill Livingstone, London.

Kapila, C. C., Kaul, S. and Chatterjee, B. C. (1956). Glycogen storage disease of the liver. *Br. Med. J.* **1**, 893–7.

Lampert, F., Mayer, H., Tocci, P. M. and Nyman, W. L. (1967). Fanconi syndrome in glycogen storage disease. In *Amino acid metabolism and genetic variation,* ed. Nyhan, W. L., p. 353. McGraw-Hill, New York.

Negishi, H., Morishata, Y., Kodama, S. and Matsuo, T. (1974). Platelet glucose-6-phosphatase activity in patients with von Gierke's disease and their parents. *Clin. Chim. Acta* **53**, 175–81.

Pompe, J. C. (1932). Over idiopatische hypertrofie van het hart. *Nederl. T, Geneesk.* **76**, 304–11.

Sarmiento, P. J. and Cortes Mendoza, E. (1974). Tres casos de hepatomegalia policórica o enfermedad de von Gierke. *Rev. Fac. Med. Bogotá* **15**, 531–42.

Senior, B. and Loridan, L. (1968a). Studies of liver glycogenosis, with particular reference to the metabolism of intravenously administered glycerol. *New Engl. J. Med.* **279**, 958–65.

—— and —— (1968b). Functional differentiation of glycogenoses of the liver with respect to the use of glycerol. *New Engl. J. Med.* **279**, 965–70.

Sidbury, J. B. Jr. (1965). The genetics of the glycogen storage diseases. In *Progress in medical genetics*, Vol. 4, eds. Steinberg, A. G. and Bearn, A. G., pp. 32–58. Grune & Stratton, New York.

Sokal, J. E., Fleissner, S., Sarcione, E. J. and Lowe, C. U. (1961). Blood glucose-

6-phosphate in heterozygous carriers and patients with liver glycogen disease (von Gierke's disease). *Nature* **192**, 265–6.

Spencer-Peet, J., Norman, M. E., Lake, B. D., McNamara, J. and Patrick, A. D. (1971). Hepatic glycogen storage disease. Clinical and laboratory findings in 23 cases. *Quart. J. Med.* **40**, 95–114.

Stamm, W. E. and Webb, D. I. (1975). Partial deficiency of hepatic glucose-6-phosphatase in an adult patient. *Arch. Intern. Med.* **135**, 1107–9.

Williams, H. E., Johnson, P. L., Fenster, L. F., Laster, L. and Field, J. B. (1963). Intestinal glucose-6-phosphatase in control subjects and relatives of a patient with glycogen storage disease. *Metabolism* **12**, 235–41.

4.1.2. Fabry's disease (angiokeratoma corporis diffusum)

Fabry (1898) and Anderson (1898) were the first authors to describe independently the disease subsequently known as angiokeratoma corporis diffusum or Fabry's disease. Several writers have described the clinical features, which consist of pain in the extremities or abdomen, or even angina, angiokeratomatous rash, corneal dystrophy, and impaired renal function (Wise *et al.* 1962; Colombi *et al.* 1967; Johnston *et al.* 1968). Death is most frequently due to renal failure (Parkinson and Sunshine 1961; Pabico *et al.* 1973; Sheth *et al.* 1979) but other causes include intracranial haemorrhage and cardiac failure (Wise *et al.* 1962). The mean age at death in hemizygous males is 41 years (Colombi *et al.* 1967) although much longer survival is reported (Jacob *et al.* 1953; Johnston *et al.* 1968). The disease is characterized by a marked variation in clinical features (Johnston *et al.* 1968), with some cases lacking the skin lesion (Johnston 1967; Flynn *et al.* 1972), or even showing only the corneal dystrophy. Franceschetti and colleagues (1969) demonstrated that isolated cornea verticillata in one family, previously described by Gruber (1946), was in fact a manifestation of Fabry's disease. Rosenberg and associates (1980) demonstrated that chronic airflow obstruction may occur in Fabry's disease as a result of sphingolipid deposition in epithelial cells of the respiratory tract.

Sweeley and Klionsky (1963) identified material that accumulates in tissues as a ceramide trisaccharide:globotriaosyl ceramide (Gal-Gal-Glc-Cer) along with the ceramide disaccharide:galabiosyl ceramide (Gal-Gal-Cer). They thereby identified the disorder as a sphingolipidosis with α-galactosyl (α-GAL) terminal moieties. They also demonstrated these ceramides in kidney as well as other tissues. These findings have been confirmed by several further groups of workers (Christensen-Loy 1966; Brady 1967; Schibanoff *et al.* 1969; Desnick *et al.* 1971, 1976). Kremer and Denk (1968) and Desnick and colleagues (1970) diagnosed Fabry's disease on the basis of the presence of these ceramides in urinary sediment, and Matalon and associates (1969) identified them in cultured fibroblasts from affected patients, and Vance and coworkers (1969) in plasma and red cells.

Brady and others (1967) reported the primary enzyme deficiency as a lysosomal galactosyl hydrolase, which they termed ceramide trihexosidase. They found absence of enzyme activity in intestinal biopsies from two male patients compared with control activities of 6.3 ± 0.9 nmol/mg protein/per hour, and excluded enzyme inhibition. Kint (1970) confirmed enzyme deficiency in leucocytes of male patients and, using synthetic substrates, characterized the enzyme involved as an α-galactosyl hydrolase or α-galactosidase. He also identified female carriers by enzyme assay. Dubach and others (1969) confirmed absence of enzyme activity in the kidneys. Ho and colleagues (1972) obtained a low residual activity in liver of male patients with similar K_m, pI and pH optimum to normal enzyme but with increased thermal stability. They used a 4-methyl umbelliferyl substrate and found intermediate levels of activity in female heterozygotes. Similar findings, also with 4-methyl umbelliferyl substrate, were reported by Wood and Nadler (1972) working entirely with fibroblasts. Brady and coworkers (1973) confirmed that the α-galactosidase deficiency is lysosomal and Desnick and associates (1973a) showed that it is the activity of the major thermolabile α-Galactosidase A isozyme that is deficient in Fabry's disease, whereas the thermostable B isozyme provides the residual activity in the patients. Further studies of the α-galactosidase isozymes in Fabry's disease have been reported by Sorenson and Hasholt (1980). Desnick's group reported on the use of enzyme assay in the diagnosis of both hemizygous males and heterozygous females. Rietra and associates (1974) showed that cross-reacting material to antibody against purified normal enzyme is present in the tissues of Fabry patients. Johnson and colleagues (1975) reported enzyme deficiency in tears and applied this to diagnosis in both hemizygotes and heterozygotes. Sheth and associates (1981) utilized multiple enzyme activities in the heterozygote detection. Mapes and others (1970) confirmed that plasma has α-galactosidase activity by infusing normal plasma into two patients and showing a decline in the plasma level of globotriaosyl ceramide in the patients.

As early as 1950 Scriba reported abnormal renal histology in Fabry's disease with birefringent material, on examination under polarized light, in the kidney and arterial walls. This was the earliest evidence for the deposition of a lipid in renal and other tissues. Similar observations were made by Ruiter (1957) on the kidney and by Fessas and colleagues (1955) in urinary sediment. The latter observed vacuolated cells in bone marrow, and Colley and colleagues (1958) and Wallace (1958) demonstrated similar vacuolation in the cells of the glomerular tufts and distal tubules of two first-cousin male patients, and confirmed that vacuoles contain lipid. They noted that these histological changes were associated functionally with a loss of urine-concentrating ability. They also found retrospectively similar renal histological changes in the mother of one of their patients who had died without any skin lesions. Rahman and colleagues (1961) confirmed the presence of birefringement material in glomerular epithelial cells of a female heterozygote. Parkinson and Sunshine (1961) reported a patient who presented with polyuria and a Pitressin-resistant diabetes-insipidus-like syndrome. These renal lesions are progressive, going on to involve proximal tubules as well as glomeruli and distal tubules (McNary and Lowenstein 1965), and interstitial histiocytes and fibrocytes (Rae *et al.* 1967), and continuing impairment of renal tubular function (Pabico *et al.* 1973). These lesions of the renal parenchyma and of the renal arteries and arterioles eventually lead to glomerulosclerosis and renal failure with death unless renal dialysis or transplantation is undertaken (Dubach *et al.* 1966, 1969). However, renal transplantation does not correct the metabolic defect (Spence *et al.* 1976). Hamburger and others (1964) described a family with proteinuria and renal insufficiency with similar renal histological changes. This may or may not have been Fabry's disease. Rosenmann and colleagues (1983) described a patient with both systemic lupus erythematosus glomerulo-nephritis and glomerular glycolipid storage of Fabry's disease.

The clinical, biochemical, and genetic aspects of Fabry's disease have been the subject of several good reviews (Desnick 1970; Clarke *et al.* 1971; Wallace 1973; Desnick *et al.* 1978; Desnick and Sweeley 1983).

Stiles and Optiz (1963) and Optiz and colleagues (1965) were the first to undertake a proper family study on a large family. They concluded that the disorder is X-linked and found loose linkage to the blood group Xg^a. X linkage has been confirmed by others (De Groot 1964; Johnston *et al.* 1966, 1969; Desnick *et al.* 1970; Malmqvist *et al.* 1971). However, a later study gave negative lod scores for linkage of Fabry and Xg, at all recombinant frequencies (Johnstone and Sanger 1981). Brady (1969) has pointed out that α-galactosidase A is the only one of the enzymes involved in glyocosphingolipid hydrolysis which is determined by a gene on the X chromosome. Hence genes for these hydrolases do not form a single operon. The localization of the gene for α-galactosidase A to the X chromosome has been confirmed using human–hamster somatic cell hybrids (Grzeschik *et al.* 1972; Rebourcet *et al.* 1974; Weil *et al.* 1979). Goss and Harris (1977) have extended this technique by fragmenting the X chromosomes of the human donor cells by irradiation before hybridization and have established a gene order as: phosphoglycerate kinase (PGK):α-GAL:hypoxanthine phosphoribosyl transferase (HPRT):G6PD (glucose 6-phosphate dehydrogenase). Further similar studies (Shows *et al.* 1978; Becker *et al.* 1979) extend this linkage relationship to: centromere:PGK:GLA (previously α-GAL):phosphoribosyl pyrophosphate synthetase (PRPS):HPRT:G6PD:Xqter. These studies give GLA a shortest region of overlap to the region Xq22→q23. Desnick's group have recently cloned a cDNA incorporating the GLA gene (Bishop *et al.* 1986); and Morgan and others (1987) have established linkage of the disease to the random DNA X-chromosomal probes DXS17 and DXS 87 with lod scores greater than 4.00. Desnick and colleagues (1978) in their review of Fabry's disease draw attention to the fact that in published pedigrees there are 45 known sons of affected fathers of whom none has the disease in addition to the standard pattern of maternal transmission. Furthermore, they note five instances of a women having two affected sons by different fathers. These observations leave no doubt as to the X-linked inheritance of this disease. That this gene locus is involved in X inactivation in the female was confirmed by Romeo and Migeon (1970). They obtained two cell populations, one with and the other without normal enzyme activity, on cloning cultured fibroblasts from two female heterozygotes, despite being unable to demonstrate reduced activity, using ρ-nitrophenyl substrate in uncloned cells. Furthermore, somatic cell hybridization indicates that the enzyme is a homodimer and hence is determined by a single structural gene (Grzeschik *et al.* 1972; Rebourcet *et al.* 1974; Hamers *et al.* 1977).

Desnick and colleagues (1978) estimate the incidence of the disease at 1 in 40 000 and comment on reports of its occurrence in Black, Latin American, Egyptian, and Oriental as well as Caucasian subjects.

Rahman and others (1961) noted intrafamilial variation in clinical expression and suggested that modifying genes may contribute to this variation, and Jensen (1966) noted that interfamilial variation was greater than intrafamilial. Philippart and coworkers (1969) suggested that assay of urinary glycolipids might assist in the recognition of atypical variants. Romeo and associates (1972) studied one of the two patients presenting with proteinuria and renal failure, but no skin lesions or corneal changes, previously reported by Clarke and colleagues (1971). Romeo and associates concluded that this patient differed enzymatically from classic cases. Even more striking evidence for genetic heterogeneity comes from the report of clinical Fabry's disease without α-galactosidase deficiency (Peltier *et al.* 1977).

Extensive studies of female heterozygotes have confirmed that expression may vary from biochemical and clinical normality (Avila *et al.* 1973; Rietra *et al.* 1976) through biochemical abnormality alone (Rietra *et al.* 1976; Spence *et al.* 1977), limited clinical expression, especially of corneal dystrophy (Franceschetti *et al.* 1969), wider mild clinical expression (Johnston *et al.* 1966; Burda and Winder 1967) to severe expression comparable to that in a male hemizygote (Ferrans *et al.* 1969;

Desnick *et al.* 1972). The typical glomerular renal lesion as seen on electron microscopy has been reported in a female heterozygote (Tondeur and Resibois 1969), and increased globotriaosylceramide has been observed in both plasma (Vance *et al.* 1969) and urinary sediment (Desnick and Krivit 1968). Detection of heterozygotes without going to the length of cell cloning rests on ezyme assay. Del Monte and colleagues (1976) and Libert and colleagues (1976) have used tears for this purpose, the latter recommending electron microscopy of a conjunctival biopsy as well. Rietra and associates (1976) assay enzyme activity in both plasma and leucocytes, and measure neutral glycolipds in urinary sediment. Several groups of workers have advocated assay on hair root follicles. Spence and others (1977) found, after failing to discriminate obligate heterozygotes by plasma or leucocyte enzyme assay, that the ratio of α- to β-galactosidase in hair follicles gave greatly improved discrimination. Improved hair follicle assays have been described by others (Beaudet and Caskey 1978; Ejiufor *et al.* 1978). Fenson and coworkers (1979) obtained clear segregation using the α-galactosidase A/β-galactosidase ratio on cultured skin fibroblasts, and Jongkind and others (1983) measured α-galactosidase A in single cells sorted from cultured fibroblasts on a cell sorter.

Brady and colleagues (1971) were the first group to use enzyme assay for prenatal diagnosis. This has since been performed by several further groups (Desnick and Sweeley 1971; Desnick *et al.* 1973b; Sorensen *et al.* 1974; Malouf *et al.* 1976). Galjaard and colleagues (1974a and b) have improved the speed of prenatal diagnosis by the use of microtechniques.

Recently Desnick's group have isolated a cDNA clone encoding human α-galactosidase A (Calhoun *et al.* 1986).

References

Anderson, W. (1898). A case of 'angeio-keratoma'. *Brit. J. Dermatol.* **10**, 113–17.
Avila, J. L., Convit, J. and Velazquez-Avila, G. (1973). Fabry's disease: normal α-galactosidase activity and urinary-sediment glycosphingolipid levels in two obligate heterozygotes. *Br. J. Dermatol.* **89**, 149–57.
Beaudet, A. L. and Caskey, C. T. (1978). Detection of Fabry's disease heterozygotes by hair root analysis. *Clin. Genet.* **13**, 251–8.
Becker, M. A., Yen, R. C., Itken, P., Seegmiller, J., Goss, S. J. and Bakay, B. (1979). Regional localization of the gene for human PRPP synthetase on the X chromosome. *Cytogenet. Cell Genet.* **25**, 134.
Bishop, D. F., Calhoun, D. H., Bernstein, H. S., Hantzopoulos, P., Quinn, M. and Desnick, R. J. (1986). Human α-galactosidase A: nucleotide sequence of a cDNA clone encoding the mature enzyme. *Proc. Nat. Acad. Sci.* **83**, 4859–63.
Brady, R. O. (1967). Enzymatic abnormalities in disease of sphingolipid metabolism. *Clin. Chem.* **13**, 565–77.

—— (1969). Genetics and the spingolipidoses. *Med. Clin. North Am.* **53**, 827–38.

——, Gal, A. E., Bradley, R. M., Martensson, E., Warshaw, A. L. and Laster, L. (1967). Enzymatic defect in Fabry's disease: Ceramidetrihexosidase deficiency. *New Engl. J. Med.* **276**, 1163–7.

——, Uhlendorf, B. W. and Jacobsen, C. B. (1971). Fabry's disease: antenatal detection. *Science* **172**, 174–5.

——, Tallman, J. F., Johnson, W. G., Gal, A. E., Leahy, W. R., Quirk, J. M. and Dekaban, A. S. (1973). Replacement therapy for inherited enzyme deficiency: use of purified ceramidetrihexosidase in Fabry's disease. *New Engl. J. Med.* **289**, 9–14.

Burda, C. D. and Winder, P. R. (1967). Angiokeratoma corporis diffusum universale (Fabry's disease) in female subjects. *Am. J. Med.* **42**, 293–301.

Calhoun, D. H., Bishop, D. F., Bernstein, H. S., Quinn, M., Hantzopoulos, P. and Desnick, R. J. (1985). Fabry disease: isolation of a cDNA clone encoding human α-galactosidase A. *Proc. Nat. Acad. Sci.* **82**, 7364–78.

Christensen-Lou, H. O. (1966). A biochemical investigation of angiokeratoma corporis diffusum. *Acta Pathol. Microbiol. Scand.* **68**, 332–42.

Clarke, J. T. R., Knaack, J., Crawhall, J. C. and Wolfe, L. S. (1971). Ceramide trihexosidosis (Fabry's disease) without skin lesions. *New Engl. J. Med.* **284**, 233–5.

Colley, J. R., Miller, D. L., Hutt, M. S. R., Wallace, H. J. and de Wardener, H. E. (1958). The renal lesion in angiokeratoma corporis diffusum. *Br. Med. J.* **1**, 1266–8 and special plate.

Colombi, A., Kostyal, A., Bracher, R., Gloor, F., Mazzi, R. and Tholen, H. (1967). Angiokeratoma corporis diffusum—Fabry's disease. *Helv. Med. Acta* **34**, 67–83.

Del Monte, M. A., Johnson, D. L., Cotlier, F. and Desnick, R. J. (1976). Diagnosis of inherited enzymatic deficiencies with tears: Fabry's disease. In *The eye and inborn errors of metabolism*, eds. Bergsma, D., Bron, A. J. and Collier, E. Nat. Found.-March of Dimes. Birth Defects Orig. Art. Ser. **12**(3), pp. 209–19. Alan R. Liss, New York.

Desnick, R. J. (1970). Biochemical and genetic studies of Fabry's disease. Ph.D. Thesis, University of Minnesota.

—— and Krivit, W. (1968). Fabry's disease: early detection and heterozygote identification by urine sediment glycolipid analysis. In *Proc. Am. Soc. Hum. Genet.*, 10 October 1968.

—— and Sweeley, C. C. (1971). Prenatal diagnosis of Fabry's disease. In *Antenatal diagnosis*, ed. Dorfman, A. p. 185. University of Chicago Press, Chicago.

—— and —— (1983). Fabry's disease: α-galactosidase A deficiency. Chapter 45 in *The metabolic basis of inherited disease*, 5th edn. eds. Stanbury, J. B., Wyngaarden, J. B., Frederickson, D. S., Goldstein, J. L. and Brown, M. S. pp. 906–44. McGraw-Hill, New York.

——, —— and Krivit, W. (1970). A method for the quantitative determination of the neutral glycosphingolipids in urine sediment. *J. Lipid Res.* **11**, 31–7.

——, Dawson, G., Desnick, S. J., Sweeley, C. C. and Krivit, W. (1971). Diagnosis of glycosphingolipidoses by urinary-sediment analysis. *New Engl. J. Med.* **284**,

739–44.

——, Simmons, R. L., Allen, K. Y., Woods, J. E., Anderson, C. F., Najarian, J. S. and Krivit, W. (1972). Correction of enzymatic deficiencies by renal transplantation: Fabry's disease. *Surgery* 72, 203–11.

——, Allen, K. Y., Desnick, S. J., Raman, M. K., Bernlohr, R. W. and Krivit,W. (1973a). Fabry's disease: enzymatic diagnosis of hemizygotes and heterozygotes. *J. Lab. Clin. Med.* 81, 157–71.

——, Raman, M. K., Bendel, R. P., Kersey, J., Lee, J. C., Krivit, W. and Sharp, H. L. (1973b). Prenatal diagnosis of glycosphingolipidoses: Sandhoff's (SD) and Fabry's diseases (FD). *J. Pediatr.* 83, 149–50.

——, Blieden, L. D., Sharp, H. L., Hofschire, P. J. and Moller, J. H. (1976). Cardiac valvular anomalies in Fabry's disease: clinical, morphologic and biochemical studies. *Circulation* 54, 818–25.

——, Klionsky, B. and Sweeley, C. C. (1978). Fabry's disease (α-galactosidase A deficiency). Chapter 39 in *The metabolic basis of inherited disease*, 4th edn. eds. Stanbury, J. B., Wyngaarden, J. B. and Frederickson, D. S., pp. 810–40. McGraw-Hill, New York.

Dubach, U. C. and Gloor, F. (1966). Fabry-Krankheit (Angiokeratoma corporis diffusum universale). *Dtsch. Med. Wschr.* 91, 241–5.

——, Enderlin, F. and Mannhart, M. (1969). Absent renal ceramide–trihexosidase activity in Fabry's disease. *German Medical Monthly* 14, 34–5.

Ejiufor, A., Robinson, D., Wise, D., Hamers, M. and Taber, J. M. (1978). Anderson–Fabry disease: rapid detection of carriers by hair bulb analysis. *J. Inher. Metab. Dis.* 1, 71–4.

Fabry, J. (1898). Ein Beitrag zur Kenntniss der Purpura haemorrhagica nodularis. *Arch. Dermatol. Syphilol.* 43, 187.

Fensom, A. H., Benson, P. F., Grant, A. R. and Jacobs, L. (1979). Fibroblast α-galactosidase A activity for identification of Fabry's disease heterozygotes. *J. Inher. Metab. Dis.* 2, 9–12.

Ferrans, V. J., Hibbs, R. G. and Burda, C. D. (1969). The heart in Fabry's disease: a histochemical and electron microscopic study. *Am. J. Cardiol.* 24, 95–110.

Fessas, P. Wintrobe, M. M. and Cartwright, G. E. (1955). Angiokeratoma corporis diffusum universale (Fabry): first American report of a rare disorder. *Am. Med. Assoc. Arch. Intern. Med.* 95, 469–81.

Flynn, D. M., Lake, B. D., Boothby, C. B. and Young, E. P. (1972). Gut lesions in Fabry's disease without a rash. *Arch. Dis. Child.* 47, 26–33.

Franceschetti, A. T., Philippart, M. and Franceschetti, A. (1969). A study of Fabry's disease. I. Clinical examination of a family with cornea verticillata. *Dermatologica* 138, 209–21.

Galjaard, H., Niermeijer, M. F., Hahnemann, N., Mohr, J. and Sorensen, S. A. (1974a). An example of rapid prenatal diagnosis of Fabry's disease using microtechniques. *Clin. Genet.* 5, 368–77.

——, Hoogeveen, A., Keijzer, W., de Wit-Verbeek, E. and Vlek-Noot, C. (1974b). The use of quantitative cytochemical analyses in rapid prenatal detection and somatic cell genetic studies of metabolic diseases. *Histochem. J.* 6, 491–509.

Goss, S. J. and Harris, H. (1977). Gene transfer by means of cell fusion. I. Statistical mapping of the human X-chromosome by analysis of radiation-induced gene segregation. *J. Cell Science* 25, 17–37.

Grzeschik, K. H., Grzeschik, A. M., Banhof, S., Romeo, G., Siniscalco, M., Van Someren, H., Meera Khan, P., Westerveld, A. and Bootsma, D. (1972). X-linkage of human α-galactosidase. *Nature (New Biol.)* **240**, 48–50.

De Groot, W. P. (1964). Genetic aspects of thesaurismosis lipoidica hereditaria Ruiter–Pompen–Wyers (angiokeratoma corporis diffusum Fabry). *Dermatologica* **129**, 281–2.

Gruber, M. (1946). Cornea verticillata. (Eine einfach-dominante Variante der Hornhaut des Menschlichen Anges). *Ophthalmologica* **111**, 120–9.

Hamburger, J., Dormont, J., De Montera, H. and Hinglais, M. (1964). Sur une singuliere malformation familiale de l'epithelium renal. *Schweiz. Med. Wschr.* **94**, 871–6.

Hamers, M. N., Westerveld, A., Khan, M. and Tager, J. M. (197). Characterization of α-galactosidase isozymes in normal and Fabry human–Chinese hamster somatic cell hybrids. *Hum. Genet.* **36**, 289–97.

Ho, M. W., Beutler, S., Tenmant, L. and O'Brien, J. S. (1972). Fabry's disease: evidence of a physically altered α-galactosidase. *Am. J. Hum. Genet.* **24**, 256–66.

Jacob, W., Gahlen, W. and Diekmann, H. (1953). Zur differential Diagnose des Angiokeratoma Fabry und der Periarteritisnodosa. *Arztliche Wschr.* **8**, 551–4.

Jensen, E. (1966). On the pathology of angiokeratoma corporis diffusum (Fabry). *Acta Pathol. Microbiol. Scand.* **68**, 313–31.

Johnson, D. L., Del Monte, M. A., Cotlier, E. and Desnick, R. J. (1975). Fabry disease: diagnosis by α-galactosidase A activity in tears. *Clin. Chim. Acta* **63**, 81–90.

Johnston, A. W. (1967). Fabry's disease without skin lesions (letter). *Lancet* **1**, 1277.

—— and Sanger, R. (1981). Linkage relationship of the loci for Anderson–Fabry disease and the Xg blood groups. *Ann. Hum. Genet.* **45**, 155–7.

——, Warland, B. J. and Weller, S. D. V. (1966). Genetic aspects of angiokeratoma corporis diffusum. *Ann. Hum. Genet.* **30**, 25–41.

——, Weller, S. D. V. and Warland, B. J. (1968). Angiokeratoma corporis diffusum. *Arch. Dis. Child.* **43**, 73–9.

——, Frost, P., Spaeth, G. L. and Renwick, J. H. (1969). Linkage relationships of angiokeratoma (Fabry) locus. *Ann. Hum. Genet.* **32**, 369–74.

Jongkind, J. F., Verkerk, A. and Niermeijer, M. F. (1983). Detection of Fabry's disease heterozygotes by enzyme analysis in single fibroblasts after cell sorting. *Clin. Genet.* **23**, 261–6.

Kint, J. A. (1970). Fabry's disease: alpha-galactosidase deficiency. *Science* **167**, 1268–9.

Kremer, G. J. and Denk, R. (1968). Angiokeratoma corporis diffusum (Fabry). Lipoid Chemische Untersuchungen des Harnsediments. *Klin. Wschr.* **46**, 24–6.

Libert, J., Tondeur, M. and Van Hoof, F. (1976). The use of conjunctival biopsy and enzyme analysis in tears for the diagnosis of homozygotes and heterozygotes with Fabry disease. In *The eye and inborn errors of metabolism*, eds. Bergsma, B., Bron, A. J. and Cotlier, E., *Birth Defects Orig. Art. Ser.* **12**(3), pp. 221–39. Alan R. Liss, New York.

McNary, W. and Lowenstein, L. M. (1965). A morphological study of the renal lesion in angiokeratoma corporis diffusum universale (Fabry's disease). *J. Urol.* **93**, 641–8.

Malmqvist, E., Ivemark, B. I., Lindsten, J., Maunsbach, A. B. and Martensson, E. (1971). Pathologic lysosomes and increased urinary glycosy–ceramide excretion in Fabry's disease. *Lab. Invest.* **25**, 1–14.

Malouf, N., Kirkman, H. N. and Buchanan, P. D. (1976). Ultrastructural changes in antenatal Fabry's disease. *Am. J. Pathol.* **82**, 13a.

Mapes, C. A., Anderson, R. L., Sweeley, C. C., Desnick, R. J. and Krivit, W. (1970). Enzyme replacement in Fabry's disease, an inborn error of metabolism. *Science* **169**, 987–9.

Matalon, R., Dorfman, A., Dawson, G. and Sweeley, C. C. (1969). Glycolipid and mucopolysaccharide abnormality in fibroblasts of Fabry's disease. *Science* **164**, 1522–3.

Morgan, S. H., Cheshire, J., Wilson, T. M., MacDermot, K. and Crawfurd, M. d'A. (1987). Restriction fragment length polymorphisms (RFLPs) in Anderson-Fabry disease. *Paediatric Nephrology* (In press).

Opitz, J. M., Stiles, F. C., Wise, D., Race, R. R., Sanger, R., von Gemmingen, G. R., Kierland, R. R., Cross, E. G. and de Groot, W. P. (1965). The genetics of angio-keratoma corporis diffusum (Fabry's disease), and its linkage relations with the Xg locus. *Am. J. Hum. Genet.* **17**, 325–42.

Pabico, R. C., Atanacio, B. C., McKenna, B. A., Pamukcoglu, T. and Yodaiken, R. (1973). Renal pathologic lesions and functional alterations in a man with Fabry's disease. *Am. J. Med.* **55**, 415–25.

Parkinson, J. E. and Sunshine, A. (1961). Angiokeratoma corporis diffusum universale (Fabry) presenting as suspected myocardial infarction and pulmonary infarcts. *Am. J. Med.* **31**, 951–8.

Peltier, A., Herbeuval, E., Brondeau, M. T., Belleville, F. and Nabet, P. (1977). Pseudo-clinical Fabry's disease without alpha-galactosidase deficiency. *Bio-medicine* **26**, 194–201.

Philippart, M., Sarlieve, L. and Manacorda, A. (1969). Urinary glycolipids in Fabry's disease: their examination in the detection of atypical variants and the presymptomatic state. *Pediatrics* **43**, 201–6.

Rae, A. I., Lee, J. C. and Hopper, J. (1967). Clinical and electron microscopic studies of a case of glycolipid lipoidosis (Fabry's disease). *J. Clin. Pathol.* **20**, 21–7.

Rahman, A. N., Simeone, F. A., Hackel, D. B., Hall, P. W., Hirsch, E. Z. and Harris, J. W. (1961). Angiokeratoma corporis diffusum universale (hereditary dystopic lipidosis). *Trans. Assoc. Am. Physicians* **74**, 366–77.

Rebourcet, R., Weil, D., Van Cong, N. and Frezal, J. (1974). Localisation d'un locus de structure de l'α-galactosidase sur le chromosome X par la methode d'hybridation cellulaire homme–hamster. *C. R. Acad. Sci. (Paris).* **278**, 3379–82.

Rietra, P. J. G. M., Brouwer-Kelder, E. M., De Groot, W. P. and Tager, J. M. (1976). The use of biochemical parameters for the detection of carriers of Fabry's disease. *J. Mol. Med.* **1**, 237–55.

——, Molenaar, J. L., Hamers, M. N., Tager, J. M. and Borst, P. (1974). Investigation of the α-galactosidase deficiency in Fabry's disease using antibodies against the purified enzyme. *Eur. J. Biochem.* **46**, 89–98.

Romeo, G. and Migeon, B. R. (1970). Genetic inactivation of the α-galactosidase locus in carriers of Fabry's disease. *Science* **170**, 180–1.

——, Childs, B. and Migeon, B. R. (1972). Genetic heterogeneity of alpha-galactosidase in Fabry's disease. *FEBS Letters* **27**, 161–6.

Rosenberg, D. M., Ferrans, V. J., Fulmer, J. D., Line, B. R., Barranger, J. A., Brady, R. O. and Crystal, R. G. (1980). Chronic airflow obstruction in Fabry's disease. *Am. J. Med.* **68**, 898–905.

Rosenmann, E., Kobrin, I. and Cohen, T. (1983). Kidney involvement in systemic lupus erythematosus and Fabry's disease. *Nephron* **34**, 180–4.

Ruiter, M. (1957). Some further observations on angiokeratoma corporis diffusum. *Br. J. Derm.* **69**, 137–44.

Schibanoff, J. M., Kamoshita, S. and O'Brien, J. S. (1969). Tissue distribution of glycosphingolipids in a case of Fabry's disease. *J. Lipid Res.* **10**, 515–20.

Scriba, K. (1950). Zur Pathogenese des Angiokeratoma corporis diffusum Fabry mit Cardio-Vasorenalem Symptomenkomplex. *Verh. Dtsch. Path. Ges.* **34**, 221.

Sheth, K. J., Tang, T. T. and Good, T. A. (1979). Fabry's disease in a black kindred. *Am. J. Dis. Child.* **133**, 1178–81.

——, Good, T. A. and Murphy, J. V. (1981). Heterozygote detection in Fabry disease utilizing mutliple enzyme activities. *Am. J. Med. Genet.* **10**, 141–6.

Shows, T. B., Brown, J. A., Haley, L. L., Goggin, A. P., Eddy, R. L. and Byers, M. G. (1978). Assignment of α-galactosidase (α-GAL) to the q22→qter region of the X-chromosome in man. *Cytogenet. Cell Genet.* **22**, 541–4.

Sorenson, S. A. and Hasholt, L. (1980). α-Galactosidase isozymes in normal individuals, and in Fabry homozygotes and heterozygotes. *Ann. Hum. Genet.* **43**, 313–21.

——, Hahnemann, N. and Mohr, J. (1974). Praenatal diagnostik af enzymede-fekter belyst ved et tilfaelde af undersogelse for angiokeratoma corporis diffusum (Fabry's sygdom).*Ugeskr. Laeger.* **136**, 1636–9.

Spence, M. W., MacKinnon, K. E., Burgess, J. K., D'Entremont, D. M., Belitsky, P., Lannon, S. G. and MacDonald, A.S. (1976). Failure to correct the metabolic defect by renal allotransplantation in Fabry's disease. *Ann. Intern. Med.* **84**, 13–16.

——, Goldbloom, A. L., Burgess, J. K., D'Entremont, D., Ripley, B. A. and Weldon, K. L. (1977). Heterozygote detection in angiokeratoma corporis diffusum. (Anderson–Fabry disease). *J. Med. Genet.* **14**, 91–9.

Stiles, F. D. and Optiz, J. M. (1963). Diffuse angiokeratosis (Fabry's disease) in children (Abs.). Meeting of the Midwest Soc. Pediatric Research, Chicago, November 1963.

Sweeley, C. C. and Klionsky, B. (1983). Fabry's disease: classification as a sphingolipidosis and partial characterization of a novel glycolipid. *J. Biol. Chem.* **238**, 3148–50.

Tondeur, M. and Resibois, A. (1969). Fabry's disease in children: an electron microscopic study. *Virchow's Arch. [Zellpathol.]* **2**, 239–54.

Vance, D. E., Krivit, W. and Sweeley, C. C. (1969). Concentrations of glycosyl ceramides in plasma and red cells in Fabry's disease: a glycolipid lipidosis. *J. Lipid Res.* **10**, 188–92.

Wallace, H. J. (1958). Angiokeratoma corporis diffusum. *Br. J. Dermatol.* **70**, 354–60.

—— (1973). Anderson–Fabry disease. *Br. J. Dermatol.* **88**, 1–23.

Weil, D., Van Cong, N., Rebourcet, R., Gross, M. S. and Frezal, J. (1979). Regional mapping of enzyme loci on human chromsomes 2, 17, 5, and X by use of somatic cell hybridization. *Cytogenet. Cell. Genet.* **25**, 215–16.

Wise, D., Wallace, H. J. and Jellinek, E. H. (1962). Angiokeratoma corporis diffusum: a clinical study of eight affected families. *Quart. J. Med.* **31**, 177–206 + 6 plates

Wood, S. and Nadler, H. L. (1972). Fabry's disease: absence of an α-galactosidase isoenzyme. *Am. J. Hum. Genet.* **24**, 250–5.

4.1.3. Gangliosidoses GM₁ types 1 and 2, and GM₂ type 2

The nomenclature of the gangliosidoses is confused by the number of synonyms for the different diseases within the group. Contemporary classification is based on the type of ganglioside that accumulates in tissues. Table 4.4 lists those currently recognized with the deficient enzyme activity for each. All are inherited in an autosomal recessive manner. In addition to the classic types listed in Table 4.4 there are several unusual variants of both β-galactosidase and hexosaminidase. Renal involvement is not a feature of these rare variants so they will not be discussed. O'Brien (1978, 1983) has reviewed both the classic types and the rare variants.

Gangliosides are deposited in the kidneys, as well as other tissues, in types 1 and 2 GM_1 gangliosidosis and in type 2 GM_2 (Sandhoff's disease). These three types will be briefly discussed separately.

Table 4.4. *The gangliosidoses*

Disease	Synonyms	Enzymic defect
GM₁ gangliosidosis, type 1	Infantile generalized gangliosidosis, Pseudo-Hurler syndrome, Landing's disease	GM₁ ganglioside acid β-galactosidases A and B. (Note B is a polymer of the monomeric A.)
GM₁ gangliosidosis, type 2	Juvenile generalized gangliosidosis	Mutations are probably allelic
GM₁ gangliosidosis, type 3	Adult generalized gangliosidosis	
GM₂ gangliosidosis, type 1	Tay–Sachs disease	Hexosaminidase A
GM₂ gangliosidosis, type 2	Sandhoff's disease	Hexosaminidase A and B
GM₂ gangliosidosis, type 3	Juvenile or late onset GM₂ gangliosidosis	Hexosaminidase A partial deficiency
GM₂ gangliosidosis, type 4	Adult (or chronic) GM₂ gangliosidosis	Hexosaminidase A partial deficiency

Compared with type 1 GM_2 gangliosidosis (Tay–Sachs' disease) all three are uncommon with only 10 to 100 known patients for each disorder (O'Brien 1978, 1983).

Type 1 GM_1 gangliosidosis (infantile generalized gangliosidosis)

This type presents at, or shortly after, birth with failure to thrive, weak sucking and ineffective swallowing. There may be oedema of extremities. The infant shows laboured, irregular breathing, and recurrent chest infection is common. Crawling and sitting are delayed. Clonic–tonic convulsions often develop and, if the infant survives beyond the first year, this progresses to decerebrate rigidity with spastic quadriplegia, deafness, and blindness. Death supervenes at anything from 6 months to 2 years (O'Brien 1969).

There are coarse features with frontal bossing, depressed nasal bridge, and large low-set ears. Hepatosplenomegaly develops within a few months and so also may kyphoscoliosis. About half the children have cherry-red spots in the retina similar to that seen in Tay–Sachs' disease. X-rays reveal anterior beaking of vertebral bodies, periosteal cloaking of long bones, modelling deformities of pelvis and extremities, and generalized bone rarefaction. Pathologically foamy histiocytes are found in bone marrow, liver, spleen, lymph nodes, and most visceral organs. The foamy appearance is due to lipids, which when removed leave clear vacuoles. Similar vacuoles are seen in epithelial cells of skin biopsies (O'Brien *et al.* 1975) and in renal glomerular epithelial cells producing cytoplasmic ballooning in the latter.

The stored material appears identical to normal GM_1 ganglioside, in both this disorder and the juvenile type of GM_1 gangliosidosis, with deposits in the brain and kidneys in the juvenile type, and in the infantile type only in the liver (O'Brien 1972).

Okada and O'Brien (1986) were the first to demonstrate an enzyme deficiency in a gangliosidosis when they reported acid β-galactosidase deficiency in two patients with infantile generalized gangliosidosis. Other lysosomal enzymes showed normal or increased activity. They found about 10 per cent of normal β-galactosidase activity in brain and 5 per cent in liver, spleen, and kidney. The deficiency was not due to soluble inhibitors. These observations were confirmed in brain and liver by Norden and O'Brien (1973) who found 0.1 per cent of normal activity, and by Sloan *et al.* (1969) in cultured fibroblasts. The diagnosis of GM_1 gangliosidosis can be confirmed by assay of β-galactosidase on white cells (Singer and Schafer 1970), urine (Thomas 1969), or cultured fibroblasts (Sloan *et al.* 1969). O'Brien (1975) and Meisler and Rattazzi (1974) have used antisera to normal human β-galactosidase A to study patients with type 1 and 2 GM_1 gangliosidosis. Normal or above normal amounts of cross-reacting material were consistently found, implying mis-sense mutations of the structural gene. O'Brien (1975) has suggested that the pleiotropic effects of a single gene mutation in GM_1 gangliosidosis may be due to impairment of the activity of the enzyme product against different substrates, that is, against β-D linked galactose in a variety of glycosaminoglycans, glycoproteins, and asialoconjugates. This would apply to both β-galactosidase A, the monomeric form of the enzyme, and the polymeric B form (Norden *et al.* 1974; O'Brien and Norden 1977).

The activity of acid β-galactosidase A and B is deficient in both types 1 and 2 GM_1 gangliosidosis. Contrary to early reports the activity of neutral β-galactosidase is normal in both disorders.

Heterozygotes have levels of enzyme activity intermediate between those of normal and affected homozygotes (Singer and Schafer 1970). Prenatal diagnosis based on enzyme assay of cultured amniotic fluid cells has been reported by several groups (Lowden *et al.* 1973); Kaback *et al.* 1973).

Type 2 GM$_1$ gangliosidosis (juvenile generalized gangliosidosis)

As the name implies this disease is of later onset than the infantile form. The course is also slower and less severe with normal development for up to a year and milder skeletal changes. Presentation is often with ataxia at about 1 year of age, followed by loss of speech and fine manipulative movements, and generalized muscular weakness. Subsequently there may be rapid mental and motor deterioration, progressive spasticity, the development of seizures, and eventually decerebrate rigidity. Death supervenes between 3 and 10 years of age (O'Brien 1972).

There is lymphocytic vacuolation, and foamy histiocytes similar to those of the infantile form are seen in the bone marrow and other tissues, but of milder degree than in type 1. Neuronal lipidosis and renal glomerular cytoplasmic ballooning resemble that of the infantile type 1.

Radiologically there may be mild vertebral beaking and proximal beaking of metacarpals from as early as 7 months (O'Brien 1972).

The enzyme defect, as in the infantile form, is a deficiency of acid β-galactosidase activity in the liver. The residual β-galactosidase A in one patient differed from that in other cases in that it showed an altered electrophoretic mobility, a raised Km, and cross-reacted with antibodies to the normal enzyme (Norden and O'Brien 1975). Otherwise the residual activity in type 2 is higher than in type 1 and may fall within the lower range of normal values (O'Brien *et al.* 1976). Nevertheless prenatal diagnosis based on enzyme assay of cultured amniotic fluid cells has been reported (Booth *et al.* 1973).

Each form of GM_1 gangliosidosis appears to be genetically distinct with affected sibs showing a similar phenotype. Parents of affected children have been consistently normal, and segregation analysis gives results consistent with autosomal recessive inheritance (Knudson 1965). Unlike Tay–Sachs disease the GM_1 gangliosidoses do not show any increased incidence among Ashkenazi Jews, although GM_1 type 1 is reported as showing an increased incidence in Malta (Aronson 1964). Galjaard and coworkers (1975) fused fibroblasts from patients with type 1 and type 2 and failed to obtain complementation, which provides evidence for allelic genetic heterogeneity. They did obtain complementation in a fusion of cells from type 1 and one of the rare variants of galactosidase deficiency, type 4, but the significance of this observation is still not clear. The gene for β-galactosidase A has been assigned to the short arm of chromosome 3 (Naylor *et al.* 1980).

References

Aronson, S. M. (1964). Epidemiology. In *Tay Sachs' disease* ed. Volk, B. W. p. 118. Grune & Stratton, New York.

Booth, C. W., Gerbie, A. B. and Nadler, H. L. (1973). Intrauterine diagnosis of GM_1 gangliosidosis, type 2. *Pediatrics* **52**, 521–24.

Galjaard, H., Hoogeveen, A., Keijzer, W., de Wit-Verbeek, H. A., Reuser, A. J. J., Ho, M. W. and Robinson, D. (1975). Genetic heterogeneity in GM_1 gangliosidosis. *Nature* **257**, 60–2.

Kaback, M. M., Sloan, H. R., Sonneborn, M., Herndon, R. M. and Percy, A. K. (1973). GM_1 gangliosidosis type 1 in utero: detection and fetal manifestations. *J. Pediatr.* **82**, 1037–41.

Knudson, A. G. (1965). *Genetics and disease.* p. 13. McGraw-Hill, New York.

Lowden, J. A., Cutz, E., Conen, P. E., Rudd, N. and Doran, T. E. (1973). Prenatal diagnosis of GM_1 angliosidosis. *New Engl. J. Med.* **288**, 225–8.

Meisler, M. and Rattazzi, M. C. (1974). Immunological studies of β-galactosidase in normal human liver and GM_1 gangliosidosis. *Am. J. Hum. Genet.* **26**, 683–91.

Naylor, S. L., Lalley, P. A., Elliott, R. W., Brown, J. A. and Shows, T. B. (1980). Evidence for homologous regions of human chromosome 3 and mouse chromosome 9 predicts location of human genes. *Am. J. Hum. Genet.* **32**, 159A.

Norden, A. G. W. and O'Brien, J. S. (1973). Ganglioside GM_1 β-galactosidase: studies in human liver and brain. *Arch. Biochem. Biophys.* **159**, 383–92.

—— and —— (1975). An electrophoretic variant of β-galactosidase with altered catalytic properties in a patient with GM_1 gangliosidosis. *Proc. Nat. Acad. Sci.* **72**, 240–4.

——, Tennant, L. L. and O'Brien, J. S. (1974). GM_1 ganglioside β-galactosidase A: purification and studies of the enzyme from human liver. *J. Biol. Chem.* **249**, 7969–76.

O'Brien, J. S. (1969). Generalized gangliosidosis. *Clin. Proc. Child. Hosp.* **25**, 40–52.

—— (1972). Ganglioside storage diseases. In *Advances in human genetics*, Vol. 3, eds. Harris, H. and Hirschhorn, K. pp. 39–98. Plenum Press, New York and London.

—— (1975). Molecular genetics of GM_1-β-galactosidase. *Clin. Genet.* **8**, 303–13.

—— (1978). The gangliosidoses, Chapter 40 in *The metabolic basis of inherited disease*, 4th edn. eds. Stanbury J. B., Wyngaarden, J. B. and Fredrickson, D. S. pp. 841–65. McGraw-Hill, New York.

—— (1983). The gangliosidoses, Chapter 46 in *The metabolic basis of inherited disease*, 5th edn. eds. Stanbury, J. B., Wyngaarden, J. B., Fredrickson, D. S., Goldstein, J. L. and Brown, M. S. pp. 945–69. McGraw-Hill, New York.

—— and Norden, A. G. W. (1977). Nature of the mutation in adult β-galactosidase deficient patients. *Am. J. Hum. Genet.* **29**, 184–90.

——, Bernett, J., Veath, M. L. and Paa, D. (1975). Lysosomal storage disorders: diagnosis by ultrastructural examination of skin biopsy specimens. *Arch. Neurol.* **32**, 592–9.

——, Gugler, E., Giedion, A., Wiessmann, U., Herschkowitz, N., Meier, C. and Le Roy, J. (1976). Spondyloepiphyseal dysplasia, corneal clouding, normal intelligence and β-galactosidase deficiency. *Clin. Genet.* **9**, 495–504.

Okada, S. and O'Brien, J. S. (1968). Generalized gangliosidosis: β-galactosidase deficiency. *Science* **160**, 1002–4.

Singer, H. S. and Schafer, I. A. (1970). White cell β-galactosidase activity. *New Engl. J. Med.* **282**, 571.

Sloan, H. R., Uhlendorf, B. W., Jacobson, C. B. and Fredrickson, D. S. (1969). β-Galactosidase in tissue culture derived from human skin and bone marrow: enzyme defection GM_1 gangliosidosis. *Pediatr. Res.* **3**, 532–7.

Thomas, G. H. (1969). β-D-Galactosidase in human urine: deficiency in generalised gangliosidosis. *J. Lab. Clin. Med.* **74**, 725–31.

Type 2 GM_2 gangliosidosis (Sandhoff's disease)

The onset of this form of gangliosidosis is typically under 6 months with progressive disease leading to death by the age of 3 years. The main features are progressive deterioration of both motor and mental development accompanied by blindness and a startle reaction to sound. The physical signs include macrocephaly, doll-like facies and cherry-red spots at the macula similar to those seen in Tay–Sachs disease. The pathology of the brain also resembles that of Tay–Sachs disease with lipid deposits in neurones and some vacuolization of histiocytes in other tissues. On electron microscopy, cytoplasmic lamellar lipid inclusions can be demonstrated in affected cells including renal tubular epithelial cells, especially those lining the loops of Henle, which may appear vacuolated on light microscopy (Sandhoff and Harzer (1973).

Whereas Tay–Sachs disease is due to a deficiency of hexosaminidase A activity, in Sandhoff's disease there is a deficiency of both hexosaminidase A and B in all tissues (Sandhoff and Harzer 1973), including amniotic fluid cells of affected fetuses in whom prenatal diagnosis has been made (Desnick *et al.* 1973; Harzer *et al.* 1975). Intermediate levels of enzyme activity have been reported in the parents of affected children using serum or white blood cells (Okada *et al.* 1972; Lowden *et al.* 1978).

Hexosaminidase A and B are both tetramers. Hexosaminidase A contains two α polypeptide chains and two β-chains ($\alpha_2\beta_2$), whereas hexosaminidase B consists of four β-chains ($\beta_2\beta_2$) (Geiger and Arnon 1976). The common β-chain is responsible for immunological cross-reactivity between the two forms (Carroll and Robinson 1973; Srivastava *et al.* 1974). Sandhoff's disease is due to a mutation within the β-chain locus and Tay–Sachs to a mutation of the α-chain locus. Several studies have indicated genetic heterogeneity in that some patients have material cross-reacting with anti-B antisera and others possess only A antigen (Srivastava and Beutler 1973). In another patient no A or B antigen was detectable (Carroll and Robinson 1973). Somatic cell hybridization of fibroblasts from Tay–Sachs and Sandhoff patients show complementation, confirming that the mutations in these two diseases are not allelic (Galjaard *et al.* 1974; Thomas *et al.* 1974), and indeed in human–hamster and human–mouse hybrids the loci for A and B segregated independently and were assigned to the human chromosomes 15 and 5 respectively (van Someren and van Henegouven 1973; Lalley *et al.* 1974; Gilbert *et al.* 1975). Some apparent inconsistencies in these studies with the two-locus, common-polypeptide-chain model have been shown to be due to the formation of a heteropolymer migrating close to human hexosaminidase A on electrophoresis (Hoeksema *et al.* 1977) in human–hamster hybrids. Family studies of Sandhoff's disease are consistent with autosomal recessive inheritance.

References

Carroll, M. and Robinson, D. (1973). Immunological properties of *N*-acetyl-β-D-glucosaminidase of normal human liver and of GM$_2$-gangliosidosis liver. *Biochem. J.* **131**, 91–6.

Desnick, R. J., Krivit, W. and Sharp, H. R. (1973). *In utero* diagnosis of Sandhoff's disease. *Biochem. Biophys. Res. Commun.* **81**, 20–6.

Galjaard, H., Hoogeveen, A., de Wit-Verbeek, H. A., Reuser, A. J. J., Keijzer, W., Westerveld, A. and Bootsma, D. (1974). Tay–Sachs' and Sandhoff's disease: intergenic complementation after somatic cell hybridization. *Exp. Cell. Res.* **87**, 444–8.

Geiger, B. and Arnon, R. (1976). Chemical characterization and subunit structure of human *N*-acetylhexosaminidases A and B. *Biochemistry* **15**, 3484–93.

Gilbert, F., Kucherlapati, R., Creagan, R. P., Murnane, M. J., Darlington, G. J. and Ruddle, F. H. (1975). Tay–Sachs and Sandhoff's disease: the assignment of genes for hexosaminidases A and B to individual human chromosomes. *Proc. Nat. Acad. Sci.* **72**, 263–7.

Harzer, K., Stengel-Rutkowski, S., Gley, E. O., Albert, A., Murken, J.-D., Zahr, V. and Henkel, K. P. (1975). Pranatale diagnose der GM$_2$ gangliosidose typ 2 (Sandhoff–Jatzkewitz–Krankheit). *Dtsch. Med. Wschr.* **100**, 106–8.

Hoeksema, H. L., Reuser, A. J. J., Hoogeveen, A., Braidman, I. and Westerveld, A. (1977). Characterization of β-D-N-acetylhexosominidase isoenzymes in man–Chinese hamster somatic cell hybrids. *Am. J. Hum. Genet.* **29**, 14–23.

Inui, K., Wenger, D. A., Furukawa, M., Suehara, N., Yutaka, Y., Okada, S., Tanizawa, O. and Yabuuchi, H. (1986). Prenatal diagnosis of GM$_2$ gangliosidoses using a fluorogenic-sulfated substrate. *Clin. Chim. Acta* **154**, 145–50.

Lalley, P. A., Rattazzi, M. C. and Shows, T. B. (1974). Human β-D-N-acetylhexosominidase A and B: expression and linkage relationships in somatic cell hybrids. *Proc. Nat. Acad. Sci.* **71**, 1569–73.

Lowden, J. A., Ives, E. J., Keene, D. L., Burton, A. L., Skomorowski, M. A. and Howard, F. (1978). Carrier detection in Sandhoff's disease. *Am. J. Hum. Genet.* **30**, 38–45.

Okada, S., McCrea, M. and O'Brien, J. S. (1972). Sandhoff's disease (GM$_2$ gangliosidosis type 2): clinical, chemical, and enzyme studies in five patients. *Pediatr. Res.* **6**, 606–15.

Sandhoff, K. and Harzer, K. (1973). Total hexosaminidase deficiency in Tay–Sachs' disease (variant O). In *Lysosomes and storage diseases*, eds. Hers, H. G. and Van Hoof, F. p. 345. Academic Press, New York.

Van Someren, H. and Van Henegouven, H. B. (1973). Independent loss of human hexosaminidases A and B in man–Chinese hamster somatic cell hybrids. *Humangenetik* **18**, 171–4.

Srivastava, S. K. and Beutler, E. (1973). Hexosaminidase A and hexosaminidase B: studies in Tay–Sachs' and Sandhoff's disease. *Nature* **241**, 463.

——, Yoshida, A., Awasthi, Y. C. and Beutler, E. (1974). Studies on human β-D-N-acetylhexosaminidases. II. Kinetic and structural properties. *J. Biol. Chem.* **249**, 2049–53.

Thomas, G. H., Taylor, H. A., Miller, C. S., Axelman, J. and Migeon, B. R. (1974). Genetic complementation after fusion of Tay–Sachs and Sandhoff cells. *Nature* **250**, 580–2.

4.1.4. Cystinosis

This disorder is distinct from cystinuria. The latter is a primary renal tubular transport defect, whereas cystinosis is a disorder in which there is excessive storage of free cystine within lysosomes of many different cell types (Schulman *et al.* 1969; States *et al.* 1974). That it is essentially a cellular defect is confirmed by the observation that renal transplants do not develop the pathological changes associated with the disease (Mahoney *et al.* 1970), and that the disorder is not due to increased intestinal absorption of cystine, an elevated serum level, nor impaired renal handling (Scriver and Rosenberg 1973).

Three clinical phenotypes have been recognized (Schneider 1973): an infantile or nephropathic (type 1), a benign or adult form (type 2)

(Schneider *et al.* 1968 and 1978; Seegmiller *et al.* 1968), and an intermediate or adolescent form (type 3) (Lietman *et al.* 1966; Goldman *et al.* 1971; Kroll and Lichte 1973).

In the nephropathic form polyuria, polydipsia, and recurring bouts of fever associated with dehydration are present from about 6 months to 1 year of age owing to impaired water reabsorption resulting from renal tubular damage. By 1 year there is also a Fanconi syndrome (Worthen and Good 1960) (see Chapter 6, p. 236) but without the generalized dibasic aminoaciduria seen in cystinuria. Excretion of cystine is in proportion to that of other amino acids and renal cystine stones are rare. Rickets and other skeletal abnormalities as well as growth retardation also ensue by 1 year of age. Subsequently there is in addition progressive evidence of glomerular damage and often electrolyte disturbances, especially hypokalaemia with acute prostration and even sudden fatal cardiovascular collapse. These electrolyte disturbances may lead to confusion with Bartter's syndrome. Other features include hypothyroidism, photophobia, and a relative lack of skin and hair pigmentation. Crystalline deposits are detectable on slit-lamp examination of the conjunctiva and cornea (Francois *et al.* 1972), and also on electron microscopic study (Wong *et al.* 1970; Kenyon and Sensenbrenner 1974). There is also irregular peripheral retinal depigmentation and pigment clumping (Wong *et al.* 1967; Francois *et al.* 1972). The progressive renal failure leads eventually to uraemia and death before puberty. Mental development is normal, but hydrocephalus can develop. Some benefit is claimed from treatment with cysteamine (da Silva *et al.* 1985).

The benign or adult form is symptomless and without retinopathy or renal disturbance. Patients do show crystalline deposits in the cornea and other tissues (Cogan *et al.* 1958; Lietman *et al.* 1966; Brubaker *et al.* 1970).

In the adolescent or juvenile form there is considerable variation in symptoms and signs, with onset from 18 months to 17 years, often incomplete Fanconi syndrome, slower progression of renal insufficiency, and variable retinal involvement. Nevertheless renal failure may ensue (Langman *et al.* 1985). The picture varies less within than between families.

Pathologically the characteristic finding is deposition of cystine crystals in leucocytes, bone-marrow cells, liver, spleen, and lymphatic tissue, ocular tissues, kidney and cultured fibroblasts. There may also be cerebral atrophy (Cochat *et al.* 1986). The concentration of free cystine in leucocytes is greatly increased over normal levels (Schneider *et al.* 1967a). The pathological changes in the kidney were reviewed by Spear (1974). The 'swan-neck' deformity of the proximal convoluted tubules, which is also seen in other forms of Fanconi syndrome, appears within the first year of life (Teree *et al.* 1970). In the late uraemic stage of the disease the kidneys show non-specific glomerular scarring, tubular degeneration, and interstitial nephritis with cystine crystals detectable in all three renal components (Jackson *et al.* 1962; Mahoney *et al.* 1970; Spear *et al.* 1971b; Spear 1974). However, despite increased free cystine content the tissues of a 23-week cystinotic fetus did not reveal cystine crystals (Schneider *et al.* 1974). A more characteristic feature is a giant-cell transformation of the visceral glomerular epithelium (Spear *et al.* 1971a), also seen in the adolescent form (Spear *et al.* 1971a; Zimmerman *et al.* 1974).

Types 1 and 2, and probably type 3, are inherited in an autosomal recessive manner (Seegmiller *et al.* 1968; Bois *et al.* 1976; Schneider *et al.* 1978). Parental consanguinity has been reported in both type 1 (Schneider *et al.* 1978) and type 2 (Lietman *et al.* 1966). The genetic relationship of the three types is unclear although McKusick (1978) has suggested that types 1 and 2 are allelic and type 3 is the double hetero-zygous compound. Steinherz and colleagues (1981) reported the curious observation that although the cystinosis gene is not linked to the HLA gene complex, nevertheless there is a positive association with HLA-B7, and a negative one with HLA-A9.

The possibility of early prenatal diagnosis was suggested by Schneider and colleagues' (1974) observation, mentioned above, of increased free cystine in the tissues of an affected fetus. Using the pulse-labelling technique of Schulman and coworkers (1970), Schneider and colleagues (1978) have undertaken prenatal diagnosis of 28 at-risk pregnancies. In three they found greatly increased radioactivity in the cystine of the amniotic fluid cells and confirmed raised free cystine in the tissues of the fetuses from the two pregnancies that were terminated. They were unable to distinguish between normal and heterozygous fetuses. A modification of this method has been described (States *et al.* 1975).

Heterozygotes for the infantile form show neither renal impairment nor deposition of cystine crystals in tissues. Until recently the most successful method of detecting heterozygotes for the infantile form had proved to be the measurement of the free cystine content of the white blood cells (Schneider *et al.* 1967a, 1968). Cultured fibroblasts have been used in a similar manner but are less reliable (Schneider *et al.* 1967b, 1968, 1978). However, both methods may give results within the normal range in known heterozygotes. Indeed Gahl and colleagues (1984), using white cells, found that 13 out of 20 obligate heterozygotes had cystine levels within two standard deviations of the normal mean. Both methods discriminate between homozygous affected individuals for the benign and adolescent forms, and the detection of heterozygotes for these forms follows a similar pattern to the infantile form (Goldman *et al.* 1971; Schneider *et al.* 1978). Recent studies by several groups have aimed at clarifying the mechanism of intralysosomal cystine accumulation. They have examined the kinetics of cellular and lysosomal uptake and extrusion, in normal, cystinotic, and in some cases heterozygous subjects. The main pathway of normal cystine uptake by the cell appears to involve plasma membrane transport rather than pinocytosis (Bannai and Kitamura 1980; Danpure *et al.* 1984a), followed by rapid reduction of the cystine to cysteine within the cytosol fraction of the cell. Either the uptake, efflux, or reduction of cystine would appear to be altered in cystinosis as the cellular cysteine:cystine ratio is reduced in cystinotic cells (Steinherz *et al.* 1982a). The cysteine is then transported into the lysosomes where in cystinotic cells it is reoxidized to cystine (Danpure *et al.* 1984a). When cystine translocation into isolated lysosomes is studied in the presence of saturating external concentrations of cystine it is found that normal, but not cystinotic, lysosomes take up cystine (Gahl *et al.* 1983) and that obligate heterozygotes lysosomes take up about half the normal amount (Gahl *et al.* 1984). However this method requires large amounts of white cells, obtained from 35–50 ml of blood and the use of a large amount of radioactive label. Furthermore, absolute uptake varies from one experiment to another, necessitating comparison with normal controls assayed simultaneously on each occasion, an observation that must leave some uncertainty about its reliability. It has also been demonstrated that the presence of chloroquine enhances lysosomal cystine accumulation in cystinotic, but not normal, cultured fibroblasts (Danpure and Fyfe 1980; Danpure 1981). The mechanism of this enhancement is unclear, and the findings in heterozygotes have not yet been reported. Danpure has suggested the chloroquine may enhance the rate of fusion between endocytic vesicles and lysosomes in cystinotics (Danpure *et al.* 1984b). Subsequently efflux of cystine from the lysosome, which is adenosine triphosphate (ATP) dependent, is impaired in cystinotic white cells (Gahl *et al.* 1982b; Jonas *et al.* 1982a), with intermediate values, with some overlap, in heterozygotes (Gahl *et al.* 1982a). Similarly efflux of cystine from the whole cell is reduced in cystinosis, with intermediate values in heterozygotes (Jonas *et al.* 1982b; Steinherz *et al.* 1982a and b). These studies suggest a possible defect involving a lysosomal membrane transport protein for cystine involved in the maintenance of the equilibrium between the intralysomal and cytosol concentrations of cystine. None of these approaches has yet provided an ideal method of heterozygote detection, nor established the nature of the basic defect.

References

Bannai, S. and Kitamura, E. (1980). Transport interaction of L-cystine and L-glutamate in human diploid fibroblasts in culture. *J. Biol. Chem.* **255**, 2372–6.
Bois, E., Feingold, J., Frenay, P. and Briard, M.-L. (1976). Infantile cystinosis in

France: genetics, incidence, geographic distribution. *J. Med. Genet.* **13**, 434–8.

Brubaker, R. F., Wong, V. G., Schulman, J. D., Seegmiller, J. E. and Kuwabara, T. (1970). Benign cystinosis. The clinical biochemical and morphologic findings in a family with two affected sibs. *Am. J. Med.* **49**, 546–50.

Cochat, P., Drachman, R., Gagnadoux, M.-F., Pariente, D. and Broyer, M. (1986). Cerebral atrophy and nephropathic cystinosis. *Arch. Dis. Child* **61**, 401–3.

Cogan, D. G., Kuwabara, T., Hurlbut, C. S. and McMurray, V. (1958). Further observations on cystinosis in the adult. *JAMA* **166**, 1725–6.

da Silva, V. A., Zurbrügg, R. P., Lavanchy, P., Blumberg, A., Suter, H., Wyss, S. R., Luthy, C. M. and Oetliker, O. H. (1985). Long-term treatment of infantile nephropathic cystinosis with cysteamine. *New Engl. J. Med.* **313**, 1460–3.

Danpure, C. J. (1981). The effect of chloroquine on the metabolism of [^{35}S]cystine in normal and cystinotic human skin fibroblasts. *Biochem. J.* **200**, 555–63.

—— and Fyfe, D. A. (1980). The effect of chloroquine on the intralysosomal accumulation of cystine in cystinotic and normal fibroblasts. *Biochem. Soc. Trans.* **8**, 571.

——, Jennings, P. R., Halsall, S. and Peters, T. J. (1984a). Mechanism of uptake and intracellular translocation of [^{35}S]cystine in cystinotic fibroblasts. *Biochem. Soc. Trans.* **12**, 857.

——, ——, Fyfe, D. A., Halsall, S. and Peters, T. J. (1984b). Mechanism of chloroquine-induced inhibition and stimulation of the labelling of the intra-lysosomal cystine pool in cystinotic fibroblasts. *Biochem. Soc. Trans.* **12**, 1037–9.

Francois, J., Hanssens, M., Coppieters, R. and Evens, L. (1972). Cystinosis: a clincal and histopathologic study. *Am. J. Ophthalmol.* **73**, 643–50.

Gahl, W. A., Bashan, N., Tietze, F., Bernardini, I. and Schulman, J. D. (1982a). Cystine transport is defective in isolated leukocyte lysosomes from patients with cystinosis. *Science* **217**, 1263–5.

——, Tietze, F., Bashan, N., Steinherz, R. and Schulman, J. D. (1982b). Defective cystine exodus from isolated lysosome-rich fractions of cystinotic leukocytes. *Science* **217**, 1263–5.

——, ——, ——, Bernardini, I., Raiford, D. and Schulman, J. D. (1983). Charac-teristics of cystine counter-transport in normal and cystinotic lysosome-rich leucocyte granular fractions. *Biochem. J.* **216**, 393–400.

——, Bashan, N., Tietze, F. and Schulman, J. D. (1984). Lysosomal cystine counter-transport in heterozygotes for cystinosis. *Am. J. Hum. Genet.* **36**, 277–82.

Goldman, H., Scriver, C. R., Aaron, K., Delvin, E. and Canlas, Z. (1971). Adolescent cystinosis: comparisons with infantile and adult forms. *Pediatrics* **47**, 979–88.

Jackson, J. D., Smith, F. G., Litman, N. N., Yuile, C. L. and Latta, H. (1962). The Fanconi syndrome with cystinosis: electron microscopy of renal biopsy specimens from five patients. *Am. J. Med.* **33**, 893–910.

Jonas, A. J., Smith, M. L. and Schneider, J. A. (1982a). ATP-dependent lysosomal cystine efflux is defective in cystinosis. *J. Biol. Chem.* **257**, 13185–8.

——, Greene, A. A., Smith, M. L. and Schneider, J. A. (1982b). Cystine accumulation and loss in normal, heterozygous, and cystinotic fibroblasts. *Proc. Nat. Acad. Sci.* **79**, 4442–5.

Kenyon, K. R. and Sensenbrenner, J. A. (1974). Electron microscopy of cornea and conjunctiva in childhood cystinosis. *Am. J. Ophthalmol.* **78**, 68–76.

Kroll, W. and Lichte, K.-H. (1973). Cystinosis: a review of the different forms and of recent advances. *Humangenetik* **20**, 75–87.

Langman, C. B., Moore, E. S., Thoene, J. G. and Schneider, J. A. (1985). Renal failure in a sibship with late-onset cystinosis. *J. Pediatr.* **107**, 755–6.

Lietman, P. S., Frazier, P. D., Wong, V. G., Shotton, D. and Seegmiller, J. E. (1966). Adult cystinosis—a benign disorder. *Am. J. Med.* **40**, 511–17.

McKusick, V. A. (1978). *Mendelian inheritance in man*, 5th edn. p. 469. Johns Hopkins Univ. Press, Baltimore and London.

Mahoney, C. P., Striker, G. E., Hickman, R. O., Manning, G. B. and Marchioro, T. L. (1970). Renal transplantation for childhood cystinosis. *New Engl. J. Med.* **283**, 397–402.

Schneider, J. A. (1973). *Clincal aspects of cystinosis.* p. 11. National Institute of Health, Publication 72–249.

——, Bradley, K. and Seegmiller, J. E. (1967a). Increased cystine in leukocytes from individuals homozygous and heterozygous for cystinosis. *Science* **157**, 1321–2.

——, Rosenbloom, F. M., Bradley, K. H. and Seegmiller, J. E. (1967b). Increased free-cystine content of fibroblasts cultured from patients with cystinosis. *Biochem. Biophys. Res. Commun.* **29**, 527–31.

——, Wong, V. G., Bradley, K. and Seegmiller, J. E. (1968). Biochemical comparisons of the adult and childhood forms of cystinosis. *New Engl. J. Med.* **279**, 1253–7.

——, Verroust, F. M., Kroll, W. A., Garvin, A. J., Horger, E. O., Wong, V. G., Spear, G. S., Jacobson, C., Pellett, O. L. and Becker, F. L. A. (1974). Prenatal diagnosis of cystinosis. *New. Engl. J. Med.* **290**, 878–82.

——, Schulman, J. D. and Seegmiller, J. E. (1978). Cystinosis and the Fanconi syndrome. Chapter 72 in *Metabolic basis of inherited disease*, 4th edn. ed. Stanbury, J. B., Wyngaarden, J. B. and Fredrickson, D. S. p. 1664. McGraw-Hill, New York.

Schulman, J. D., Bradley, K. H. and Seegmiller, J. E. (1969). Cystine: compartmentalization within lysozomes in cystinotic leukocytes. *Science* **166**, 1152–4.

——, Fujimoto, W. Y., Bradley, K. H. and Seegmiller, J. E. (1970). Identification of heterozygous genotype for cystinosis in utero by a new pulse-labelling technique: preliminary report. *J. Pediatr.* **77**, 468–70.

Scriver, C. R. and Rosenberg, L. E. (1973). Cystonisis. In *Amino acid metabolism and its disorders.* Chapter 11. p. 222. W. B. Saunders, Philadelphia.

Seegmiller, J. E., Friedmann, T., Harrison, H. E., Wong, V. and Schneider, J. A. (1968). Cystinosis. *Ann. Intern. Med.* **68**, 883–905.

Spear, G. S. (1974). Pathology of the kidney in cystinosis. In *Pathology annual* ed. Sommers, S. C. p. 81. Appleton-Century-Crofts, New York.

——, Slusser, R. J., Shulman, J. D. and Alexander, F. (1971a). Polykaryocytosis of the visceral glomerular epithelium in cystinosis with description of an unusual clinical variant. *Johns Hopkins Med. J.* **129**, 83–99.

——, ——, Tousimis, A. J., Taylor, C. G. and Schulman, J. D. (1971b). Cystinosis. An ultrastructural and electron-probe study of the kidney with unusual findings. *Arch. Pathol.* **91**, 206–21.

States, B., Harris, D. and Segal, S. (1974). Uptake and utilization of exogenous cystine by cystinotic and normal fibroblasts. *J. Clin. Invest.* **53**, 1003–16.

——, Blazer, B., Harris, D. and Segal, S. (1975). Prenatal diagnosis of cystinosis. *J. Pediatr.* **87**, 558–62.

Steinherz, R., Raiford, D., Mittal, K. K. and Schulman, J. D. (1981). Association of certain human leukocyte antigens with nephropathic cystinosis in the absence of linkage between these loci. *Am. J. Hum. Genet.* **33**, 227–33.

——, Tietze, F., Gahl, W. A., Triche, T. J., Chiang, H., Modesti, A. and Schulman, J. D. (1982a). Cystine accumulation and clearance by normal and cystinotic leukocytes exposed to cystine dimethyl ester. *Proc. Nat. Acad. Sci.* **79**, 4446–50.

——, ——, Triche, T., Modesti, A., Gahl, W. A. and Schulman, J. D. (1982b). Heterozygote detection in cystinosis using leukocytes exposed to cystine dimethyl ester. *New Engl. J. Med.* **306**, 1468–70.

Teree, T. M., Friedman, A. B., Kest, L. M. and Fetterman, G. H. (1970). Cystinosis and proximal tubular nephropathy in siblings. Progressive development of the physiological and anatomical lesion. *Am. J. Dis. Child.* **119**, 481–7.

Wong, V. G., Lietman, P. S. and Seegmiller, J. E. (1967). Alterations of pigment epithelium in cystinosis. *Arch. Ophthalmol. (Chicago)*, **77**, 361–9.

——, Kuwabara, T., Brubaker, R., Olson, W., Schulman, J. and Seegmiller, J. E. (1970). Intralysosomal cystine crystals in cystinosis. *Invest. Ophthalmol.* **9**, 83–8.

Worthen, H. G. and Good, R. A. (1960). The de Toni–Fanconi syndrome with cystinosis: clinical and metabolic study of two cases in a family and a critical review of the nature of the syndrome. *Am. J. Dis. Child.* **100**, 653–88.

Zimmerman, T. J., Hood, C. I. and Gasset, A. R. (1974). 'Adolescent' cystinosis: a case presentation and review of the recent literatures. *Arch. Ophthalmol.* **92**, 265–8.

4.1.5. Wilson's disease (hepatolenticular degeneration)

Hepatolenticular degeneration is named after Kinnear Wilson who gave a definitive clinical description of a patient with this disorder in 1912. He recognized earlier reports in the literature of patients who must have had the same disorder and also recognized its familial occurrence, but not its inheritance.

The time of onset is typically adolescence to early adulthood but the disease has been reported as early as 4 years and as late as the forties (Fitzgerald *et al.* 1975). Clinically it is characterized by a neurological syndrome, cirrhosis of the liver, and the pathognomonic sign of Kayser–Fleischer rings. The neurological syndrome observed by Wilson and later workers is that of lenticular degeneration. It is, however, a relatively uncommon manifestation of the disease with spasticity, rigidity, dysarthria, dysphagia, and drooling of saliva. There are painful spasms and eventually contractures. Progression is steady, with acute febrile episodes in the terminal stage leading to death within as little as a year in some cases (Sass-Korsak and Bearn 1978). The neurological disorder previously known as *pseudosclerosis* (Westphal 1883), in which there is a flapping tremor of the wrists and shoulders, is also a manifestation of Wilson's disease (Stadler 1939). Psychiatric symptoms are also common with an aggressive personality change or childish euphoria as the most frequent, and schizophrenia or hysteria as rare, disturbances.

The earliest sign of liver involvement is hepatosplenomegaly, and the earlier the onset the more likely the presentation is to be one of hepatic symptoms (Strickland *et al.* 1973). Subsequently a picture of subacute or chronic hepatitis develops. This may be associated with jaundice, or with ascites and oedema, and may progress to hepatic cirrhosis and eventually failure within weeks to years (Silverberg and Gellis 1962). The classical triad of features that includes neurological and hepatic involvement is completed by the Kayser–Fleischer ring, generally regarded as the one pathognomonic sign. This sign had been described earlier by Kayser (1902) in a patient diagnosed as having multiple sclerosis, and by Fleischer (1903) in a patient with a neurological disorder and cirrhosis. Fleischer (1912) prophetically suggested that the eye, brain and, liver changes were all due to a common metabolic defect. The Kayser–Fleischer ring consists of a golden-brown to greenish ring at the outer margin of the cornea due to deposition of copper granules in Descemet's membrane lining the inner surface of the cornea. However, the rings are not necessarily present in asymptomatic patients (Wiebers *et al.* 1977). Another ocular lesion is the 'sunflower' cataract (Wiebers *et al.* 1977). These eye lesions are well illustrated in papers by Cairns and coworkers (1969) and Walshe (1970).

Poor growth and acidosis due to renal disease may be the presenting features in Wilson's disease, and laboratory evidence of renal involvement is common. Uzman and Denny-Brown (1948) first reported aminoaciduria, confirmed by Uzman (1953) and Stein and colleagues (1954). Others have reported impaired renal function or mild haematuria (Hodges *et al.* 1956; Bearn *et al.* 1957; Wolfe 1964; Reynolds *et al.* 1966). Renal tubular function is more markedly affected than glomerular function, with reduced concentrating power and a tubular proteinuria (Peterson *et al.* 1969), and clearance of uric acid (Bishop *et al.* 1954; Mahoney *et al.* 1955; Bearn *et al.* 1957), and a reduced urate pool (Mahoney *et al.* 1955; Sorensen and Kappas 1966). There may also be a reduced maximal tubular reabsorption of glucose and hyperphosphaturia (Bearn *et al.* 1957), hypercalciuria (Finby and Bearn 1958; Litin *et al.* 1959; Randall *et al.* 1966), and even renal stones (Wiebers *et al.* 1979) or a urine acidification defect (Fulop *et al.* 1968; Walshe 1968). Wilson and Goldstein (1973, 1974) have questioned whether the uricosuria is due solely to impaired proximal tubular reabsorption of urate. The assumption that these disturbances of renal function are due to the excess copper deposition in the kidney is supported by the observation that the removal of this excess copper by penicillamine therapy eventually restores renal function to normal (Fulop *et al.* 1968; Walshe 1968; Leu *et al.* 1970b; Schonheyder *et al.* 1971). Since penicillamine therapy may itself prove toxic to the kidney it is important to assess renal function prior to starting treatment.

Another occasional clinical feature is episodes of acute haemolytic anaemia, which may be the presenting symptom, seen only in untreated patients and associated with markedly increased serum and urine copper (McIntyre *et al.* 1967). Finby and Bearn (1958) described a variety of bone lesions in Wilson's disease and Aksoy and others (1972) found intrafamilial similarity in the type of bone lesion. Vitamin-D-resistant rickets is a rare complication which has been reported predominantly from India (Dastur *et al.* 1968; Joshua 1973) and which it has been suggested may be a genetic variant of the disease (Dastur *et al.* 1968). An unusual physical sign which may, however, be of value when present is a blueish colour to the base of the finger nails, *azure linulae* (Bearn and McKusick 1958).

An important clinical observation is the virtual inability of women with untreated Wilson's disease to carry pregnancy through successfully to term (Walshe 1977). Some even miscarry during the presymptomatic stage of the disease. Klee (1979) has described one such patient who had miscarriages before the onset of the disease. Hence Wilson's disease is probably the only recognized monogenic maternal disorder causing spontaneous abortion.

Glazebrook (1945) was the first to establish clearly a role for copper in the pathogenesis of Wilson's disease, although earlier papers had implicated copper in 'pseudosclerosis'. Glazebrook found high levels of copper in the liver and brain of a patient. This observation has been confirmed for these tissues, and for kidney and cornea, by other groups (Perman *et al.* 1979). During the presymptomatic phase hepatic copper is deposited diffusely in the cytoplasm of parenchymal cells but may later become localized to lysosomes (Goldfischer and Sternlieb 1968). Copper deposition in the kidneys appears to remain diffuse. In the brain maximal deposition is found in the basal ganglia and the cortex, predominantly in glial cells. It is associated non-specifically with various copper-binding proteins in the brain, especially the major component cerebrocuprein I, which is not itself increased (Porter 1968). This protein has been identified as cytocuprein or superoxide dismutase (Carrico and Deutsch 1969; McCord and Fridovich (1969). Serum copper is typically low in Wilson's disease although the non-caeruloplasmin-bound fraction is increased (Cartwright *et al.* 1954). Exceptionally the non-bound fraction may be so high as to give a normal or elevated total serum copper. In presymptomatic patients the unbound fraction is not yet increased and, as caeruloplasmin is clearly decreased, total serum copper is low. Mandelbrote and colleagues (1948) were the first to report increased urinary copper excretion in Wilson's disease. This increased copper excretion is augmented by protein intake and is paralleled by amino-aciduria (Bearn and Kunkel 1952). Following both oral and intravenous administration of radioisotope-labelled copper there is a higher than normal rise and a slower fall of serum copper (Cartwright *et al.* 1954; Sternlieb *et al.* 1961; Smallwood *et al.* 1971), and the normal secondary rise at 4–6 hours fails to occur, associated with a failure to incorporate the copper into caeruloplasmin even when the plasma caeruloplasmin level is normal (Bearn and Kunkel 1954; Sternlieb *et al.* 1961; Gibbs and Walshe 1971; Vierling *et al.* 1978; Sternlieb and Scheinberg 1979). With intravenous injection of radiocopper there is also reduced and slower hepatic uptake in Wilson's disease, little or no subsequent release, and reduced faecal but increased urinary excretion (Strickland *et al.* 1972).

The first biochemically characteristic finding in Wilson's disease is a low or absent serum caeruloplasmin level (Bearn and Kunkel 1952; Scheinberg and Gitlin 1952). This is a consistent finding except in patients with severe or active liver disease, and in pregnancy or oestrogen administration (Walshe and Briggs 1962; Scheinberg and Sternlieb 1963). Sass-Kortak and Bearn (1978) have compared caerulo-plasmin levels in 230 patients and 309 controls. Ninety-six per cent of patients had levels below 20 mg/100 ml and the remaining 4 per cent fell within the 95 per cent confidence limits for the controls. Second and most definitive in establishing the diagnosis is the failure of incorpora-tion of radiocopper into caeruloplasmin mentioned above. Third is a reduction in the rate of biliary excretion of copper (Strickland *et al.* 1972; Gibbs and Walshe 1980). A variety of hypotheses have been proposed regarding the basic defect in Wilson's disease. An early suggestion was that synthesis of caeruloplasmin is reduced. This idea is incompatible with the variation in caeruloplasmin level in Wilson's disease and the lack of correlation of the level with the degree of copper deposition in tissues, including the fact that the caeruloplasmin level often falls further on treatment whereas all other parameters of disease improve. Another proposal was that the caeruloplasmin present is abnormal (Scheinberg and Sternlieb 1965) but peptide map and physico-chemical comparison have either shown no differences from normal caeruloplasmin (Holtzman *et al.* 1967) or variable differences (Needleman *et al.* 1970; Neifakh *et al.* 1972). In contrast Walshe and Carpenter (1965) found differences in the behaviour of caeruloplasmin from Wilson's disease and normal subjects in the presence of inhibitors. This does not, of course, necessarily imply that the difference lies in the caeruloplasmin. On the basis of a finding of normal serum concentrations of apocaeruloplasmin in Wilson's disease, Holtzman and coworkers suggested that the defect lies in a failure of the mechanism of incorporation of copper into newly synthesized apocaeruloplasmin (Holtzman *et al.* 1967; Holtzman and Gaumnitz 1970a and b; Matsuda *et al.* 1974). On the basis of finding a reduced activity of cytochrome oxidase in patients, and to a lesser extent heterozygotes, Shokeir and Shreffler (1969) suggested that caeruloplasmin may play a role in the transfer of copper to such copper-containing enzymes. Other hypotheses involve proteins that are unrelated to caeruloplasmin. Uzman suggested that the defect involves an increased affinity of an intracellular copper-binding protein in liver and other tissues with copper deposition in Wilson's disease (Uzman *et al.* 1956; Iber *et al.* 1957). For some years there was no evidence forthcoming to support this idea but in 1973 Evans and his coworkers purified a low molecular weight protein, probably a metallothionein, from the livers of Wilson's disease and biliary cirrhosis patients. The protein from both groups had a similar number of copper-binding sites but that from the Wilson's disease patients had a greater copper-binding constant. This metallothionein may be identical to the 'copper-associated protein' of Sherlock's group (Evans *et al.* 1980) found in hepatic lysosomes (Goldfischer and Sternlieb 1968). Another hypothesis proposes that the primary defect is the reduced biliary excretion of copper resulting in a positive copper balance not compensated by the increased renal excretion of copper. One suggestion is that a carrier protein that transfers copper to both caeruloplasmin and to the bile is defective (Saas-Kortsak 1965; Cox *et al.* 1972). Such a carrier might be Evans' metallothionein, the hepatic lysosomal copper-binding protein L-6D discovered by Sternlieb *et al.* (1973), or some other unknown carrier. Epstein and Sherlock (1981) point out that the normal infant is born with high levels of hepatic copper and low serum copper and caeruloplasmin (Shokeir 1971). They go on to propose that the mutation in Wilson's disease involves a controller gene that switches copper metabolism from a fetal to a postnatal form. However, this hypothesis has been criticized by Matsuda (1981) who points out that apocaeruloplasmin levels in Wilson's disease resembles those of the normal adult rather than the lower values of the neonate. None of these hypotheses is supported by sufficient evidence to be regarded as anything more than working hypotheses. The abnormal metallothionein and other hypotheses have been discussed in a recent leading article in the *Lancet* (1981).

Following Wilson's observation of familial occurrence of the disease in his original report the first evidence that this had an inherited basis came from the studies of Hall (1921) who noted affected sibs, unaffected parents, and parental consanguinity. Subsequent studies have amply confirmed an autosomal recessive mode of inheritance (Kehrer 1930; Andre and van Bogaert 1950), as have the later studies of Bearn (1953, 1960) on 30 American families, of Arima and Kurumada (1962, 1963) (who like Bearn found a high rate of parental consanguinity) on 18 Japanese families, of Wald (1962) on 21 Polish families, and of Tu (1963) on nine Chinese families, Strickland *et al.* (1973) on Taiwanese families, and Passwell *et al.* (1977) in Israel, and Fukuda (1965) and Saito (1983) in Japan. Arima and colleagues have estimated the heterozygote frequence of Mikura to be as high as 0.01 (Arima and Kurumada 1962; Arima *et al.* 1963, 1964; Arima and Sano 1968). Earlier estimates of the disease prevalence were generally lower than for Mikura in Japan but have shown an increase with time, due to improved ascertainment, from about 5 to 30 per million (Saito 1981; Scheinberg 1983). The latter estimate would imply a heterozygote frequency of 0.0109, similar to that for Mikura. These estimates take account of the likelihood that only about a quarter of all affected patients are diagnosed as having Wilson's disease (Scheinberg 1982).

The higher prevalance estimate of 30 per million has received support from more recent studies, especially those of Bachmann and colleagues in East Germany (1979) whose data give an estimate of gene frequency of 0.0053, and hence of carrier frequency of 0.0106. Scheinberg and Sternlieb (1984) in a recent monograph on Wilson's disease have reviewed the evidence for this relatively high prevalence; and Parkes (1984) points out that this incidence if applied to Britain would imply up to 1500 patients, most of whom would be unrecognized. Walshe (1984), commenting on Parkes' article, presents further data on the disease prevalence in East Anglia supporting an estimate of around 30 per million, especially in the age range of 16 to 34 years in which ascertainment is likely to be maximal. These figures, with their evidence for substantial underdiagnosis of the disease, present a major challenge to clinicians—the difficulties of which are highlighted by the experience of Downie (1984), a neurologist in Aberdeen, who despite a personal interest in diagnosing the disease has failed to detect a single new case over the last 19 years.

The extent of genetic heterogeneity among cases of Wilson's disease is a moot point. Two family studies have given some indication of such heterogeneity in terms both of the geographical origin of the gene concerned and of the clinical course of the disease, although they do not appear to point in quite the same directions. Bearn (1953, 1960) undertook a formal genetic analysis of 30 American families. Thirteen of these families had originated from Eastern Europe and all of their affected members had shown a late onset with only mild neurological signs. Cox and colleagues (1972) studied 28 Canadian families. Like Walshe (1967) in England they found a relatively low rate of parental consanguinity compared with Bearn's New York families and Arima and Kurumada's Japanese families. They claimed to recognize at least three different forms of the disease, two of which they termed 'typical' and one 'atypical'. In their two typical forms heterozygotes have normal caeruloplasmin levels but show delayed reappearance of copper into serum and caeruloplasmin. The two forms differ in their clinical course. One, which they term the 'Slavic type', from the origin of the families, is of late onset, like Bearn's East European families, and has mainly neurological features. The other typical form, termed the 'juvenile type', is of West European origin, has an onset under 16 years of age, and is more often hepatic in symptomatology. Their atypical form shows a common German–Mennite origin and is characterized by a half-normal level of caeruloplasmin in heterozygotes. Passwell *et al.* (1977) observed striking differences between Jewish and Arab patients in Israel. How far these variations in geographical origin, age of onset, and natural history of the disease can by accepted as representing distinct genetic forms, rather than constituting a spectrum of expression of a single genetic defect, as in one large Japanese family (Arima and Sano 1968), is for the present conjectural.

For the purpose of genetic counselling it is helpful to be able to diagnose the presymptomatic patient and the unaffected heterozygote. Diagnosis of the presymptomatic homozygote is important because treatment at this stage will prevent the development of symptoms (Levi *et al.* 1967; Sternlieb and Scheinberg 1968). Over 90 per cent of such patients can be detected by assay of the serum caeruloplasmin level at any time beyond infancy. Caution must be exercised in the use of this test in the asymptomatic sib of a known patient as a small proportion of heterozygotes do have a low serum caeruloplasmin (Gibbs and Walshe 1979; and see Cox *et al.* 1972). As this change tends to segregate within families, assay of parents and other sibs will in most cases resolve the uncertainty.

A study of 37 parents of Wilson's disease patients found a low serum caeruloplasmin in 6 per cent (Cox *et al.* 1972) and in all instances but one these clustered in three of the 26 families studied. These three families constituted the authors' 'atypical' group. This study confirmed similar obseravtions of earlier studies (Bearn 1953, 1957; Bickel *et al.* 1957; Sass-Kortsak *et al.* 1961; Sternlieb *et al.* 1961; Sternlieb and Scheinberg 1968). The liver copper content in heterozygotes is not a very useful test as although it tends to be increased the range overlaps with those of both normals and patients (Sternlieb and Scheinberg 1968). A slight increase in muscle copper (Leu *et al.* 1970a), of copper excretion after administration of penicillamine (Tu and Blackwell 1967; Gibbs *et al.* 1978), and some disturbance of renal tubular function (Leu and Strickland 1972) have all been reported as inconsistent findings in heterozygotes.

Early reports of a low rate of incorporation of oral ^{64}Cu into caeruloplasmin in heterozygotes (Sass-Kortsak *et al.* 1961; Sternlieb *et al.* 1961) were not confirmed in a more extensive study (Sternlieb and Scheinberg 1972). However, Cox and his colleagues measured plasma total and caeruloplasmin-bound radioactive copper in several samples following intravenous injection in normals, patients, and heterozygotes. Fourteen out of 16 obligate heterozygotes gave levels for both total and caeruloplasmin-bound copper intermediate between their lower limits of normal and upper limit for patients. Their two exceptions fell within the normal range (Cox *et al.* 1972). An alternative method is to measure the duration of total body retention of radiocopper following injection of a single dose. This too gives intermediate degrees of prolongation between normals and patients in heterozygotes but again with overlap (O'Reilly *et al.* 1969, 1971a; Strickland *et al.* 1972; Robinson *et al.* 1974; Willvonsender *et al.* 1974). Poor discrimination has also been obtained using the reduced rate of discharge of copper from the liver following the initial uptake by heterozygotes (Osborn and Walshe 1961, 1969; Strickland *et al.* 1972). Values for heterozygotes intermediate between those of patients and normals have also been obtained for 5-day faecal excretion of ^{67}Cu (O'Reilly *et al.* 1971b; Strickland *et al.* 1972), and for urinary excretion after intravenous radiocopper (Gibbs *et al.* 1978).

A recent study from Czechoslovakia reports the findings in 16 children of 10 patients with Wilson's disease (Maracek and Nevsimalova 1984). They found low serum copper and caeruloplasmin levels and high urinary copper excretion following penicillamine administration— findings that differed from those in adult heterozygotes. They also observed EEG and clinical neurological abnormalities in some of the children.

Another recent observation, that may eventually prove useful in pre- or postnatal diagnosis and perhaps in heterozygote detection, is that of increased levels of copper in fibroblasts cultured from Wilson's disease patients (Goka *et al.* 1976; Camarakis *et al.* 1980; Chan *et al.* 1980). The fibroblast model will also be valuable in further studies on the basic defect, as will the animal model of the disease reported by Su and colleagues (1982) in Bedlington terriers. In the meantime wholly reliable discrimination of heterozygotes still eludes us. Nevertheless, the observations of impaired body handling of administered copper by heterozygotes are clearly significant and point strongly to the basic defect lying in this area. It may well be that further study of fibroblasts or other features in heterozygotes may elucidate the basic defect.

A step towards the molecular definition of the disease has been taken with the demonstration of probable linkage of the Wilson's disase gene to the esterase D locus on chromosome 13 (Fryman *et al.* 1985). These workers obtained a lod score of 3.21 at $\theta = 0.06$. Esterase D is also linked to the gene for hereditary retinoblastoma and has been assigned to 13q14.

References

Aksoy, M., Camli, N., Dicol, K., Erdem, S. and Akgün, T. (1972). Osseous changes in Wilson's disease: a radiological study of nine patients. *Radiology* **102**, 505–9.

André, M. J. and van Bogaert, L. (1950). L'hérédité dans la dégénérescence hépato-lenticulaire et le probleme des rapports intrinseques de la pseudo-sclérose de Westphal-Strumpell et de la maladie de Wilson. La situation nosologique de l' "abdominal-Wilson" de Kehrer au sein de la D.H.L. *Encéphale* **39**, 1–54.

Arima, M. and Kurumada, T. (1962). Genetical studies of Wilson's disease in childhood. I. Clinical and biochemical analyses of sixteen families. II. Mode of inheritance and gene frequency in Japan. *Paediatr. Univ. Tokyo* **7**, 1–12,

—— and Sano, I. (1968). Genetic studies of Wilson's disease in Japan. *Birth Defects* **4**(2), 54–9.

——, Kurumada, T. and Kamoshita, S. (1963). Genetic studies on Wilson's disease. II. Model of inheritance, geographical distribution and gene frequency. *Brain and Nerve* **15**, 29–35.

——, Kamoshita, S., Komiya, H. and Murokawa, H. (1964). Genetical studies of Wilson's disease. III. Genetical and epidemiological studies of Wilson's disease in Mikura Island. *Paediatr. Univ. Tokyo* **10**, 5–10.

Bachmann, H., Lossner, J., Gruss, B. and Ruchholtz, U. (1979). Die epidemiologie der Wilsonschen Erkrankung in der DDR und die derzeitige Problematik einer population-genetischen Bearbeitung. *Psychiatr. Neurol. Med. Psychol.* **31**, 393–400.

Bearn, A. G. (1953). Genetic and biochemical aspects of Wilson's disease. *Am. J. Med.* **15**, 442–9.

—— (1957). Wilson's disease: an inborn error of metabolism with multiple manifestations. *Am. J. Med.* **22**, 747–57.

—— (1960). A genetical analysis of thirty families with Wilson's disease (hepatolenticular degeneration). *Ann. Hum. Genet.* **24**, 33–43.

—— and Kunkel, H. G. (1952). Biochemical abnormalities in Wilson's disease (abs.). *J. Clin. Invest.* **31**, 616.

—— and —— (1954). Localization of ^{64}Cu in serum fractions following oral administration: an alteration in Wilson's disease. *Proc. Soc. Exp. Biol. Med.* **85**, 44–8.

—— and McKusick, V. A. (1958). Azure lunulae. An unusual change in the fingernails in two patients with hepatolenticular degeneration (Wilson's disease). *JAMA* **166**, 904–6.

——, Yü, T. F. and Gutman, A. B. (1957). Renal function in Wilson's disease. *J. Clin Invest.* **36**, 1107–14.

Bickel, H., Neale, F. C. and Hall, G. (1957). A clinical and biochemical study of hepatolenticular degeneration (Wilson's disease). *Quart. J. Med.* **26**(NS), 527–58.

Bishop, C., Zimdahl, W. T. and Talbott, J. H. (1954). Uric acid in two patients with Wilson's disease (hepatolenticular degeneration). *Proc. Soc. Exp. Biol. Med.* **86**, 440–1.

Cairns, J. E., Williams, H. P. and Walshe, J. M. (1969). 'Sunflower cataract' in Wilson's disease. *Br. Med. J.* **3**, 95–6 and colour plate facing p. 97.

Carmarakis, J., Ackland, L. and Danks, D. M. (1980). Abnormal copper metabolism in cultured fibroblasts from patients with Wilson's disease. *J. Inher. Metab. Dis.* **3**, 155–7.

Carrico, R. J. and Deutsch, H. F. (1970). The presence of zinc in human cytocuprein and some properties of the apoprotein. *J. Biol. Chem.* **245**, 723–7.

Cartwright, G. E., Hodges, R. E., Gubler, C. J., Mahoney, J. P., Daum, K., Wintrobe, M. M. and Bean, W. B. (1954). Studies on copper metabolism. XIII. Hepatolenticular degeneration. *J. Clin. Invest.* **33**, 1487–501.

Chan, W.-Y., Cushing, W., Coffman, M. A. and Rennert, O. M. (1980). Genetic expression of Wilson's disease in cell culture: a diagnostic marker. *Science* **208**, 299–300.

Cox, D. W., Fraser, F. C. and Sass-Kortsak, A. (1972). A genetic study of Wilson's disease: evidence for heterogeneity. *Am. J. Hum. Genet.* **24**, 646–66.

Dastur, D. K., Manghani, D. K. and Wadia, N. H. (1968). Wilson's disease in India. I. Geographic, genetic, and clinical aspects in 16 families. *Neurology* **18**, 21–31.

Downie, A. W. (1984). Wilson's disease (letter). *Br. Med. J.* **288**, 1915.

Epstein, O. and Sherlock, S. (19981). Is Wilson's disease caused by a controller gene mutation resulting in perpetuation of the fetal mode of copper metabolism into childhood? *Lancet* **1**, 303–5.

Evans, G. W., Dubois, R. S. and Hambidge, K. M. (1973). Wilson's disease: identification of an abnormal copper-binding protein. *Science* **181**, 1175–76.

Evans, J., Newman, S. P. and Sherlock, S. (1980). Observations on copper associated protein in childhood liver disease. *Gut* **21**, 970–6.

Finby, N. and Bearn, A. G. (1958). Roentgenographic abnormalities of the skeltal system in Wilson's disease (hepatolenticular degeneration). *Am. J. Roentgenol. Radium. Ther. Nucl. Med.* **79**, 603–11.

Fitzgerald, M. A., Gross, J. B., Goldstein, N. P., Wahrer, H. W. and McCall, J. T. (1975). Wilson's disease (hepatolenticular degeneration) of late adult onset: report of a case. *Mayo Clin. Proc.* **50**, 438–42.

Fleischer, B. (1903). Zwei weitere Fälle von grunlicher Verfärbung der Kornea. *Klin. Monatsbl. Augenheilkd.* **41**, 489–91.

—— (1912). Uber einer der 'Pseudoskerlose' nahestehende bisher unbekannte Krankheit (gekennzeichnet durch Tremor, psychiche Störungen, bräunliche Pigmentierung bestimmter Gewebe, insbesondere auch der Hornhaut periphertie, Leber cirrhose). *Dtsch. Z. Nervenheilk.* **44**, 179–201.

Fryman, M., Bonne-Tamir, B., Farrer, L. A., Conneally, P. M., Magazanik, A., Ashbel, S. and Goldwitch, Z. (1985). Assignment of the gene for Wilson disease to chromosome 13: linkage to the esterase D locus. *Proc. Nat. Acad. Sci.* **82**, 1819–21.

Fukuda, K. (1965). Genetic aspects of Wilson's disease in Japan. *Tohoku J. Exp.*

Med. **85**, 115–19.

Fulop, M., Sternlieb, I. and Scheinberg, I. H. (1968). Defective urinary acidification in Wilson's disease. *Ann. Intern. Med.* **68**, 770–7.

Gibbs, K. and Walshe, J. M. (1971). Studies with radioactive copper (^{64}Cu and [67]Cu); the incorporation of radioactive copper into caeruloplasmin in Wilson's disease and in primary biliary cirrhosis. *Clin. Sci.* **41**, 189–202.

—— and —— (1979). A study of ceruloplasmin concentrations found in 75 patients with Wilson's disease, their kinships and various control groups. *Quart. J. Med.* **48**, 447–63.

—— and —— (1980). Biliary excretion of copper in Wilson's disease. *Lancet* **2**, 538.

——, Hanka, R. and Walshe, J. M. (1978). The urinary excretion of radiocopper in presymptomatic and symptomatic Wilson's disease, heterozygotes and controls: its significance in diagnosis and management. *Quart. J. Med.* **47**, 349–64.

Glazebrook, A. J. (1945). Wilson's disease. *Edinburgh Med. J.* **52**, 83–7.

Goka, T. J., Stevenson, R. E., Heffernan, P. M. and Howell, R. R. (1976). Menkes' disease a biochemical abnormality in cultured human fibroblasts. *Proc. Nat. Acad. Sci.* **73**, 604–6.

Goldfischer, S. and Sternlieb, I. (1968). Changes in the distribution of hepatic copper in relation to progression of Wilson's disease (hepatolenticular degeneration). *Am. J. Pathol.* **53**, 883–901.

Hall, H. C. (1921). La dégénérescence hépato-lenticulaire; maladie de Wilson, pseudo-sclérose. pp. 190–2. Masson, Paris.

Hodges, R. E., Kirkendall, W. M. and Gubler, C. J. (1956). Some aspects of kidney function in hepatolenticular degeneration (Wilson's disease). *J. Lab. Clin. Med.* **47**, 337–42.

Holtzman, N. A. and Gaumnitz, B. M. (1970a). Identification of an apoceruloplasmin-like substance in the plasma of copper-deficient rats. *J. Biol. Chem.* **245**, 2350–3.

—— and —— (1970b). Studies on the rate of release and turnover of ceruloplasmin and apoceruloplasmin in rat plasma. *J. Biol. Chem.* **245**, 2354–8.

——, Naughton, M. A., Iber, F. L. and Gaumnitz, B. M. (1967). Ceruloplasmin in Wilson's disease. *J. Clin. Invest.* **46**, 993–1002.

Iber, F. L., Chalmers, T. C. and Uzman, L. L. (1957). Studies of protein metabolism in hepatolenticular degeneration. *Metabolism* **6**, 388–96.

Joshua, G. E. (1973). Hepatolenticular degeneration (Wilson's disease) and rickets in children. *Indian J. Med. Res.* **61**, 1876–84.

Kayser, B. (1902). Uber einen Fall von angeborener grunlicher Verfärbung der Kornea. *Monatsbl. Augenheilkd.* **40**, 22–5.

Kehrer, F. (1930). Zur Atiologie und Nosologie der Pseudosklerose Westphal–Wilson. *Z. Neurol. Psychiatr.* **129**, 488–542.

Klee, J. G. (1979). Undiagnosed Wilson's disease as cause of unexplained miscarriage. *Lancet* **2**, 423.

Lancet (1981). Wilson's disease and copper-associated protein. *Lancet* **1**, 644–6.

Leu, M.-L. and Strickland, G. T. (1972). Renal function in heterozygotes for Wilson's disease. *Am. J. Med. Sci.* **263**, 19–24.

——, ——, Beckner, W. M., Chen, T. S. M., Wang, C. C. and Yeh, S. J. (1970a). Muscle copper, zinc, and manganese levels in Wilson's disease: studies with the use of neutron-activation analysis. *J. Lab. Clin. Med.* **76**, 432–8.

——, —— and Gutman, R. A. (1970b). Renal function in Wilson's disease: response to penicillamine therapy. *Am. J. Med. Sci.* **260**, 381–98.

Levi, A. J., Sherlock, S., Sheuer, P. J. and Cumings, J. N. (1967). Presymptomatic Wilson's disease. *Lancet* **2**, 575–9.

Litin, R. B., Randall, R. V., Goldstein, N. P., Power, M. H. and Diessner, G. R. (1959). Hypercalciuria in hepatolenticular degeneration (Wilson's disease). *Am. J. Med. Sci.* **238**, 614–20.

McCord, J. M. and Fridovich, I. (1969). Superoxide dismutase: an enzymic function for erythrocuprein (hemocuprein). *J. Biol. Chem.* **244**, 6049–55.

McIntyre, N., Clink, H. M., Levi, A. J., Cumings, J. N. and Sherlock, S. (1967). Hemolytic anemia in Wilson's disease. *New Engl. J. Med.* **276**, 439–44.

Mahoney, J. P., Sandberg, A. A., Gubler, C. J., Cartwright, G. E. and Wintrobe, M. M. (1955). Uric acid metabolism in hepatolenticular degeneration. *Proc. Soc. Exp. Biol. Med.* **88**, 427–30.

Mandelbrote, B. M., Stanier, M. W., Thompson, R. H. S. and Thurston, M. N. (1948). Studies on copper metabolism in demyelinating diseases of the central nervous system. *Brain* **71**, 212–28.

Marecek, Z. and Nevsimalova, S. (1984). Biochemical and clinical changes in Wilson's disease heterozygotes. *J. Inher. Metab. Dis.* **7**, 41–5.

Matsuda, I. (1981). Apocaeruloplasmin in Wilson's disease (letter). *Lancet* **1**, 666.

——, Pearson, T. and Holtzman, N. A. (1974). Determination of apoceruloplasmin by radioimmunoassay in nutritional copper deficiency, Menkes' kinky hair syndrome, Wilson's disease, and umbilical cord blood. *Pediatr. Res.* **8**, 821–4.

Needleman, S. B., Sahgal, V. and Boshes, B. (1970). Studies on the biochemical characterization of human ceruloplasmin. *Experientia* **26**, 495–6.

Neifakh, S. A., Vasiletz, I. M. and Shavlovsky, M. M. (1972). Molecular pathology of ceruloplasmin. *Biochem. Genet.* **6**, 231–8.

O'Reilly, S., Weber, P., Pollycove, M. and Shipley, L. (1969). Detection of the heterozygote of Wilson's disease. *J. Nucl. Med.* **10**, 143–4.

——, Strickland, G. T. Jr., Weber, P. M., Beckner, W. M. and Shipley, L. (1971a). Abnormalities of the physiology of copper in Wilson's disease. I. The whole-body turnover of copper. *Arch Neurol.* **24**, 385–90.

——, Weber, P. M., Oswald, M. and Shipley, L. (1971b). Abnormalities of the physiology of copper in Wilson's disease. III. The excretion of copper. *Arch. Neurol.* **25**, 28–32.

Osborn, S. B. and Walshe, J. M. (1961). Copper uptake by the liver: study of a Wilson's disease family. In *Wilson's disease: some current concepts*, eds. Walshe, J. M. and Cumings, J. N. pp. 141–50. Blackwell Scientific, Oxford.

—— and —— (1969). The influence of genetic and acquired liver defects on radiocopper turnover in Wilson's disease. *Lancet* **2**, 17–20.

Parkes, D. (1984). Wilson's disease (leading article). *Br. Med. J.* **288**, 1180–1.

Passwell, J., Adam, A., Garfinkel, D., Streiffler, M. and Cohen, B. E. (1977). Heterogeneity of Wilson's disease in Israel. *Israel J. Med. Sci.* **13**, 15–19.

Perman, J. A., Werlin, S. L., Grand, R. J. and Watkins, J. B. (1979). Laboratory measures of copper metabolism in the differentiation of chronic active hepatitis and Wilson's disease in children. *J. Pediatr.* **94**, 564–8.

Peterson, P. A., Evrin, P.-E. and Bergeard, I. (1969). Differentiation of glomerular tubular and normal proteinuria: determination of urinary excretion of β_2-microglobulin, albumin and total protein. *J. Clin. Invest.* **48**, 1189–98.

Porter, H. (1968). Copper proteins in brain and liver in normal subjects and in cases of Wilson's disease. *Birth Defects* **4**(2), 23–8.

Randall, R. V., Goldstein, N. P., Gross, J. B. and Rosevear, J. W. (1966). Hypercalciuria in hepatolenticular degeneration (Wilson's disease). *Am. J. Med. Sci.* **252**, 715–20.

Reynolds, E. S., Tanner, R. L. and Tyler, H. R. (1966). The renal lesion in Wilson's disease. *Am. J. Med.* **40**, 518–27.

Robinson, A., Aspin, N. and Sass-Kortsak, A. (1974). Total body retention of a single i.v. dose of ^{67}Cu. In Sass-Kortsak, A. Hepatolenticular degeneration (Kinnear Wilson's disease), in *Handbuch der inneren Medizin*, ed. Schweigk, H. Vol. 1, Pt. 1, p. 651. Springer, Berlin.

Saito, T. (1981). An assessment of efficiency in potential screening for Wilson's disease. *J. Epidemiol. Community Health* **35**, 274–80.

—— (1983). Evaluation of segregation ratio in Wilson's disease. *J. Med. Genet.* **20**, 271–5.

Sass-Kortsak, A. (1965). Copper metabolism. *Advances in Clin. Chem.* **8**, 1–67.

—— and Bearn, A. G. (1978). Hereditary disorders of copper metabolism. In *The metabolic basis of inherited disease*, 4th edn. eds. Stanbury, J. B., Wyngaarden, J. B. and Fredrickson, D. S. pp. 1099–126. McGraw-Hill, New York.

——, Glatt, B. S., Cherniak, M. and Cederlund, I. (1961). Observations on copper metabolism in homozygotes and heterozygotes of Wilson's disease. In *Wilson's disease: some current concepts*, eds. Walshe, J. M. and Cumings, J. N. pp. 151–67. Blackwell Scientific, Oxford.

Scheinberg, I. H. (1982). Penicillamine in Wilson's disease. *Lancet* **1**, 1469.

—— (1983). Investigating diseases no one's got. *New Engl. J. Med.* **309**, 918–19.

—— and Gitlin, D. (1952). Deficiency of ceruloplasmin in patients with hepato-lenticular degeneration (Wilson's disease). *Science* **116**, 484–5.

—— and Sternlieb, I. (1963). Wilson's disease and the concentration of caerulo-plasmin in serum. *Lancet* **1**, 1420–1.

—— and —— (1965). Wilson's disease. *Ann. Rev. Med.* **16**, 119–34.

—— and —— (1984). *Wilson's disease: major problems in internal medicine.* W. B. Saunders, Philadelphia.

Schonheyder, F., Gregersen, G., Hansen, H. E. and Skov, P. E. (1971). Renal clearances of different aminoacids in Wilson's disease before and after treatment with penicillamine. *Acta Med. Scand.* **190**, 395–9.

Shokeir, M. H. K. (1971). Investigations on the nature of ceruloplasmin deficiency in the new born. *Clin. Genet.* **2**, 223–7.

—— and Shreffler, D. C. (1969). Cytochrome oxidase deficiency in Wilson's disease: a suggested ceruloplasmin function. *Proc. Nat. Acad. Sci.* **62**, 867–72.

Silverberg, M. and Gellis, S. S. (1962). The liver in juvenile Wilson's disease. *Pediatrics* **30**, 402–13.

Smallwood, R. A., McIlveen, B., Rosenoer, V. M. and Sherlock, S. (1971). Copper kinetics in liver disease. *Gut* **12**, 139–44.

Sorensen, L. B. and Kappas, A. (1966). The effects of penicillamine therapy on uric acid metabolism in Wilson's disease. *Trans. Assoc. Am. Physicians* **79**, 157–64.

Stadler, H. (1939). Die Erkrankungen der Westphal–Wilson chen Pseudosklerose auf ground austomischer, klinischer und erbbiologischer Untersuchungen. *J. Neurol. Psychiatr.* **164**, 583–643.

Stein, W. H., Bearn, A. G. and Moore, S. (1954). The aminoacid content of the blood and urine in Wilson's disease. *J. Clin. Invest.* **33**, 410–19.

Sternlieb, I. and Scheinberg, I. H. (1972). Radiocopper in diagnosing liver disease. *Semin. Nucl. Med.* **2**, 176–88.

—— and —— (1968). Prevention of Wilson's disease in asymptomatic patients. *New Engl. J. Med.* **278**, 352–9.

—— and —— (1979). The role of radiocopper in the diagnosis of Wilson's disease. *Gastroenterology* **77**, 138–42.

——, Morell, A. G., Bauer, C. D., Combes, B., De Bobes-Sternberg, S. and Scheinberg, I. H. (1961). Detection of the heterozygous carrier of the Wilson's disease gene. *J. Clin. Invest.* **40**, 707–15.

——, van den Hamer, C. J. A., Morell, A. G., Alpert, S., Gregoriadis, G. and Scheinberg, I. H. (1973). Lysosomal defect of hepatic copper excretion in Wilson's disease (hepatolenticular degeneration). *Gastroenterology* **64**, 99–105.

Strickland, G. T., Beckner, W. M. and Leu, M.-L. (1972). Absorption of copper in homozygotes and heterozygotes for Wilson's disease and controls: isotope tracer studies with ^{67}Cu and ^{64}Cu. *Clin. Sci.* **43**, 617–25.

——, Frommer, D., Leu, M.-L., Pollard, R., Sherlock, S. and Cummings, J. N. (1973). Wilson's disease in the United Kingdom and Taiwan. I. General characteristics of 142 cases and prognosis. II. A genetic analysis of 88 cases. *Quart. J. Med.* **42**, 619–38.

Su, L.-C., Ravanshad, S., Owen, C. A., McCall, J. T., Zollman, P. E. and Hardy, R. M. (1982). A comparison of copper-loading disease in Bedlington terriers and Wilson's disease in humans. *Am. J. Physiol.* **243**, G226–30.

Tu, J.-B. (1963). A genetical biochemical and clinical study of Wilson's disease among Chinese in Taiwan. *Acta Paediatr. Sinica*, **4**, 81–104.

—— and Blackwell, R. Q. (1967). Studies on levels of penicillamine-induced cupriuresis in heterozygotes of Wilson's disease. *Metabolism* **16**, 507–13.

Uzman, L. L. (1953). On the relationship of urinary copper excretion to amino-aciduria in Wilson's disease (hepatolenticular degeneration). *Am. J. Med. Sci.* **226**, 645–52.

—— and Denny-Brown, D. (1948). Amino-aciduria in hepatolenticular degeneration (Wilson's disease). *Am. J. Med. Sci.* N.S. **215**, 599–611.

—— Iber, F. L., Chalmers, T. C. and Knowlton, M. (1956). The mechanism of copper deposition in the liver in hepatolenticular degeneration (Wilson's disease). *Am. J. Med. Sci.* **231**, 511–18.

Vierling, J. M., Shrager, R., Rumble, W. F., Aamodt, R., Berman, M. D. and Jones, E. A. (1978). Incorporation of radiocopper into ceruloplasmin in normal subjects and in patients with primary biliary cirrhosis and Wilson's disease. *Gastroenterology* **74**, 652–60.

Ward, I. (1962). A genetical analysis of hepato-lenticular degeneration (abs.). *Folia Biol. (Warsaw)* **10**, 321.

Walshe, J. M. (1967). The physiology of copper in man and its relation to Wilson's disease. *Brain* **90**, 149–76.

—— (1968). Effect of penicillamine on failure of renal acidification in Wilson's disease. *Lancet* **1**, 775–8.

—— (1970). Wilson's disease: its diagnosis and management. *Br. J. Hosp. Med.* **4**, 90–8.

—— (1977). Pregnancy in Wilson's disease. *Quart. J. Med.* **46**, 73–83.

—— (1984). Wilson's disease (letter). *Br. Med. J.* **288**, 1689.

—— and Briggs, J. (1962). Ceruloplasmin in liver disease: a diagnostic pitfall. *Lancet* **2**, 263–5.

—— and Carpenter, R. G. (1965). Abnormal behaviour of Wilson's disease ceruloplasmin in the presence of enzyme inhibitors (abs.). *Gastroenterology* **48**, 499.

Westphal, C. F. O. (1883). Uber eine dem Bilde der cerebrospinalen grauen Degeneration ähnliche Erkrankung des centralen Nervensystems ohne anatomischen Befund nebst einigen Bemerkungen über paradoxe Contraction. *Arch. Psychiatr.* **14**, 87–134.

Wiebers, D. O., Hollenhorst, R. W. and Goldstein, N. P. (1977). The ophthalmologic manifestation of Wilson's disease. *Mayo Clin. Proc.* **52**, 409–23.

——, Wilson, D. M., McLeod, R. A. and Goldstein, N. P. (1979). Renal stones in Wilson's disease. *Am. J. Med.* **67**, 249–54.

Willvonseder, R., Goldstein, N. P. and Tauxe, W. N. (1974). Long-term body retention of radiocopper (^{67}Cu) and the diagnosis of Wilson's disease. *Mayo Clin. Proc.* **49**, 387–93.

Wilson, D. M. and Goldstein, N. P. (1973). Renal urate excretion in patients with Wilson's disease. *Kidney Int.* **4**, 331–6.

—— and —— (1974). Evidence for a urate, reabsorptive defect in patients with Wilson's disease. *Adv. Exp. Med. Biol.* **41**, 729–37.

Wilson, S. A. K. (1912). Progressive lenticular degeneration: a familial nervous disease associated with cirrhosis of the liver. *Brain* **34**, 295–509.

Wolff, S. M. (1964). Renal lesions in Wilson's disease. *Lancet* **1**, 843–5.

4.1.6. The hereditary amyloidoses

Although amyloidosis is commonly seen as an acquired pathological response there are several inherited forms. These may be generalized or localized to particular tissues. It is only in the generalized types that renal involvement occurs, whether it be the predominant feature, nephropathic amyloidosis, or only a minor secondary feature as in the neuropathic or cardiopathic types. Indeed renal insufficiency is the most frequent cause of death among patients with generalized amyloidosis as a whole (Cohen 1967; Brandt *et al.* 1968). Renal involvement usually presents as proteinuria and this may persist for years without further symptoms (Sohar *et al.* 1967), but may progress to nephrotic syndrome. Such proteinuria is associated with glomerular amyloid deposition, especially in the mesangial area (Brandt *et al.* 1968), but vascular infiltration may also be prominent. Interstitial and tubular basement membrane infiltration may also be seen in late cases (Hepinstall and Joekes 1960) and less commonly medullary infiltration may lead to polyuria (Carone and Epstein 1960). In neuropathic amyloidosis infiltration of motor nerves to

Table 4.5. *Generalized hereditary amyloidoses*

Type according to: McKusick (1978 & 1983)	Glenner *et al.* (1978)	Urinary tract involvement	Mode of inheritance	Reference
Nephropathic:				
Amyloidosis VIII, familial visceral amyloidosis	Amyloidopathy of Ostertag	Progressive early nephropathy	AD	Weiss & Page (1973)
Familial Mediterranean fever	Familial Mediterranean fever	Proteinuria, leading late in the disease, to nephropathy	AR	Meyerhoff (1980)
(Hyperimmunoglobulin D with period fever)		Cells and casts in urine progressing to renal amyloidosis	AD	van der Meer *et al.* (1984)
Urticaria, deafness and amyloidosis	Amyloid nephropathy with deafness, urticaria and limb pains (Muckle Wells syndrome)	Nephrotic syndrome late in the disease	AD	Prost *et al.* (1976)
Cold hypersensitivity	—	Nephropathy a frequent cause of death	AD	Doeglas & Bleumink (1974)
Neuropathic:				
Amyloidosis I (Swedish type[1])	Type I, Portuguese or Andrade	Neuropathic bladder and occasional reports of nephropathy[2]	AD	Andrade *et al.* (1969)
Amyloidosis II	Type II, Indiana or Rukavina	Histological renal amyloid deposition only	AD	Rukavina *et al.* (1956)
Amyloidosis IV	Type III, Iowa or Van Allen	Nephropathy late in the disease	AD	Gimeno *et al.* (1974)

Amyloidosis V	Type IV, Finland or Meretoja	May develop nephrotic syndrome and renal failure	AD	Meretoja (1973)
Amyloidosis VII, Ohio type (Texan, late onset type with similarities to McKusick type VII)	—	Not reported	AD	Goren et al. (1980)
		Neuropathic bladder with amyloid infiltration and secondary infection leading to renal failure in one patient only	AD	Libbey et al. (1984)
Cardiopathic: Amyloidosis III	Amyloid cardiomyopathy, Denmark	Not reported	AD	Frederiksen et al. (1962)
	Amyloid cardiomyopathy with persistent atrial standstill [3]	Not reported	AD	Allensworth et al. (1969) Harrison & Derrick (1969)
Amyloidosis VI, cerebral arterial or Iceland type	—	Not reported	AD	Gudmundsson et al. (1972)
Cutaneous: Amyloidosis IX, primary cutaneous or familial lichen amyloidosis	—	Not reported	AD	Sagher & Shanon (1963)

[1] McKusick lists a Swedish type, described by Benson & Cohen (1977) under a separate catalogue number, but not as certainly distinct. It is similar to type I and may be identical to it, just as other reported families have been so accepted.
[2] Zalin et al. (1974) reported 3 brothers, with a form of neuropathic amyloidosis similar to the Andrade type, in one of whom there was also renal impairment.
[3] McKusick describes this condition under the same heading as the Denmark type.

the bladder and of the detrusor muscles may cause overflow incontinence from a neuropathic bladder and lead on to urinary infection (Andersson and Hofer 1974).

The one common feature of the amyloidoses, inherited and acquired, is the extracellular deposition of amyloid: a fibrillar protein with a β-pleated sheet secondary structure. The protein forming this amyloid deposit varies, being in some acquired forms derived from immunoglobulin light chain and in some others a serum protein of unidentified origin designated AA, or serum amyloid protein A. The origin in inherited types of amyloidosis is known for some. For example, amyloid protein AA has been identified in familial Mediterranean fever; and different variant prealbumins have been isolated from amyloid in the familial polyneuropathic amyloidoses, including the Portuguese, or type I amyloidosis, with an antigenically similar protein detected in the serum of patients (Costa and Andrade 1975; Skinner and Cohen 1981; Dwulet and Benson 1984; Wallace *et al.* 1986). It is tempting to speculate that in one or more of the nephropathic forms the deposited amyloid might be related to the amyloid P protein found in normal glomerular basement membrane.

Unfortunately different authors have adopted conflicting classifications. Gafni and colleagues (1964) divided the generalized hereditary amyloidoses into three groups: nephropathic with a perireticular distribution of amyloid deposition, and neuropathic or cardiopathic with a pericollagenous distribution. It is difficult to fit all of the more recently described types into this classification and it does not take into account the renal involvement that may be seen in the types that are not predominantly nephropathic. The currently recognized forms, as designated by Glenner (Glenner *et al.* 1978; Glenner 1980), and by McKusick (1978, 1983) are listed in Table 4.5 along with an indication of the type and extent of urinary tract involvement. With the exception of familial Mediterranean fever, which is autosomal recessive, all the disorders listed are inherited in an autosomal dominant manner. The nephropathic forms and Glenner and colleagues types I and III neuropathic forms will now be described in greater detail.

References

Allensworth, D. C., Rice, G. J. and Lowe, G. W. (1969). Persistent atrial standstill in a family with myocardial disease. *Am. J. Med.* **47**, 775–84.

Andersson, R. and Hofer, P. A. (1974). Genito urinary disturbances in familial and sporadic cases of primary amyloidosis with polyneuropathy. *Acta Med. Scand.* **195**, 49–58.

Andrade, C., Canijo, M., Klein, D. and Kaelin, A. (1969). The genetic aspect of the familial amyloidotic polyneuropathy. Portuguese type of paramyloidosis. *Humangenetik* **7**, 163–75.

Benson, M. D. and Cohen, A. S. (1977). Generalized amyloid in a family of Swedish origin: a study of 426 family members in seven generations of a new kinship with neuropathy, nephropathy, and central nervous system involvement. *Ann. Intern. Med.* **86**, 419–24.

Brandt, K., Cathcart, E. S. and Cohen, A. S. (1968). A clinical analysis of the course and prognosis of forty-two patients with amyloidosis. *Am. J. Med.* **29**, 539–44.

Carone, F. A. and Epstein, F. H. (1960). Nephrogenic diabetes insipidus caused by amyloid disease. *Am. J. Med.* **29**, 539–44.

Cohen, A. S. (1967). Amyloidosis. *New Engl. J. Med.* **277**, 522–30, 574–83, and 628–38.

Costa, P. and Andrade, C. (1975). Personal communication to Glenner *et al.* (1978). q.v.

Doeglas, H. M. G. and Bleumink, E. (1974). Familial cold urticaria: clinical findings. *Arch. Dermatol.* **110**, 382–8.

Dwulet, F. E. and Benson, M. D. (1984). Primary structure of an amyloid prealbumin and its plasma precursor in a heredo-familial polyneuropathy of Swedish origin. *Proc. Nat. Acad. Sci.* **81**, 694–8.

Frederiksen, T., Gotzsche, H., Harboe, N., Kiaer, W. and Mellemgaard, K. (1962). Familial primary amyloidosis with severe amyloid heart disease. *Am. J. Med.* **33**, 328–48.

Gafni, J., Sohar, E. and Heller, H. (1964). The inherited amyloidoses: their clinical and theoretical significance. *Lancet* **1**, 71–4.

Gimeno, A., Garcia-Alix, D., Segovia de Arana, J. M., Mateos, F. and Sotelo, M. T. (1974). Amyloidotic polyneuritis of Type VII (Iowa-Van Allen). *Eur. Neurol.* **11**, 48–57.

Glenner, G. (1980). Amyloid deposits and amyloidosis. *New Engl. J. Med.* **302**, 1282–92, 1333–43.

——, Ignaczak, T. F. and Page, D. L. (1978). The inherited systemic amyloidoses and localized amyloid deposits. Chapter 4 in *The metabolic basis of inherited disease*, 4th edn. eds. Stanbury, J. B., Wyngaarden, J. B. and Fredrickson, D. S. pp. 1308–39. McGraw-Hill, New York.

Goren, H., Steinberg, M. C. and Farboody, G. H. (1980). Familial oculoleptomeningeal amyloidosis. *Brain* **103**, 473–95.

Gudmundsson, G., Hallgrimsson, J., Jonasson, T. A. and Bjarnason, O. (1972). Hereditary cerebral haemorrhage with amyloidosis. *Brain* **95**, 387–404.

Harrison, W. H. and Derrick, J. R. (1969). Atrial standstill. A review, and presentation of two new cases of familial and unusual nature with reference to epicardial pacing in one. *Angiology* **20**, 610–17.

Heptinstall, R. H. and Joekes, A. M. (1960). Renal amyloid: a report on 11 cases proven by renal biopsy. *Ann. Rheum. Dis.* **19**, 126–34.

Libbey, C. A., Rubinow, A., Shirahama, T., Deal, C. and Cohen, A. S. (1984). Familial amyloid polyneuropathy: demonstration of prealbumin in a kinship of German/English ancestry with onset in the seventh decade. *Am. J. Med.* **76**, 18–24.

McKusick, V. A. (1978). *Mendelian inheritance in man*, 5th edn. Johns Hopkins University Press, Baltimore and London.

—— (1983). *Mendelian inheritance in man*, 6th edn. Johns Hopkins University Press, Baltimore and London.

Van der Meer, J. W. M., Vossen, J. M., Radl, J., van Nieuwkoop, J. A., Meyer, C. J.

L. M., Lobatto, S. and van Furth, R. (1984). Hyperimmunoglobulinaemia D and periodic fever: a new syndrome. *Lancet* **1**, 1087–90.

Meretoja, J. (1973). Genetic aspects of familial amyloidosis with corneal lattice dystrophy and cranial neuropathy. *Clin. Genet.* **4**, 173–85.

Meyerhoff, J. (1980). Familial Mediterranean fever: report of a large family, review of the literature and discussion of the frequency of amyloidosis. *Medicine* **59**, 66–77.

Prost, A., Barriere, H., Legent, F., Cottin, S. and Wally, B. (1976). Rhumatisme intermittent revelaateur d'un syndrome familial arthritis, eruption urticarienne, surdite: syndrome de Muckle et Wells sans amylose renale. *Rev. Rheum.* **43**, 201–8.

Rukavina, J. G., Block, W. D., Jackson, C. E., Falls, H. F., Carey, J. H. and Curtis, A. C. (1956). Primary systemic amyloidosis: a review and an experimental genetic and clinical study of 29 cases with particular emphasis on the familial form. *Medicine* **35**, 239–334.

Sagher, F. and Shanon, J. (1963). Amyloidosis cutis: familial occurrence in three generations. *Arch. Dermatol.* **87**, 171–5.

Sohar, E., Gafni, J., Pras, M. and Heller, H. (1967). Familial Mediterranean fever. A survey of 470 cases and review of the literature. *Am. J. Med.* **43**, 227–53.

Skinner, M. and Cohen, A. S. (1981). The prealbumin nature of the amyloid protein in familial amyloid polyneuropathy (FAP)—Swedish variety. *Biochem. Biophys. Res. Commun.* **99**, 1326–32.

Wallace, M. R., Dwulet, F. E., Conneally, P. M. and Benson, M. D. (1986). Biochemical and molecular genetic characterization of a new variant pre-albumin associated with hereditary amyloidosis. *J. Clin. Invest.* **78**, 6–12.

Weiss, S. W. and Page, D. L. (1973). Amyloid nephropathy of Ostertag with special reference to renal glomerular giant cells. *Am. J. Pathol.* **72**, 447–60.

Zalin, A., Darby, A., Vaughan, S. and Raftery, E. B. (1974). Primary neuropathic amyloidosis in three brothers. *Br. Med. J.* **1**, 65–6.

Nephropathic hereditary amyloidoses

Amyloid nephropathy of Ostertag (familial visceral amyloidosis) This disease was described by Ostertag in 1932 and 1950 in three generations of a single family. Further families have been reported by Weiss and Page (1973, 1974), by Maxwell and Kimbell (1936) with a follow-up by McKusick (1978), and by Alexander and Atkins (1975). The clinical picture in these families was of a nephrotic syndrome progressing to hypertension and renal failure, and after a course of about a decade to death in the fourth to early sixth decade. Pathologically amyloid deposits were found in the kidneys, adrenals, and liver. The renal amyloid had infiltrated glomeruli, around tubules, in the interstitial tissue of the medulla, and within vessel walls.

In all of these families at least three generations must be presumed to have been affected with an autosomal dominant pattern of transmission. The basic defect is unknown and the gene responsible has not been assigned to any one chromosome.

References

Alexander, F. and Atkins, E. L. (1975). Familial renal amyloidosis. Case reports, literature review and classification. *Am. J. Med.* **59**, 121–8.

McKusick, V. A. (1978). *Mendelian inheritance in man*, 5th edn. pp. 23–5, 73, 257–8, and 383. Johns Hopkins University Press, Baltimore.

Maxwell, E. S. and Kimbell, I. (1936). Familial amyloidosis with case reports. *Med. Bull. Vet. Admin.* **12**, 365–9.

Ostertag, B. (1932). Demonstration einer, eigenartigen familiaeren Paramyloidose. *Zentbl. Path.* **56**, 253–4.

—— (1950). Familiaere Amyloid-erkrankung. *Z. Menschl. Vererb. Konstitutionsl.* **30**, 105–15.

Weiss, S. W. and Page, D. L. (1973). Amyloid nephropathy of Ostertag with special reference to renal glomerular giant cells. *Am. J. Pathol.* **72**, 447–60.

—— and Page, D. L. (1974). Amyloid nephropathy of Ostertag: report of a kindred. In *Clinical delineation of birth defects. XVI. Urinary system and others*, ed. Bergsma, D. *Birth Defects Orig. Art. Series* **10**(4), 67–8.

Familial Mediterranean fever   The first description of this disease is usually credited to Siegal (1945) who further reviewed 50 American cases, mainly in Ashkenazic Jews (1964). However, an earlier report by Janeway and Mosenthal (1908) was probably of the same disorder. Further case surveys have come from Lebanon, in Armenians (Reimann *et al.* 1954; Armenian and Kachadurian 1973) among whom amyloidosis is rare; from Israel among Armenians and Jews, predominantly Sephardic (Heller *et al.* 1958; Sohar *et al.* 1967); from Lebanon among Arabs (Barakat *et al.* 1986); and from California among Armenians (Schwabe *et al.* 1977). Meyerhoff (1980) analysed 1327 cases and found that half were Sephardic Jews, 22 per cent were Armenians, 11 per cent were Arabs, 7 per cent were Turkish, and 5 per cent were Ashkenazi Jews.

The typical clinical presentation is with acute feverish attacks lasting 1–2 days. Onset may be as early as the first year and in the great majority of patients is under 20 years (Siegal 1964; Sohar *et al.* 1967). The attacks are frequently associated with pain, which may be abdominal due to peritonitis (Heller *et al.* 1961), pleuritic (Siegal 1964), or synovial (Sohar *et al.* 1967), or may be accompanied by an erysipelas-like erythema. The earlier the age of clinical onset the more that physical signs of disease tend to be present (Cattan *et al.* 1984).

In a proportion of cases, especially among Jewish patients, generalized amyloidosis with prominent renal involvement is a serious complication. As early as 1952 Mamou and Cattan recognized nephropathy as a complication and later Mamou (1955) demonstrated that this was due to amyloidosis. Sohar's group in particular have studied amyloid disease describing its perireticular distribution and a progression from a pre-clinical stage, through proteinuria and nephrosis to death from renal failure, over a period of 3 to 13 years from the onset of proteinuria (Heller *et al.* 1961; Sohar *et al.* 1967). Levin and coworkers (1972) have sequenced the amino acids of the major fibrillar protein from amyloid of a patient with familial Mediterranean fever and shown it to be identical to the amyloid A protein of patients with acquired secondary amyloidosis. Elevated levels of this protein in serum of these patients has also been reported (Rosenthal and Franklin 1975). Knecht and colleagues (1985) found serum amyloid A protein to be elevated in patients with familial Mediterranean fever compared with controls, and to be higher in those with nephropathy than without, and also higher at the onset of an acute attack than between attacks. Derosena and colleagues (1975) and Neale (1976) have reported the finding of amyloid fibrils in urinary sediment of patients with renal amyloidosis by electron microscopy. Nimoityn and associates (1976) used this method, in preference to renal biopsy, to diagnose renal amyloidosis in a patient with familial Mediterranean fever. The likely role of a circulating protein in the formation of renal amyloidosis is reinforced by the observation of amyloid deposition in transplanted kidneys (Benson *et al.* 1977; Jones *et al.* 1977), and the effective treatment of acute attacks by haemodialysis (Rubinger *et al.* 1979).

Familial Mediterranean fever typically shows autosomal recessive inheritance as exemplified by the Israeli patients of Sohar and his colleagues (Sohar *et al.* 1961; Heller *et al.* 1964; Sohar *et al.* 1967). They analysed 229 family pedigrees and estimated a gene frequency in Sephardic Jews of 0.22. Kachadurian and Armenian (1974) likewise found recessive inheritance in Lebanon and this has also been the pattern in American cases. There have been a number of reports of families with affected members in more than one generation. Reimann *et al.* (1954) described 20 affected members of a family over five generations but this may possibly be accounted for by inbreeding. However in several other reports, involving three or more generations, there has been no evidence of consanguinity (Bouroncle and Doan 1957; Sohar *et al.* 1961; Bergman and Warmenius 1968; Reich and Franklin 1970). In view of these reports it cannot be excluded that in a minority of families inheritance may be autosomal dominant. Even among recessive families the consistent rarity of amyloidosis in Armenian cases, whether in the Middle East or in the USA, suggests the possibility of further genetic heterogeneity. Genetic analysis has been hampered by the fact that up to the present there has been no specific test for the diagnosis of the disorder, which has had to be purely clinical. If the observation of Barakat and colleagues (1984a and b), that metaraminol infusion provokes a mild catecholamine-induced attack of pain, is confirmed then this situation will be remedied. However, it is not yet clear whether this test gives a positive result in young presymptomatic patients.

Despite the occurrence of sacro-iliitis in younger patients (Brodey and Wolff 1975) no association with the HLA-B27 phenotype has been observed (Lehman *et al.* 1978).

Since the basic defect remains unknown it is not surprising that prenatal diagnosis and carrier detection have not been reported.

Hyperimmunoglobulinaemia D with periodic fever This is a newly recognized disorder reported in Dutch patients. It resembles familial Mediterranean fever in presenting with periodic fever, though not fixed periodicity. Abdominal pain does occur but is less marked than with familial Mediterranean fever. There is a high level of serum IgD and large numbers of plasma cells with cytoplasmic IgD in the bone marrow (van der Meer *et al.* 1984). Three of the six patients reported by van der Meer and colleagues had a positive family history, two of the reported patients being brother and sister and another patient having an affected mother and two affected maternal uncles. Whilst these familial occurrences suggest autosomal dominant inheritance definition of the mode of inheritance must await full family studies.

One of these patients had a history of red and white cells and red-cell casts in the urine, but further urological investigation was not reported. The only evidence of amyloidosis in this disorder is the report that one of the affected uncles of the patient whose mother was affected had had a renal transplant for renal amyloidosis.

The authors found a raised serum IgD in only one of eight patients they investigated with classic familial Mediterranean fever.

References

Armenian, H. K. and Kachadurian, A. K. (1973). Familial paroxyomal poly-serositis: clinical and laboratory findings in 120 cases. *Leban. Med. J.* **26**, 605–14.

Barakat, M. H., EL-Khawad, A. O., Gumaa, K. A., EL-Sobki, N. I. and Fenech, F. F. (1984a). Metaraminol provocative test: a specific diagnostic test for familial Mediterranean fever. *Lancet* **1**, 656–7.

——, EL-Sobki, N. I., EL-Khawad, A. O., Gumma, K. A. and Fenech, F. F. (1984b). Diagnosing familial Mediterranean fever. *Lancet* **2**, 41–2.

——, Karnik, A. M., Majeed, H. W. A., EL-Sobki, N. I. and Fenech, F. F. (1986). Familial Mediterranean fever (recurrent hereditary polyserositis) in Arabs—a study of 175 patients and review of the literature. *Quart. J. Med.* **60**, 837–47.

Benson, M. D., Skinner, M. and Cohen, A. S. (1977). Amyloid deposition in a renal transplant in familial Mediterranean fever. *Ann. Intern. Med.* **87**, 31–4.

Bergman, F. and Warmenius, S. (1968). Familial perireticulin amyloidosis in a

Swedish family. *Am. J. Med.* **45**, 601–6.

Bouroncle, B. A. and Doan, C. A. (1957). 'Periodic fever': occurrence in five generations. *Am. J. Med.* **23**, 502–6.

Brodey, P. A. and Wolff, S. M. (1975). Radiographic changes in the sacrocliac joints in familial Mediterranean fever. *Radiology* **114**, 331–3.

Cattan, D., Dervichian, M., Courillon, A. and Nurit, Y. (1984). Metaraminol provocation test for familial Mediterranean fever. *Lancet* **1**, 1130–1.

Derosena, R., Koss, M. N. and Pirani, C. L. (1975). Demonstration of amyloid fibrils in urinary sediments. *New Engl. J. Med.* **293**, 1131–3.

Heller, H., Sohar, E. and Sherf, L. (1958). Familial Mediterranean fever. *Arch. Intern. Med.* **102**, 50–71.

——, ——, Gafni, J. and Heller, J. (1961). Amyloidosis in familial Mediterranean fever. *Arch. Intern. Med.* **107**, 539–50.

——, —— and —— (1964). Classification of amyloidosis with special regard to the genetic types. *Pathol. Microbiol.* **27**, 833–40.

Janeway, T. C. and Mosenthal, H. O. (1908). An unusual paroxysmal syndrome, probably allied to recurrent vomiting, with a study of the nitrogen of metabolism. *Trans. Assoc. Am. Physicians* **23**, 504–18.

Jones, M. B., Adams, J. M. and Passer, J. A. (1977). Amyloidosis in a renal allograft in familial Mediterranean fever. *Ann. Intern. Med.* **87**, 579–80.

Kachadurian, A. K. and Armenian, H. K. (1974). Familial paroxysmal polyserositis (familial Mediterranean fever): incidence of amyloidosis and mode of inheritance. *Birth Defects Orig. Art. Series* **10**(6), 62–6.

Knecht, A., de Beer, F. C. and Pras, M. (1985). Serum amyloid A protein in familial Mediterranean fever. *Ann. Intern. Med.* **102**, 71–2.

Lehman, T. J. A., Hanson, V., Kornreich, H., Peters, R. S. and Schwabe, A. D. (1978). HLA-B27 negative sacroiliitis: a manifestation of familial Mediterranean fever in childhood. *Pediatrics* **61**, 423–6.

Levin, M., Franklin, E. C., Frangione, B. and Pras, M. (1972). The amino acid sequence of a major nonimmunoglobulin component of some amyloid fibrils. *J. Clin. Invest.* **51**, 2773–6.

Mamou, H. (1955). Maladie périodique amylogene. *Sem. Hôp. Paris.* **31**, 388–91.

—— and Cattan, R. (1952). La maladie périodique (sur 14 cas personnels dont 8 compliqués de néphropathies). *Sem. Hôp. Paris.* **28**, 1062–6.

van der Meer, J. W. M., Vossen, J. M., Radl, J., van Nieuwkoop, J. A., Meyer, C. J. L. M., Lobatto, S. and van Furth, R. (1984). Hyperimmunoglobulinaemia D and periodic fever: a new syndrome. *Lancet* **1**, 1087–90.

Meyerhoff, J. (1980). Familial Mediterranean fever: report of a large family, review of the literature, and discussion of the frequency of amyloidosis. *Medicine* **59**, 66–77.

Neale, T. J. (1976). Amyloid fibrils in urinary sediment. *New Engl. J. Med.* **294**, 444–5.

Nimoityn, P., Lasker, N. and Soriano, R. Z. (1976). Detection of urinary amyloid in familial Mediterranean fever. *Br. Med. J.* **2**, 284.

Reich, C. B. and Franklin, E. C. (1970). Familial Mediterranean fever in an Italian family. *Arch. Intern. Med.* **125**, 337–40.

Reimann, H. A., Moadié, J., Semerdjian, S. and Sahyoun, P. F. (1954). Periodic peritonitis—hereditary and pathology. Report of seventy-two cases. *JAMA* **154**, 1254–9.

Rosenthal, C. J. and Franklin, E. C. (1975). Variation with age and disease of an amyloid A protein-related serum component. *J. Clin. Invest.* **55**, 746–53.

Rubinger, D., Friedlander, M. M. and Popovtzer, M. M. (1979). Amelioration of familial Mediterranean fever during haemodialysis. *New Engl. J. Med.* **301**, 142–4.

Schwabe, A. D., Terasaki, P. I., Barnett, E. V., Territo, M. C., Klinenberg, J. R. and Peters, R. S. (1977). Familial Mediterranean fever—recent advances in pathogenesis and management. *West. J. Med.* **127**, 15–23.

Siegal, S. (1945). Benign paroxysmal peritonitis. *Ann. Intern. Med.* **23**, 1–21.

—— (1964). Familial paroxysmal polyserositis: analysis of fifty cases. *Am. J. Med.* **36**, 893–918.

Sohar, E., Pras, M., Heller, J. and Heller, H. (1961). Genetics of familial Mediterranean fever (FMF). *Arch. Intern. Med.* **107**, 529–38.

——, Gafni, J., Pras, M. and Heller, H. (1967). Familial Mediterranean fever. A survey of 470 cases and review of the literature. *Am. J. Med.* **43**, 227–53.

Amyloid nephropathy with urticaria and deafness (Muckle–Wells syndrome), and cold urticaria A syndrome of progressive nerve deafness, urticaria and nephropathy due to amyloidosis was first described in five generations of a family by Muckle and Wells in 1962. Inheritance followed an autosomal dominant pattern. Autopsy on two affected members of the family demonstrated the amyloidosis and also atrophy of the cochlear nerve and absence of the organ of Corti. Onset of deafness is typically in childhood, with attacks of urticaria associated with fever, malaise, and limb pains supervening in adolescence and signs of nephrotic syndrome in middle age leading to uraemic death. However, there was considerable clinical variation within this family.

Further families (Black 1969; Lagrue *et al.* 1972) and sporadic cases (Kennedy *et al.* 1966; Anderson *et al.* 1967) have been reported, and Prost and colleagues (1976) have reported a family with a similar syndrome except that they did not observe renal amyloidosis.

This syndrome is presumably distinct from cold urticaria, or cold hypersensitivity, without deafness described by McKusick and Goodman (1962), being accompanied by renal amyloidosis. The renal pathology in this latter syndrome, which also shows autosomal dominant inheritance, has been described in detail by Shephard (1971). Further studies have been reported by Derbes and Coleman (1972), and by Doeglas and colleagues in a large family in which they were unable to detect any linkage to genetic markers (Doeglas 1973; Doeglas and Bleumink 1974; Doeglas *et al.* 1974), and others.

References

Andersen, V., Buch, N. H., Jensen, M. K. and Killman, S.-A. (1967). Deafness, urticaria and amyloidosis. *Am. J. Med.* **42**, 449–56.

Black, J. T. (1969). Amyloidosis, deafness, urticaria and limb pains: a hereditary syndrome. *Ann. Intern. Med.* **70**, 989–94.

Derbes, V. J. and Coleman, W. P. (1972). Familial cold urticaria. *Ann. Allergy* **30**, 335–41.

Doeglas, H. M. G. (1973). Familial cold urticaria (letter). *Arch. Derm.* **107**, 136–7.

—— and Bleumink, E. (1974). Familial cold urticaria: clinical findings. *Arch. Derm.* **110**, 382–8.

——, Bernini, L. F., Fraser, G. R., van Loghem, E., Meera Khan, P., Nyenhuis, L. E. and Pearson, P. L. (1974). A kindred with familial cold urticaria: linkage analysis. *J. Med. Genet.* **11**, 31–4.

Kennedy, D. D., Rosenthal, F. D. and Sneddon, I. B. (1966). Amyloidosis presenting as cold urticaria. *Br. Med. J.* **1**, 31–2.

Lagrue, G., Vernant, J. P., Revuz, J., Touraine, R. and Weil, B. (1972). Syndrome de Muckle et Wells. Cinquieme observation familiale. *Nouv. Presse Med.* **1**, 2223–6.

McKusick, V. A. and Goodman, R. M. (1962). Pinnal calcification. Observations in systemic diseases not associated with disordered calcium metabolism. *JAMA* **179**, 230–2.

Muckle, T. J. and Wells, M. (1962). Urticaria, deafness and amyloidosis: a new heredo-familial syndrome. *Quart. J. Med.* **31**, 235–48.

Prost, A., Barriere, H., Legent, F., Cottin, S. and Wally, B. (1976). Rhumatisme intermittent revalaateur d'un syndrome familial arthritis, eruption urticarienne, surdité syndrome de Muckle et Wells sons amylose renale. *Rev. Rheum.* **43**, 201–8.

Shephard, M. (1971). Cold hypersensitivity. *Birth Defects* **5**(pt.12), 352.

Neuropathic hereditary amyloidoses

Hereditary amyloidosis I (Portuguese or Andrade type)   Andrade (1952) described a peripheral neuropathy endemic to northern coastal regions of Portugal, affecting primarily the legs. It is known locally as 'foot disease', starts at between 20 and 30 years of age and runs a course of 7–10 years. A similar neuropathy occurs among Portuguese immigrants in Brazil (Mello 1959) and elsewhere and also among non-Portuguese subjects in Japan (Araki *et al.* 1968; Kito *et al.* 1973), Sweden (Andersson 1970; Andersson and Hofer 1974a), and many other countries. Inheritance is autosomal dominant (Klein 1963; Andrade *et al.* 1969). The amyloid deposition is pericollagenous and is seen in blood vessels of all tissues, in nerves, and as vitreous opacities (Kaufman and Thomas 1959; Silva Horta *et al.* 1964). On electron microscopy the lesion in peripheral nerves involves Schwann cells with myelin degeneration, with amyloid deposition apparently secondary to the consequent axonomic degeneration (Coimbra and Andrade 1971).

Renal amyloid deposition limited to the interstitial tissue of the papillae is common, but glomerular involvement is rare (Silva Horta *et al.* 1964). Symptoms of nephropathy, especially proteinuria, have occasionally been reported but not as the cause of death. However, urinary incontinence from a neuropathic bladder may develop in the later stages of the disease (Andersson and Hofer 1974b). Glenner and associates (1978) quote work of Costa and Andrade (1975) on the isolation of a protein from amyloid fibrils which is distinct from that of amyloid of immunogenic origin and from the AA protein. The neuropathic amyloidosis described by Benson and Cohen (1977) in a Swedish family, which may or may not be identical to Andrade's type, certainly did involve nephropathy in affected members of the family.

The English family described by Zalin and associates (1974), although regarded by them as more like the Andrade type than any other, differed from the Andrade type in age of onset and in the pattern of familial occurrence. In Zalin's family three brothers were affected, one with renal impairment, three sisters were unaffected, and the apparently unaffected parents had died at 84 and 78 years. This would appear to be a genetically distinct form.

Two groups of workers have cloned human pre-albumin cDNA and have used detection of a variant in the diagnosis of familial amyloid polyneuropathy (Whitehead *et al.* 1984; Mita *et al.* 1986). The former group assigned the gene to chromosome 18.

References

Andersson, R. (1970). Hereditary amyloidosis with polyneuropathy. *Acta Med. Scand.* **188**, 85–94.

—— and Hofer, P. A. (1974a). Primary amyloidosis with polyneuropathy: some aspects on the histopathological diagnosis antemortem based on studies of biopsy specimens from 30 familial and non-familial cases. *Acta Med. Scand.* **196**, 115–20.

—— and —— (1974b). Genitourinary disturbances in familial and sporadic cases of primary amyloidosis with polyneuropathy. *Acta Med. Scand.* **195**, 49–58.

Andrade, C. (1952). A peculiar form of peripheral neuropathy: familial atypical generalised amyloidosis with special involvement of peripheral nerves. *Brain* **75**, 408–27.

——, Canijo, M., Klein, D. and Kaelin, A. (1969). The genetic aspect of the familial amyloidotic polyneuropathy. Portuguese type of paramyloidosis. *Humangenetik* **7**, 163–175.

Araki, S., Mawatari, S., Ohta, M., Nakajima, A. and Kuroiwa, Y. (1968). Polyneuritic amyloidosis in a Japanese family. *Arch. Neurol.* **18**, 593–602.

Benson, M. D. and Cohen, A. S. (1977). Generalized amyloid in a family of Swedish origin: a study of 426 family members in seven generations of a new kinship with neuropathy, nephropathy, and central nervous system involvement. *Ann. Intern. Med.* **86**, 419–24.

Coimbra, A. and Andrade, C. (1971). Familial amyloid polyneuropathy: an electron microscope study of the peripheral nerve in five cases. I. Interstitial changes. II. Nerve fibre changes. *Brain* **94**, 199–206 and 207–12.

Costa, P. and Andrade, C. (1975). Personal communication to Glenner *et al.* (1978) q.v.

Glenner, G. G., Ignaczak, T. F. and Page, D. L. (1978). The inherited systemic amyloidoses and localized amyloid deposits. Chapter 4 in *The metabolic basis of inherited disease*, 4th edn. eds. Stanbury, J. B., Wyngaarden, J. B. and Frederickson, D. S. pp. 1308–39. McGraw-Hill, New York.

Kaufman, H. E. and Thomas, L. B. (1959). Vitreous opacities diagnostic of familial primary amyloidosis. *New Engl. J. Med.* **261**, 1267–71.

Kito, S., Fujimori, N., Yamamoto, M., Itoga, E. and Toyoizum, Y. (1973). A new focus of familial amyloid neuropathy. *Nippon Rinsho* **31**, 170–82.

Klein, D. (1963). La polyneuropathie amyloide héréditaire. *Acta Neuropathol.* Suppl. **2**, 49–53.

Mello, A. R. (1959). Polineuropatia amyloidotica familial. *J. Bras. Med.* **1**, 161–218.

Mita, S., Maeda, S., Ide, M., Tsuzuki, T., Shimada, K. and Araki, S. (1986). Familial amyloidotic polyneuropathy diagnosed by cloned human prealbumin cDNA. *Neurology* **36**, 298–301.

Silva Horta, J. da., Filipe, I. and Duarte, S. (1964). Portuguese polyneuritic familial type of amyloidosis. *Pathol. Microbiol (Basel)* **27**, 809–25.

Whitehead, A. S., Skinner, M., Bruns, G. A. P., Costello, W., Edge, M. D., Cohen, A. S. and Sipe, J. D. (1984). Cloning of human prealbumin complementary DNA. Localization of the gene to chromosome 18 and detection of a variant prealbumin allele in a family with familial amyloid polyneuropathy. *Mol. Biol. Med.* **2**, 411–23.

Zalin, A., Darby, A., Vaughan, S. and Raftery, E. B. (1974). Primary neuropathic amyloidosis in three brothers. *Br. Med. J.* **1**, 65–6.

Hereditary amyloidosis III (Iowa or Van Allen type, McKusick type IV) Van Allen and coworkers (1968) reported a single family from Iowa, in which eight members from two generations were affected. This family included father to son transmission, with neuropathy early in the disease but nephropathy supervening later on. The average age of onset was about 35 years and survival about 12 years, with death from renal amyloidosis. Several affected individuals also had cataracts, some had peptic ulceration, and others hearing loss. The renal amyloid deposition may predominantly involve the renal arteries leading to small shrunken kidneys, but more extensive glomerular infiltration was seen in some cases.

The family reported by Gimeno and colleagues (1974) could be another example of this type. Inheritance in Van Allen's family was clearly autosomal dominant, and probably so in Gimeno's.

References

Gimeno, A., Garcia-Alix, D., Segovia de Arana, J. M., Mateos, F. and Sotelo, M. T. (1974). Amyloidotic polyneuritis of Type VII (Iowa-Van Allen). *Eur. Neurol.* **11**, 48–57.

Van Allen, M. W., Frohlich, J. A. and Davis, J. R. (1968). Inherited predisposition to generalized amyloidosis: clinical and pathological studies of a family with neuropathy, nephropathy and peptic ulcer. *Neurology* **19**, 10–25.

4.1.7. Glutamyl ribose 5-phosphate storage disease

This disease was recently described by Williams and colleagues (1984) from Houston, Texas, in a 6-year-old boy. The disorder belongs to the group of lysosomal storage diseases in which there is a defect in the degradation of the carbohydrate moiety of glycoproteins. This group includes mannosidosis, fucosidosis, sialidosis, and aspartylglyco-saminuria and has recently been reviewed by Beaudet (1983).

The propositus was the first child of unrelated parents of European origin, and was normal at birth and for his first 2 years of life. Subsequently his speech deteriorated and he developed *grand mal* epilepsy. When seen by the authors, at nearly 6 years of age he was microcephalic with developmental delay, course facies, optic atrophy, generalized hypotonia, muscle wasting, and frequent seizures. Both the electroencephalogram and the electroretinogram were abnormal. He had proteinuria, and a renal biopsy showed focal segmental and global glomerulosclerosis with negative immunofluorescence.

Within less than a year he had deteriorated further with only single word speech, increased hypotonia and decreased tendon reflexes, nystagmus, and severe optic atrophy. The degree of proteinuria had almost doubled, there was a generalized aminoaciduria, and creatinine clearance was impaired. His deterioration continued with death at the age of 8 years.

Earlier investigations had excluded mucopolysaccharidosis, known gangliosidoses, and organic acidurias. A range of lysosomal enzymes had all given normal results. Electron microscopy of a conjuctival biopsy revealed lysosomes containing granular and multilamellar material. Sequential renal biopsies had shown progressive glomerulosclerosis, interstitial fibrosis, tubular atrophy, and eventually occasional foamy glomerular epithelial cells. The autopsy findings were characteristic of end-stage renal disease, and showed diffuse cortical atrophy of the brain with prominent ventricles and neuronal loss.

Biochemically β-mannosidose, sialidase, and aspartylglycosaminidase activities, in addition to those of the more commonly assayed lysosomal enzymes, were all normal. Thin-layer chromatography of brain ganglio-sides was normal, but chromatography of acetic acid extracts of kidney and brain demonstrated an abnormal carbohydrate-containing peak, which was shown to be due to glutamyl ribose 5-phosphate. This glyco-peptide is known to be involved in post-translational adenosine diphosphate (ADP)-ribosylation of histones and other proteins, which in turn is implicated in the regulation of gene expression and DNA repair. The authors propose that the accumulation of glutamyl ribose 5-phosphate is due to deficiency of an ADP-ribose protein hydrolase.

In addition to the propositus there was a history of a maternal uncle who developed seizures at 9 months of age, and developed deterioration of speech and vision with optic atrophy and severe retardation, followed by nephrotic syndrome and death from renal failure. The authors reasonably suggest that this new disease is inherited in an X-linked recessive manner.

References

Beaudet, A. L. (1983). Disorders of glycoprotein degradation: mannosidosis, fucosidosis, sialidosis, and aspartylglycosaminuria. In *The metabolic basis of inherited disease*, 5th edn. eds. Stanbury, J. B., Wyngaarden, J. B., Frederickson, D. S., Goldstein, J. C. and Brown, M. S. pp. 788–802. McGraw-Hill, New York.
Williams, J. C., Butler, I. J., Rosenberg, H. S., Verani, R., Scott, C. I. and Conley, S. B. (1984). Progressive neurological deterioration and renal failure due to storage of glutamyl ribose 5-phosphate. *New Engl. J. Med.* **311**, 152–5.

4.1.8. Hurler's disease (mucopolysaccharidosis type I H)

Symptomatic renal disease in this autosomally recessively inherited disorder is rare. Nephrotic syndrome has been recorded in at least three patients (Schimke *et al.* 1974; Taylor *et al.* 1986), associated with hypertension in the two patients reported by Taylor and associates.

Renal histopathological changes in Hurler's disease were first described by Kressler and Aegerter (1938) who reported finding storage material and vacuoles in renal cells at autopsy. A decade later Lindsay and colleagues (1948) described the autopsy findings in the kidneys in eight out of the 12 cases reviewed by them. In five out of these eight cases renal abnormalities were detected, including non-specific glomerular proliferative and interstitial changes, and the characteristic distension of glomerular and tubular cells with granular material and vacuoles. These last abnormalities were noted in four of the cases. Taylor and associates (1986) studied the kidneys from their two nephrotic cases confirming swelling and vacuolation of glomerular epithelial cells and of tubules. They also demonstrated acid mucopolysaccharides in cytoplasm of podocytes, and on electron microscopy found that the podocyte vacuoles were filled with a fine granular material.

Thus there is clearly deposition of mucopolysaccharide material within vacuoles, presumably lysosomes as in other tissues, in renal epithelial cells, and it would appear that this may exceptionally lead to nephrotic syndrome.

References

Kressler, R. J. and Aegerter, E. E. (1938). Hurler's syndrome (Gargoylism). A summary of the literature and a report of a case with autopsy findings. *J. Pediatr.* **12**, 579.

Lindsay, S., Reilly, W. A., Gotham, T. J. and Skahen, R. (1948). Gargoylism. II. Study of pathologic lesions and clinical review of twelve cases. *Am. J. Dis. Child.* **76**, 239–306.

Schimke, R. N., Horton, W. A., King, C. R. and Martin, N. L. (1974). Chondroitin-6-sulfate mucopolysaccharidosis in conjunction with lymphopenia, defective cellular immunity and the nephrotic syndrome. *Birth Defects* **10**(12), 258–66.

Taylor, J., Thorner, P., Geary, D. F., Baumal, R. and Balfe, J. W. (1986). Nephrotic syndrome and hypertension in two children with Hurler's syndrome. *J. Pediatr.* **108**, 726–9.

4.2. DISEASES WITH SECONDARY RENAL DAMAGE

4.2.1. Due to exercise-induced myoglobinuria

Myoglobinuria following severe muscular exertion has been recognized for over a century (Fleischer 1881). This phenomenon is also associated with traumatic injury or metabolic disease of muscle and has been termed *rhabdomyolysis*. The causes and pathogenesis of rhabdomyolysis, the consequent myoglobinuria, and the ensuing acute renal failure have been fully reviewed by Knockel (1981, 1982). It has been shown that the plasma concentration of myoglobin must exceed 1.5 mg/100 ml before myoglobinuria will occur, the myoglobin probably being reabsorbed in the proximal tubule at lower concentrations. Myoglobin is bound to plasma proteins but saturation does not occur until a plasma concentration of 23 mg/100 ml is reached, above which myoglobin is excreted quantitatively (Kagen 1971). Knockel (1981, 1982) discusses three possible mechanisms of acute renal failure in patients with myoglobinuria. These are: tubular obstruction due to myoglobin precipitation, decreased renal blood flow and glomerular filtration rate leading to renal ischaemia, and direct toxic injury to the renal tubular epithelium from myoglobin or other metabolites released in rhabdomyolysis. The relative importance of these factors is uncertain but the evidence seems to favour myoglobin nephrotoxicity, especially in the presence of an acid urine, as a major contributor. Under acid conditions myoglobin dissociates into globin and ferrihaemate, which has been implicated in nephrotoxicity (Braun *et al.* 1970).

The inherited disorders in which myoglobinuria is a known complication are listed in Table 4.2 and include several glycogen storage diseases, which will now be discussed in turn. Myoglobinuria is also listed by Knockel (1982) as occuring in glucose phosphate isomerase deficiency, an autosomal recessive haemolytic anaemia; and in malignant hyperpyrexia, an autosomal dominant myopathy that is usually symptomless except under certain forms of anaesthesia. These two disorders will not be discussed further, except to mention that acute renal failure has been described in one of three patients with rhabdomyolysis due to factors other than anaesthesia found to have malignant hyperpyrexia (Denborough *et al.* 1984).

References

Braun, S. R., Weiss, F. R., Keller, A. I., Ciccone, J. R. and Preuss, H. G. (1970). Evaluation of renal toxicity of heme proteins and their derivatives: a role in the genesis of acute tubule necrosis. *J. Exp. Med.* **131**, 443–60.

Denborough, M. A., Collins, S. P. and Hopkinson, K. C. (1984). Rhabdomyolysis and malignant hyperpyrexia. *Br. Med. J.* **288**, 1878.

Fleischer, R. (1881). Ueber eine neue Form von Haemoglibinurie beim Menschen. *Berl. Klin. Wschr.* **18**, 691.

Kagen, L. J. (1971). Myoglobinemia and myoglobinuria in patients with myositis. *Arthritis Rheum.* **14**, 457–64.

Knockel, J. P. (1981). Rhabdomyolysis and myoglobinuria. In *The kidney in systemic disease,* 2nd edn. eds. Suki, W. N. and Eknoyan, G. pp. 263–84. John Wiley, New York.

—— (1982). Rhabdomyolysis and myoglobinuria. *Ann. Rev. Med.* **33**, 435–43.

McArdle's disease (glycogenosis type V)

This disorder is one of a small group of glycogen storage diseases, involving skeletal muscle, in which myoglobinuria with acute renal failure is occasionally seen.

McArdle (1951) first described this disease in a patient in whom pain and stiffness in skeletal muscles had followed even moderate exercise from childhood. He showed that these symptoms were due to a myopathy with defective breakdown of muscle glycogen. A similar patient, who became more severely affected after adolescence, was reported by Schmid and Mahler (1959). Their patient was the first of many patients with this disease in whom myoglobinuria in association with muscle cramps is recorded. Typically there are no symptoms or abnormal physical signs at rest and specifically there is no hepatomegaly, hypoglycaemia, nor cardiac symptoms, although electrocardiographic changes have been reported (Pearson *et al.* 1961; Salter 1968). Schmid and Mahler (1959) defined three phases in the natural history of the disease: the first in childhood and adolescence with increased fatigability, the second from 20–40 years of age with severe painful muscle cramp and myoglobinuria on exertion, and the third in later life when weakness and muscle wasting become gradually more prominent. Pearson and colleagues (1961) and Mellick and colleagues (1962) reported further sporadic cases, which in the latter case may be a variant of the disease in the earlier reports. Further evidence for genetic heterogeneity comes from the two unrelated patients described by Grünfeld and his coworkers (1972), one of which had no detectable myophosphorylase activity and no cross-reacting material in muscle to an antiserum to the enzyme; and the other in which 10–15 per cent of normal, but unstable, activity was detected by both methods. Similar findings were reported by Dreyfus and colleagues (1974), and two other families with an unusually severe form with death in infancy have been reported (Di Mavro and Hartlage 1978; Miranda *et al.* 1979; De la Marza *et al.* 1980). Acute renal failure associated with myoglobinuria following excessive exercise was first reported in two patients with McArdle's disease by Grünfeld and coworkers (1972) with two further cases being described by Bank and colleagues (1972).

Histologically there is excess glycogen in the intermyofibrillar space with, on electron microscopy, myofibrillar disorganization (Schotland *et al.* 1965).

McArdle's (1951) suggestion of a defect in muscle glycogen break-down was confirmed by Schmid and Mahler (1959) who observed a five-fold increase in muscle glycogen and an absence of myophosphorylase activity in their patient. This absence of myophosphorylase activity was rapidly confirmed in further patients (Mommaerts *et al.* 1959; Pearson *et al.* 1961; Schmid and Hammaker 1961; Mellick *et al.* 1962). It is presumed that both the active *a* and the inactive *b* precursor forms are defective, but in many cases a defect of myophosphorylase kinase cannot be altogether excluded. However, some groups have found low, rather than absent, enzyme activity (Dreyfus and Alexandre 1971; Bank *et al.* 1972) or even normal activity (Feit and Brooke 1976; Cerri and Willner 1981). Hence the disease is almost certainly genetically heterogeneous. Recently an absence of functional messenger RNA for glycogen myophosphorylase was found in muscle from two unrelated patients and a decreased amount in one obligate and one possible heterozygote among their relatives (Daegelen *et al.* 1983).

Three affected sibs out of a family of children born to first-cousin parents were described by Schmid and Hammaker (1961). They concluded from this family that the disease is due to a single rare mutant gene with autosomal recessive inheritance. Further instances of families with affected sibs have been reported by Rowland and colleagues (1966) and by Dawson and colleagues (1968) and by Cochrane and coworkers (1973), leaving little doubt that the inheritance is indeed autosomal recessive. Dawson's group observed cramps after exercise in members of their family who could have been heterozygotes. The evidence for genetic heterogeneity quoted above leaves it unknown whether such heterogeneity is due to different autosomal genes, as for example for phosphorylase b or for phosophorylase kinase, or is allelic with perhaps different mutations of the phosphorylase gene.

Lebo and colleagues (1984) have assigned the gene for myo-phosphorylase to the chromosome 11 long arm or proximal short arm (11p 13–11 qter), using a novel method. They sorted chromosomes from a normal human cell line stained with chromomycin A3 and DIPI, using a fluorescence-activated cell sorter with a dual laser, directly onto a nitrocellulose filter. Hybridization of a DNA probe for the 3′ end of the gene was demonstrated to a spot containing chromosomes 10, 11, and 12. Regional localization was obtained using a cell line containing a translocation between chromosomes 4 and 11.

References

Bank, W. J., Di Mauro, S. and Rowland, L. P. (1972). Renal failure in McArdle's disease (letter). *New Engl. J. Med.* **287**, 1102.

Cerri, C. G. and Willner, J. H. (1981). Phosphorylation of McArdle phosphory-lase induces activity. *Proc. Nat. Acad. Sci.* **78**, 2688–92.

Cochrane, P., Hughes, R. R., Buxton, P. H. and Yorke, R. A. (1973). Myo-phosphorylase deficiency (McArdle's disease) in two interrelated families. *J. Neurol. Neurosurg. Psychiatry.* **36**, 217–24.

Daegelen, D., Munnich, A., Levin, M. J., Girault, A., Goasguen, J., Kahn, A. and Dreyfus, J. C. (1983). Absence of functional messenger RNA for glycogen phosphorylase in the muscle of two patients with McArdle's disease. *Ann. Hum. Genet.* **47**, 107–15.

Daegelen-Proux, D., Kahn, A., Marie, J. and Dreyfus, J. C. (1981). Research on molecular mechanisms of McArdle's disease (muscle glycogen phosphorylase deficiency). Use of new protein mapping and immunological techniques. *Ann. Hum. Genet* **45**, 113–20.

De La Marza, M., Patten, B. M., Williams, J. C. and Chambers, J. P. (1980). Myophosphorylase deficiency: a new cause of infantile hypotonia simulating infantile muscular atrophy (abs.). *Neurology* **30**, 402.

Dawson, D. M., Spong, F. L. and Harrington, J. F. (1968). McArdle's disease: lack of muscle phosphorylase. *Ann. Intern. Med.* **69**, 229–35.

Di Mavro, S. and Hartlage, P. L. (1978). Fatal infantile form of muscle phosphorylase deficiency. *Neurology* **28**, 1124–9.

Dreyfus, J. C. and Alexandre, Y. (1971). Immunological studies on glycogen storage diseases type III and V. Demonstration of the presence of an immunoreactive protein in one case of muscle phosphorylase deficiency. *Biochem. Biophys, Res. Commun.* **44**, 1364–70.

——, Proux, D. and Alexandre, Y. (1974). Molecular studies on glycogen storage diseases. *Enzyme* **18**, 60–72.

Feit, H. and Brooke, M. H. (1976). Myophosphorylase deficiency: two different molecular etiologies. *Neurology* **26**, 963–7.

Grünfeld, J.-P., Ganeval, D., Chanard, J., Fardeau, M. and Dreyfus, J.-C. (1972). Acute renal failure in McArdle's disease. *New. Engl. J. Med.* **286**, 1237–41.

Lebo, R. V., Gorin, F., Fletterick, R. J., Kao, F.-T., Cheung, M.-C., Bruce, B. D. and Kan, Y. W. (1984). High resolution chromosome sorting and DNA spotblot analysis assign McArdle's syndrome to chromosome 11. *Science* **225**, 57–9.

Miranda, A. F., Nette, E. G., Hartlage, P. L. and Di Mauro, S. (1979). Phosphorylase isoenzymes in normal and myophosphorylase-deficient human heart. *Neurology* **29**, 1538–41.

McArdle, B. (1951). Myopathy due to a defect in muscle glycogen breakdown. *Clin. Sci.* **10**, 13–35.

Mellick, R. S., Mahler, R. F. and Hughes, B. P. (1962). McArdle's syndrome. Phosphorylase-deficient myopathy. *Lancet* **1**, 1045–8.

Mommaerts, W. F. H. M., Illingworth, B., Pearson, C. M., Guillory, R. J. and Seraydarian, K. (1959). A functional disorder of muscle associated with the absence of phosphorylase. *Proc. Nat. Acad. Sci.* **45**, 791–7.

Pearson, C. M., Rimer, D. G. and Mommaerts, W. F. H. M. (1961). A metabolic myopathy due to absence of muscle phosphorylase. *Am. J. Med.* **30**, 502–17.

Rowland, L. P., Lovelace, R. E., Schotland, D. L., Araki, S. and Carmel, P. (1966). The clinical diagnosis of McArdle's disease. Identification of another family with deficiency of muscle phosphorylase. *Neurology* **16**, 93–100.

Salter, R. H. (1968). The muscle glycogenoses. *Lancet* **1**, 1301–4.

Schmid, R. and Hammaker, L. (1961). Hereditary absence of muscle phosphorylase (McArdle's syndrome). *New Engl. J. Med.* **264**, 223–5.

—— and Mahler, R. (1959). Chronic progressive myopathy with myoglobinuria: demonstration of a glycogenolytic defect in the muscle. *J. Clin. Invest.* **38**, 2044–58.

Schotland, D. L., Spiro, D., Rowland, L. P. and Carmel, P. (1965). Ultrastructural studies of muscle in McArdle's disease. *J. Neuropath. Exp. Neurol.* **24**, 629–44.

Glycogenosis type VII

This disorder presents a clinical picture similar to McArdle's syndrome with easy fatigability, but with the addition of a mild haemolytic anaemia. The first report was from Japan of a family with three affected sibs, one of whom had had myoglobinuria (Tarui *et al.* 1965; Okuno *et al.* 1966). As in McArdle's disease there is no rise in venous lactate on ischaemic exercise but patients differed in having only 1–3 per cent of normal activity of muscle phosphofructokinase. They also had erythrocyte phosphofructokinase levels only half that of normal. Tarui and colleagues (1969) have shown that the enzyme in red cells normally has two components, half the activity being due to an enzyme identical to that in muscle and half to a different enzyme. Layzer and colleagues (1969) showed that the muscle and erythrocyte enzymes are related immunologically but not identical. Vora and associates (1980) demonstrated five isozymes formed by polymerization of two subunits, M (muscle) and L (liver) to form all possible tetramers. In a patient studied by them the red-cell phosphofructokinase was entirely of the L type. The gene locus for the muscle type has been assigned to chromosome 1 (Vora *et al.* 1981). A case with myoglobinuria also, reported from the United States, showed a lack of cross-reacting material to an antibody to normal enzyme, as well as deficient activity (Layzer *et al.* 1967).

The occurrence in sibs and an instance of parenteral consanguinity (Tarui *et al.* 1965) suggest autosomal recessive inheritance, and this is confirmed by the observation of intermediate levels of enzyme activity in the parents of the patient reported by Layzer and colleagues (1967).

References

Layzer, R. B., Rowland, L. P. and Ranney, H. M. (1967). Muscle phosphofructokinase deficiency. *Arch. Neurol.* **17**, 512–23.
——, —— and Bank, W. J. (1969). Physical and kinetic properties of human phosphofructokinase from skeletal muscle and erythrocytes. *J. Biol. Chem.* **244**, 3823–31.
Okuno, G., Hizukuri, S. and Nishikawa, M. (1966). Activities of glycogen synthetase and UDPG-pyrophosphorylase in muscle of a patient with a new type of muscle glycogenosis caused by phosphofructokinase deficiency. *Nature* **212**, 1490–1.
Tarui, S., Okuno, G., Ikura, Y., Tanaka, T., Suda, M. and Nishikawa, M. (1965). Phosphofructokinase deficiency in skeletal muscle: a new type of glycogenosis. *Biochem. Biophys. Res. Commun.* **19**, 517–23.
——, Kono, N., Nasu, T. and Nishikawa, M. (1969). Enzymatic basis for the coexistence of myopathy and hemolytic disease in inherited muscle phosphofructokinase deficiency. *Biochem. Biophys. Res. Commun.* **34**, 77–83.
Vora, S., Corash, L., Engel, W. K., Durham, S., Seaman, C. and Piomelli, S. (1980). The molecular mechanism of the inherited phosphofructokinase deficiency associated with hemolysis and myopathy. *Blood* **55**, 629–35.
——, Durham, S., De Martinville, B. and Francke, U. (1981). Assignment of the genes for liver type phosphofructokinase (PFKL) to chromosome 21 and for muscle type (PFKM) to region p32–q32 of chromosome 1. *Human Gene Mapping Workshop 6, Oslo, 1981.*

Forbes' or Cori's disease (limit dextrinosis, glycogenosis type III)

This is another glycogenosis in which patients develop a myopathy and show a lack of increase in blood lactate on the ischaemic exercise test, although the clinical picture generally resembles von Gierke's disease (type I). The earliest report of this disorder was that of Oliner and colleagues in 1961. Biochemical and histochemical studies of both liver and skeletal muscle biopsies showed an excess of limit dextrin and a lack of amylo-1,6-glucosidase activity. Patients show hepatomegaly, especially in childhood, and a tendency to hypoglycaemia. As in type II (Pompe's disease) heart muscle is also involved but usually only to a relatively mild degree, leading at most to moderate cardiomegaly (Levin *et al.* 1967). The myopathic picture is seen mainly in older patients (Brunberg *et al.* 1971; Murase *et al.* 1973), and exercise may induce weakness rather than cramps. Myoglobinuria is a rare complication (Knockel 1981) and, unlike type I, renal enlargement is not a feature, but renal acidosis has been reported (Cohen and Friedman 1979).

   On the basis of enzyme assays with different substrates Hers and van Hoof (Hers 1960; van Hoof and Hers 1967) have defined several biochemical subtypes designated IIIA to F, indicative of genetic hetero-geneity. Daegelen-Proux and colleagues (1981) have confirmed hetero-geneity by protein mapping and immunoreactivity.

   There is abundant evidence for autosomal recessive inheritance including affected sibs, parental consanguinity, and intermediate enzyme levels in erythrocytes of parents (Williams *et al.* 1963; Williams and Field 1968; Waaler *et al.* 1970). The disease is rare except among non-Ashkenazi Jews of North African origin and it is therefore the most common form of glycogenosis in Israel (Levin *et al.* 1967). It has also been reported from the USSR (Rosenfeld *et al.* 1976) and among Faeroe Islanders (Cohn *et al.* 1975). Attempts at carrier detection using leucocytes have yielded conflicting results but red blood cells have given better discrimination.

References

Brunberg, J. A., McCormick, W. F. and Schocket, S. S. Jr. (1971). Type III glyco-genosis. An adult with diffuse weakness and muscle wasting. *Arch. Neurol.* **25**, 171–8.

Cohen, J. and Friedman, M. (1979). Renal tubular acidosis associated with type III glycogenosis. *Acta Paediatr. Scand.* **68**, 779–82.

Cohn, J., Wang, P., Hauge, M., Henningsen, K., Jensen, B. and Svejgaard, A. (1975). Amylo-1,6-glucosidase deficiency (glycogenosis type III) in the Faeroe Islands. *Hum. Hered.* **25**, 115–26.

Daegelen-Proux, D., Kahn, A., Marie, J. and Dreyfus, J. C. (1981). Research on molecular mechanisms of McArdle's disease (muscle glycogen phosphorylase deficiency). Use of new protein mapping and immunological techniques. *Ann. Hum. Genet.* **45**, 113–20.

Hers, H. G. (1960). Amylo-1,6-glucosidase activity in tissues of children with glycogen storage diseases. *Biochem. J.* **76**, 69.

van Hoof, F. and Hers, H. G. (1967). The subgroups of type III glycogenosis. *Eur. J. Biochem.* **2**, 265–70.

Knockel, J. P. (1981). Rhabdomyolysis and myoglobinuria. In *The kidney in systemic disease*, 2nd edn. eds. Suki, W. N. and Eknoyani, G. pp. 263–84. John Wiley, New York.

Levin, S., Moses, S. W., Chayoth, R., Jagoda, N. and Steinitz, K. (1967). Glycogen storage disease in Isreal. A clinical, biochemical and genetic study. *Isreal J. Med. Sci.* **3**, 397–410.

Murase, T., Ikeda, H., Muro, T., Nakao, K. and Sugita, H. (1973). Myopathy associated with type III glycogenosis. *J. Neurol. Sci.* **20**, 287–95.

Oliner, L., Schulman, M. and Larner, J. (1961). Myopathy associated with glycogen deposition resulting from generalized lack of amylo-1,6-glucosidase. *Clin. Res.* **9**, 243.

Rosenfeld, E. L., Popova, I. A. and Chibisov, I. V. (1976). Some cases of type III glycogen storage disease. *Clin. Chim. Acta* **67**, 123–30.

Waaler, P. E., Garatun-Tjeldsto, O. and Moe, P. J. (1970). Genetic studies in glycogen storage disease type III. *Acta Paediatr. Scand.* **57**, 529–35.

Williams, C. and Field, J. B. (1968). Studies in glycogen storage disease. III Limit dextrinosis: a genetic study. *J. Pediatr.* **72**, 214–21.

Williams, H. E., Kendig, E. M. and Field, J. B. (1963). Leukocyte debranching enzyme in glycogen storage disease. *J. Clin. Invest.* **42**, 656–60.

Glycogenosis type II (Pompe's disease)

The classical form of this disease, the infantile form, presents with profound hypotonia and cardiomegaly. Death ensues from cardiac failure within the first year (Pompe 1932). There are also less severe early childhood or juvenile and adult forms of the disease. In the early childhood form, also with hypotonia, organ involvement is variable but death still ensues before adult life (Gambetti *et al.* 1971; Engel *et al.* 1973; Tanaka *et al.* 1979). The less common adult form presents with muscular weakness and very slow progression (Zellweger *et al.* 1965; Roth and Williams 1967; Hudgson *et al.* 1968; Angelini *et al.* 1972; Engel *et al.* 1973), in the course of which myoglobinuria may occur (Knockel 1981).

In all three clinical forms there is an absence of tissue lysosomal α-1,4-glucosidase (acid maltase) (Hers 1963; Koster *et al.* 1972). The acid maltase of kidney differs from the enzyme which is deficient in Pompe's disease and renal activity and urinary excretion of the enzyme in the patients are normal (Steinitz and Rutenberg 1967). This excludes the assay of acid maltase in the amniotic fluid supernatant as a possible method of prenatal diagnosis. In the infantile form an inactive enzyme which shows cross-reaction with an antibody to the normal enzyme has been identified, but in the adult form there appears to be a reduced amount of enzyme (Beratis *et al.* 1978).

Leucocyte enzyme activity is variable, especially in the adult form, as a variable proportion of renal isozyme of α-1,4-glucosidase is present in white blood cells (Dreyfus and Poënaru 1978). Diagnosis is best made on assay of glycogen and enzyme activity from a muscle biopsy, from placenta in the new-born, or by enzyme assay on cultured fibroblasts (Angelini *et al.* 1972; Reuser *et al.* 1978). Alternatively the renal isozyme can be removed from leucocyte preparations by isoelectric precipitation of pH 5.0, which may then be used for diagnosis (Broadhead and Butterworth 1978).

Family studies indicate that inheritance is autosomal recessive. This includes the adult form in which affected sibs have been observed (Zellweger *et al.* 1965). Reduced enzyme levels of α-1,4-glucosidase have been observed in heterozygotes in cultured fibroblasts (Nitowsky and Grunfeld 1967). Reuser and colleagues (1978) found no evidence of non-allelism of the three different clinical forms of the disease in complementation studies with fused fibroblasts. This does not preclude the possibility that some cases may be compound heterozygotes. Cultured amniotic fluid cells are reported to be reliable for prenatal diagnosis (Butterworth and Broadhead 1977). The acid α-1,4-glucosidase locus shows normal polymorphic variation (Swallow *et al.* 1975; Beratis *et al.* 1980) and has been assigned to chromosome 17, in the 17q22–q25 region (D'Ancona *et al.* 1979; Soloman *et al.* 1979).

References

Angelini, C., Engel, A. G. and Titus, J. L. (1972). Adult acid maltase deficiency. Abnormalities of fibroblasts cultured from patients. *New Engl. J. Med.* **287**, 948–51.

Beratis, N. G., Labadie, G. U. and Hirshhorn, K. (1978). Characterization of the molecular defect in infantile and adult acid α-glucosidase deficiency fibroblasts. *J. Clin. Invest.* **62**, 1264–74.

——, —— and —— (1980). An isozyme of acid α-glucosidase with reduced catalytic activity for glycogen. *Am. J. Hum. Genet.* **32**, 137–49.

Broadhead, D. M. and Butterworth, J. (1978). α-Glucosidase in Pompe's disease. *J. Inher. Metab. Dis.* **1**, 153–4.

Butterworth, J. and Broadhead, D. M. (1977). Diagnosis of Pompe's disease in cultured skin fibroblasts and primary amniotic fluid cells using 4-methyl-umbelliferyl-α-D-glucopyranoside as substrate. *Clin. Chim. Acta* **78**, 335–42.

D'Ancona, G. G., Wurm, J. and Croce, C. M. (1979). Genetics of type II glycogenosis: assignment of the human gene for acid alpha-glucosidase to chromosome 17. *Proc. Nat. Acad. Sci.* **76**, 4528–9.

Dreyfus, J. C. and Poënaru, L. (1978). Alpha glucosidases in white blood cells, with reference to the detection of acid α-1,4-glucosidase deficiency. *Biochem. Biophys. Res. Commun.* **85**, 615–22.

Engel, A. G., Gomez, M. R., Seybold, M. E. and Lambert, E. U. (1973). The spectrum and diagnosis of acid maltase deficiency. *Neurology* **23**, 95–106.

Gambetti, P., Di Mauro, S. and Baker, L. (1971). Nervous system in Pompe's disease: ultrastructure and biochemistry. *J. Neuropathol. Exp. Neurol.* **30**, 412–430.

Hers, H. G. (1963). α-Glucosidase deficiency in generalized glycogen-storage disease (Pompe's disease). *Biochem. J.* **86**, 1–6.

Hudgson, P., Gardner-Medwin, D., Worsfold, M., Pennington, R. J. T. and Walton, J. N. (1968). Adult myopathy from glycogen storage disease due to acid maltase deficiency. *Brain* **91**, 635–62.

Knockel, J. P. (1981). Rhabdomyolysis and myoglobinuria. In *The kidney in systemic disease*, 2nd edn. eds. Suki, W. N. and Eknoyan, G. pp. 263–84. John Wiley, New York.

Koster, J. F., Slee, R. G. and Hülsmann, W. C. (1972). The use of leukocytes as an aid in the diagnosis of a variant of glycogen storage disease type II (Pompe's disease). *Eur. J. Clin. Invest.* **2**, 467–71.

Nitowsky, H. M. and Grunfeld, A. (1967). Lysosomal α-glucosidase in type II glycogenosis; activity in leukocytes and cell cultures in relation to genotype. *J. Lab. Clin. Med.* **69**, 472–84.

Pompe, J. C. (1932). Over idopatische hypertrofie van het hart. *Ned. Tijdschr. Geneeskd.* **76**, 304–11.

Reuser, A. J. J., Koster, J. F., Hoogeveen, A. and Galjaard, H. (1978). Biochemical, immunological and cell genetic studies in glycogenosis type II. *Am. J. Human Genet.* **30**, 132–43.

Roth, J. C. and Williams, H. E. (1967). The muscular variant of Pompe's disease. *J. Pediatr.* **71**, 567–73.

Solomon, E., Swallow, D., Burgess, S. and Evans, L. (1979). Assignment of the human acid α-glucosidase gene (GLU) to chromosome 17 using somatic cell hybrids. *Ann. Hum. Genet.* **42**, 273–81.

Steinitz, K. and Rutenberg, A. (1967). Tissue α-glucosidase activity and glycogen content in patients with generalized glycogenosis. *Israel J. Med. Sci.* **3**, 411–21.

Swallow, D. M., Corney, G., Harris, H. and Hirschhorn, R. (1975). Acid α-glucosidase: a new polymorphism in man demonstrable by affinity electrophoresis. *Ann. Hum. Genet.* **38**, 391–406.

Tanaka, K., Shimazu, S., Oya, N., Tomisawa, M., Kusunoki, T., Soyama, K. and Ono, E. (1979). Muscular form of glycogenosis type II (Pompe's disease). *Pediatrics* **63**, 124–9.

Zellweger, H., Brown, B-I., McCormick, W. F. and Jun-Bi, T. (1965). A mild form of muscular glycogenosis in two brothers with α-1,4-glucosidase deficiency. *Ann. Paediatr.* **205**, 413–37.

4.2.2. Diseases with secondary renal damage from other metabolites

Hereditary fructose intolerance

This disorder must be distinguished from the benign condition of essential fructosuria due to hepatic fructokinase deficiency, and also from heriditary fructose 1,6-diphosphatase deficiency in which there is hepatomegaly and episodes of ketotic hypoglycaemia with lactic acidosis but apparently no renal involvement. A possible case of hereditary fructose intolerance was described by Chambers and Pratt in 1956 but the first description of the typical syndrome was that of Froesch and his colleagues in 1957, who reported an affected brother and sister. The symptoms of the disorder are entirely related to ingestion of fructose.

Acute symptoms appearing in the infant on initial or subsequent ingestion of fructose or sucrose are largely attributable to hypoglycaemia and include sweating, nausea and vomiting which may be protracted, dizziness, and even coma. In addition to hypoglycaemia there is fructosaemia and fructosuria, and hypophosphataemia (Froesch *et al.* 1957, 1959; Bergstrom *et al.* 1968). The acute episode is associated with proteinuria and aminoaciduria (Froesch *et al.* 1957, 1959; Dubois *et al.* 1961; Jeune *et al.* 1961; Lelong *et al.* 1962), and renal tubular acidosis (Dubois *et al.* 1961; Levin *et al.* 1963; Mass *et al.* 1966). The aminoaciduria may present as an acute tyrosyluria (Lindemann *et al.* 1969). Morris has studied the renal tubular acidosis of hereditary fructose intolerance and shown that it is promptly corrected on withdrawal of fructose (Morris 1968a and b). He also demonstrated the primary enzyme deficiency in the kidney itself (Morris *et al.* 1967), and showed that the renal dysfunction is modulated by circulating parathyroid hormone (Morris *et al.* 1971). The childhood clinical picture is reviewed by Baerlocher and colleagues (1978) and by Odievre and associates (1978).

The picture of chronic fructose intolerance is one of failure to thrive and eventually cachexia, hepatomegaly progressing to cirrhosis with jaundice and hyperbilirubinaemia, protracted vomiting and dehydration, peripheral oedema and ascites, attacks of hypoglycaemic coma (Bergstrom *et al.* 1968), and impaired renal function, in particular a loss of the ability to acidify urine. Many of these children develop a strong aversion to the foods containing fructose or sucrose. Levin and colleagues (1963) introduced the term 'fructosaemia' for the disorder and drew attention to the renal acidosis. The severity of the condition does vary, with an occasional asymptomatic case, even within the same family as a typical case (Perheentupa and Pitkanen 1962), or adult case (Froesch *et al.* 1963; Swales and Smith 1966).

Hers and Joassin (1961) found that fructose-1,6-diphosphate aldolase in the liver was only about a quarter of the normal activity. However the primary enzyme defect has been shown to involve fructose 1-phosphate aldolase B with hepatic levels only 0–15 per cent of normal (Schapira *et al.* 1961/2; Perheentupa *et al.* 1962; Froesch *et al.* 1963; Schapira and Dreyfus 1967; Schapira *et al.* 1974; Steinmann and Gitzelmann 1981). There is evidence that the two aldolase activities may be properties of the same enzyme molecule (Gürtler and Leuthardt 1970; Koster *et al.* 1975).

Surprisingly, in view of the confirmation of autosomal recessive inheritance (Dubois *et al.* 1961; Cornblath *et al.* 1963; Levin *et al.* 1968; Perheentupa *et al.* 1972; Steinmann *et al.* 1975), hepatic levels of the enzyme activity in parents, who must be heterozygotes, have been found to be normal (Raivio *et al.* 1967), although this was questioned by Beyreiss and colleagues (1968).

The disorder is seen primarily in Caucasian populations but has also been diagnosed in an Indian (Sitadevi *et al.* 1968). An incidence of 1 in 20 000 was estimated in Switzerland (Cornblath & Schwartz 1976) but is almost certainly an underestimate.

The mutation is probably a point (mis-sense) mutation as evidenced by a less marked reduction in antibody reaction than in enzymatic activity (Nordmann *et al.* 1968). Gitzelmann and coworkers (1974) produced evidence for genetic heterogeneity on the basis of finding antibody activation of mutant enzyme in some patients but not others. Other reports lend support to the idea of genetic heterogeneity. Levin and associates (1968) found a normal ratio of fructose 1-phosphate aldolase to the diphosphate aldolase in one case. Koster and colleagues (1975) observed differing Km values for the enzyme in different patients. Lamiere and others (1978) reported a 21-year-old male with severe illness induced by fructose who had 30 per cent of normal fructose 1-phosphate aldolase activity and normal diphosphate aldolase activity. It is not clear as to whether this was due to a 'mild' allele in a homozygote, or to exceptional provocation of intolerance in a hetero-zygote. Grégori and colleagues (1982), in a study of 15 patients, found levels of cross-reacting material (CRM) varying between 3 and 100 per cent of control levels, and also differences in molecular charge of the enzyme.

Finally although in the great majority of reported families the pattern of inheritance with affected sibs, with frequent parental consanguinity and concordance of monozygotic twins (Morris *et al.* 1971; Rampa and Froesch 1981), is entirely consistent with autosomal recessive inheritance there are exceptional families. Typical of the recessive pattern is the very large family of Froesch and colleagues (1963) with four interrelated kindreds with respectively one, three, three, and one affected child, and all with consanguineous parents. The exceptional families all appear to demonstrate autosomal dominant inheritance, but this is in many, if not all, cases pseudodominance due to one homo-zygous parent and one undiagnosed heterozygous parent. In the family of Wolf *et al.* (1959) a father and son were affected but the mother may have been heterozygous. However, Froesch (1972) has reported two apparently dominant families including one in which both father and child had the typical syndrome, but again a homozygous and a hetero-zygous parent cannot be excluded. Schulte and Lenz (1977) reported a couple, both affected, with four children all affected, confirming recessive inheritance.

References

Baerlocher, K., Gitzelmann, R., Steinmann, B. and Gitzelmann-Cumarasamy, N. (1978). Hereditary fructose intolerance in early childhood: a major diagnostic challenge: survey of 20 symptomatic cases. *Helv. Paediatr. Acta* **33**, 465–87.

Bergström, J., Hultman, E. and Roch-Norlund, A. E. (1968). Lactic acid accumulation in connection with fructose administration. *Acta Med. Scand.* **184**, 359–64.

Beyreiss, K., Willgerodt, H. and Theile, H. (1968). Untersuchungen bei heterozygoten Merkmalsträgern fur Fructoseintoleranz. *Klin. Wschr.* **46**, 465–8.

Chambers, R. A. and Pratt, R. T. C. (1956). Idiosyncrasy to fructose. *Lancet* **2**, 340.

Cornblath, M. and Schwartz, R. (1976). *Disorders of carbohydrate metabolism in infancy,* edn. 2. Vol. 3 in the series of *Major Problems in Clinical Paediatrics.* W. B. Saunders, Philadelphia.

——, Rosenthal, I. M., Reisner, S. H., Wybregt, S. H. and Crane, R. K. (1963). Hereditary fructose intolerance. *New. Engl. J. Med.* **269**, 1271–8.

Dubois, R., Loeb, H., Ooms, H. A., Gillet, P., Bartman, J. and Champenois, A. (1961). Etude d'un cas d'hypoglycémie fonctionelle par intolerance au fructose. *Helv. Paediatr. Acta* **16**, 90–6.

Froesch, E. R. (1972). Essential fructosuria and hereditary fructose intolerance. In *The metabolic basis of inherited disease,* 3rd edn. eds. Stanbury, J. B., Wyngaarden, J. B. and Frederickson, D. S. pp. 136–48. McGraw-Hill, New York.

——, Prader, A., Labhart, A., Stuber, H. W. and Wolf, H. P. (1957). Die hereditäre Fructoseintoleranz, eine bisher nicht bekannte kongenitale Stoffwech-selstörung. *Schweiz. Med. Wschr.* **87**, 1168–71.

——, ——, Wolf, H. P. and Labhart, A. (1959). Die hereditäre Fructoseintoleranz. *Helv. Paediatr. Acta* **14**, 99–112.

——, Wolf, H. P., Baitsch, H., Prader, A. and Labhart, A. (1963). Hereditary fructose intolerance: an inborn defect of hepatic fructose 1-phosphate splitting aldolase. *Am. J. Med.* **34**, 151–67.

Gitzelmann, R., Steinmann, B., Bally, C. and Lebherz, H. G. (1974). Antibody activation of mutant human fructose diphosphate aldolase B in liver extracts of patients with hereditary fructose intolerance. *Biochem. Biophys. Res. Commun.* **59**, 1220–77.

Grégori, C., Schapira, F., Kahn, A., Delpech, M. and Dreyfus, J.-C. (1982). Molecular studies of liver aldolase B in hereditary fructose intolerance using blotting and immunological techniques. *Ann. Hum. Genet.* **46**, 281–92.

Gürtler, B. and Leuthardt, F. (1970). Ueber die Heterogenität der Aldolasen. *Helv. Chim. Acta.* **53**, 654–8.

Hers, H. G. and Joassin, G. (1961). Anomalie de l'aldolase hépatique dans l'intolerance au fructose. *Enzymol. Biol. Clin.* **1**, 4–14.

Jeune, M., Planson, E., Cotte, J., Bonnefoy, S., Nivelon, J. L. and Skosowsky, J. (1961). L'intolerance héréditaire au fructose, a propos d'un cas. *Pédiatrie* **16**, 605–26.

Koster, J. F., Slee, R. G. and Fernandes, J. (1975). On the biochemical basis of hereditary fructose intolerance. *Biochem. Biophys. Res. Commun.* **64**, 289–94.

Lamiere, N., Mussche, M., Baele, G., Kint, J. and Ringoir, S. (1978). Hereditary fructose intolerance: a difficult diagnosis in an adult. *Am. J. Med.* **65**, 416–23.

Lelong, M., Alagille, D., Gentil, C., Colin, J., Tupin, J. and Bougier, J. (1962). Cirrhose hépatique et tubulopathie par absence congenitale de l'aldolase hépatique: intolerance héréditaire au fructose. *Bull. Soc. Med. Hop. (Paris)* **113**, 58.

Levin, B., Oberholzer, V. G., Snodgrass, G. J. A. I., Stimmler, L. and Wilmers, M. J. (1963). Fructosaemia: an inborn error of fructose metabolism. *Arch. Dis. Child.* **38**, 220–30.

——, Snodgrass, G. J. A. I., Oberholzer, V. G., Burgess, E. A. and Dobbs, R. H. (1968). Fructosaemia: observations on seven cases. *Am. J. Med.* **45**, 826–38.

Lindemann, R., Gjessing, L. R., Merton, B. and Halvorsen, S. (1969). Fructosaemia 'acute tyrosinosis'. *Lancet* **1**, 891.

Mass, R. E., Smith, W. R. and Walsh, J. R. (1966). The association of hereditary fructose intolerance and renal tubular acidosis. *Am. J. Med. Sci.* **251**, 516–23.

Morris, R. C. Jr. (1968a). An experimental renal acidification defect in patients with hereditary fructose intolerance. I. Its resemblance to renal tubular acidosis. *J. Clin. Invest.* **47**, 1389–98.

—— (1968b). An experimental renal acidification defect in patients with hereditary fructose intolerance. II. Its distinction from classical renal tubular acidosis; its resemblance to the renal acidification defect associated with the Fanconi syndrome of children with cystinosis. *J. Clin. Invest.* **47**, 1648–63.

——, Ueki, I., Loh, D., Eanes, R. Z. and McLin, P. (1967). Absence of renal fructose-1-phosphate aldolase activity in hereditary fructose intolerance. *Nature* **214**, 920–1.

——, McSherry, E. and Sebastian, A. (1971). Modulation of experimental renal dysfunction of hereditary fructose intolerance by circulating parathyroid hormone. *Proc. Nat. Acad. Sci.* **68**, 132–5.

Nordmann, Y., Schapira, F. and Dreyfus, J. C. (1968). A structurally modified liver aldolase in fructose intolerance: immunological and kinetic evidence. *Biochem. Biophys. Res. Commun.* **31**, 884–9.

Odievre, M., Gentil, C., Gautier, M. and Alagille, D. (1978). Hereditary fructose intolerance in childhood: diagnosis, management, and course in 55 patients. *Am. J. Dis. Child.* **132**, 605–8.

Perheentupa, J. and Pitkänen, E. (1962). Symptomless hereditary fructose intolerance (letter). *Lancet* **1**, 1358–9.

——, ——, Nikkilä, E. A., Somersalo, O. and Hakasalo, J. (1962). Hereditary fructose intolerance, a clinical study of 4 cases. *Ann. Paediatr. Fenn.* **8**, 221–35.

——, Raivio, K. O. and Nikkilä, E. A. (1972). Hereditary fructose intolerance. *Acta. Med. Scand.* Suppl. **542**, 65–75.

Raivio, K., Perheentupa, J. and Nikkilä, E. A. (1967). Aldolase activities in the liver in parents of patients with hereditary fructose intolerance. *Clin. Chim. Acta.* **17**, 275–9.

Rampa, M. and Froesch, E. R. (1981). Eleven cases of hereditary fructose intolerance in one Swiss family with a pair of monozygotic and dizygotic twins. *Helv. Paediatr. Acta.* **36**, 317–24.

Schapira, F. and Dreyfus, J. C. (1967). L'Aldolase hepatique dans l'intolerance au fructose. *Rev. Fr. Étude Clin. Biol.* **12**, 486–9.

——, Schapira, G. and Dreyfus, J. C. (1961/62). La lésion enzymatique de la fructosurie bénign. *Enzymol. Biol. Clin. (Basel),* **1**, 170–5.

——, Hatzfeld, A. and Gregori, C. (1974). Studies on liver aldolases in hereditary fructose intolerance. *Enzyme* **18**, 73–83.

Schulte, M.-J. and Lenz, W. (1977). Fatal sorbitol infusion in patient with fructose–sorbitol intolerance. *Lancet* **2**, 188.

Sitadevi, C., Ramaiah, Y. and Askari, Z. (1968). Fructose intolerance associated with congenital cataract. *Ind. J. Pediatr.* **35**, 496–8.

Steinmann, B. and Gitzelmann, R. (1981). The diagnosis of hereditary fructose intolerance. *Helv. Paediatr. Acta* **36**, 297–316.

——, Baerlocher, K. and Gitzelmann, R. (1975). Hereditäre Storungen des Fruktosestoff-wechsels: Belastungs proben mit Frukose, Sorbitol und Dihydroxyaceton. *Nutr. Metab.* **18**, (Suppl. 1), 115–32.

Swales, J. D. and Smith, A. D. M. (1966). Adult fructose intolerance. *Quart. J. Med.* **35**, 455–73.

Wolf, H. P., Zschokke, D., Wedermeyer, F. W. and Hubner, W. (1959). Angeborene hereditäre Fructose-Intoleranz. *Klin. Wschr.* **37**, 693–6.

Galactosaemia

The earliest description of a patient with galactosaemia was probably that of Goppert (1917). The first account from Britain was given by Bray and his colleagues (1952); and Komrower and Lee (1970) reviewed the long term follow-up of 60 British cases. Further studies of large numbers of patients have been reported by Hsia and Walker (1961), Donnell and colleagues (1961, 1969), Nadler and associates (1969) and Fishler and coworkers (1980). The disease classically presents with failure to thrive, vomiting and liver enlargement associated with high galactose levels and galactosuria. Without treatment jaundice, cirrhosis, cataracts, and developmental retardation appear and an aminoaciduria (Holzel *et al.* 1952; Cusworth *et al.* 1955), as well as glycosuria, proteinuria (Holzel *et al.* 1957), and renal tubular acidosis (Komrower *et al.* 1956), is found culminating in death in infancy. Dietary restriction of galactose leads to disappearance of the renal, as well as other, abnormalities (Komrower *et al.* 1956). Schwartz and associates (1956, 1961) demonstrated that following a milk feed the red cells of galactosaemic children accumulated galactose 1-phosphate but not glucose 1-phosphate.

The mechanism of renal damage is very similar to that in hereditary fructose intolerance. Both galactose 1-phosphate (Schwarz 1960) and galactitol (Quan-Ma *et al.* 1966) have been detected in the kidneys of patients with galactosaemia. Aminoaciduria is not seen in patients with galactokinase deficiency who excrete large amounts of galactitol (Gitzelmann 1967) but is seen in both human subjects (Fox *et al.* 1964) and rats (Rosenberg *et al.* 1961) administered galactose, as well as galactosaemic patients. Further evidence that it is the galactosaemia itself that causes renal damage comes from the observation that kidney cortex slices incubated with galactose show impaired accumulation of amino acids by the tubule cells (Thier *et al.* 1964).

Kalckar, Anderson and Isselbacher showed the primary enzyme defect to involve galactose 1-phosphate uridyltransferase in both red cells (Isselbacher *et al.* 1956; Kalckar *et al.* 1956) and liver (Anderson *et al.* 1957). This enzyme catalyses the first step in the conversion of galactose 1-phosphate to glucose 1-phosphate, and activity in affected homozygotes is virtually undetectable. That defective enzyme is present is shown by cross-reaction to antibody for the normal enzyme (Tedesco and Mellman 1971; Tedesco *et al.* 1975a; Banroques *et al.* 1983), implying a structural gene mutation. Tedesco (1972) likewise obtained a band of complete identity to normal enzyme on immune precipitation with red-cell extracts from the Duarte variant described below. Dale and Popjak (1976) isolated transferase-deficient enzyme by affinity chromatography and obtained similar peptide maps to those of normal enzyme. Both mutant and normal enzymes have a dimeric structure.

Cox and Pugh (1954) noted a high proportion of patients with affected sibs and also parental consanguinity. They considered the familial pattern to be consistent with autosomal recessive inheritance. Holzel and Komrower (1955) studied five families and in each found at least one parent with an abnormal galactose tolerance but only one in which both parents gave an abnormal result. In one of their families the parents were cousins. Six clinically normal sibs also gave an abnormal result. Hsia and others (1958) found that about half of the obligate heterozygotes could be detected by enzyme assay on red cells. This incomplete detection of heterozygotes, by both Hsia and Holzel and Komrower, was almost certainly due to the relative insensitivity of their methods as improved methods of enzyme assay have subsequently consistently found levels of about 50 per cent of normal activity and have confirmed the autosomal recessive pattern of inheritance (Kirkman and Bynum 1959; Donnel *et al.* 1960; Hugh-Jones *et al.* 1960; Gitzelman and Hadorn 1961; Schwarz *et al.* 1961; Walker *et al.* 1962; Robinson 1963; Beutler *et al.* 1964; Ng *et al.* 1964). Russell and De Mars (1967) obtained clear segregation of normal, heterozygous, and galactosaemic enzyme levels in stationary phase fibroblast cultures. Mellman and Tedesco (1969) were able to discriminate between normal and heterozygous leucocytes or cultured fibroblasts using the transferase/galactokinase ratio. There is considerable genetic heterogeneity in galactose 1-phosphate uridyltransferase deficiency. Apart from classic severe galactosaemia with profound transferase deficiency several variant forms of the disorder have been described. The first such variant reported was the Negro variant in which galactose $1\text{-}^{14}C$ is converted to $^{14}CO_2$ at normal rates despite absence of red-cell activity (Topper *et al.* 1962; Mellman *et al.* 1965; Segal *et al.* 1965; Baker *et al.* 1966; Hsia 1967; Segal and Cuatrecasas 1968; Segal 1969) and white-cell activity (Mellman *et al.* 1965), and only 10 per cent of normal transferase activity in the intestine (Rogers *et al.* 1970) and liver (Segal *et al.* 1971). Heterozygotes have normal levels of enzyme activity in leucocytes (Mellman *et al.* 1965) but reduced levels in red cells. One of the patients with the Negro variant of Segal's group (Segal *et al.* 1965) had been the subject of one of the earliest clinical reports as a case of chronic galactosaemia (Mason and Turner 1935). The clinical phenotype in patients with this variant varies from a symptomless state (Baker *et al.* 1966; Hsia 1967) to the chronic disease of Mason and Turner's patient, or the typical galactosaemia seen by Mellman and colleagues (1965). The genetic basis of this variant has not been established.

Another mutation of the transferase gene, the Duarte variant (Beutler *et al.* 1965; Beutler 1969) is usually symptomless, although jaundice and hepatomegaly in the neonatal period have been reported (Kelly *et al.* 1972). The transferase activity of red cells from homozygotes for the Duarte variant is 50 per cent of normal. The enzyme differs from normal enzyme in migrating faster on starch-gel electrophoresis (Mathai and Beutler 1966) but is identical in kinetic properties, pH optimum, and thermal stability (Beutler and Baluda 1966). In addition to faster migration the Duarte enzyme produces two bands (Ng *et al.* 1969) and, as would be expected, obligate heterozygotes produce three bands and show 75 per cent of normal activity. The genetic determination of this variant as an allele of the normal and the classical galactosaemia genes is well established on the basis of double heterozygotes for the classical galactosaemic and Duarte variants (Beutler *et al.* 1966; Gitzelmann *et al.* 1967; Mellman *et al.* 1968). Such double heterozygotes are again symptomless and without galactosuria, despite having only 25 per cent of normal transferase activity, and are the variants most commonly detected in new-born screening programmes (Levy *et al.* 1978).

A symptomatic galactosaemia, with a residual enzyme activity (7 per cent) higher than in the classic form, has been reported in sibs in a Congolese family and designated the Rennes variant (Schapira and Kaplan 1969). The enzyme here migrates more slowly than normal on starch-gel electrophoresis. A single probably double heterozygote for the classic and Rennes variants has been reported (Hammersen *et al.* 1975). The Rennes variant enzyme has an increased negative charge (Banroques *et al.* 1983).

The Indiana variant is associated with an enzyme giving 75 per cent of normal activity but showing marked instability, and in heterozygotes slow migration on electrophoresis. A child doubly heterozygous for this variant and the classic variant, in whom the Indiana variant was first identified, had classical galactosaemia which in a sib who died had been thought to be the classic form (Chacko *et al.* 1971).

A further variant, Los Angeles, has been detected in six families (Ng *et al.* 1973). This is associated with higher than normal activity of an enzyme with similar electrophoretic migration to the Duarte variant, but giving three bands, and is symptomless. Heterozygosity for the Los Angeles variant was detected in 4.5 per cent of a group of 418 Caucasian adults. Within the families of these heterozygotes others were found, including some individuals doubly heterozygous for Los Angeles and either the Duarte or classic variant. A further family has been reported (Ibarra *et al.* 1979).

Other new variants include Chicago, a probable genetic compound with 27 per cent of normal red-cell activity and fast electrophoretic mobility (Chacko *et al.* 1977); and a German variant from Münster with 30 per cent of normal red-cell activity and product inhibition (Matz *et al.* 1975; Lang *et al.* 1980).

The properties of these variants are summarized in Table 4.6.

Brandt *et al.* (1963) observed levels of transferase activity in red cells of patients with Down's syndrome 50 per cent higher than those of normal blood donors. They suggested that the galactosaemia gene locus may be on chromosome number 21. Rosner *et al.* (1965) confirmed high red-cell transferase in Down's patients and Hsia *et al.* (1964) found it raised in white, but not red, blood cells of Down's patients. However, other enzyme levels are also increased in Down's syndrome white cells (Mellman *et al.* 1964; Krone *et al.* 1965). This suggested gene assignment has been disproved by direct assignment to the chromosome number 9 short arm using human–mouse somatic cell hybrids (Mohandas *et al.* 1977, 1979; Benn *et al.* 1979; Sparkes *et al.* 1979, 1980a). The assignment to chromosome 9 also resolves earlier tentative assignments to chromosome 2, 3, and 9. The same group (Sparkes *et al.* 1980b) narrowed the assignment to the short arm of 9 (9cen → 9p22). Mulcahy and Wilson (1980) further narrowed it to 9p13 → p22 and Bricarelli and colleagues (1981) by deletion mapping put it at 9p21.

There is probably further genetic heterogeneity among patients with classic galactosaemia. Evidence for this comes from Nadler and colleagues' (1970) study in which they produced somatic cell hybrids between cell lines established from different galactosaemic patients. They obtained complementation with three out of the 21 hybrid clones formed from the seven primary abnormal lines. The enzyme obtained from one of these complementing hybrids differed from the normal in level of specific activity, V_{max}, and thermostability. They suggest that their observations are evidence for interallelic complementation but recognize

Variant	Clinical phenotype	Enzyme activity (% normal rbc's)	Electrophoretic mobility	Other enzyme findings
Classic				
homozygotes	Severe	0	Not detectable	—
heterozygotes	Normal	50	Normal	—
Negro				
homozygotes	Mild to normal	0	Not detectable	Activity in liver and intestine 10% of normal
heterozygotes	Normal	25	—	Normal activity in leucocytes
Duarte				
homozygotes	Normal	50	Fast: 2 bands	—
heterozygotes	Normal	75	Fast: 2 bands and normal: 1 band	—
Rennes				
homozygotes	Severe	7	Slow	—
double heterozygote with classic variant	Normal	10	Slow	—
Indiana				
heterozygotes	Normal	75	Slow and normal	Unstable
double heterozygote with classic variant	Severe	35	Not detectable	—
Los Angeles				
homozygotes	Normal	140	Fast: 3 bands	—
heterozygotes	Normal		Fast and normal: 3 bands	—
Chicago				
heterozygotes	—	27	Fast	—
Munster				
homozygotes	Severe	30	Not detectable	Substrate inhibition

that if different subunits were involved it could be intergenic. On either hypothesis at least three different mutations must be involved.

Estimates of the frequency of the classic mutation vary. Birth incidence in Britain has been estimated at 1 in 70 000 (Schwarz *et al.* 1961). American estimates from infant screening programmes are 1 in 35 000 in New York State (Kelly *et al.* 1970 and 1 in 190 000 in Massachusetts (Shih *et al.* 1971). Prevalance estimates found on detection of heterozygotes suggest that between 0.9 and 1.25 per cent of the populations of Europe and America are heterozygous, giving an estimate of galactosaemia prevalance of 1 in 18 000 to 1 in 180 000 (Hansen *et al.* 1964; Beutler *et al.* 1966; Brandt 1967; Gitzelmann *et al.* 1967; McGuiness and Saunders 1967; Tedesco *et al.* 1975b). Heterozygotes for the Duarte variant amount to 8–13 per cent of the population (Mellman *et al.* 1968).

Nadler (1968) reported finding transferase deficiency in cultured amniotic fluid cells obtained at an amniocentesis of 33 weeks gestation, and Fensom and colleagues (1974) diagnosed an affected fetus following amniocentesis at 13 weeks, and excluded deficiency in another case with amniocentesis at 15 weeks. The same group diagnosed a heterozygote by fetal blood enzyme assay at 20 weeks (Fensom *et al.* 1979), and reviewed the results in these three families with the addition of a further three, two of which were diagnosed as heterozygotes and one as a double heterozygote for classic and Duarte variants (Benson *et al.* 1979). The last of these families is the subject of a separate report (Christensen and Brandt 1978). Ng and associates (1977) and Schapira and coworkers (1978) have also reported prenatal diagnosis of galactosaemia. Holton's group in Bristol have also made several such diagnoses and in two with an affected fetus have shown that the amniotic fluid galactitol is markedly raised (Monk and Holton 1976; Allen *et al.* 1980). Nyhan's group at La Jolla, California, have developed this approach further, and have shown that a stable isotope dilution assay for galactitol provides a rapid and accurate method of prenatal diagnosis for galactosaemia (Jakobs *et al.* 1984). Shin and colleagues (1983) at Munich have reported the results of prenatal diagnosis for classical galactosaemia in nine families with affected homozygotes detected in two cases, and heterozygosity in four.

References

Allen, J. T., Gillett, M., Holton, J. B., King, G. S. and Pettit, B. R. (1980). Evidence of galactosaemia in utero. *Lancet* **1**, 603.

Anderson, E. P., Kalckar, H. M. and Isselbacher, K. J. (1957). Defect in uptake of galactose-1-phosphate into liver nucleotides in congenital galactosemia. *Science* **112**, 113–14.

Baker, L., Mellman, W. J., Tedesco, T. A. and Segal, S. (1966). Galactosemia:

symptomatic and asymptomatic homozygotes in one Negro sibship. *J. Pediatr.* **68**, 551–8.

Banroques, J., Schapira, F., Gregori, C. and Dreyfus, J.-C. (1983). Molecular studies on galactose-1-phosphate uridyl transferase from normal and mutant subjects. An immunological approach. *Ann. Hum. Genet.* **47**, 177–85.

Benn, P. A., D'Ancona, G. G., Groce, M. M., Shows, T. B. and Mellman, W. J. (1979). Confirmation of the assignment of the gene for galactose-1-phosphate uridyltransferase (E.C. 2.7.7.12) to human chromosome 9. *Cytogenet. Cell Genet.* **24**, 37–41.

Benson, P. F., Brandt, N. J., Christensen, E. and Fensom, A. H. (1979). Prenatal diagnosis of galactosaemia in six pregnancies—possible complications with rare alleles of the galactose 1-phosphate uridyl transferase locus. *Clin. Genet.* **16**, 311–16.

Beutler, E. (1969). The Duarte variant in galactosemia. In *Galactosemia*, ed. Hsia, D. Y. Y. p. 163. Charles C. Thomas, Springfield, Illinois.

—— and Baluda, M. C. (1966). Biochemical properties of human red cell galactose-1-phosphate uridyl transferase (UDP glucose: α-D galactose-1-phosphate uridyl transferase (E.C. 2.7.7.12) from normal and mutant subjects. *J. Lab. Clin. Med.* **67**, 947–54.

——, —— and Donnell, G. N. (1964). A new method for the detection of galactosemia and its carrier state. *J. Lab. Clin. Med.* **64**, 694–705.

——, ——, Sturgeon, P. and Day, R. W. (1965). A new genetic abnormality resulting in galactose-1-phosphate uridyl transferase deficiency. *Lancet* **1**, 353–4.

——, ——, —— and —— (1966). The genetics of galactose-1-phosphate uridyl transferase deficiency. *J. Lab. Clin. Med.* **68**, 646–58.

Brandt, N. J. (1967). Frequency of heterozygotes for hereditary galactosemia in a normal population. *Acta Genet. (Basel)* **17**, 289–98.

——, Froland, A., Mikkelsen, M., Nielsen, A. and Tolstrup, N. (1963). Galactosaemia locus and the Down's chromosome. *Lancet* **2**, 700–3.

Bray, P. T., Isaac, R. J. and Watkins, A. G. (1952). Galactosaemia. *Arch. Dis. Child.* **27**, 341–7.

Bricarelli, F. D., Magnani, M., Arslanian, A., Camera, G., Coviello, D. A., Di Pietro, P. and Dallapiccola, B. (1981). Expression of GALT in two unrelated 9p− patients. Evidence for the assignment of the GALT locus to the 9p21 band. *Hum. Genet.* **59**, 112–14.

Chacko, C. M., Christian, J. C. and Nadler, H. L. (1971). Unstable galactose-1-phosphate uridyl transferase: a new variant of galactosemia. *J. Pediatr.* **78**, 454–60.

——, Wappner, R. S., Brandt, I. K. and Nadler, H. L. (1977). The Chicago variant of clincal galactosaemia. *Humangenetik* **37**, 261–70.

Christensen, E. and Brandt, N. J. (1978). Prenatal and postnatal diagnostic difficulties in a family with rare alleles of the galactose-1-phosphate uridyl transferase locus. *J. Inher. Metab. Dis.* **1**, 167–9.

Cox, P. J. N. and Pugh, R. J. P. (1954). Galactosaemia. *Br. Med. J.* **2**, 613–18.

Cusworth, D. C., Dent, C. E. and Flynn, F. V. (1955). The aminoaciduria in galactosaemia. *Arch. Dis. Child.* **30**, 150–4.

Dale, G. L. and Popják, G. (1976). Purification of normal and inactive galactosemic galactose-1-phosphate uridyl transferase from human red cells. *J.*

Biol. Chem. **251**, 1057–63.

Donnell, G. N., Bergren, W. R., Bretthauer, M. S. and Hansen, R. G. (1960). The enzymatic expression of heterozygosity in families of children with galactosemia. *Pediatrics* **25**, 572–81.

——, Collado, M. and Koch, R. (1961). Growth and development of children with galactosemia. *J. Pediatr.* **58**, 836–44.

——, Koch, R. and Bergren, W. R. (1969). Observations on results of management of galactosemic patients. In *Galactosemia*, ed. Hsia, D. Y. Y. p. 247. Charles C. Thomas, Springfield, Illinois.

Fensom, A. H., Benson, P. F. and Blunt, S. (1974). Prenatal diagnosis of galactosaemia. *Br. Med. J.* **4**, 386–7.

——, ——, Rodeck, C. H., Campbell, S. and Gould, J. D. M. (1979). Prenatal diagnosis of galactosaemia heterozygote by a fetal blood enzyme assay. *Br. Med. J.* **1**, 21–2.

Fishler, K., Koch, R., Donnell, G. N. and Wenz, E. (1980). Developmental aspects of galactosemia from infancy to childhood. *Clin. Pediatr.* **19**, 38–44.

Fox, M., Thier, S., Rosenberg, L. and Segal, S. (1964). Impaired renal rubular function induced by sugar infusion in man. *J. Clin. Endocrinol.* **24**, 1318–27.

Gitzelmann, R. (1967). Hereditary galactokinase deficiency, a newly recognised cause of juvenile cataracts. *Pediatr. Res.* **1**, 14–23.

—— and Hadorn, R. (1961). Zur biochemischen Genetik der Galaktosamie. *Helv. Paediatr. Acta* **16**, 1–16.

——, Poley, J. R. and Prader, A. (1967). Partial galactose-1-phosphate uridyltransferase deficiency due to a variant enzyme. *Helv. Paediatr. Acta* **22**, 252–7.

Göppert, F. (1917). Galaktosurie nach Milchzuckergabe bei angeborenem, familiärem, chronischem Leberleiden. *Berl. Klin. Wschr.* **54**, 473–7.

Hammersen, G., Houghton, S. and Levy, H. L. (1975). Rennes-like variant of galactosemia: clinical and biochemical studies. *J. Pediatr.* **87**, 50–7.

Hansen, R. G., Bretthauer, R. K., Mayes, J. and Nordin, J. H. (1964). Estimation of frequency of occurrence of galactosemia in the population. *Proc. Soc. Exp. Biol. Med.* **115**, 560–4.

Holzel, A. and Komrower, G. M. (1955). A study of the genetics of galactosaemia. *Arch. Dis. Child.* **30**, 155–9.

——, —— and Schwartz, V. (1957). Galactosemia. *Am. J. Med.* **22**, 703–11.

——, —— and Wilson, V. K. (1952). Aminoaciduria in galactosaemia. *Br. Med. J.* **1**, 194–5.

Hsia, D. Y.-Y. (1967). Clinical variants of galactosemia. *Metabolism* **16**, 419–37.

—— and Walker, F. A. (1961). Variability in the clinical manifestations of galactosemia. *J. Pediatr.* **59**, 872–83.

——, Huang, I. and Driscoll, S. G. (1958). The heterozygous carrier in galactosaemia. *Nature* **182**, 1389–90.

——, Inouye, T., Wong, P. and South, A. (1964). Studies on galactose oxidation in Down's syndrome. *New Engl. J. Med.* **270**, 1085–8.

Hugh-Jones, K., Newcombe, A. L. and Hsia, D. Y.-Y. (1960). The genetic mechanism of galactosaemia. *Arch. Dis. Child.* **35**, 521–8.

Ibarra, B., Vaca, G., Sánchez-Corona, J., Hernández, A., Ramirez, M. L. and Cantú, J. M. (1979). Los Angeles variant of galactose-1-phosphate uridyltransferase (E.C. 2.7.7.12) in a Mexican family. *Hum. Genet.* **48**, 121–4.

Isselbacher, K. J., Anderson, E. P., Kurahaski, K. and Kalckar, H. M. (1956).

Congenital galactosemia, a single enzymatic block in galactose metabolism. *Science* **123**, 635–6.

Jakobs, C., Warner, T. G., Sweetman, L. and Nyhan, W. L. (1984). Stable isotope dilution analysis of galactitol in amniotic fluid: an accurate approach to the prenatal diagnosis of galactosemia. *Pediatr. Res.* **18**, 714–18.

Kalckar, H. M., Anderson, E. P. and Isselbacher, K. J. (1956). Galactosemia, a congenital defect in a nucleotide transferase. *Biochem. Biophys. Acta* **20**, 262–8.

Kelly, S., Katz, S., Burns, J. and Boylan, J. (1970). Screening for galactosemia in New York State. *Public Health Rep.* **85**, 575–8.

——, Desjardins, L. and Khera, S. A. (1972). A Duarte variant with clinical signs. *J. Med. Genet.* **9**, 129–31.

Kirkman, H. N. and Bynum, E. (1959). Enzymic evidence of a galactosemic trait in parents and galactosemic children. *Ann. Hum. Genet.* **23**, 117–26.

Komrower, G. M. and Lee, D. H. (1970). Long term follow-up of galactosaemia. *Arch. Dis. Child.* **45**, 367–73.

——, Schwarz, V., Holzel, A. and Goldberg, L. (1956). A clinical and biochemical study of galactosaemia: a possible explanation of the nature of the biochemical lesion. *Arch. Dis. Child.* **31**, 254–64.

Krone, W., Wolf, U., Goedde, H. W. and Baitsch, H. (1965). Untersuchungen uber des Aktivitat der Galaktokinase in Blut von Normal-personen und von Patienten mit G_{DO}-Trisomie. *Hum. Genet.* **1**, 279–88.

Lang, A., Groebe, H., Hellkuhl, B. and Von Figura, K. (1980). A new variant of galactosaemia: galactose-1-phosphate uridyltransferase sensitive to product inhibition by glucose-1-phosphate. *Pediatr. Res.* **14**, 729–34.

Levy, H. L., Sepe, S. J., Walton, D. S., Shih, V. E., Hammersen, G., Houghton, S. and Beutler, E. (1978). Galactose-1-phosphate uridyltransferase deficiency due to Duarte/galactosemia combined variation: clinical and biochemical studies. *J. Pediatr.* **92**, 390–3.

McGuinness, R. and Saunders, R. A. (1967). Erthrocyte galactose-1-phosphate uridyltransferase and glucose-6-phosphate dehydrogenase activity in the population of the Rhondda Fach. *Clin. Chim. Acta* **46**, 221–6.

Mason, H. H. and Turner, M. E. (1935). Chronic galactemia: Report of a case with studies on carbohydrates. *Am. J. Dis. Child.* **50**, 359–74.

Mathai, C. K. and Beutler, E. (1966). Electrophoretic variation in galactose-1-phosphate uridyltransferase. *Science* **154**, 1179–80.

Matz, D., Enzenauer, J. and Menne, F. (1975). Uber einen Fall von atypischer Galaktosämie. *Humangenetik* **27**, 309–13.

Mellman, W. J., Oski, F. A., Tedesco, T. A., Maciera-Coelho, A. and Harris, H. (1964). Leucocyte enzymes in Down's syndrome. *Lancet* **2**, 674–5.

——, Tedesco, T. A. and Baker, L. (1965). A new genetic abnormality (letter). *Lancet* **1**, 1395–6.

——, —— and Feigl, P. (1968). Estimation of the gene frequency of the Duarte variant of galactose-1-phosphate uridyl transferase. *Ann. Hum. Genet.* **32**, 1–8.

Mohandas, T., Sparkes, R. S., Sparkes, M. C. and Shulkin, J. D. (1977). Assignment of the human gene for galactose-1-phosphate uridyltransferase to chromosome 9: studies with Chinese hamster–human somatic cell hybrids. *Proc. Nat. Acad. Sci.* **74**, 5628–31.

——, ——, ——, ——, Toomey, K. E. and Funderburk, S. J. (1979). Regional localization of human gene loci on chromosome 9: studies of somatic cell hybrids containing human translocations. *Am. J. Hum. Genet.* **31**, 586–600.

Monk, A. M. and Holton, J. B. (1976). Galactose-1-phosphate uridyltransferase in cultured cells. *Clin. Chim. Acta* **73**, 537–46.

Mulcahy, M. T. and Wilson, R. G. (1980). Where is the gene for GALT? (letter). *Hum. Genet.* **54**, 129–30.

Nadler, H. L. (1968). Antenatal detection of hereditary disorders. *Pediatrics* **42**, 912–18.

——, Chacko, C. M. and Rachmeler, M. (1970). Interallelic complementation in hybrid cells derived from human diploid strains deficient in galactose-1-phosphate uridyltransferase activity. *Proc. Nat. Acad. Sci.* **67**, 976–82.

——, Inouye, T. and Hsia, D. Y.-Y. (1969). Clinical galactosemia: a study of fifty-five cases. In *Galactosemia*, ed. Hsia, D. Y.-Y. p. 127. Charles C. Thomas, Springfield, Illinois.

Ng, W. G., Bergren, W. R. and Donnell, G. N. (1964). Galactose-1-phosphate uridyltransferase assay by use of radioactive galactose-1-phosphate. *Clin. Chim. Acta* **10**, 337–43.

——, ——, Fields, M. and Donnell, G. N. (1969). An improved electrophoretic procedure for galactose-1-phosphate uridyltransferase: demonstration of multiple activity bands with the Duarte variant. *Biochem. Biophys. Res. Commun.* **37**, 354–62.

——, —— and Donnell, G. N. (1973). A new variant of galactose-1-phosphate uridyltransferase in man: the Los Angeles variant. *Ann. Hum. Genet.* **37**, 1–8.

——, Donnell, G. N., Bergren, W. R., Alfi, O. and Golbus, M. S. (1977). Prenatal diagnosis of galactosaemia. *Clin. Chim. Acta* **74**, 227–35.

Quan-Ma, R., Wells, H. J., Wells, W., Sherman, F. E. and Egan, T. J. (1966). Galactitol in the tissues of a galactosemic child. *Am. J. Dis. Child.* **112**, 477–8.

Robinson, A. (1963). The assay of galactokinase and galactose-1-phosphate uridyl transferase activity in human erythrocytes: a presumed test for hetero-zygous carriers of the galactosemic defect. *J. Exp. Med.* **118**, 359–70.

Rogers, S., Holtzapple, P. G., Mellman, W. J. and Segal, S. (1970). Characteristics of galactose-1-phosphate uridyltransferase in intestinal mucosa of normal and galactosemic humans. *Metabolism* **19**, 701–8.

Rosenberg, L. E., Weinberg, A. N. and Segal, S. (1961). The effect of high galactose diets on urinary excretion of amino-acids in the rat. *Biochim. Biophys. Acta* **48**, 500–5.

Rosner, F., Ong, B. H., Paine, R. S. and Mahanand, D. (1965). Biochemical differentiation of trisomic Down's syndrome (mongolism) from that due to translocation. *New Engl. J. Med.* **273**, 1356–61.

Russel, J. D. and De Mars, R. (1967). UDP-Glucose: αD-Galactose-1-phosphate uridyltransferase activity in cultured human fibroblasts. *Biochemical Genetics* **1**, 11–24.

Schapira, F. and Kaplan, J. C. (1969). Electrophoretic abnormality of galactose-1-phosphate uridyltransferase in galactosemia. *Biochem. Biophys. Res. Commun.* **35**, 451–5.

——, Gregori, C., Boue, J., Henrion, R., Vigneron, C. and Vidailhet, M. (1978). Prenatal diagnosis of galactosaemia. *Biomedicine* **29**, 136–8.

Schwarz, V. (1960). The value of galactose phosphate determinations in the treatment of galactosaemia. *Arch. Dis. Child.* **35**, 428–32.

——, Goldberg, L., Komrower, G. M. and Holzel, A. (1956). Some disturbances of erythrocyte metabolism in galactosaemia. *Biochem. J.* **62**, 34–40.

——, Wells, A. R., Holzel, A. and Komrower, G. M. (1961). A study of the genetics of galactosaemia. *Ann. Hum. Genet.* **25**, 179–88.

Segal, S. (1969). The Negro variant of congenital galactosemia. In *Galactosemia*, ed. Hsia, D. Y.-Y. p. 176. Charles C. Thomas, Springfield, Illinois.

—— and Cuatrecasas, P. (1968). The oxidation of ^{14}C galactose by patients with congenital galactosemia. Evidence for a direct oxidative pathway. *Am. J. Med.* **44**, 340–7.

——, Blair, A. and Roth, H. (1965). The metabolism of galactose by patients with congenital galactosemia. *Am. J. Med.* **38**, 62–70.

——, Rogers, S. and Holtzapple, P. G. (1971). Liver galactose-1-phosphate uridyltransferase: activity in normal and galactosemic subjects. *J. Clin. Invest.* **50**, 500–6.

Shih, V. E., Levy, H. L., Karolkewicz, V., Houghton, S., Efron, M. L., Isselbacher, K. J., Beutler, E. and MacCready, R. A. (1971). Galactosemia screening of newborns in Massachusetts. *New Engl. J. Med.* **284**, 753–7.

Shin, Y. S., Endres, W., Rieth, M. and Schaub, J. (1983). Prenatal diagnosis of galactosemia and properties of galactose-1-phosphate uridyltransferase in erythrocytes of galactosemic variants as well as in human fetal and adult organs. *Clin. Chim. Acta* **128**, 271–81.

Sparkes, R. S., Sparkes, M. C., Funderburk, S. J. and Moedjono, S. (1979). Expression of galactose-1-P uridyltransferase in patients with chromosome alterations affecting 9p: assignment of the locus to p11–22 (abs.). *Cytogenet. Cell Genet.* **25**, 209.

——, Epstein, P. A., Kidd, K. K., Klisak, I., Sparkes, M. C., Crist, M. and Morton, L. A. (1980a). Probable linkage between the human galactose-1-P uridyl transferase locus and 9qh. *Am. J. Hum. Genet.* **32**, 188–93.

——, Sparkes, M. C., Funderburk, S. J. and Moedjono, S. (1980b). Expression of GALT in 9p chromosome alterations: assignment of GALT locus to 9 cen→9p22. *Ann. Hum. Genet.* **43**, 343–7.

Tedesco, T. A. (1972). Human galactose-1-phosphate uridyltransferase: purification, antibody production, and comparison of the wild type, Duarte variant, and galactosemic gene products. *J. Biol. Chem.* **247**, 6631–6.

—— and Mellman, W. J. (1969). Galactose-1-phosphate uridyl transferase and galctokinase activity in cultured human diploid fibroblasts and peripheral blood leukocytes. I. Analysis of transferase genotypes by the ratio of the activities of the two enzymes. *J. Clin. Invest.* **48**, 2390–7.

—— and —— (1971). Galactosemia: evidence for a structural gene mutation. *Science* **172**, 727–8.

——, Miller, K. L., Rawnsley, B. E., Mennuti, M. T., Spielman, R. S. and Mellman, W. J. (1975b). Human erythrocyte galactokinase and galactose-1-phosphate uridyltransferase: a population survey. *Am. J. Hum. Genet.* **27**, 737–47.

——, Wu, J. W., Boches, F. S. and Mellman, W. J. (1975a). The genetic defect in galactosemia. *New Engl. J. Med.* **292**, 737–40.

Thier, S., Fox, M., Rosenberg, L. and Segal, S. (1964). Hexose inhibition of amino acid uptake in the rat-kidney-cortex slice. *Biochim. Biophys. Acta* **93**, 106–15.

Topper, Y. J., Laster, L. and Segal, S. (1962). Galactose metabolism: phenotype

differences among tissues of a patient with congenital galactosemia. *Nature* **196**, 1106.
Walker, F. A., Hsia, D. Y.-Y., Slatis, H. M. and Steinberg, A. G. (1962). Galactosemia: a study of 27 kindreds in North America. *Ann. Hum. Genet.* **25**, 287–311.

Hereditary tyrosinaemia I (hepatorenal type or tyrosinosis)

There are a number of disorders of tyrosine catabolism including a transient, harmless tyrosinaemia of the new-born and several inherited diseases including a form of tyrosinosis reported by Medes (1932) in a single patient previously diagnosed as having myasthenia gravis. She postulated that *p*-hydroxyphenylpyruvic acid oxidase was deficient, but La Du and Gjessing (1972) have argued that a tyrosine aminotransferase defect is more likely. Cytosol tyrosine aminotransferase is certainly defective in tyrosinaemia II (Richner–Henhart syndrome), the form of tyrosinaemia associated with skin and corneal lesions and mental subnormality, but without liver or renal disease (Wadman *et al.* 1968; Fellman *et al.* 1969; Kennaway and Buist 1971; Goldsmith *et al.* 1973). Tyrosinaemia may also be secondary to liver disease of any cause.

Hereditary tyrosinaemia of hepato-renal type (tyrosinosis or tyrosinaemia I) is distinct from all of the above disorders. The earliest description was probably that of Baber (1956). Further reports followed from Sakai and colleagues (1957a and b, 1959), Lelong and coworkers (1961, 1963), Gentz and fellow researchers (Fritzell *et al.* 1964; Gentz *et al.* 1965), Scriver and coauthors (1967), and many others. Over 100 case reports were reviewed by La Du and Gjessing (1978).

The clinical picture is of a child with failure to thrive, diarrhoea and vomiting, hepatosplenomegaly, and later rickets. Mental subnormality of mild degree has been observed in only some cases. A more acute onset within the first months of life has also been reported (Gjessing and Halvorsen 1965; Gaull *et al.* 1968) but typically onset is later and of slower progression. Some cases develop acute porphyria-like clinical attacks and biochemical changes (Strife *et al.* 1977).

Investigation reveals nodular cirrhosis of the liver which may progress to malignant hepatoma (Lelong *et al.* 1963; Weinber *et al.* 1976), and a Fanconi-like renal tubular defect with hypophosphataemia, hyperphosphaturia and rickets, aminoaciduria, glycosuria, and proteinuria (Gentz *et al.* 1965). There is tyrosinaemia and tyrosyluria, and also methioninaemia and marked excretion of *p*-hydroxyphenyllactic acid *p*-hydroxyphenyl pyruvic acid. On histology of the kidneys there is swelling and degeneration of renal tubular cells, and in one case hyperplasia and hypertrophy of the juxtaglomerular apparatus (Jevtic *et al.* 1974).

Numerous studies have found reduced activity of *p*-hydroxyphenylpyruvate oxidase in the liver (Sakai *et al.* 1959; Gentz *et al.* 1965; La Du 1967; Scriver *et al.* 1967), but this is probably not the primary defect (Woolf 1976; Gaull *et al.* 1968, 1970; La Du and Gjessing 1972). Lindblad and colleagues (1977) have postulated a deficiency of fumaryl-acetoacetate hydrolase as the primary defect on the basis of increased serum and urinary succinylacetoacetate and succinylacetone. Succinyl-acetone is a known inhibitor of porphobilinogen synthetase. Deficient hepatic activity of fumarylacetoacetate hydrolase has been confirmed by several workers (Kvittingen *et al.* 1981; Furukawa *et al.* 1984; Gray *et al.* 1981; Stoner *et al.* 1984). Furukawa and colleagues reported one case in which hepatic enzyme activity was normal, but activity in the kidney was deficient, suggesting genetic heterogeneity. Stoner and colleagues observed hepatic and erythrocytic glutathione deficiency in their patient, presumably secondary to interaction of glutathione with the excess fumarylacetoacetate.

The acute and chronic forms of hereditary tyrosinaemia occur within the same family and show an autosomal recessive pattern of inheritance (Gentz *et al.* 1965; Dallaire 1967). The frequency of the disease in the Chicoutimi–Lac St Jean district of Quebec has been estimated at 14.6 cases per 10 000 population, giving a carrier frequency of 1 in 14 (Bergeron *et al.* 1974). Consanguinity was frequent among the parents of affected children in this French-Canadian population and the authors produce evidence for a founder effect. Despite the recent claims that the basic enzymatic defect involves fumarylacetoacetate hydrolase there are not as yet any reports of the use of enzyme assay in carrier detection. Gagne and associates (1982) reported prenatal diagnosis from measurement of succinylacetone in amniotic fluid. Pettit and coworkers (1984) reported using gas chromatography–mass spectrometry to assay succinylacetone in urine for the diagnosis and monitoring of type 1 hereditary tyrosinaemia, and suggested that similar assays on amniotic fluid could be used for prenatal diagnosis. Malpuech and colleagues (1981) reported the disease in a child with partial deletion of the short arm of one chromosome 4 and suggest that the gene for *p*-hydroxy-phenylpyruvate oxidase is on 4p.

References

Baber, M. D. (1956). A case of congenital cirrhosis of the liver with renal tubular defects akin to those in the Fanconi syndrome. *Arch. Dis. Child.* **31**, 335–9.

Bergeron, P., Laberge, C. and Grenier, A. (1974). Hereditary tyrosinemia in the province of Quebec: prevalence at birth and geographic distribution. *Clin. Genet.* **5**, 157–62.

Dallaire, L. (1967). Genetic aspects of tyrosinemia. *Can. Med. Assoc. J.* **97**, 1098–9.

Fellman, J. H., Vanbellinghen, P. J., Jones, R. T. and Koler, R. D. (1969). Soluble and mitochondrial forms of tyrosine transaminase: relationship to human tyrosinemia. *Biochemistry* **8**, 615–22.

Fritzell, S., Jagenburg, O. R. and Schnürer, L. B. (1964). Familial cirrhosis of the liver, renal tubular defects with rickets and impaired tyrosine metabolism. *Acta Paediatr.* **53**, 18–32.

Furukawa, N., Hayano, T., Sato, N., Inoue, F., Machida, Y., Kinugasa, A., Imashuku, S., Kusunoki, T. and Takamatisu, T. (1984). The enzyme defects in hereditary tyrosinaemia type I. *J. Inher. Metab. Dis.* **7** (Suppl. 2), 137–8.

Gagné, R., Lescault, A., Grenier, A., Laberge, C., Mélancon, S. B. and Dallaire, L. (1982). Prenatal diagnosis of hereditary tyrosinaemia: measurement of succinylacetone in amniotic fluid. *Prenatal Diagnosis* **2**, 185–8.

Gaull, G. E., Rassin, D. K. and Sturman, J. A. (1968). Significance of hypermethionaemia in acute tyrosinosis (letter). *Lancet* **1**, 1318–19.

——, ——, Solomon, G. E., Harris, R. C. and Sturman, J. A. (1970). Biochemical observations on so-called hereditary tyrosinemia. *Pediatr. Res.* **4**, 337–44.

Gentz, J., Jagenburg, R. and Zetterstrom, R. (1965). Tyrosinemia. An inborn error of tyrosine metabolism with cirrhosis of the liver and multiple renal tubular defects (de Toni–Debré–Fanconi syndrome). *J. Pediatr.* **66**, 670–96.

Gjessing, L. R. and Halvorsen, S. (1965). Hypermethioninaemia in acute tyrosinosis (letter). *Lancet* **2**, 1132–3.

Goldsmith, L. A., Kang, E., Bienfang, D. C., Jimbow, K., Gerald, P. and Baden, H. P. (1973). Tyrosinemia with plantar and palmar keratosis and keratitis. *J. Pediatr.* **83**, 798–805.

Gray, R. G. F., Patrick, A. D., Preston, F. E. and Whitefield, M. F. (1981). Acute hereditary tyrosinaemia type I: clinical biochemical and haematological studies in twins. *J. Inher. Metab. Dis.* **4**, 37–40.

Jevtic, M. M., Thorp, F. K. and Hruban, Z. (1974). Hereditary tyrosinemia with hyperplasia and hypertrophy of juxtaglomerular apparatus. *Am. J. Clin. Pathol.* **61**, 423–37.

Kennaway, N. G. and Buist, N. R. M. (1971). Metabolic studies in a patient with hepatic cytosol tyrosine aminotransferase deficiency. *Pediatr. Res.* **5**, 287–97.

Kvittingen, E. A., Jellum, E. and Stokke, O. (1981). Assay of fumarylacetoacetate fumarylhydrolase in human liver—deficient activity in a case of hereditary tyrosinemia. *Clin. Chim. Acta* **115**, 311–19.

La Du, B. N. (1967). The enzymatic deficiency in tyrosinemia. *Am. J. Dis. Child.* **113**, 54–7.

—— and Gjessing, L. R. (1972). Tyrosinosis and tyrosinemia. In *The metabolic basis of inherited disease*, 3rd edn. eds. Stanbury, J. B., Wyngaarden, J. B. and Fredrickson, D. S. pp. 256–67. McGraw-Hill, New York.

—— and —— (1978). Tyrosinosis and tyrosinemia. In *The metabolic basis of inherited disease*, 4th edn. eds. Stanbury, J. B., Wyngaarden, J. B. and Frederickson, D. S. p. 256. McGraw-Hill, New York.

Lelong, M., Algagille, D., Le Tan Vinh, Colin, J., Roux, M., Gentil, C. and Gabilan, J.-C. (1961). Cirrhose congénitale et familiale, rachitisme vitamino-résistant avec diabete glucophosphoaminé, hépatome terminal. *Pédriatrie* **16**, 221–9.

——, ——, Gentil, C. I., Colin, J., Le Tan Vinh and Gabilan, J.-C. (1963). Cirrhose congénitale et familiale avec diabete phospho-gluco-aminé, rachitisme vitamine-D résistant et tyrosinurie massive. *Rev. Fr. Étude Clin. Biol.* **8**, 37–50.

Lindblad, B., Lindstedt, S. and Steen, G. (1977). On the enzymic defects in hereditary tyrosinemia. *Proc. Nat. Acad. Sci.* **74**, 4641–5.

Malpuech, G., Mattei, J. F., Gaulme, J., Palcoux, J. B., Lesec, G. and Vanlieferinghen, P. (1981). Association, chez le meme sujet, d'une deletion du bras court du chromosome 4 (4p−) et d'un deficit complet en parahydroxy-phenylpyruvate oxydase hepatique (tyrosinase). *J. Genet. Hum.* **29**, 455–61.

Medes, G. (1932). A new error of tyrosine metabolism: tyrosinosis. The intermediary metabolism of tyrosine and phenylalanine. *Biochem. J.* **26**, 917–40.

Pettit, B. R., MacKenzie, F., King, G. S. and Leonard, J. V. (1984). The antenatal diagnosis and aid to the management of hereditary tyrosinaemia by use of a specific GC-MS assay for succinylacetone. *J. Inher. Metab. Dis.* **7** (Suppl. 2), 135–6.

Sakai, K. and Kitagawa, T. (1957a). An atypical case of tyrosinosis. Part I. Clinical and laboratory findings. *Jikeikai Med. J.* **4**, 1.

—— and —— (1957b). An atypical case of tyrosinosis. II. A research on the metabolic block. *Jikeikai Med. J.* **4**, 11.

——, —— and Yoshioka, K. (1959). An atypical case of tyrosinosis. III. The outcome of the patient: pathological and biochemical observations on the organ tissues. *Jikeikai Med. J.* **6**, 15–24.

Scriver, C. R., Larochelle, J. and Silverberg, M. (1967). Hereditary tyrosinemia and tyrosyluria in a French-Canadian geographic isolate. *Am. J. Dis. Child.* **113**, 41–6.

Stoner, E., Starkman, H., Wellner, D., Wellner, V. P., Sassa, S., Rifkind, A. B., Grenier, A., Steinherz, P. G., Meister, A., New, M. I. and Levine, L. S. (1984). Biochemical studies of a patient with hereditary hepatorenal tyrosinemia: evidence of glutathione deficiency. *Pediatr. Res.* **18**, 1332–6.

Strife, C. F., Zuroweste, E. L. Emmett, E. A., Finelli, V. N., Petering, H. G. and Berry, H. K. (1977). Tyrosinemia with acute intermittent porphyria: amino-levulinic acid dehydratase deficiency related to elevated urinary aminolevulinic acid levels. *J. Pediatr.* **90**, 400–4.

Wadman, S. K., Van Sprang, F. J., Maas, J. W. and Ketting, D. (1968). An exceptional case of tyrosinosis. *J. Ment. Defic. Res.* **12**, 269–81.

Weinber, A. G., Mize, C. E. and Worthen, H. G. (1976). Occurrence of hepatoma in chronic form of hereditary tyrosinemia. *J. Pediatr.* **88**, 434–8.

Woolf, L. I. (1966). Inborn hepato-renal dysfunction. In *Symposium on tyrosinosis in honour of Dr Grace Medes*, 2–3 June, 1965, ed. Gjessing, L. R. pp. 82–91. Universitetsforlaget, Oslo.

Familial lecithin: cholesterol acyltransferase deficiency (Norum's disease)

This is a rare disorder of lipid metabolism many cases of which have been reported from a single isolated area of Norway. The first reported family with this disorder consisted of three affected sisters described by Norum and Gjone (Norum and Gjone 1967; Gjone and Norum 1968; Torsvik *et al.* 1968). Subsequently three further Norwegian (Norum *et al.* 1970; Gjone *et al.* 1974a and b, 1981) and a Swedish family (Hamnstrom *et al.* 1969) have been reported. The disease is characterized clinically by corneal opacities in the form of a peripheral arcus of fine dots (Gjone and Bergaust 1969); normochromic anaemia with reduced red-cell half-life, increased lecithin and unesterified cholesterol content, and target-cell appearance (Gjone *et al.* 1968; Gjone 1974); sea-blue histiocytes with a lamellar ultrastructure (Jacobsen *et al.* 1972); early atherosclerosis (Gjone 1974); and renal disease.

On lipid electrophoresis the pre-β-lipoprotein band is absent and the α_1-band absent or faint. In most patients there is hypertriglyceridaemia, and in all there is low plasma cholesteryl ester and lysolethicin, high unesterified cholesterol and lecithin, and increased heterogeneity of lipoprotein fractions (Glomset *et al.* 1973).

Deficient activity of plasma lecithin: cholesterol acyltransferase (LCAT) was reported in the original family (Norum and Gjone 1967; Torsvik *et al.* 1968), and is not due to inhibitors (Norum and Gjone 1967), nor to any lack of activators of LCAT (Alaupovic *et al.* 1974). Glomset and colleagues (1980) have made a detailed study of the lipo-protein changes (Glomset *et al.* 1980; Mitchell *et al.* 1980).

The initial renal abnormality is proteinuria, often associated with red cells and hyaline casts in the urine, detectable from early in life. This proteinuria persists at a moderate degree until, typically in the fourth–fifth decades, there is a marked increase in proteinuria accompanied by a falling serum albumin and deteriorating renal function (Gjone 1974). On renal biopsy foam cells are observed in the glomerular tufts, associated with increased amounts of unesterified cholesterol and phospholipid in the glomeruli (Stokke *et al.* 1974). In addition there are abnormalities of the capillary wall and of the renal arterioles and arteries including lipid accumulation (Hovig and Gjone 1973, 1974). Gjone and his co-authors (1978) have pointed out that similar renal changes have been reported in association with the relative LCAT deficiency of obstructive jaundice (Blomhoff *et al.* 1975). Renal transplantation will restore renal function for at least several years (Flatmark *et al.* 1977) but does not raise plasma LCAT levels.

The pattern of affected sibs and the common ancestral origins of the Norwegian families strongly suggest autosomal recessive inheritance. The pattern of inheritance in other parts of the world is also consistent with autosomal recessive determination (Utermann *et al.* 1972; Bethel *et al.* 1975; Bron *et al.* 1975; Salmon *et al.* 1976; Chevet *et al.* 1978; Fröhlich *et al.* 1978; Iwamoto *et al.* 1978). In Norway a single mutational event occurring earlier than the year 1700 is indicated, leading to a con-temporary gene frequency, in the region of the country involved, of about 0.02, and a carrier frequency of 4 per cent (Teisberg and Gjone 1974; Teisberg *et al.* 1975). The same authors have detected close linkage of the LCAT deficiency gene to the haptoglobin gene with a lod score of

3.41 at $\theta = 0.000$ and linkage disequilibrium with an association of the LCAT deficiency allele with the Hp[IS] allele. This close linkage implies that the LCAT gene is on chromosome 16, through the existing assignment of haptoglobin.

Albers and colleagues have studied the relationship of LCAT mass to activity in Sardinian families, and have obtained evidence that this varies between different LCAT-deficient families, indicating interallelic genetic heterogeneity (Albers *et al.* 1981a and b; Albers and Utermann 1981; Utermann *et al.* 1981). They have also demonstrated reduced LCAT activity in heterozygotes, although other workers have failed to do so in families from other areas. Frohlich and co-authors (1982) identified heterozygotes in a Canadian family. Teisberg and Gjone (1981) have also produced evidence of genetic heterogeneity.

References

Alaupovic, P., McConathy, W. J., Curry, M. D., Magnani, H. N., Torsvic, H., Berg, K. and Gjone, E. (1974). Apoliproproteins and lipoprotein families in familial lecithin: cholesterol acyltransferase deficiency. *Scand. J. Clin. Lab. Invest.* **33**, Suppl. 137, 83–7.

Albers, J. J. and Utermann, G. (1981). Genetic control of lecithin: cholesterol acyltransferase: measurement of LCAT mass in a large kindred with LCAT deficiency. *Am. J. Hum. Genet.* **33**, 702–8.

——, Adolphson, J. L. and Chen, C. H. (1981a). Radioimmunoassay of human plasma lecithin: cholesterol acyltransferase. *J. Clin. Invest.* **67**, 141–8.

——, Chen, C.-H. and Adolphson, J. L. (1981b). Familial lecithin: cholesterol acyltransferase: identification of heterozygotes with half-normal enzyme activity and mass. *Hum. Genet.* **58**, 306–9.

Bethell, W., McCullough, C. and Ghosh, M. (1975). Lecithin: cholesterol acyltransferase deficiency. Light and electron microscopic findings from two corneas. *Can. J. Ophthalmol.* **10**, 494–501.

Blomhoff, J. P., Holme, R., Hovig, T., Flatmark, A. and Gjone, E. (1975). Lipid deposition in the kidneys in hepatorenal syndrome. A pathogenic factor? (abs.). *Digestion* **12**, 250–1.

Bron, A. F., Lloyd, J. K., Forsbrooke, A. S., Winder, A. F. and Tripathi, R. C. (1975). Primary L.C.A.T.-deficiency disease (letter). *Lancet* **1**, 928–9.

Chevet, D., Ramée, P. L., Le Pogamp, P., Thomas, R., Garré, M. and Alcindor, L. G. (1978). Hereditary lecithin: cholesterol acyltransferase deficiency: report of a new family with two afflicted sisters. *Nephron* **20**, 212–19.

Flatmark, A. L., Hovig, T., Myhre, E. and Gjone, E. (1977). Renal transplantation in patients with familial lecithin: cholesterol-acyltransferase deficiency. *Transplant. Proc.* **9**, 1665–71.

Frohlich, J., Godolphin, W. J., Reeve, C. E. and Evelyn, K. (1978). Familial LCAT deficiency. Report of two patients from a Canadian family of Italian and Swedish descent. *Scand. J. Clin. Lab. Invest.* **38**, Suppl. 150, 156–61.

——, Hon, K. and McLeod, R. (1982). Detection of heterozygotes for familial lecithin: cholesterol acyltransferase (LCAT) deficiency. *Am. J. Hum. Genet.* **34**, 65–72.

Gjone, E. (1974). Familial lecithin: cholesterol acyltransferase deficiency: a clinical survey. *Scan. J. Clin. Lab. Invest.* **33**, Suppl. 137, 73–82.

—— and Bergaust, B. (1969). Corneal opacity in familial plasma cholesterol ester deficiency. *Acta Ophthalmol.* **47**, 222–7.

—— and Norum, K. R. (1968). Familial serum cholesterol ester deficiency. A clinical study of a patient with a new syndrome. *Acta. Med. Scand.* **183**, 107–12.

——, Torsvik, H. and Norum, K. R. (1968). Familial Plasma cholesterol ester deficiency: a study of the erythrocytes. *Scand. J. Clin. Lab. Invest.* **21**, 327–32.

——, Skarbovik, A. J., Blomhoff, J. P. and Teisberg, P. (1974a). Familial lecithin: cholesterol acyltransferase deficiency: report of a third Norwegian family with two affected members. *Scand. J. Clin. Lab. Invest.* **33**, Suppl. 137, 101–8.

——, Blomhoff, J. P. and Skarbovik, A. J. (1974b). Possible association between an abnormal low density lipoprotein and nephropathy in lecithin: cholesterol acyltransferase deficiency. *Clin. Chim. Acta* **54**, 11–18.

——, Norum, K. R. and Glomset, J. A. (1978). Familial lecithin: cholesterol acyltransferase deficiency. In *The metabolic basis of inherited disease*, 4th edn. eds. Stanbury, J. B., Wyngaarden, J. B. and Fredrickson, D. S. pp. 589–603. McGraw-Hill, New York.

——, Blomhoff, J. P., Holme, R., Hovig, T., Olaisen, B., Skarbovik, A. J. and Teisberg, P. (1981). Familial lecithin: cholesterol acyltransferase deficiency: report of a fourth family from North Western Norway. *Acta Med. Scand.* **210**, 3–6.

Glomset, J. A., Nichols, A. V., Norum, K. R., King, W. and Forte, I. (1973). Plasma lipoproteins in familial lecithin: cholesterol acyltransferase deficiency: further studies of very low density lipoprotein abnormalities. *J. Clin. Invest.* **52**, 1078–92.

——, Applegate, K., Forte, T., King, W. C., Mitchell, C. D., Norum, K. R. and Gjone, E. (1980). Abnormalities in lipoproteins of $d < 1.006$ g/ml in familial lecithin: cholesterol acyltransferase deficiency. *J. Lipid Res.* **21**, 1116–27.

Hamnstrom, B., Gjone, E. and Norum, K. R. (1969). Familial plasma lecithin: cholesterol acyltransferase deficiency. *Br. Med. J.* **2**, 283–6.

Hovig, T. and Gjone, E. (1973). Familial lecithin: cholesterol acyltransferase (LCAT) deficiency: ultrastructural aspects of a new syndrome with particular reference to lesions in the kidneys and spleen. *Acta Pathol. Microbiol. Scand.* **81**, 681–97.

—— and —— (1974). Familial lecithin: cholesterol acyltransferase deficiency: ultrastructural studies on lipid deposition and tissue reactions. *Scand. J. Clin. Invest.* **33**, Suppl. 137, 135–46.

Iwamoto, A., Naito, C., Teramoto, T., Katu, H., Kako, M., Kariya, T., Shimizu, T., Oka, H. and Oda, T. (1978). Familial lecithin: cholesterol acyltransferase deficiency complicated with unconjugated hyperbilirubinemia and peripheral neuropathy. The first reported cases in the Far East. *Acta Med. Scand.* **204**, 219–27.

Jacobsen, C. D., Gjone, E. and Hovig, T. (1972). Sea-blue histiocytes in familial lecithin: cholesterol acyltransferase deficiency. *Scand. J. Haematol.* **9**, 106–13.

Mitchell, C. D., King, W. C., Applegate, K. R., Forte, T., Glomset, J. A., Norum,

K. R. and Gjone, E. (1980). Characterization of apolipoprotein in E-rich high density lipoproteins in familial lecithin: cholesterol acyltransferase deficiency. *J. Lip. Res.* **21**, 625–34.

Norum, K. R. and Gjone, E. (1967). Familial plasma lecithin: cholesterol acyltransferase deficiency: biochemical study of a new inborn error of metabolism. *Scand. J. Clin. Lab. Invest.* **20**, 231–43.

——, Borsting, S. and Grundt, I. (1970). Familial lecithin: cholesterol acyltransferase deficiency. *Acta Med. Scand.* **188**, 323–6.

Salmon, S., Alcindor, L.-G., Beucler, I., Ayrault-Jarrier, M., Infante, R., Chevet, D. and Polonovski, J. (1976). Etude immunoelectrophorique des lipoproteines plasmatiques dans un cas de deficience familiale en lecithine–cholesterol acyltransferase. *Clin. Chim. Acta* **66**, 311–18.

Stokke, K. T., Bjerve, K. S., Blomhoff, J. P., Oystese, B., Flatmark, A., Norum, K. R. and Gjone, E. (1974). Familial lecithin: cholesterol acyltransferase deficiency: studies on lipid compositions and morphology of tissues. *Scand. J. Clin. Invest.* **33**, Suppl. 137, 93–100.

Teisberg, P. and Gjone, E. (1974). Probable linkage of LCAT locus in man to the haptoglobin locus on chromosome 16. *Nature* **249**, 550–1.

—— and —— (1981). Genetic heterogeneity in familial lecithin: cholesterol acyltransferase (LCAT) deficiency. *Acta Med. Scand.* **210**, 1–2.

——, —— and Olaisen, B. (1975). Genetics of LCAT (lecithin: cholesterol acyltransferase) deficiency. *Ann. Hum. Genet.* **38**, 327–31.

Torsvik, H., Gjone, E. and Norum, K. R. (1968). Familial plasma cholesterol ester deficiency: clinical studies in a family. *Acta Med. Scand.* **183**, 387–91.

Utermann, G., Schoenborn, W., Langer, K. H. and Diecker, P. (1972). Lipoproteins in LCAT deficiency. *Humangenetik* **16**, 295–306.

——, Menzel, H. J., Diecker, P., Langer, K. H. and Fiorelli, G. (1981). Lecithin-cholesterol–acyltransferase deficiency: autosomal recessive transmission in a large kindred. *Clin. Gent.* **19**, 448–55.

Hypophosphatasia

Hypophosphatasia is a rare familial disease first described under this name by Rathbun (1948), although his is not the first description of the disease. Historical reviews have been provided by several authors (Fraser 1957; Rasmussen 1983). Fraser estimated the incidence at 1 in 100 000 live births.

Fraser and subsequent workers recognized three clinical variants of hypophosphatasia. Type 1, the infantile and most common type, shows perinatal onset, failure to thrive, severe rickets with gross bone disorganization, craniostenosis, hypercalcaemia, and death in more than half of cases within the first year or two. Type 2, the childhood type, shows a later more gradual onset with premature loss of deciduous teeth and less severe rackitic changes. Type 3, the adult type, may be a chance asymptomatic biochemical finding or there may be a history of childhood rickets (Bethune and Dent 1960). Pseudohypophosphatasia with the characteristic skeletal changes but normal biochemical findings has been reported in the same family as patients with true hypophosphatasia (Méhes *et al.* 1972), suggesting that it is a variant of the same genetic defect.

Patients, especially those with the infantile type, with hypercalcaemia may develop evidence of renal failure and of nephrocalcinosis (Chown 1935/1936; Engfeldt and Zetterstrom 1954). It is one of several inherited disorders in which nephrocalcinosis occurs, listed in Table 4.7.

Biochemically alkaline phosphatase levels in serum and tissues are low (Rathbun 1948). There is some dispute as to exactly which tissue alkaline phosphatases are deficient, partially due to the fact that different tissues contain differing mixtures of isoenzymes. One isoenzyme common to liver, bone, spleen and kidney shows immunological identity (Boyer 1963), and it is these tissues that principally show deficiency. The

Table 4.7. *Inherited diseases with nephrocalcinosis*

Disease	Primary defect	Mode of inheritance	Page no.
Hypophosphatasia	Serum and tissue alkaline phosphatase deficiency	AR	167
Hyperoxaluria, type 1	Peroxisomal alanine: glyoxylate aminotransferase deficiency, at least in pyridoxine-resistant form	AR	188
Hyperoxaluria, type 2	D-glyceric dehydrogenase deficiency	AR	191
Arthrogryposis multiplex with renal and hepatic abnormality	?	XR	272
Renal tubular acidosis, type I:			
(a) San Francisco syndrome	Distal tubular acidification defect	AD	279
(b) Philadelphia syndrome	Distal tubular acidification defect with hypocitratruria	AD	279
(c) Atlanta syndrome	Distal tubular hypercalciuria	AD	279
(d) Oklahoma syndrome	?	AD	279

Table 4.7.—*Continued*

Disease	Primary defect	Mode of inheritance	Page no.
Renal tubular acidosis with nerve deafness	Distal tubular defect, possibly associated in some families with a carbonic anhydrase defect	AR (genetically heterogeneous)	285
Renal tubular magnesium defect	?	Prob. AR	287
Blue diaper syndrome with hypercalcaemia	Defect in intestinal transport of tryptophan, with unknown cause of hypercalcaemia	Prob. AR	297
Nephrocalcinosis and azotaemia	?	AD or XD	382
Amelogenesis imperfecta and nephrocalcinosis	?	AR	384
Severe juvenile arterial sclerosis	?	AR	448
Williams syndrome	?	Prob. AD with variable penetrance	564

alkaline phosphatases of intestine and placenta appear not to be defective (Danovitch *et al.* 1968; Rattenbury *et al.* 1976). However, this enzyme deficiency is not necessarily the primary defect. The second main biochemical abnormality is excessive excretion of phosphoethanolamine (Fraser *et al.* 1955; McCance *et al.* 1955), and raised plasma phosphoethanolamine (Fraser *et al.* 1955).

The pathogenesis appears to involve poor calcification of cartilage (Fraser and Yendt 1955), and to be a local tissue defect unrelated to any serum factor (Engfeldt and Zetterstrom 1954; McCance *et al.* 1956), presumably involving a deficiency of bone alkaline phosphatase. In normal bone mineralization alkaline phosphatase is present within matrix vesicles and calcification proceeds within these vesicles. It is as yet unclear whether the failure of mineralization in hypophosphatasia is due to an absence of matrix vesicles or whether the vesicles are present but lack alkaline phosphatase and thus do not accumulate phosphate necessary for the function of calcium phosphate (Rasmussen 1983).

Evidence in favour of a defective alkaline phosphatase as the primary defect, in at least some cases, comes from the observation of enzyme with an altered Km for phosphorylethanolamine and increased heat lability in a patient with pseudohypophosphatasia (Scriver and Cameron 1969). The increased excretion of phosphoethanolamine, and also of inorganic pyrophosphate (Russel 1965; Bongionvanni *et al.* 1968), indicates that these substances are natural substrates for alkaline phosphatase. However, the cause of the hypercalcaemia and hyper-calcinuria seen in some patients is still obscure.

A number of family studies have confirmed the autosomal recessive inheritance of hypophosphatasia on the basis of measurements of serum alkaline phosphatase and of urinary excretion of phosphoethanolamine and pyrophosphate (Fraser and Yendt 1955; McCance *et al.* 1956; Harris and Robson 1959; Rathbun *et al.* 1961; Pimstone *et al.* 1966; Bongiovanni *et al.* 1968; Rasmussen 1968; Méhes *et al.* 1972; Rubecz *et al.* 1974). Normal serum alkaline phosphatase levels alone do not exclude an affected homozygote (Pimstone *et al.* 1966; Eisenberg and Pimstone 1967; Scriver and Cameron 1969; Méhes *et al.* 1972).

Genetic heterogeneity is suggested by reports of the milder, childhood and adult, forms of the disease occuring in two to three generations suggestive of autosomal dominant inheritance (Silverman 1962; Pimstone *et al.* 1966; Poland *et al.* 1972; Whyte *et al.* 1979). Hetero-geneity is also reported by the finding of higher levels of alkaline phosphatase activity in less clinically severe cases (Fraser 1957; Blau *et al.* 1978.

Heterozygote detection is unreliable because of the varied factors that can cause increased phosphoethanolamine excretion (Whyte *et al.* 1979) and the fact, mentioned above, that serum alkaline phosphatase may be normal even in affected subjects. Nevertheless in typical families for type 1 heterozygotes have low serum alkaline phosphatase (Rathbun *et al.* 1961).

Prenatal diagnosis has been reported on the basis of ultrasound assess-ment of fetal bone calcification, especially of the skull (Beratis *et al.* 1976; Rudd *et al.* 1976), or of the measurement of alkaline phosphatase in amniotic fluid, or more reliably cultured amniotic fluid cells (Beratis *et al.* 1976; Hoar and Rudd 1976; Rattenbury *et al.* 1976; Rudd 1976; Blau *et al.* 1977; Blau *et al.* 1978; Mulivor *et al.* 1978; Osang *et al.* 1979). Both Blau and colleagues and Mulivor and others found that the skull was ill-defined on ultrasound scanning at 16 weeks, in the presence of normal amniotic fluid α-fetoprotein in the latter study, and that alkaline phosphatase of cultured amniotic fluid cells was low whereas that of the supernatant fluid was unhelpful.

References

Benzie, R., Doran, T. A., Escoffery, W., Gardner, H. A., Hoar, D. I., Hunter, A., Malone, R., Miskin, M. and Rudd, N. L. (1976). Prenatal diagnosis of hypophosphatasia. *Birth Defects Orig. Art. Series.* **12**(6), 271–82.

Beratis, N. G., Kaffe, S., Aron, A. M. and Hirschhorn, K. (1976). Alkaline phosphatase activity in cultured skin fibroblasts from fibrodysplasia ossificans progressiva. *J. Med. Genet.* **13**, 307–9.

Bethune, J. E. and Dent, C. E. (1960). Hypophosphatasia in the adult. *Am. J. Med.* **28**, 615–22.

Blau, K., Hoar, D. I., Rattenbury, J. M. and Rudd, N. L. (1977). Prenatal diagnosis of hypophosphatasia. *Lancet* **2**, 1139.

——, Rattenbury, J. M., Pryse-Davies, J., Clark, P. and Sandler, M. (1978). Prenatal detection of hypophosphatasia: cytological and genetic considerations. *J. Inher. Metab. Dis.* **1**, 37–9.

Bongiovanni, A. M., Album, M. M., Root, A. W., Hope, J. W., Marino, J. and Spencer, D. M. (1968). Studies in hypophosphatasia and response to high phosphate intake. *Am. J. Med. Sci.* **255**, 120–63.

Boyer, S. H. (1963). Human organ alkaline phosphatases: discrimination by several means including starch gel electrophoresis of antienzyme–enzyme supernatant fluids. *Am. NY Acad. Sci.* **103**, 938–51.

Chown, B. (1935/1936). Renal rickets and dwarfism: a pituitary disease. *Br. J. Surg.* **23**, 552–66.

Danovitch, S. H., Baer, P. N. and Laster, L. (1968). Intestinal alkaline phosphatase activity in familial hypophosphatasia. *New. Engl. J. Med.* **278**, 1253–60.

Eisenberg, E. and Pimstone, B. (1967). Hypophosphatasia in an adult. *Clin. Orthop.* **52**, 199–212.

Engfeldt, B. and Zetterstrom, R. (1954). Osteo-dysmetamorphosis fetalis: clinical–pathological study of congenital skeletal disease with retarded growth, hypophosphatemia and renal damage. *J. Pediatr.* **45**, 125–40.

Fraser, D. (1957). Hypophosphatasia. *Am. J. Med.* **22**, 730–46.

—— and Yendt, E. R. (1955). Metabolic abnormalities in hypophosphatasia. *Am. J. Dis. Child.* **90**, 552–4.

——, —— and Christie, F. H. (1955). Metabolic abnormalities in hypophosphatasia. *Lancet* **1**, 286.

Harris, H. and Robson, E. B. (1959). A genetical study of ethanolamine phosphate excretion in hypophosphatasia. *Ann. Hum. Genet.* **23**, 421–41.

Hoar, D. I. and Rudd, N. L. (1976). Prenatal diagnosis of hypophosphatasia. *Lancet* **1**, 1194.

McCance, R. A., Morrison, A. B. and Dent, C. E. (1955). The excretion of phosphoethanolamine and hypophosphatasia. *Lancet* **1**, 131.

——, Fairweather, D. V. I., Barrett, A. M. and Morrison, A. B. (1956). Genetic, clinical, biochemical and pathological features of hypophosphatasia. *Quart. J. Med.* **25**, 523–7.

Méhes, K., Klujber, L., Lassu, G. and Kajtar, P. (1972). Hypophosphatasia: screening and family investigations in an endogamous Hungarian village. *Clin. Genet.* **3**, 60–6.

Mulivor, R. A., Mennoti, M., Zackai, E. H. and Harris, H. (1978). Prenatal diagnosis of hypophosphatasia, genetics, biochemical and clinical studies. *Am. J. Hum. Genet.* **30**, 271–82.

Osang, M., Santer, R., Zahn, V. and Schaub, J. (1979). Prenatal diagnosis of hypophosphatasia (abst.). *Eur. J. Pediatr.* **130**, 225.

Pimstone, B., Eisenberg, E. and Silverman, S. (1966). Hypophosphatasia: genetic and dental studies. *Ann. Intern. Med.* **65**, 722–9.

Poland, C., Eversole, L. R., Bixler, D. and Christian, J. C. (1972). Histochemical observations of hypophosphatasia. *J. Dent. Res.* **51**, 333–8.

Rasmussen, K. (1968). Phosphorylethanolamine and hypophosphatasia. *Dan. Med. Bull.* **15**, Suppl. 2: 1–112.

—— (1983). Hypophosphatasia. Chapter 68 in *The metabolic basis of inherited disease*, 5th edn. eds. Stanbury, J. B., Wyngaarden, J. B., Fredrickson, D. S., Goldstein, J. L. and Brown, M. S. pp. 1497–507. McGraw-Hill, New York.

Rathbun, J. C. (1948). Hypophosphatasia, a new developmental anomaly. *Am. J. Dis. Child* **75**, 822–31.

——, MacDonald, J. W., Robinson, H. M. C. and Wanklin, J. M. (1961). Hypophosphatasia: a genetic study. *Arch. Dis. Child.* **36**, 540–2.

Rattenbury, J. M., Blau, K., Sandler, M., Pryse-Davies, J., Clark, P. J. and Pooley, S. S. F. (1976). Prenatal diagnosis of hypophosphatasia. *Lancet* **1**, 306.

Rubecz, I., Méhes, K., Klujber, L., Bozzay, L., Weisenbach, J. and Fenyvesi, J. (1974). Hypophosphatasia: screening and family investigation. *Clin. Genet.* **6**, 155–9.

Rudd, N. L., Miskin, M., Hoar, D. I., Benzie, R. and Doran, T. A. (1976). Prenatal diagnosis of hypophosphatasia. *New Engl. J. Med.* **295**, 146–8.

Russel, R. G. G. (1965). Excretion of inorganic pyrophosphate in hypophosphatasia. *Lancet* **2**, 461–4.

Scriver, C. R. and Cameron, D. (1969). Pseudohypophosphatasia. *New Engl. J. Med.* **281**, 604–6.

Silverman, J. L. (1962). Apparent dominant inheritance of hypophosphatasia. *Arch. Intern. Med.* **110**, 191–8.

Whyte, M. P., Teitelbaum, S. L., Murphy, W. A., Bergfeld, M. A. and Avioli, L. V. (1979). Adult hypophosphatasia. *Medicine* **58**, 329–47.

4.2.3. Cause unknown

Cerebro-hepato-renal (Zellweger) syndrome

This curious disorder, which has been recently reviewed by Kelley (1983) and by Wilson and colleagues (1986), combines dysmorphic features with an inborn error of metabolism, and was first described by Zellweger and his colleagues (Bowen *et al.* 1964). They reported two pairs of sibs but it was subsequently suggested that only one of these pairs, that contributed by Zellweger, had the cerebro-hepato-renal syndrome (Opitz *et al.* 1969). The disorder was independently described by Smith and coworkers (1965) in a brother and sister. These latter authors, along with Passarge and McAdams (1967) and Opitz and colleagues (1969), established the main clinical features. These are gross hypotonia; failure to thrive with death within 2 to 3 years and usually within 6 months; a characteristic craniofacial dysmorphology with dolicocephaly, a prominent high forehead, narrow palatal arch, and in some cases epicanthic folds and malformed auricles; hepatomegaly; ocular changes and minor skeletal defects such as camptodactyly, and restricted movement of the knee and elbow joints. Ocular abnormalities reported include optic atrophy and retinal degeneration with extinction of the electroretinogram and, in at least one case, asymmetrical visually evoked responses (Stanescu and Dralands 1972), lenticular changes with cataracts in the lens cortex, and, on electron microscopy, inclusion bodies in the lens fibres and abnormal mitochondrial proliferation in the lens epithelium (Hittner *et al.* 1981). These authors also demonstrated condensations in the cortical region in the lenses of the parents. Protein-uria but normal renal function may be noted during life, and other variable findings include congenital iron overload with deposition in the reticuloendothelial system (Opitz *et al.* 1969; Vitale *et al.* 1969; Jan *et al.* 1970), hypoglycaemia (Patton *et al.* 1972; Vincens *et al.* 1973), and hypoprothrombinaemia (Jan *et al.* 1970). Gilchrist and colleagues (1976) in a follow-up study found that the elevated serum iron and iron deposition tend to correct spontaneously in those children who survive beyond 6 months. A characteristic radiographic finding has been punctuate chondral calcification, giving a stippled appearance to the patellae and the acetabular cartilage at the hip (Opitz *et al.* 1969; Poznanski *et al.* 1970; Williams *et al.* 1972). The investigation of infants suspected of having Zellweger syndrome was reviewed by Gilchrist *et al.* 1975).

A wide spectrum of pathological changes have been noted. The outstanding changes are in the central nervous system with microgyria of the cortex and hypoplasia of the cerebellum, pons, and medulla. Histo-logically there is irregular neuronal stratification in the cortex and fibrillary astrogliosis of the cortex, cerebellum, midbrain, pons, medulla, and spinal cord (Danks *et al.* 1975; Friedman *et al.* 1980), and also gross demyelination (Gatfield *et al.* 1968). A common finding is intrahepatic cholestasis, which may or may not be associated with a fine nodular periportal cirrhosis and heavy iron deposition (Smith *et al.* 1965; Jan *et al.* 1970; Danks *et al.* 1975; Mathis *et al.* 1978; Friedman *et al.* 1980). Another frequent observation is the presence of renal cortical cysts of Bowman's capsule or the renal tubules resembling Potter's type 4 cysts associated with lower urinary tract obstruction. These are usually small, up to a few millimeters in diameter, although larger cysts are occasionally seen (Smith *et al.* 1965; Passarge and McAdams 1967; Jan *et al.* 1970; Poznanski *et al.* 1970; Danks *et al.* 1975; Friedman *et al.* 1980). The renal abnormalities in this disease are of interest but are not clinically of great importance. Other pathological findings include thymic hypoplasia (Patton *et al.* 1972; Gilchrist *et al.* 1974) or even aplasia (Friedman *et al.* 1980).

The basic pathogenetic defect appears to involve cellular respiration. The evidence for this comes from two main lines of observation: a disorder of pipecolic acid metabolism, and disturbances of the two main organelles of cellular respiration—the mitochondria and the peroxisomes. Gatfield and colleagues (1968) reported a child with neuropathy and hepatomegaly and a raised blood pipecolic acid. There was no further rise on lysine loading and no delay in clearing lysine. There are two alternative pathways of lysine degradation in mammals. L-lysine is readily converted via saccharopine and α-amino-adipic semi-aldehyde to α-amino-adipic acid by isolated mammalian liver or kidney mitochondria, whereas D-lysine is only very slowly catabolized. However, intact animals catabolize DL lysine via pipecolic acid, with the greater part of the latter being formed from D-lysine (Grove and Henderson 1968; Grove *et al.* 1969). Both D- and L-lysine, when injected into the rat brain, are metabolized mainly via L-pipecolic acid but there is a blood–brain barrier for the latter (Chang 1976, 1978a and b). Thus if the handling of lysine in humans is the same as in the rat the sacharopine pathway of degradation is used by liver and kidney mitochondria and the pipecolic acid pathway by the brain. The presumption must be that in Zellweger syndrome there is some disturbance of lysine metabolism in the central nervous system. Gatfield and colleagues observations were confirmed by Danks and coworkers (1975) in four patients with typical Zellweger syndrome in whom they found excess urinary excretion of pipecolic acid and raised serum levels. Further confirmation comes from other groups (Thomas *et al.* 1976; Trijbels *et al.* 1979; Arneson and Ward 1981; Burton *et al.* 1981). Trijbels and colleagues gave patients and controls an oral load of DL pipecolic acid and observed a slower return to fasting levels in the patients and a failure of the normal increase in excretion of α-amino-adipic acid. They also confirmed that oral lysine did not increase serum pipecolic acid in patients. Arneson and Ward obtained similar results. Whilst these studies clearly implicate a block in pipecolic acid metabolism in Zellweger's syndrome, at least some of the catabolic enzymes for which are mitochondrial, they do not pinpoint the exact site of the block, nor do they indicate whether this is primary or secondary.

The second line of work on the pathogenesis of the disease was initiated by Goldfischer and coworkers (1973) who studied liver biopsies from two patients and kidney and muscle from one of them. A combination of electron microscopical, histochemical, and biochemical findings indicated major defects of the organelles of cellular respiration.

Neither peroxisomes nor the peroxisomal enzyme catalase could be detected in liver or proximal renal tubules. Mitochondria from liver, and from cortical astrocytes showed a distorted appearance. Oxygen consumption of mitochondria of brain and liver was markedly diminished with succinate and substrates reducing nicotinamide-adenine dinucleotide (NAD), but not with ascorbate and tetramethylphenylenediamine, suggesting a defect in electron transport prior to cytochrome and probably in the region of non-heme protein. These observations were confirmed and extended by others (Versmold *et al.* 1977; Mathis *et al.* 1978; Friedman *et al.* 1980; Trijbels *et al.* 1981). Kelley and Corkey (1983) have pinpointed the defect in electron transport more precisely by showing that antimycin A, an inhibitor of the cytochrome bc_1 complex (complex III), inhibits the growth of fibroblasts from patients far more than those from controls, whereas inhibitors of other steps in the respiratory chain act equally on patient and control fibroblasts. Their findings do not exclude the possibility that this defect is secondary to the absence of peroxisomes (Kelley 1983). Zellweger syndrome shares a generalized defect of peroxisomes with infantile Refsum's disease, rhizomelic chondrodysplasia punctata (Wanders *et al.* 1986), and adrenoleucodystrophy (Rocchiccioli *et al.* 1986).

Mathis and colleagues, using gas chromatography and mass spectroscopy, confirmed an earlier report (Eyssen *et al.* 1972) that a precursor of cholic acid, non-sulphated trihydroxycoprostanic acid, which requires mitochondrial oxidation for its conversion to cholic acid, was present in excess in the bile and urine of a patient. Others have shown very long chain fatty acids generally to be elevated (Brown *et al.* 1982; Moser *et al.* 1984; Govaerts *et al.* 1985), have measured precursors of bile salts that require mitochondrial oxidation for their metabolism and found similar excess to that of cholic acid in patients (Hanson *et al.* 1979; Monnens *et al.* 1980; Gustafsson *et al.* 1983), or have reported organic aciduria with excretion of abnormal dicarboxylic acids (Chalmers *et al.* 1980; Rocchiccioli *et al.* 1986). The membrane phospholipids phosphatidylethanolamine plasmalogen and phosphatidylcholine plasmalogen have been shown to be present at greatly reduced concentration in the tissues of patients (Heymans *et al.* 1983), and the membrane-bound peroxisomal enzyme dihydroxy-acetone phosphate acyltransferase activity in liver homogenates and cultured fibroblasts of patients to be only 5–10 per cent that of control tissues. This enzyme deficiency has been confirmed in cultured fibroblasts from three patients, and the presence of activity in cultured normal amniotic fluid cells demonstrated (Datta *et al.* 1984). Deficiency of other enzymes of peroxisomal β-oxidation has also been reported (Suzuki *et al.* 1986; Wanders *et al.* 1986). These findings point to a possible primary defect in a peroxisomal enzyme and suggest that the highly pleomorphic effects of the gene mutation in this disease are possibly all mediated through the defects in mitochondria and peroxisomes. However, sibs with typical Zellweger syndrome have been reported as having normal peroxisomes and catalase (Burton *et al.* 1981). The relationship between the mitochondrial and peroxisomal defects remains to be demonstrated, and the nature of the underlying molecular defect leading to the enzyme deficiency and the absence of the peroxisomes is also still unknown.

The numerous reports of the disease in sibs (Bowen *et al.* 1964; Smith *et al.* 1965; Passarge and McAdams 1967; Jan *et al.* 1970; Poznanski *et al.* 1970; Danks *et al.* 1975; Gustafsson *et al.* 1983) and also reports of parental consanguinity (Poznanski *et al.* 1970; Williams *et al.* 1972; Danks *et al.* 1975) leave little doubt that Zellweger syndrome is inherited in an autosomal recessive manner. Danks and colleagues estimated an incidence of 1 in 100 000 live births.

Methods of prenatal diagnosis are currently under development. Moser and colleagues (Moser *et al.* 1984; Powers *et al.* 1985) have demonstrated increased levels of the very long chain fatty acids, hexacosanoic, and hexacosenoic acids in cultured amniotic fluid cells or cultured chorionic villus fibroblasts from pregnancies with an affected fetus. They have also reported confirmatory findings on four fetuses from pregnancies terminated because of the prenatal diagnosis of an affected fetus (Powers *et al.* 1985; Solish *et al.* 1985). Björkhem and coworkers (1984) have made similar observations on amniotic fluid from an affected pregnancy. Schutgens and associates (1983, 1984) have shown that dihydroxy-acetone phosphate acyltransferase, a peroxisomal enzyme involved in the synthesis of ethanolamine plasmalogens, is grossly deficient in liver or fibroblast homogenates from patients, and in cultured amniotic fluid cells from affected fetuses. They have also demonstrated enzyme activity in normal chorionic villi, and Carey and others (1986) reported the use of this method for the prenatal diagnosis of an affected male from chorionic villi. Both Moser's group (Schutgens *et al.* 1985) and Roscher and colleagues (1985) have used the assay of impaired plasmalogen synthesis for prenatal diagnosis.

Moser's group have also reported that the demonstration of a deficiency of acyl-CoA: dihydroxyacetone phosphate acyltransferase in thrombocytes provides a simple postnatal diagnostic test (Wanders *et al.* 1985).

References

Arneson, D. W. and Ward, J. C. (1981). Pipecolic acid (PA) loading studies on an infant with cerebro-hepato-renal syndrome. *Am. J. Hum. Genet.* **33**, 35A.

Björkhem. I., Sisfontes, L., Bostrom, B., Kase, F., Hagenfeldt, L. and Blomstrand, R. (1984). Possibility of prenatal diagnosis of Zellweger syndrome. *Lancet* **1**, 1234–5.

Bowen, P., Lee, C. S. N., Zellweger, H. and Lindenberg, R. (1964). A familial syndrome of multiple congenital defects. *Bull. Johns Hopkins Hosp.* **114**, 402–14.

Brown, F. R., McAdams, A. J., Cummins, J. W., Konkol, R., Singh, I., Moser, A. B. and Moser, H. W. (1982). Cerebro-hepato-renal (Zellweger) syndrome and neonatal adrenoleukodystrophy: similarities in phenotype and accumulation of very long chain fatty acids. *Johns Hopkins Med. J.* **151**, 344–51.

Burton, B. K., Reed, S. P. and Remy, W. T. (1981). Hyperpipecolic acidemia: clinical and biochemical observations on two male siblings. *J. Pediatr.* **99**, 729–34.

Carey, W. F., Robertson, E. F., Van Crugten, C., Poulos, A., Nelson, P. V. and Finiriotis, G. (1986). Short communication: prenatal diagnosis of Zellweger's syndrome by chorionic villus sampling—and a caveat. *Prenatal Diagnosis* **6**, 227–9.

Chalmers, R. A., Purkiss, P. and Watts, R. W. E. (1980). Screening for organic acidurias and aminoacidopathies in newborns and children. *J. Inher. Metab. Dis.* **3**, 27–43.

Chang, Y.-F. (1976). Pipecolic acid pathway: the major lysine metabolic route in the rat brain. *Biochem. Biophys. Res. Commun.* **69**, 174–80.

—— (1978a). Lysine metabolism in the rat brain: the pipecolic acid-forming pathway. *J. Neurochem.* **30**, 347–54.

—— (1978b). Lysine metabolism in the rat brain: blood brain carrier transport, formation of pipecolic acid and human hyperpipecolatemia. *J. Neurochem.* **30**, 355–60.

Danks, D. M., Tippett, P., Adams, C. and Campbell, P. (1975). Cerebro-hepato-renal syndrome of Zellweger. *J. Pediatr.* **86**, 382–7.

Datta, N. S., Wilson, G. N. and Hajra, A. K. (1984). Deficiency of enzymes catalyzing the biosynthesis of glycerol–ether lipids in Zellweger syndrome. *New. Engl. J. Med.* **311**, 1080–3.

Eyssen, H., Parmentier, G., Compernolle, F., Boon, J. and Eggermont, E. (1972). Trihydroxycoprostanic acid in the duodenal fluid of two children with intra-hepatic bile duct anomalies. *Biochim. Biophys. Acta.* **273**, 212–21.

Friedman, A., Bethzhold, J., Hong, R., Gilbert, E. F., Viseskul, C. and Opitz, J. M. (1980). Clinicopathologic conference: a three-month old infant with failure to thrive, hepatomegaly and neurological impairment. *Am. J. Med. Genet.* **7**, 171–86.

Gatfield, P. D., Taller, E., Hinton, G. G., Wallace, A. C., Abdelnour, G. M. and Haust, M. D. (1968). Hyperpipecolataemia: a new metabolic disorder associated with neuropathy and hepatomegaly. *Can. Med. Assoc. J.* **99**, 1215–33.

Gilchrist, K. W., Opitz, J. M., Gilbert, E. F., Tsang, W. and Miller, P. (1974). Immunodeficiency in the cerebro-hepato-renal syndrome of Zellweger. *Lancet* **1**, 164–5.

——, Gilbert, E. F., Shahidi, N. T. and Opitz, J. M. (1975). The evaluation of infants with the Zellweger (cerebro-hepato-renal) syndrome. *Clin. Genet.* **7**, 413–16.

——, ——, Goldfarb, S., Goll, U., Spranger, J. W. and Opitz, J. M. (1976). Studies of malformation syndromes of man. X1B: the cerebro-hepato-renal sydrome of Zellweger: comparative pathology. *Eur. J. Pediatr.* **121**, 99–118.

Goldfischer, S., Moore, C. L., Johnson, A. B., Spiro, A. J., Valsamis, M. P., Wisniewski, H. K., Ritch, R. H., Norton, W. T., Rapin, I. and Gartner, L. M. (1973). Peroxisomal and mitochondrial defects in the cerebro-hepato-renal syndrome. *Science* **182**, 62–4.

Govaerts, L., Bakkeren, J., Monnens, L., Maas, J., Trijbels, F. and Kleijer, W. (1985). Disturbed very long chain (C24–C26) fatty acid pattern in fibroblasts of patients with Zellweger's syndrome. *J. Inher. Metab. Dis.* **8**, 5–8.

Grove, J. and Henderson, L. M. (1968). The metabolism of D- and L-lysine in the intact rat, perfused liver and liver mitochondria. *Biochim. Biophys. Acta* **165**, 113–20.

——, Gilbertson, T. J., Hammerstedt, R. H. and Henderson, L. M. (1969). The metabolism of D- and L-lysine specifically labelled with ^{15}N. *Biochim. Biophys. Acta* **184**, 329–37.

Gustafsson, J., Gustavson, K.-H., Karlaganis, G. and Sjövall, J. (1983). Zellweger's cerebro-hepato-renal syndrome—variations in expressivity and in defects of bile acid synthesis. *Clin. Genet.* **24**, 313–19.

Hanson, R. F., Szczepanik-Van Leeuwen, P., Williams, G. C., Grabowski, G. and Sharp, H. L. (1979). Defects of the bile acid synthesis in Zellweger's syndrome. *Science* **203**, 1107–8.

Heymans, H. S. A., Schutgens, R. B. H., Tan, R., van den Bosch, H. and Borst, P. (1983). Severe plasmalogen deficiency in tissues of infants without peroxisomes (Zellweger syndrome). *Nature* **306**, 69–70.

Hittner, H. M., Kretzer, F. L. and Mehta, R. S. (1981). Zellweger syndrome: lenticular opacities indicating carrier status and lens abnormalities characteristic of homozygotes. *Arch. Ophthal.* **99**, 1977–82.

Jan, J. E., Hardwick, D. F., Lowry, R. B. and McCormick, A. Q. (1970). Cerebro-hepato-renal syndrome of Zellweger. *Am. J. Dis. Child.* **119**, 274–7.

Kelley, R. I. (1983). Review: the cerebrohepatorenal syndrome of Zellweger, morphologic and metabolic aspects. *Am. J. Med. Genet.* **16**, 503–17.

—— and Corkey, B. E. (1983). Increased sensitivity of cerebrohepatorenal syndrome fibroblasts to antimycin A. *J. Inher. Metab. Dis.* **6**, 158–62.

Mathis, R. K., Lott, I. T., Szczepanik, P. and Watkins, J. B. (1978). Cholestasis in the cerebro-hepato-renal (CHR) syndrome: bile acid and mitochondrial abnormalities. *Pediatr. Res.* **12**, 439.

Monnens, L., Bakkeren, J., Parmentier, G., Janssen, G., van Haelst, U., Trijbels, F. and Eyssen, H. (1980). Disturbances in bile acid metabolism of infants with the Zellweger (cerebro-hepato-renal) syndrome. *Eur. J. Pediatr.* **133**, 31–5.

Moser, A. B., Singh, I. S., Brown, F. R., Solish, G. I., Kelley, R. I., Benke, P. J. and Moser, H. W. (1984). The cerebrohepatorenal (Zellweger) syndrome: increased levels and impaired degradation of very-long-chain fatty acids and their use in prenatal diagnosis. *New Engl. J. Med.* **310**, 1141–6.

Opitz, J. M., Zurhein, G. M., Vitale, L., Shahidi, N. T., Howe, J. J., Chou, S. M., Shanklin, D. R., Sybers, H. D., Dood, A. R. and Gerritsen, T. (1969). The Zellweger syndrome (cerebro-hepato-renal syndrome). *The clinical delineation of birth defects. II. Malformation syndromes. Birth Defects Orig. Art. Ser.* **5**(2), 144–60.

Passarge, E. and McAdams, A. J. (1967). Cerebro-hepato-renal syndrome. A newly recognized hereditary disorder of multiple congenital defects, including sudanophilic leukodystrophy, cirrhosis of the liver and polycystic kidneys. *J. Pediatr.* 71, 691–702.

Patton, R. G., Christie, D. L., Smith, D. W. and Beckwick, J. B. (1972). Cerebro-hepato-renal syndrome of Zellweger. *Am. J. Dis. Child.* 124, 840–4.

Powers, J. M., Moser, H. W., Moser, A. B., Upshur, J. K., Bradford, B. F., Pai, S. G., Kohn, P. H., Frias, J. and Tiffany, C. (1985). Fetal cerebrohepatorenal (Zellweger) syndrome: dysmorphic, radiologic, biochemical, and pathologic findings in four affected fetuses. *Hum. Pathol.* 16, 610–20.

Poznanski, A. K., Nosanchuk, J. S., Baublis, J. and Holt, J. F. (1970). The cerebro-hepato-renal syndrome (CHRS): (Zellweger's syndrome). *Am. J. Roentgen.* 109, 313–22.

Rocchiccioli, F., Aubourg, P. and Bougneres, P. F. (1986). Medium- and long-chain dicarboxylic aciduria in patients with Zellweger syndrome and neonatal adrenoleukodystrophy. *Pediatr. Res.* 20, 62–6.

Roscher, A., Molzer, B., Bernheimer, H., Stocker, S., Mutz, I. and Paltauf, F. (1985). The cerebrohepatorenal (Zellweger) syndrome: an improved method for the biochemical diagnosis and its potential value for prenatal detection. *Pediatr. Res.* 19, 930–3.

Schutgens, R. B. H., Purvis, R., Romeyn, G. J., Heymans, H. S. A. and Van den Bosch, H. (1983). Zellweger (cerebro-hepato-renal) syndrome: pre- and postnatal diagnosis by quantitative analysis of ethanolamine plasmalogens. *Proc. II Internat. Sympos. on Monoclonal Antibodies and Inborn Errors of Metabolism,* Brugge, 20–22 Oct. 1983, Belgian Soc. for Clin. Chem., abs. No. 113.

——, Heymans, H. S. A., Wanders, R. J. A., Van den Bosch, H. and Schrakamp, G. (1984). Prenatal detection of Zellweger syndrome. *Lancet* 2, 1339–40.

——, Schrakamp, G., Wanders, R. J. A., Heymans, H. S. A., Moser, H. W., Moser, A. E., Tager, J. M., Bosch, H. V. D. and Aubourg, P. (1985). The cerebro-hepato-renal syndrome: prenatal detection based on impaired biosynthesis of plasmalogens. *Prenatal Diagnosis* 5, 337–44.

Smith, D. W., Opitz, J. M. and Inhorn, S. L. (1965). A syndrome of multiple developmental defects including polycystic kidneys and intrahepatic biliary dysgenesis in two siblings. *J. Pediatr.* 67, 617–24.

Solish, G. I., Moser, H. W., Ringer, L. D., Moser, A. E., Tiffany, C. and Schutta, E. (1985). Prenatal diagnosis of the cerebro-hepato-renal syndrome of Zellweger. *Prenatal Diagnosis* 5, 27–34.

Stanescu, B. and Dralands, L. (1972). Cerebro-hepato-renal (Zellweger's) syndrome, ocular involvement. *Arch. Ophthalmol.* 87, 590–2.

Suzuki, Y., Orii, T., Masataka, M., Tatibana, M. and Hashimoto, T. (1986). Deficient activities and proteins of peroxisomal β-oxidation enzymes in infants with Zellweger syndrome. *Clin. Chim. Acta.* 156, 191–6.

Thomas, G. H., Haslam, R. H. A., Batshaw, M. L., Capute, A. J., Neidengard, L., and Ransom, J. L. (1976). Hyperpipecolic acidemia associated with hepatomegaly, mental retardation, optic nerve dysplasia and progressive neurological disease. *Clin. Genet.* 8, 376–82.

Trijbels, J. M. F., Monnens, L. A. H., Bakkeren, J. A. J. M., Van Raay-Selten, A. H. J. and Cortiaensen, J. M. B. (1979). Biochemical studies in the cerebro-hepato-renal syndrome of Zellweger: a disturbance in the metabolism of pipecolic acid. *J. Inher. Metab. Dis.* **2**, 39–42.

——, ——, ——, Willems, J. L. and Sengers, R. C. A. (1981). Mitochondrial abnormalities in the cerebro-hepato-renal syndrome of Zellweger. In *Mitochondria and muscular diseases*, eds. Busch, H. F. M., Jennekens, F. G. I. and Scholte, H. R. pp. 187–90. Beetsterzwaag, Holland, Mefar b.v.

Versmold, H. T., Bremer, H. J., Herzog, V., Siegel, G., Bassewitz, D. B., Irle, U., Voss, H., Lombeck, I. and Brauser, B. (1977). A metabolic disorder similar to Zellweger syndrome with hepatic acatalasia and absence of peroxisomes, altered content and redox state of cytochrome, and infantile cirrhosis with hemosiderosis. *Eur. J. Pediatr.* **124**, 261–75.

Vincens, A., Guillat, J.-C., Gatin, G., Rodier, J. and Graveleau, D. (1973). A propos d'un cas de syndrome de Zellweger (Syndrome Hépato-cérébro-rénal). *Sem. Hôp. (Paris).* **49-26**, 553–560.

Vitale, L., Opitz, J. M. and Shahidi, N. T. (1969). Congenital and familial iron overload. *New. Engl. J. Med.* **280**, 642–5.

Wanders, R. J. A., van Roermund, C. W. T., de Vries, C. T., van den Bosch, H., Schrakamp, G., Tager, J. M., Schram, A. W. and Schutgens, R. B. H. (1986). Peroxisomal β-oxidation of palmitoyl-CoA in human liver homogenates and its deficiency in the cerebro-hepato-renal (Zellweger) syndrome. *Clin. Chim. Acta* **159**, 1–10.

——, van Weringh, G., Schrakamp, G., Tager, J. M., Van den Bosch, H. and Schutgens, R. B. H. (1985). Deficiency of acyl-CoA: dihydroxyacetone phosphate acyltranferase in thrombocytes of Zellweger patients: a simple postnatal diagnostic test. *Clin. Chim. Acta* **151**, 217–21.

——, Saelman, D., Heymans, H. S. A., Schutgens, R. B. H., Westerveld, A., Poll-Thé, B. T., Saudubray, J. M., Van den Bosch, H., Strijland, A., Schram, A. W. and Tager, J. M. (1986). Genetic relationship between the Zellweger syndrome, infantile Refsum's disease and rhizomelic chondrodysplasia punctata. *New Engl. J. Med.* **314**, 787–8.

Williams, J. P., Secrist, L., Fowler, G. W., Gwinn, J. L. and Dumars, K. C. (1972). Roentgenographic features of the cerebro-hepato-renal syndrome of Zellweger. *Am. J. Roentgenol. Rad. Ther. Nucl. Med.* **115**, 607–10.

Wilson, G. N., Holmes, R. G., Custer, J., Lipkowitz, J. L., Stover, J., Datta, N. and Hajra, A. (1986). Zellweger syndrome: diagnostic assays, syndrome delineation, and potential therapy. *Am. J. Med. Genet.* **24**, 69–82.

Nephrosialidosis

Maroteaux and colleagues have described a form of sialidosis with dysmorphic features and renal involvement (Le Sec *et al.* 1978; Maroteaux 1978; Maroteaux *et al.* 1978). There is early and severe mental subnormality, dysmorphic facies, skeletal abnormalities, and a glomerular nephropathy. Foam cells can be demonstrated in bone marrow and the development of a cherry-red spot on direct ophthalmoscopy is a late feature. The nephropathy is of early onset and leads to death within the first decade.

Leucocytes are deficient in α-(2-6) neuraminidase, as is also found in several other sialidoses. Inheritance is autosomal recessive but it is not yet established whether this and the other disorders of neuraminidase activity are allelic. Spranger (1981) refers to this type as sialidosis I; and mucolipidosis I, Goldberg disease (combined neuraminididase and β-galactosidase deficiency), and cherry-red spot myoclonus syndrome as sialidosis II, III, and IV respectively.

A variant of this syndrome with congenital ascites, hepatospleno-megaly, growth failure, delayed development, dysmorphic changes, and pericardial effusion and nephrotic syndrome leading to death at 22 months has been reported (Aylsworth *et al.* 1979). There was a gross deficiency of neuraminidase activity in cultured fibroblasts from the patient, with intermediate levels of activity in cells from the parents.

References

Aylsworth, A. S., Thomas, G. H. and Hood, J. L. (1979). The severe infantile form of neuraminidase deficiency. *Am. J. Hum. Genet.* **31**, 68A.

Le Sec, G., Stanescu, R. and Lyon, G. (1978). Un nouveau type de sialidose avec atteinte renale: la nephrosialidose. II. Etude anatomique. *Arch. Fr. Pédiatr.* **35**, 830–44.

Maroteaux, P. (1978). Les sialidoses par deficit en α-(2-6) neuraminidase: un groupe heterogene. *Arch. Fr. Pédiatr.* **35**, 815–18.

——, Humbel, R., Strecker, G., Michalski, J.-C. and Mande, R. (1978). Un nouveau type de sialidose avec atteinte renale: la nephrosialidose. I. Etude clinique, radiologique et nosologique. *Arch. Fr. Pédiatr.* **35**, 819–29.

Spranger, J. (1981). Advances in bone dysplasias. Sixth Internat. Congr. Hum. Genet., Jerusalem.

Glutaricaciduria type II

This disorder was first described, and distinguished from glutaricaciduria type I which has a different clinical picture arising from a deficiency of glutaryl-CoA dehydrogenase, by Przyrembel and colleagues (1976). They described a boy who developed metabolic acidosis and hypo-glycaemia within hours of birth. Despite vigorous treatment he became hypothermic, developed seizures and died at 70 hours. There was a strong odour of sweaty feet. Further cases have been reported which clinically fall into two groups: patients similar to that of Pryzrembel and colleagues with immediate postnatal onset of metabolic acidosis, hyper-ammonaemia, and hypoglycaemia leading to early death (Gregersen *et al.* 1980; Sweetman *et al.* 1980; Coude *et al.* 1981), and a milder form with transient hypoglycaemia (Dusheiko *et al.* 1979; Mantagos *et al.* 1979; Goodman *et al.* 1980).

In the severe form, termed glutaricaciduria IIA by Coude and colleagues, there is a complex pattern of organic aciduria associated with raised plasma glutaric acid and other dicarboxylic acids, hydroxy acids, and long chain fatty acids. There may also be an aminoaciduria not associated with comparable elevation of plasma amino acids, suggestive of a secondary renal tubular damage.

As in glutaricaciduria type I there is a deficiency of glutaryl-CoA dehydrogenase, but unlike type I several other CoA dehydrogenases are also deficient (Sweetman *et al.* 1980). The basic defect leading to this multiple CoA dehydrogenase defect is unknown, although one suggestion is a defect of an electron transferring flavoprotein (Goodman *et al.* 1980; Rhead *et al.* 1980). Vamecq and associates (1985) demonstrated that the glutaryl-CoA dehydrogenase reaction in the liver is a peroxisomal one. This suggests that glutaricaciduria type II may be another peroxisomal disorder like Zellweger's syndrome, adrenoleuco-dystrophy, infantile Refsum's syndrome, and rhizomelic chondro-dysplasia punctata. That glutaricaciduria type II is distinct from isovaleric acidaemia is confirmed by the observation of complementation in heterokaryons of cell lines from the two disorders (Dubiel *et al.* 1983).

Further possible clinical heterogeneity is added by the observation that several reported infants with the severe form have had dysmorphic features and polycystic kidneys (Sweetman *et al.* 1980, case 1; Lehnert *et al.* 1982 and Böhm *et al.* 1982; Goodman *et al.* 1983; Boué *et al.* 1984). The renal cysts are described as microcysts of the cortex and medulla (Goodman *et al.* 1983). The other dysmorphic features reported have varied but in the case reported by Goodman and coworkers (1983) they included hypospadias with chordee. Hypospadias was also present in the patient reported by Boué and others (1984). This association of a metabolic defect involving peroxisomal enzymes, dysmorphic features, and cystic kidneys is again reminiscent of Zellweger syndrome.

In the mild type, termed glutaricaciduria IIB by Coude and colleagues and ethylmalonic-adipic aciduria by Goodman and coworkers (1983), the organic aciduria is less severe but ethylmalonic and adipic acids as well as glutaric acid are characteristically present. Nevertheless there is a similar multiple CoA dehydrogenase deficiency.

Glutaricaciduria type II has to be distinguished not only from type I and isovaleric acidaemia but also from oxoglutaric aciduria. The latter was described as a progressive neurodegenerative disorder occuring in sibs with consanguineous parents. Both affected sibs excreted a great excess of 2-oxoglutaric acid in their urine and had a greatly reduced 2-oxoglutarate dehydrogenase activity in cultured fibroblasts (Kohls-chütter *et al.* 1982).

The genetics of glutaricaciduria type II poses problems. Clearly types IIA and IIB with their differing clinical course and metabolic picture are genetically distinct. There is evidence of possible further heterogeneity within each type. All the reported cases of type IIA have been boys, with two exceptions: the girl reported by Gregersen and colleagues (1980) who died in coma at 3 days, and the female fetus from the terminated pregnancy reported by Boué and associates (1984). All of the other reported cases have not only been male but in many cases there have been brothers who have died from unidentified causes, or normal sisters. In the family reported by Coude and others (1981) there were five proved or presumed cases related through five presumptive female carriers. Thus the pedigree evidence suggests that both X-linked and autosomal recessive forms exist. All of the reported cases with renal cysts and dysmorphic features are consistent with X-linked recessive inheritance except for that of Boué and associates where the proband was male and a subsequent affected fetus female. It remains unclear how much further genetic heterogeneity arises from this clinical heterogeneity.

Even among the cases of type IIB there is one case with an atypical picture: a 19-year-old female with repeated hypoglycaemic attacks, raised serum concentrations of free fatty acids, fatty infiltration of the liver, and a proximal myopathy (Dusheiko *et al.* 1979). All the reported cases are consistent with autosomal recessive inheritance, but whether or not the patient of Dusheiko and colleagues is distinct from the others is not clear. In one case both parents had reduced levels of enzyme activities (Mantagos *et al.* 1979).

Prenatal diagnosis has been reported on the basis of assay of amniotic fluid glutaric acid level by gas chromatography/mass spectrometry in two cases (Mitchell *et al.* 1983; Boué *et al.* 1984).

References

Böhm, N., Uy, J., Kiebling, M. and Lehnert, W. (1982). Multiple acyl-CoA dehydrogenation deficiency (glutaric aciduria type II), congenital polycystic kidneys, and symmetric warty dysplasia of the cerebral cortex in two newborn brothers. II. Morphology and pathogenesis. *Eur. J. Pediatr.* **139**, 60–5.

Boué, J., Chalmers, R. A., Tracey, B. M., Watson, D., Gray, R. G. F., Keeling, J. W., King, G. S., Pettit, B. R., Lindenbaum, R. H., Rocchiccioli, F. and Saudubray, J.-M. (1984). Prenatal diagnosis of dysmorphic neonatal-lethal type II glutaricaciduria. *Lancet* **1**, 846–7.

Coude, F. X., Ogier, H., Charpentier, C., Thomassin, G., Checoury, A., Amedee-Manesme, O., Saudubray, J. M. and Frezal, J. (1981). Neonatal glutaric aciduria type II: an X-linked recessive inherited disorder. *Hum. Genet.* **59**, 263–5.

Dubiel, B., Dabrowski, C., Wetts, R. and Tanaka, K. (1983). Complementation studies of isovaleric acidemia and glutaric aciduria type II using cultured skin fibroblasts. *J. Clin. Invest.* **72**, 1543–52.

Dusheiko, G., Kew, M. C., Joffe, B. I., Lewin, J. R., Mantagos, S. and Tanaka, K. (1979). Glutaric aciduria type II: a cause of recurrent hypoglycemia in an adult. *New Engl. J. Med.* **301**, 1405–9.

Goodman, S. I., McCabe, E. R. B., Fennessey, P. V. and Mace, J. W. (1980).

Multiple acyl-CoA dehydrogenase deficiency (glutaric aciduria type II) with transient hypersarcosinemia and sarcosinuria; possible inherited deficiency of an electron transfer flavoprotein. *Pediatr. Res.* **14**, 12–17.

——, Reale, M. and Barlow, S. (1983). Glutaric aciduria type II: a form with deleterious intrauterine effects. *J. Pediatr.* **102**, 411–13.

Gregersen, N., Kolveraa, S., Rasmussen, K., Christensen, E., Brandt, N. J., Ebbesen, F. and Hanse, F. E. (1980). Biochemical studies in a patient with defects in metabolism of acyl CoA and sarcosine: another possible cause of glutaric aciduria type II. *J. Inher. Metab. Dis.* **3**, 67–72.

Kohlschütter, A., Behbehani, A., Langenbeck, U., Albani, M., Heidemann, P., Hoffmann, G., Kleinecke, J., Lehnert, W. and Wendel, U. (1982). A familial progressive neurodegenerative disease with 2-oxoglutaric aciduria. *Eur. J. Pediat.* **138**, 32–7.

Lehnert, W., Wendel, V., Lindenmeier, S. and Böhm, M. (1982). Multiple acyl-CoA dehydrogenation deficiency (glutaric aciduria type II), congenital polycystic kidneys, and symmetric warty dysplasia of the cerebral cortex in two brothers. I. Clinical, metabolic and biochemical findings. *Eur. J. Pediatr.* **132**, 56–9.

Mantagos, S., Genel, M. and Tanaka, K. (1979). Ethylmalonic adipic aciduria: *in vivo* and *in vitro* studies indicating deficiency of activities of multiple acyl-CoA dehydrogenases. *J. Clin. Invest.* **64**, 1580–9.

Mitchell, G., Saudubray, J. M., Benoit, Y., Rocchiccioli, F., Charpentier, C., Ogier, H. and Boué, J. (1983). Antenatal diagnosis of glutaricaciduria type II. *Lancet* **1**, 1099.

Przyrembel, H., Wendel, U., Becker, K., Bremer, H. J., Bruinvis, L., Ketting, D. and Wadman, S. K. (1976). Glutaric aciduria type II: Report on a previously undescribed metabolic disorder. *Clin. Chim. Acta* **66**, 227–39.

Rhead, W., Mantagos, S. and Tanaka, K. (1980). Glutaric aciduria type II: *in vitro* studies on substrate oxidation, acyl-CoA dehydrogenases, and electron transferring flavoprotein in cultured skin fibroblasts. *Pediatr. Res.* **14**, 1339–42.

Sweetman, L., Nyhan, W. L., Trauner, D. A., Merritt, T. A. and Singh, M. (1980). Glutaric aciduria type II. *J. Pediatr.* **96**, 1020–6.

Vamecq, J., de Hoffmann, E. and van Hoof, F. (1985). Mitochondrial and peroxisomal metabolism of glutaryl-CoA. *Eur. J. Biochem.* **146**, 663–9.

5. Urolithiasis and crystalluria

5.1. SPECIFIC INHERITED DISORDERS

Several mendelian disorders producing renal stones of specific chemical composition are discussed in this section. Cystinuria will be discussed in Chapter 6 under renal tubular disorders.

5.1.1. Familial hyperparathyroidism and multiple endocrine adenomatosis

Hyperparathyroidism is usually non-familial, even in its primary form. The frequency of familial primary hyperparathyroidism has been estimated at 0.13 or 0.14 per thousand (Jackson and Boonstra 1967; Christensson 1976).

Despite the overall rarity of familial hyperparathyroidism it does occur in a bewildering variety of syndromes whose relationship one to another is not altogether clear. It may occur either in isolation or, in about a sixth of cases, as part of multiple endocrine adenomatosis (Boey *et al.* 1975), and there is also a neonatal form. In contrast to the non-familial form the usual histological change is a primary chief-cell hyperplasia rather than parathyroid adenomata in both isolated familial hyperparathyroidism and in endocrine adenomatosis.

Isolated familial hyperparathyroidism with chief-cell hyperplasia has been described showing an autosomal dominant pattern of inheritance (Cutler *et al.* 1964; Cameron *et al.* 1966; Peters *et al.* 1966; Marsden *et al.* 1971). A less common form with multiple parathyroid adenomata has also been reported as showing dominant inheritance (Cassidy and Anderson 1960; Jackson *et al.* 1960). The relationship of this form in particular to multiple endocrine adenomatosis is obscure but has been discussed by Jackson and Boonstra (1967).

Hyperparathyroidism is a common feature of familial multiple endocrine adenomatosis, which is also autosomal dominant, and in which adenomata of other endocrine glands, especially of pancreatic islet cells, occurs along with carcinoid tumours. In one variety, Zollinger–Ellinson syndrome or multiple endocrine adenomatosis type I, intractable peptic ulceration is a further feature and this distinction appears to run true within individual families (Johnson *et al.* 1967; Friesen *et al.* 1972; Betts

185

et al. 1980). Marx and colleagues (1986) have reported their assessment of laboratory tests in the detection of affected members of a large family.

Parathyroid adenoma is also seen in multiple endocrine adenomatosis type 2, or Sipple syndrome (Urbanski 1967; Steiner *et al.* 1968). In this form there is phaeochromocytoma associated with an amyloid-producing medullary thyroid carcinoma (Schimke and Hartmann 1965). As with type 1, inheritance is autosomal dominant. Parathyroid disturbance has not been reported in the variant of multiple endocrine adenomatosis termed type 3 or type 2B (Carney *et al.* 1980). Schimke (1984) has recently reviewed the multiple endocrine adenomatoses. It is claimed that whereas nephrolithiasis is a common complication of multiple endocrine adenomatosis with hyperparathyroidism it is unusual in isolated familial hyperparathyroidism (Marx *et al.* 1977). Goldsmith and colleagues (1976) also concluded that isolated familial hyperparathyroidism is a distinct disorder.

Hillman and associates (1964) reported neonatal primary hyperparathyroidism in two brothers, the sons of first-cousin parents, and a further pair of affected brothers were described by Thompson and colleagues (1978). However, the presumption of autosomal recessive inheritance in this latter family is thrown into doubt by the finding that the asymptomatic father had hypercalcaemia requiring parathyroidectomy for correction. Spiegel and coworkers (1977) described a further case in a new-born girl whose family on investigation contained 15 hypercalcaemic relatives, all with low to low normal serum phosphate and six of whom had increased urinary cyclic adenosine 3′,5′-monophosphate (AMP) excretion. These latter two families suggest that severe neonatal cases may occur in families of typical autosomal dominant familial hyperparathyroidism. It is not of course strictly analogous to neonatal myotonic dystrophy in which the neonatal cases are associated with the adult onset form in the mother. Nor is genetic heterogeneity with a truly recessive neonatal form excluded. Whether infants with sporadic neonatal hyperparathyroidism might represent single cases of a recessive form is also unclear.

References

Betts, J. B., O'Malley, B. P. and Rosenthal, F. D. (1980). Hyperparathyroidism: a prerequisite for Zollinger–Ellison syndrome in multiple endocrine adenomatosis type 1—report of a further family and a review of the literature. *Quart. J. Med.* **49**, 69–76.

Boey, J. H., Gilbert, J. M., Cooke, T. J. C., Sweeney, E. C. and Taylor, S. (1975). Occurrence of other endocrine tumours in primary hyperparathyroidism. *Lancet* **2**, 781–4.

Cameron, K. M., Ogg, C. S. and Harrison, A. R. (1966). Familial hyperparathyroidism. *Lancet* **2**, 1006–7.

Carney, J. A., Roth, S. I., Heath, H., Sizemore, G. W. and Hayes, A. B. (1980). The parathyroid glands in multiple endocrine neoplasia type 2b. *Am. J. Pathol.* **99**, 387–98.

Cassidy, C. E. and Anderson, A. S. (1960). A familial occurrence of hyperparathyroidism caused by multiple parathyroid adenomas. *Metabolism* **9**, 1152–8.

Christensson, T. (1976). Familial hyperparathyroidism (letter). *Ann. Intern. Med.* **85**, 614–15.

Cutler, R. E., Reiss, E. and Ackerman, L. V. (1964). Familial hyperparathyroidism: a kindred involving eleven cases, with a discussion of primary chief-cell hyperplasia. *New Engl. J. Med.* **270**, 859–65.

Friesen, S. R., Schimke, R. N. and Pearse, A. G. E. (1972). Genetic aspects of the Z-E syndrome: prospective studies in two kindred: antral gastrin cell hyperplasia. *Ann. Surg.* **176**, 370–83.

Goldsmith, R. E., Sizemore, G. W., Chen, I. W., Zalme, E. and Altemeier, W. A. (1976). Familial hyperparathyroidism: description of a large kindred with physiologic observations and a review of the literature. *Ann. Intern. Med.* **84**, 36–43.

Hillman, D. A., Scriver, C. R., Pedvis, S. and Shragovitch, I. (1964). Neonatal familial primary hyperparathyroidism. *New Engl. J. Med.* **270**, 483–90.

Jackson, C. E. and Boonstra, C. E. (1967). The relationship of hereditary hyperparathyroidism to endocrine adenomatosis. *Am. J. Med.* **43**, 727–34.

——, Talbert, P. C. and Taylor, H. D. (1960). Hereditary hyperparathyroidism. *J. Indiana Med. Assoc.* **53**, 1313–16.

Johnson, G. J., Summerskill, W. H. J., Anderson, V. E. and Keating, F. R. (1967). Clinical and genetic investigation of a large kindred with multiple endocrine adenomatosis. *New Engl. J. Med.* **277**, 1379–85.

Marsden, P., Anderson, J., Doyle, D., Morris, B. A. and Burns, D. A. (1971). Familial hyperparathyroidism. *Br. Med. J.* **3**, 87–90.

Marx, S. J., Spiegel, A. M., Brown, E. M. and Aurbach, G. D. (1977). Family studies in patients with primary parathyroid hyperplasia. *Am. J. Med.* **62**, 698–706.

——, Vinik, A. I., Santen, R. J., Floyd, J. C., Mills, J. L. and Green, J. (1986). Multiple endocrine neoplasia type I: assessment of laboratory tests to screen for the gene in a large kindred. *Medicine* **65**, 226–41.

Peters, N., Chalmers, T. M., Truscott, B. McN., Rack, J. H. and Adams, P. H. (1966). Familial hyperparathyroidism. *Postgrad. Med. J.* **42**, 228–33.

Schimke, R. N. (1984). Genetic aspects of multiple endocrine neoplasia. *Ann. Rev. Med.* **35**, 25–31.

—— and Hartmann, W. H. (1965). Familial amyloid-producing medullary thyroid carcinoma and pheochromocytoma, a distinct genetic entity. *Ann. Intern. Med.* **63**, 1027–39.

Spiegel, A. M., Marx, S. J., Brown, E. M. and Aurbach, G. D. (1977). Neonatal primary hyperparathyroidism with autosomal dominant inheritance. *J. Pediatr.* **90**, 269–72.

Steiner, A. L., Goodman, A. D. and Powers, S. R. (1968). Study of a kindred with pheochromocytoma, medullary thyroid carcinoma, hyperparathyroidism and Cushing's disease: multiple endocrine neoplasia, type II. *Medicine* **47**, 371–409.

Thompson, N. W., Carpenter, L. C. and Kessler, D. L. (1978). Hereditary neo-natal hyperparathyroidism. *Arch. Surg.* **113**, 100–3.
Urbanski, F. X. (1967). Medullary thyroid carcinoma, parathyroid adenoma, and bilateral pheochromocytoma: an unusual triad of endocrine tumors. *J. Chronic Dis.* **20**, 627–36.

5.1.2. Hyperoxaluria

The formation of calcium oxalate renal stones is common throughout the world but is usually associated with normal urinary oxalate excretion. Familial aggregations have been reported in some cases suggestive of autosomal dominant inheritance (Gram 1932; Shepard *et al.* 1960), but the evidence suggests that the genetic influence on oxalate stone function is polygenic (Resnick *et al.* 1968). In rare instances hyperoxaluria is due to increased metabolic production of oxalate (Archer *et al.* 1957) and may result in either calcium oxalate stone formation or in nephro-calcinosis. It is only one of many genetic causes of nephrocalcinosis, discussed in several chapters, and these are listed in Table 4.7. Two types of such oxalosis or primary hyperoxaluria, both with autosomal recessive inheritance, have been described: type I, glycolic aciduria; and type II, L-glyceric aciduria (Williams and Smith 1978). In both types there is renal deposition of calcium oxalate. The earliest report of oxalosis was an autopsy finding of calcium oxalate crystals in bones and kidney of a child who died of renal failure at 12 years of age following recurrent renal stones and nephrocalcinosis (Davis *et al.* 1950). Newns and Black (1953) reported primary oxaluria during life and Aponte and Fetter (1954) described the condition in identical twins. Over 100 cases were reviewed in 1964 (Hockaday *et al.* 1964).

Hyperoxaluria (or oxalosis) type I, glycolicaciduria
Onset is typically within the first half decade with renal colic or haematuria, and less typically with uraemia. The great majority die from renal failure within the first two decades. There may be a secondary hyperuricaemia, and even joint pain (Aponte and Fetter 1954). A less common symptom is heart block due to oxalosis of the conducting tissue of the heart (Coltart and Hudson 1971).

Pathologically there is nephrolithiasis, hydronephrosis, and pyelo-nephritis with or without nephrocalcinosis. Renal damage may be due to nephrocalcinosis but in many cases is wholly or partially secondary to obstruction or infection. At autopsy the kidneys are usually shrunken and scarred (Scowen *et al.* 1959) with, on microscopy, refractile crystals in the convoluted tubules and sometimes also within the interstitial spaces. Glomeruli are largely spared. Extrarenal deposition of calcium oxalate is most prominent in bone and heart.

The immediate precursors of oxalate in humans are ascorbate and glyoxylate. Atkins and colleagues (1965) found normal metabolism of ascorbate in two patients. Glycolic acid and glyoxylate excretion are increased (Chisholm and Heard 1962; Hockaday *et al.* 1964). The catabolism of glyoxylate is diminished with increased excretion as oxalate or glycolate in patients (Crawhall *et al.* 1959; Hockaday *et al.* 1865a and b), and catabolism is less markedly reduced in presumed heterozygotes (Frederick *et al.* 1963). A similar defect in glyoxylate metabolism was demonstrated in kidney homogenates by Dean and coworkers (1966). A diminution in the catabolism of glycolate has also been observed (Hockaday *et al.* 1964). The activity of soluble α-ketoglutarate:glyoxylate carboligase, has been reported as being markedly reduced in tissues from liver, spleen, or kidney of affected patients (Koch *et al.* 1967; Williams and Smith 1968a). The mitochondrial isozyme is not affected. This enzyme catalyses the conversion of glyoxylate and α-ketoglutarate to α-keto-β-hydroxy adipic acid, and is one pathway of glyoxylate catabolism. Glycine is a major precursor of glyoxylate in a reaction which in the reverse direction is dependent on pyridoxine. Although the conversion to glyoxylate is largely carried out by glycine oxidase the reverse reaction is catalysed by transaminases, whose activity was found to be normal in patients (Hockaday *et al.* 1965b; Williams *et al.* 1967).

The early observations of carboligase deficiency in type I hyperoxaluria were questioned by Bourke and associates (1972) who found normal activity of this enzyme in muscle from a patient. Unfortunately they did not assay the enzyme in liver, kidney, or spleen. The doubts raised by this observation have been reinforced by further recent research which indeed necessitates a radical revision of the traditional views. Danpure and colleagues (1986) have shown that the 'soluble' form of α-ketoglutarate:glyoxylate carboligase is merely an artefact due to release of the mitochondrial enzyme into the cystol owing to *in vitro* mitochondrial damage. They found that carboligase of non-mitochondrial origin was virtually undetectable in both normal and hyperoxaluric human liver, and concluded that deficiency of a soluble form could not be the primary defect in type I hyperoxaluria.

This focuses attention back to transamination of glyoxylate to glycine as the possible site of the block. It is of great interest that an early study reported that alanine was an equally effective amino donor as glutamic acid for transamination by the soluble fraction of human liver cells, but a very much more efficient donor for the particulate fraction (Williams *et al.* 1967). The authors also demonstrated normal transamination, with both alanine and glutamic acid, by the soluble fraction from hyper-oxaluric patients, but did not undertake the assay on the particulate fraction from patients, presumably because they had previously reported the apparent carboligase deficiency. Other workers had found normal activity of either soluble (Hockaday *et al.* 1965b), or mitochondrial transaminase (Crawhall and Watts 1962a and b) in hyperoxaluric patients. Danpure and his associates have now demonstrated that there is a total deficiency of peroxisomal alanine:glyoxylate aminotransferase activity in the liver of two patients with type I hyperoxaluria, at least one of whom was pyridoxine resistant (Danpure and Jennings 1986).

Oxalate dynamics have been studied sequentially in a series of patients by Watts and colleagues. They have shown that patients have a raised plasma oxalate concentration, and a grossly increased oxalate metabolic pool especially in renal failure. They found that haemodialysis is the most efficient method of removing oxalate but nevertheless eventually fails to keep pace with tissue oxalate accumulation (Watts *et al.* 1982, 1983, 1984). The high urinary excretion of oxalate cannot be readily modified (Watts *et al.* 1979) except that the administration of pyridoxine has been found to decrease urinary oxalate excretion, plasma oxalate concentration, and metabolic pool size in some patients (Smith and Williams 1967; Gibbs and Watts 1970; Watts *et al.* 1985a; Yendt and Cohanim 1985). More recently a child treated from the age of 8 weeks is reported to have shown a marked fall in urinary oxalate by 7 months and to be still well at 1 year (Rose *et al.* 1982); another infant, similarly treated, was also well at 1 year despite earlier transient pyridoxine neurotoxicity (de Zegher *et al.* 1985). However an elder sib of this latter child had died from oxalosis at 6 months, despite pyridoxine therapy. Renal transplantation does not provide a cure as the transplanted kidney becomes affected by oxalosis (Klauwers *et al.* 1969). An alternative approach which has been attempted is combined renal and hepatic transplantation (Watts *et al.* 1985b).

Hockaday and coworkers (1964) reviewed at least 16 families with two or more sibs affected with type I hyperoxaluria and with no evidence of the disease in their parents. Of 13 families for which information was available there were 30 affected to 29 unaffected, a ratio which allowing for ascertainment bias is consistent with autosomal recessive inheritance. Furthermore the incidence of parental consanguinity was over tenfold greater than in the general population. Lindenmayer (1970) managed to trace the ancestry of three affected sibships to a common ancestral couple born in the eighteenth century. It would seem reasonable to conclude that in at least some cases of the pyridoxine-resistant form of type I hyperoxaluria there is autosomal recessive inheritance of deficient activity of peroxisomal alanine:glyoxylate aminotransferase. Whether this is so for all such cases, and for pyridoxine-sensitive cases, remains to be seen. There is as yet no method of prenatal diagnosis. Measurement of oxalate and glycolate is not reliable (Leumann *et al.* 1986).

Hyperoxaluria (or oxalosis) type II, glycericaciduria

Williams and Smith (1986b) reported a new variant of primary hyper-oxaluria in three sibs and a fourth unrelated patient. These patients had a milder form of disease with presentation with haematuria or renal colic at anything from 18 months to 24 years of age, and without progression to renal failure. Metabolic studies have shown increased oxalate excretion as in type I but normal glycolate and glyoxylate excretion and markedly increased urinary excretion of L-glyceric acid (Hockaday *et al.* 1964; Williams and Smith 1968b). Williams and Smith (1968b) demonstrated that the enzyme deficiency in this form, assayed in leuco-cytes, involves D-glyceric dehydrogenase, which converts hydroxy-pyruvate to D-glycerate. They later suggested that the high blood levels of hydroxypyruvate, that result from this metabolic block, stimulate oxidation of glycolate to oxalate and decrease reduction of glyoxylate to glycolate (Williams and Smith 1971).

Inheritance of this form of primary hyperoxaluria is probably auto-somal recessive in view of its occurrence in three sibs and leucocyte enzyme activities in the mother that were reduced and in the father at the lower range of normal (Williams and Smith 1968b). However, further families will need to be studied before the mode of inheritance can be confirmed.

Atypical primary hyperoxaluria

Watts and colleagues (1983) described two differing atypical cases, one with onset at 44 years with renal stones, sustained hyperoxaluria but normal glycolate excretion; and the other with recurring oxalate stones, hyperglycollic aciduria, and a urinary oxalate excretion, which although initially raised has gradually declined to normal on a low dietary oxalate intake.

References

Aponte, G. E. and Fetter, T. R. (1954). Familial idiopathic oxalate nephro-calcinosis. *Am. J. Clin. Pathol.* **24**, 1363–73.

Archer, H. E., Dormer, A. E., Scowen, E. F. and Watts, R. W. E. (1957). Primary hyperoxaluria. *Lancet* **2**, 320–2.

Atkins, G. L., Dean, B. M., Griffin, W. J., Scowen, E. F. and Watts, R. W. E. (1965). Quantitative aspects of ascorbic acid metabolism in patients with primary hyperoxaluria. *Clin. Sci.* **29**, 305–14.

Bourke, E., Frindt, G., Flynn, P. and Schreiner, G. E. (1972). Primary hyperoxaluria with normal alpha-ketoglutarate:glyoxylate carboligase activity. Treatment with isocarboxid. *Ann. Intern. Med.* **76**, 279–84.

Chisholm, G. D. and Heard, B. E. (1962). Oxalosis, *Br. J. Surg.* **50**, 78–92.

Coltart, D. J. and Hudson, R. E. B. (1971). Primary oxalosis of the heart: a cause of heart block. *Br. Heart J.* **33**, 315–19.

Crawhall, J. C. and Watts, R. W. E. (1962a), The metabolism of glyoxylate by human- and rat-liver mitochondria. *Biochem. J.* **85**, 163–71.

—— and —— (1962b). The metabolism of [1-^{14}C] glyoxylate by the liver mitochondria of patients with primary hyperoxaluria and non-hyperoxaluric subjects. *Clin. Sci.* **23**, 163–8.

——, Scowen, E. F. and Watts, R. W. E. (1959). Conversion of glycine to oxalate in primary hyperoxaluria. *Lancet* **2**, 806–9.

Danpure, C. J. and Jennings, P. R. (1986). Peroxisomal alanine:glyoxylate aminotransferase deficiency in primary hyperoxaluria type I. *FEBS Lett.,* **201**, 20–4.

——, Purkiss, P., Jennings, P. R. and Watts, R. W. E. (1986). Mitochondrial damage and the subcellular distribution of 2-oxoglutarate:glyoxylate carboligase in normal human and rat liver and in the liver of a patient with primary hyperoxaluria type I. *Clin. Sci.* **70**, 417–25.

Davis, J. S., Klingberg, W. G. and Stowell, R. E. (1950). Nephrolithiasis and nephrocalcinosis with calcium oxalate crystals in kidneys and bones. *J. Pediatr.* **36**, 323–34.

Dean, B. M., Griffin, W. J. and Watts, R. W. E. (1966). Primary hyperoxaluria. The demonstration of a metabolic abnormality in kidney tissue. *Lancet* **1**, 406.

Frederick, E. W., Rabkin, M. T., Richie, R. H. and Smith, L. H. Jr. (1963). Studies in primary hyperoxaluria. I. *In vivo* demonstration of a defect in glyoxylate metabolism. *New Engl. J. Med.* **269**, 821–9.

Gibbs, D. A. and Watts, R. W. E. (1970). The action of pyridoxine in primary hyperoxaluria. *Clin. Sci.* **38**, 277–86.

Gram, H. C. (1932). The heredity of oxalic urinary calculi. *Acta Med. Scand.* **78**, 268–81.

Hockaday, T. D. R., Clayton, J. E., Frederick, E. W. and Smith, L. H. Jr. (1964). Primary hyperoxaluria. *Medicine* **43**, 315–45.

——, Frederick, E. W., Clayton, J. E. and Smith, L. H. Jr. (1965a). Studies on primary hyperoxaluria. II. Urinary oxalate, glycolate, and glyoxylate measurements by isotope dilution method. *J. Lab. Clin. Med.* **65**, 677–87.

——, Clayton, J. E. and Smith, L. H. Jr. (1965b). The metabolic error in primary hyperoxaluria. *Arch. Dis. Child.* **40**, 485–91.

Klauwers, J., Wolf, P. L. and Cohn, R. (1969). Renal transplantation in primary oxalosis. *JAMA* **209**, 551.

Koch, J., Stokstad, E. L., Williams, H. E. and Smith, L. H. Jr. (1967). Deficiency of 2-oxo-glutarate:glyoxylate carboligase activity in primary hyperoxaluria. *Proc. Nat. Acad. Sci.* **57**, 1123–9.

Leumann, E., Matasovic, A. and Niederwieser, A. (1986). Primary hyperoxaluria type I: oxalate and glycolate unsuitable for prenatal diagnosis. *Lancet* **2**, 340.

Lindenmeyer, J. P. (1970). L'hérédité dans l'oxalose familiale. *J. Génét. Hum.* **18**, 31–44.

Newns, G. H. and Black, J. A. (1953). A case of calcium oxalate nephrocalcinosis. *Great Ormond St. J.* **5**, 40–4.

Resnick, M., Pridgen, D. B. and Goodman, H. O. (1968). Genetic predisposition to calcium oxalate renal calculi. *New Engl. J. Med.* **278**, 1313–18.

Rose, G. A., Arthur, L. J. H., Chambers, T. L., Kasidas, G. P. and Scott, I. V. (1982). Successful treatment of primary hyperoxaluria in a neonate. *Lancet* **1**, 1298–9.

Scowen, E. F., Stansfield, A. G. and Watts, R. W. E. (1959). Oxalosis and primary hyperoxaluria. *J. Pathol. Bact.* **77**, 195–205.

Shepard, T. H. Jr., Lee, L. W. and Krebs, E. G. (1960). Primary hyperoxaluria. II. Genetic studies in a family. *Pediatrics* **25**, 869–71.

Smith, L. H. Jr. and Williams, H. E. (1967). Treatment of primary hyperoxaluria. *Mod. Treat.* **4**, 522–30.

Watts, R. W. E., Chalmers, R. A., Gibbs, D. A., Lawson, A. M., Purkiss, P. and Spellacy, E. (1979). Studies on some possible biochemical treatment of primary hyperoxaluria. *Quart. J. Med.* **48**, 259–72.

——, Veall, N. and Purkiss, P. (1982). Simultaneous oxalate and ^{99m}Tc-DTPA clearances and spaces in primary hyperoxaluria. *Clin. Sci.* **63**, 43P.

——, —— and —— (1984). Oxalate dynamics and removal rates during haemodialysis and peritoneal dialysis in patients with primary hyperoxaluria and severe renal failure. *Clin. Sci.* **66**, 591–7.

——, —— and —— (1983). Sequential studies of oxalate dynamics in primary hyperoxaluria. *Clin. Sci.* **65**, 627–33.

——, ——, ——, Mansell, M. and Haywood, E. F. (1985a). The effect of pyridoxine on oxalate dynamics in three cases of primary oxaluria (with glycollic aciduria). *Clin. Sci.* **69**, 87–90.

——, Calne, R. Y., Williams, R., Mansell, M. A., Veall, N., Purkiss, P. and Rolles, K. (1985b). Primary hyperoxaluria (type 1): attempted treatment by combined hepatic and renal transplantation. *Quart. J. Med.* **57**, 697–703.

Williams, H. E. and Smith, L. H. Jr. (1968a). Disorders of oxalate metabolism. *Am. J. Med.* **45**, 715–35.

—— and —— (1968b). L-glyceric aciduria: a new genetic variant of primary hyperoxaluria. *New Engl. J. Med.* **278**, 233–9.

—— and —— (1971). Hyperoxaluria in L-glyceric aciduria: possible pathogenetic mechanism. *Science* **171**, 390–1.

—— and —— (1978). Primary hyperoxaluria. Chapter 9 in *The metabolic basis of inherited disease*, 4th edn. eds. Stanbury, J. B., Wyngaarden, J. B. and Fredrickson, D. S. pp. 182–204. McGraw-Hill, New York.

——, Wilson, M. and Smith, L. H. (1967). Studies on primary hyperoxaluria. III. Transamination reactions of glyoxylate in human tissue preparations. *J. Lab. Clin. Med.* **70**, 494–502.

Yendt, E. R. and Cohanim, M. (1985). Response to a physiologic dose of pyridoxine in type I primary hyperoxaluria. *New Engl. J. Med.* **312**, 953–7.

de Zegher, F., Przyrembel, H., Chalmers, R. A., Wolff, E. D. and Huijmans, J. G. M. (1985). Successful treatment of infantile type I primary hyperoxaluria complicated by pyridoxine toxicity. *Lancet* **2**, 392–3.

5.1.3. Lesch–Nyhan disease and partial hypoxanthine phosphoribosyltranferase deficiency

This disorder was originally described as one characterized by spastic cerebral palsy, choreoathetosis, mental retardation, self-multilation, and hyperuricaemia with excess excretion of uric acid (Lesch and Nyhan 1964). This clinical picture has been generally accepted up to the present day. However a critical assessment of a series of patients over a period of 10 years by R. W. E. Watts' group has led to a refinement of the clinical features (Watts *et al.* 1982). Because of the severe neurological deficit with dysarthria, movement incoordination, and behavioural disturbance, communication is grossly impaired in these children and psychological tests are very difficult to interpret. However, there is only doubtful evidence of intellectual impairment, and indeed this remains clearly normal in many severely handicapped patients. The apparent spastic cerebral palsy and choreoathetosis are in fact a marked hypotonia super-imposed on torsion dystonia with ridigity, rather than spasticity, postural distortion, and dysarthria. These abnormalities prevent the child developing normal speech and locomotion. The most striking feature is the self-mutilation consisting mainly in biting of the fingers, lips and buccal mucosa, but also head banging and scratching. This biting is a compulsive disorder which the patients cannot help yet fear. It may be externalized as aggressive behaviour, which likewise they regret.

The hyperuricaemia is associated with increased purine synthesis leading to excess uric acid production (Michener 1967; Rosenberg *et al.* 1967). The increased uric acid excretion leads in most patients to crystal-luria at some time (Hoefnagal *et al.* 1965), and may progress to symptomatic uric acid or xanthine urolithiasis with eventual urinary tract obstruction and even renal failure as the cause of death. At autopsy the kidneys are shrunken and contain deposits of monosodium urate and uric acid (Crussi *et al.* 1969). Two of the eight patients followed by Watts *et al.* (1982) developed renal stones but none developed obstructive uropathy. In adequately treated patients urinary tract obstruction due to stones is an avoidable complication, but in earlier case studies is relatively common.

The disease was shown to be associated typically with virtually complete deficiency in the activity of the purine salvage pathway enzyme hypoxanthine–quanine phosphoribosyltransferase (HGPRT) by Seegmiller and colleagues (Seegmiller *et al.* 1967) in red cells and cultured fibroblasts. The enzyme deficiency has subsequently been confirmed in other tissues including liver and brain (Rosenbloom *et al.* 1967a; Kelley 1968; Watts *et al.* 1982). This complete deficiency has to be distinguished from the partial deficiency of the same enzyme seen in a rare form of gout (Kelley *et al.* 1967, 1969). Nevertheless even among patients with Lesch–Nyhan syndrome there is evidence for variation in the enzyme defect. In some patients there are variably low levels of activity rather than complete absence (Fujimoto and Seegmiller 1970; Kelley and Meade 1971; McDonald and Kelley 1971), but within a single family levels of activity vary very little. Thermal stability of HGPRT may be either reduced (Kelley *et al.* 1967; Sperling *et al.* 1972) or increased (Kelley *et al.* 1967). It may show altered electrophoretic mobility (Kelley *et al.* 1969; Bakay and Nyhan 1972a and b) and further differences in kinetic and other properties suggesting at least 10 or 12 different defective variants (Willers *et al.* 1977; Kelley and Wyngaarden 1983). Even among those cases without measureable HGPRT activity there is variation as to immunological cross-reactivity with antisera to the normal enzyme, the majority being cross-reacting material negative (CRM⁻) but with CRM⁺ patients exhibiting an amount of cross-reacting protein comparable to the amount of enzyme protein in normal individuals (Arnold *et al.* 1972; Muller and Stermberger 1974; Yip *et al.* 1974; Ghangas and Milman 1975; Upchurch *et al.* 1975; Watts *et al.* 1982).

Wilson and colleagues (1981, 1982) have purified HGPRT from several unrelated patients and partially characterized five distinct mutant enzymes: HGPRT Toronto, HGPRT London, HGPRT Kinston, HGPRT Munich, and HGPRT Ann Arbor. More recently they have published the complete amino acid sequence of the normal protein (Wilson *et al.* 1983a), and described an amino acid substitution in one mutant form (Wilson *et al.* 1983b). Even more recently the HGPRT gene has been cloned and sequenced (Jolly *et al.* 1983) and recombinant DNA studies using radiolabelled HGPRT-cDNA probes have confirmed genetic heterogeneity with evidence for gene mutation in some cases (Wilson and Kelley 1983; Wilson *et al.* 1983c and d), and gene deletion in others (Yang *et al.* 1984). A three-allele restriction fragment length polymorphism defined by the restriction enzyme BamHI has been detected within the HGPRT gene (Jolly *et al.* 1983; Nussbaum *et al.* 1983), and has proved useful in prenatal diagnosis and heterozygote detection (Gibbs *et al.* 1986). Others have reported a variety of mutations and deletions in the HGPRT gene (Patel *et al.* 1986; Wilson *et al.* 1986).

Patients with the Lesch–Nyhan syndrome have all been boys, with only a single exception (Hara *et al.* 1982). X linkage was first suggested by Hoefnagel and colleagues (Hoefnagel *et al.* 1965) who noted that transmission was through unaffected females. This view has been fully supported by later family studies (Shapiro *et al.* 1966; Nyhan *et al.* 1967). In the presumed allelic disorder of partial HGPRT deficiency with gout no male-to-male transmission has been observed (Kelley *et al.* 1969), confirming X linkage. Furthermore the assignment of the HGPRT locus to the X chromosome (Nabholz *et al.* 1969), and the observation of two cell populations in fibroblast cultures from obligate heterozygotes (Rosenbloom *et al.* 1967b; Migeon *et al.* 1968; Salzmann *et al.* 1968; Migeon 1970), provide further confirmation. The latter observation, based on autoradiographic demonstration of uptake of labelled hypoxanthine by some cells but not others, also establishes that the HGPRT locus is subject to normal X inactivation. In mouse–human somatic cell hybrids the HGPRT consistently segregates with glucose 6-phosphate dehydrogenase (G6PD) activity, indicating synteny for these loci on the X chromosome (Ruddle 1971) and a regional assignment to the long arm (Shows and Brown 1975). Goss and Harris (1977) using cell hybrids in which the human parental cell line had been irradiated established a gene order of PGK:a-GAL:HGPT:G6PD. However, although HGPRT and G6PD are assigned close to one another they are not closely linked, as in one family in which both HGPRT and G6PD deficiency were segregating there were two recombinants out of four (Nyhan *et al.* 1970).

Heterozygotes cannot be detected by red-cell enzyme assay as these cells may not contain any of the mutant enzyme (McDonald and Kelley 1972), and this also appears to be true of peripheral lymphocytes (Dancis *et al.* 1968). This is probably due to progenitor cells with normal enzyme having a growth advantage *in vivo* (McKeran *et al.* 1975). Heterozygote detection therefore depends on the demonstration of mosaicism for normal and mutant enzyme activity in cultured skin fibroblasts or hair roots (Gartler *et al.* 1971; Silvers *et al.* 1972; McKeran *et al.* 1975; Watts *et al.* 1982). Such methods have been used to determine the frequency of fresh mutation in sporadic cases by estimating the proportion of such cases with homozygous normal mothers. Francke and coworkers (1976) found a much lower proportion of fresh mutations than the expected one-third, and Watts *et al.* (1982) found that in only one of their eight cases was the mother not a heterozygote. This may be due to a higher mutation rate in males than females, disturbed segregation, or increased fitness of female heterozygotes (Winter 1980). The enzymatic and molecular studies discussed above bare witness to the extreme genetic heterogeneity of mutations at the HGPRT locus. Enzyme assay on cultured amniotic fluid cells permits the prenatal diagnosis of the heterozygous (Fujimoto *et al.* 1968) or hemizygous state (DeMars *et al.* 1969). Prenatal diagnosis of the hemizygote with subsequent termination was first made by Boyle and colleagues (1970) and is now an established procedure. A recent paper has reported prenatal diagnosis by chorionic villus biospy (Gibbs *et al.* 1984).

The partial enzyme deficiency, mentioned earlier, has been frequently reported with a variable clinical picture (Kelley *et al.* 1967, 1969; Sweetman *et al.* 1978; Kelley and Wyngaarden 1983). Most of these patients show nephropathy and gout. In about one fifth of these there are mild to severe neurological abnormalities but no self-mutilation (Kelley *et al.* 1969; Dancis *et al.* 1973; Emmerson and Thompson 1973; de Bruyn 1976). In one family, without neurological involvement but with

HGPRT levels about 5–12 per cent of normal assayed against hypoxanthine, the K_m of the residual enzyme for phosphoribosyl pyrophosphate (PP-ribose-P) was elevated 10- to 20-fold and showed increased thermal lability (Synder *et al.* 1984). As mentioned above, Wilson and colleagues (1983b) have reported a point mutation of the enzyme, with a single amino acid substitution, in a patient with partial enzyme deficiency and gout. Partial HGPRT deficiency with gout, or hyperuricaemia, and renal failure has also been reported in infancy (Rosenthal *et al.* 1964; Holland *et al.* 1983; Lorentz *et al.* 1984).

References

Arnold, W. J., Meade, J. C. and Kelley, W. N. (1972). Hypoxanthine–guanine phosphoribosyltransferase: characteristics of the mutant enzyme in erythrocytes from patients with the Lesch–Nyhan syndrome. *J. Clin. Invest.* **51**, 1805–12.

Bakay, B. and Nyhan, W. L. (1972a). Activation of variants of hypoxanthine–guanine phosphoribosyltransferase by the normal enzyme. *Proc. Nat. Acad. Sci.* **69**, 2523–7.

—— and —— (1972b). Electrophoretic properties of hypoxanthine–guanine phosphoribosyl transferase in erythrocytes of subjects with Lesch–Nyhan syndrome. *Biochem. Genet.* **6**, 139–46.

Boyle, J. A., Raivio, K. O., Astrin, K. H., Shulman, J. D., Graf, M. L., Seegmiller, J. E. and Jacobson, C. B. (1970). Lesch–Nyhan syndrome: preventive control by prenatal diagnosis. *Science* **169**, 688–9.

Crussi, F. G., Robertson, D. M. and Hiscox, J. L. (1969). The pathological condition of the Lesch–Nyhan syndrome. *Am. J. Dis. Child.* **118**, 501–6.

Dancis, J., Berman, P. H., Jansen, V. and Balis, M. E. (1968). Absence of mosaicism in the lymphocyte in X-linked congenital hyperuricosuria. *Life Sci.* **7**, 587–91.

——, Yip, L. C., Cox, R. P., Piomelli, S. and Balis, M. E. (1973). Disparate enzyme activity in erythrocytes and leukocytes. *J. Clin. Invest.* **52**, 2068–74.

de Bruyn, G. (1976). Hypoxanthine–guanine phosphoribosyl transferase deficiency. *Hum. Genet.* **31**, 127–50.

DeMars, R., Sarto, G., Felix, J. S. and Benke, P. (1969). Lesch–Nyhan mutation: prenatal detection with amniotic fluid cells. *Science* **164**, 1303–5.

Emmerson, B. T. and Thompson, L. (1973). The spectrum of hypoxanthine–guanine phosphoribosyl transferase deficiency. *Quart. J. Med.* **42**, 423–40.

Francke, U., Felsenstein, J., Gartler, S. M., Migeon, B. R., Dancis, J., Seegmiller, J. E., Bakay, F. and Nyhan, W. L. (1976). The occurrence of new mutants in the X-linked recessive Lesch–Nyhan disease. *Am. J. Hum. Genet.* **28**, 123–37.

Fujimoto, W. Y. and Seegmiller, J. E. (1970). Hypoxanthine–guanine phosphoribosyltransferase deficiency: activity in normal, mutant and heterozygote cultured human skin fibroblasts. *Proc. Nat. Acad. Sci.* **65**, 577–84.

——, ——, Uhlendorf, B. W., and Jacobson, C.-B. (1968). Biochemical diagnosis of an X-linked disease *in utero*. *Lancet* **2**, 511–12.

Gartler, S. M., Scott, R. C., Goldstein, J. L., Campbell, B. and Sparkes, R. (1971).

Lesch–Nyhan syndrome: rigid detection of heterozygotes by the use of hair follicles. *Science* **172**, 572–4.

Ghangas, G. S. and Milman, G. (1975). Radioimmune determination of hypoxanthine phosphoribosyltransferase cross-reacting material in erythrocytes of Lesch–Nyhan patients.

Gibbs, D. A., McFadyen, I. R., Crawfurd, M. d'A., de Muinck Keizer, E. E., Headhouse-Benson, C. M., Wilson, T. M. and Farrant, P. H. (1984). First-trimester diagnosis of Lesch–Nyhan syndrome. *Lancet* **2**, 1180–3.

——, Headhouse-Benson, C. M. and Watts, R. W. E. (1986). Family studies of the Lesch–Nyhan syndrome: the use of a restriction fragment length polymorphism (RFLP) closely linked to the disease gene for carrier state and prenatal diagnosis. *J. Inher. Metab. Dis.* **9**, 45–58.

Goss, S. J. and Harris, H. (1977). Gene transfer by means of cell fusion. I. Statistical mapping of the human X-chromosome by analysis of radiation-induced gene segregation. *J. Cell Sci.* **25**, 17–37.

Hara, K., Kashiwamata, S., Ogasawara, N., Ohishi, H., Natsume, R., Yamanaka, T., Hakamada, S., Miyazaki, S. and Watanabe, K. (1982). A female case of the Lesch–Nyhan syndrome. *Tohoku, J. Exp. Med.* **137**, 275–82.

Hoefnagal, D., Andrew, E. D., Mireault, N. G. and Berndt, W. O. (1965). Hereditary choreoathetosis, self-mutilation and hyperuricaemia in young males. *New Engl. J. Med.* **273**, 130–5.

Holland, P. C., Dillon, M. J., Pincott, J., Simmonds, H. A. and Barratt, T. M. (1983). Hypoxanthine guanine phosphoribosyltransferase deficiency presenting with gout and renal failure in infancy. *Arch. Dis. Child.* **58**, 831–3.

Jolly, D. J., Okayama, H., Berg, P., Esty, A. C., Filpula, D., Bohlen, P., Johnson, G. G., Shively, J. E., Hunkapillar, T. and Friedmann, T. (1983). Isolation and characterization of a full-length expressible cDNA for human hypoxanthine phosphoribosyltransferase. *Proc. Nat. Acad. Sci.* **80**, 477–81.

Kelley, W. N. (1968). Hypoxanthine–guanine phosphoribosyltransferase deficiency in the Lesch–Nyhan syndrome and gout. *Fed. Proc.* **27**, 1047–52.

—— and Meade, J. C. (1971). Studies on hypoxanthine–guanine phosphoribosyltransferase in fibroblasts from patients with the Lesch–Nyhan syndrome: evidence for genetic heterogeneity. *J. Biol. Chem.* **246**, 2953–8.

—— and Wyngaarden, J. B. (1983). The Lesch–Nyhan syndrome. Chapter 51 in *The metabolic basis of inherited disease,* 5th edn. eds. Stanbury, J. B., Wyngaarden, J. B., Fredrickson, D. S., Goldstein, J. L. and Brown, M. S. pp. 1115–43. McGraw-Hill, New York.

——, Rosenbloom, F. M., Henderson, J. F. and Seegmiller, J. E. (1967). A specific enzyme defect in gout associated with overproduction of uric acid. *Proc. Nat. Acad. Sci.* **57**, 1735–9.

——, Greene, M. L., Rosenbloom, F. M., Henderson, J. F. and Seegmiller, J. E. (1969). Hypoxanthine–guanine phosphoribosyltransferase deficiency in gout. *Ann. Intern. Med.* **70**, 155–206.

Lesch, M. and Nyhan, W. L. (1964). A familial disorder of uric acid metabolism and central nervous function. *Am. J. Med.* **36**, 561–70.

Lorentz, W. B., Burton, B. K., Trillo, A. and Browning, M. C. (1984). Failure to thrive, hyperuricaemia, and renal insufficiency in early infancy secondary to partial hypoxanthine–guanine phosphoribosyltransferase deficiency. *J. Pediatr.* **104**, 94–7.

McDonald, J. A. and Kelley, W. N. (1971). Lesch–Nyhan Syndrome: altered kinetic properties of the mutant enzyme. *Science* 171, 689–91.

—— and —— (1972). Lesch–Nyhan Syndrome: absence of the mutant enzyme in erythrocytes of a heterozygote for both normal and mutant hypoxanthine-guanine phosphoribosyltransferase. *Biochem. Genet.* 6, 21–6.

McKern, R. O., Andrews, T. M., Howell, A., Gibbs, D. A., Chinn, S. and Watts, R. W. E. (1975). The diagnosis of the carrier state for the Lesch–Nyhan syndrome. *Quart. J. Med.* 44, 189–206.

Michener, W. M. (1967). Hyperuricaemia and mental retardation with athetosis and self-mutilation. *Am. J. Dis. Child.* 113, 195–206.

Migeon, B. R. (1970). X-linked hypoxanthine–guanine phosphoribosyltransferase deficiency: detection of heterozygotes by selective medium. *Biochem. Genet.* 4, 377–83.

——, der Kaloustian, V. M., Nyhan, W. L., Young, W. J. and Childs, B. (1968). X-linked hypoxanthine–guanine phosphoribosyltransferase deficiency: heterozygote has two clonal populations. *Science* 160, 425–7.

Muller, M. M. and Stermberger, H. (1974). Biochemische und immunologische Untersuchungen der Hypoxanthin–guanin Phosphoribosyltransferase in der Erythrozyten von Lesch–Nyhan-Patienten. *Wien Klin. Wschr.* 86, 127–31.

Nabholz, M., Miggiano, V. and Bodmer, W. (1969). Genetic analysis with human–mouse somatic cell hybrids. *Nature* 223, 358–63.

Nussbaum, R. L., Crowder, W. E., Nyhan, W. L. and Caskey, C. T. (1983). A three-allele restriction-fragment-length polymorphism at the hypoxanthine phosphoribosyltransferase locus in man. *Proc. Nat. Acad. Sci.* 80, 4035–9.

Nyhan, W. L., Resek, J., Sweetnam, L., Carpentner, D. G. and Carter, C. H. (1967). Genetics of an X-linked disorder of uric acid metabolism and cerebral function. *Pediatr. Res.* 1, 5–13.

——, Bakay, B., Connor, J. D., Marks, J. F. and Keele, D. K. (1970). Hemizygous expression of glucose-6-phosphate dehydrogenase in erythrocytes of heterozygotes for the Lesch–Nyhan syndrome. *Proc. Nat. Acad. Sci.* 65, 214–18.

Page, T., Bakay, B., Nissinen, E. and Nyhan, W. L. (1981). Hypoxanthine–guanine phosphoribosyltransferase variants: correlation of clinical phenotype with enzyme activity. *J. Inher. Metab. Dis.* 4, 203–6.

Patel, P. I., Framson, P. E., Caskey, C. T. and Chinault, A. C. (1986). Fine structure of the human hypoxanthine phosphoribosyltransferase gene. *Mol. Cell. Biol.* 6, 393–403.

Rosenberg, D., Monnet, P., Mamelle, J. L., Colombel, M., Salle, B. and Bovier-Lapierre, M. (1967). Encephalopathie avec troubles du metabolisme des purines. *Presse Med.* 76, 2333–40.

Rosenbloom, F. M., Kelley, W. N., Miller, J., Henderson, J. F. and Seegmiller, J. E. (1967a). Inherited disorder of purine metabolism: correlation between central nervous system dysfunction and biochemical defects. *JAMA* 202, 175–7.

——, ——, Henderson, J. F. and Seegmiller, J. E. (1967b). Lyon hypothesis and X-linked disease (letter). *Lancet* 2, 305–6.

Rosenthal, I. M., Gaballah, S. and Rafelson, M. E. (1964). Gout in infancy manifested by renal failure. *Pediatrics* 33, 251–7.

Ruddle, F. H. (1971). Linkage studies employing mouse–man somatic cell hybrids. *Fed. Proc.* 30, 921–5.

Salzmann, J., de Mars, R. and Benke, P. (1968). Single allele expression at an

X-linked hyperuricaemia locus in heterozygous human cells. *Proc. Nat. Acad. Sci.* **60**, 545–52.

Seegmiller, J. E., Rosenbloom, F. M. and Kelley W. N. (1967). An enzymatic defect associated with a sex-linked human neurologic disorder and excessive purine synthesis. *Science* **155**, 1682–4.

Shapiro, S. L., Sheppard, G. L. Jr., Dreifuss, F. E. and Newcombe, D. S. (1966). X-linked recessive inheritance of a syndrome of mental retardation with hyperuricemia. *Proc. Soc. Exp. Biol. Med.* **122**, 609–11.

Shows, T. B. and Brown, J. A. (1975). Human X-linked genes regionally mapped utilizing X-autosome translocations and somatic cell hybrids. *Proc. Nat. Acad. Sci.* **72**, 2124–9.

Silvers, D. N., Cox, R. P., Balis, M. E. and Dancis, J. (1972). Detection of the heterozygote in Lesch–Nyhan disease by hair-root analysis. *New Engl. J. Med.* **286**, 390–5.

Snyder, F. F., Chudley, A. E., MacLeod, P. M., Carter, R. J., Fung, E., and Lowe, J. K. (1984). Partial deficiency of hypoxanthine–guanine phosphoribosyltransferase with reduced affinity for PP-ribose-P in four related males with gout. *Hum. Genet.* **67**, 18–22.

Sperling, O., Boer, P., Eilam, G. and De Vries, A. (1972). Altered kinetic properties of erythrocyte phosphoribosylpyrophosphate synthetase in excessive purine production. *Eur. J. Clin. Biol. Res.* **17**, 703–6.

Sweetman, L., Hock, M. A., Bakay, B., Boden, M., Lesh, P. and Nyhan, W. L. (1978). A distinct variant of hypoxanthine–guanine phosphoribosyl transferase. *J. Pediatr.* **92**, 385–9.

Upchurch, K. S., Leyva, A., Arnold, W. J., Holmes, E. W. and Kelley, W. N. (1975). Hypoxanthine phosphoribosyltransferase deficiency: association of reduced catalytic activity with reduced levels of immunologically detectable enzyme protein. *Proc. Nat. Acad. Sci.* **72**, 4142–6.

Watts, R. W. E., Spellacy, E., Gibbs, D. A., Allsop, J., McKeran, R. O. and Slavin, G. E. (1982). Clinical, postmortem, biochemical and therapeutic observations on the Lesch–Nyhan syndrome with particular reference to the neurological manifestations. *Quart. J. Med.* **51**, 43–78.

Willers, I., Held, K. R., Singh, S. and Goedde, H. W. (1977). Genetic heterogeneity of hypoxanthine- phosphoribosyltransferase in human fibroblasts of 3 families. *Clin. Genet.* **11**, 193–200.

Wilson, J. M. and Kelley, W. N. (1983). Molecular basis of hypoxanthine–guanine phosphoribosyltransferase deficiency in a patient with the Lesch–Nyhan syndrome. *J. Clin. Invest.* **71**, 1331–5.

——, Baugher, B. W., Landa, L. and Kelley, W. N. (1981). Human hypoxanthine–guanine phosphoribosyltransferase: purification and characterization of mutant forms of the enzyme. *J. Biol. Chem.* **256**, 10306–12.

——, ——, Mattes, P. M., Daddona, P. E. and Kelley, W. N. (1982). Human hypoxanthine–guanine phosphoribosyltransferase: demonstration of structural variants in lymphoblastoid cells derived from patients with a deficiency of the enzyme. *J. Clin. Invest.* **69**, 706–15.

——, Tarr, G. E. and Kelley, W. N. (1983a). Human hypoxanthine (guanine) phosphoribosyltransferase. Complete amino-acid sequence of the erythrocyte enzyme. *J. Biol. Chem.* **257**, 10978–85.

——, —— and —— (1983b). Human hypoxanthine (guanine) phosphoribosyltransferase: an amino acid substitution in a mutant form of the enzyme isolated from a patient with gout. *Proc. Nat. Acad. Sci.* **80**, 820–73.

——, Frossard, P., Nussbaum, R. L., Caskey, C. T. and Kelley, W. N. (1983c). Human hypoxanthine–guanine phosphoribosyltransferase. Detection of a mutant allele by restriction endonuclease analysis. *J. Clin. Invest.* **72**, 767–72.

——, Young, A. B. and Kelley, W. N. (1983d). Hypoxanthine–guanine phosphoribosyltransferase deficiency. The molecular basis of the clinical syndromes. *New Engl. J. Med.* **309**, 900–10.

——, Stout, J. T., Palella, T. D., Davidson, B. L., Kelley, W. N. and Caskey, C. T. (1986). A molecular survey of hypoxanthine–guanine phosphoribosyltransferase deficiency in man. *J. Clin. Invest.* **77**, 188–95.

Winter, R. M. (1980). Estimation of male to female ratio of mutation rates from carrier-detection tests in X-linked disorders. *Am. J. Hum. Genet.* **32**, 582–8.

Yang, T. P., Patel, P. I., Chinault, A. C., Stout, J. T., Jackson, L. G., Hildebrand, B. M. and Caskey, C. T. (1984). Molecular evidence for new mutation at the *hprt* locus in Lesch–Nyhan patients. *Nature* **310**, 412–14.

Yip, L. C., Dancis, J., Mathieson, B. and Balis, M. E. (1974). Age induced changes in adenosinemonophosphate: pyrophosphate phosphoribosyltransferase and inosine monophosphate: pyrophosphate phosphoribosyltransferase from normal and Lesch–Nyhan erythrocytes. *Biochemistry* **13**, 2558–61.

5.1.4. Phosphoribosylpyrophosphate synthetase overactivity

This enzyme is best known clinically for a severe deficiency associated with a rare megaloblastic anaemia, hypouricaemia, and mental deficiency (Wada *et al.* 1974). However, two families have been reported in which overactivity of this enzyme is associated with hyperuricaemia and excessive uric acid excretion. In one family studied by Sperling and his colleagues (Sperling *et al.* 1972, 1973; Zoref *et al.* 1975, 1977) clinical gout is associated with increased enzyme activity only at low concentrations of orthophosphate, and the enzyme shows reduced sensitivity to the potential feedback inhibitors ADP and guanosine diphosphate (GDP). In the mother of the male proband two cell populations were demonstrated in fibroblast culture, one mutant and the other normal. In the second family, presumably due to a different mutation, two brothers had hyperuricaemia, gout, and in one case renal colic due to urolithiasis. The enzyme was overactive at all concentrations of orthophosphate and showed normal sensitivity to ADP and GDP. In this family gout and urolithiasis were seen only in males with clinical onset at puberty or shortly thereafter, but enzyme overactivity was found in both sexes (Becker *et al.* 1973a and b). One carrier female in this family had an intermediate level of enzyme activity and on electrophoresis showed two distinct bands of enzyme activity (Yen and Becker 1977).

The assignment of the gene for this enzyme to the X chromosome long arm, between HGPRT and α-galactosidase, confirms that the disorder is inherited in an X-linked recessive manner, but clearly even with only two reported families there is genetic heterogeneity.

References

Becker, M. A., Meyer, L. J. and Seegmiller, J. E. (1973a). Gout with purine over-production due to increased phosphoribosylpyrophosphate synthetase activity. *Am. J. Med.* **55**, 223–42.

——, ——, Wood, A. W. and Seegmiller, J. E. (1973b). Purine overproduction in man associated with increased phosphoribosylpyrophosphate synthetase activity. *Science* **179**, 1123–6.

——, Yen, R. C. K., Itkin, P., Gross, S. J., Seegmiller, J. E. and Bakay, B. (1979). Regional localization of the gene for human phosphoribosylpyrophosphate synthetase on the X chromosome. *Science* **203**, 1016–19.

Sperling, O., Boer, P., Persky-Brosh, S., Kanarek, E. and De Vries, A. (1972). Altered kinetic property of erythrocyte phosphoribosylpyrophosphate synthe-tase in excessive purine production. *Eur. J. Clin. Biol. Res.* **17**, 703–6.

——, Persky-Brosh, S., Boer, P. and De Vries, A. (1973). Human erythrocyte phosphoribosylpyrophosphate synthetase mutationally altered in regulatory properties. *Biochem. Med.* **7**, 389–95.

Wada, Y., Nishimura, Y., Tanabu, M., Yoshimura, Y., Iinuma, K., Yoshida, T. and Arakawa, T. (1974). Hypouricemic, mentally retarded infant with a defect of 5-phosphoribosyl-1-pyrophosphate synthetase of erythrocytes. *Tohoku J. Exp. Med.* **113**, 149.

Yen, R. C. K. and Becker, M. A. (1977). Evidence for X-linkage of human phosphoribosylpyrophosphate (PRPP) synthetase (abs.). *Am. J. Hum. Genet.* **29**, 117A.

Zoref, E., De Vries, A. and Sperling, O. (1975). Mutant feedback-resistant phosphoribosylpyrophosphate synthetase associated with purine overproduc-tion and gout; phosphoribosylpyrophosphate and purine metabolism in cultured fibroblasts. *J. Clin. Invest.* **56**, 1093–9.

——, —— and —— (1977). Evidence for X-linkage of phosphoribosylpyro-phosphate synthetase in man: studies with cultured fibroblasts from a gouty family with mutant feedback-resistant enzyme. *Hum. Hered.* **27**, 73–80.

5.1.5. Hereditary xanthinuria

This is a rare inborn error of metabolism in which there is a defect in the conversion of xanthine to uric acid, so that the former becomes the chief end-product of purine catabolism.

The disorder may be symptomless. It may present with urinary xanthine calculi, which may be associated with complications such as haematuria or ureteric obstruction (Dent and Philpot 1954; Dickinson and Smellie 1959). Other features that have been reported include myopathy with deposition of xanthine and hypoxanthine crystals (Chalmers *et al.* 1969), and polyarthritis (Bradford *et al.* 1968).

The nature of the defect was demonstrated by the observation of the replacement of uric acid by xanthine as the end-product of purine metabolism with the excretion of 100 to over 500 mg of xanthine and hypoxanthine per day, compared with a normal of about 16 mg per day, and by the finding of raised plasma oxypurines. Watts and colleagues (Engelman *et al.* 1964; Watts *et al.* 1964a and b) demonstrated that this metabolic block was due to deficiency of xanthine oxidase, an observation later confirmed by Sperling and coworkers (1971). Watts and colleagues found less than 0.1 per cent of normal activity in jejunal mucosa and liver biopsy tissue. Earlier studies measured total oxypurines in plasma. A more recent study, using high performance liquid chromatography, reports that xanthine rather than hypoxanthine is the major oxypurine in plasma and urine of patients, and that they also have high erythrocyte xanthine concentrations (Boulieu *et al.* 1984).

The disorder has been observed in both White and Black patients. There have been reports of several families in which there have been affected sibs (Cifuentes Delatte and Castro-Mendoza 1967; Wilson and Tapia 1974; Auscher *et al.* 1977; Wyngaarden 1978). Evidence regarding expression in heterozygotes is conflicting. Most workers have found normal patterns of excretion of xanthine and uric acid, and plasma levels of urate and oxypurines in the parents and normal sibs of their patients. However, Wilson and Tapia found increased urinary oxypurine excretion in 3 out of 21 possible heterozygotes in their family; and Cifuentes, Delatte and Castro-Mendoza observed a sister of their patient who had elevated oxypurine along with substantial uric acid excretion. In one case a normal xanthine oxidase activity in jejunal mucosa was found in the mother of a patient (Engelman *et al.* 1964). There have been no other reports of assay of the enzyme in either liver or intestine of obligate heterozygotes. The above observations taken together suggest that the disorder is most probably inherited in an autosomal recessive manner but that there may well be genetic heterogeneity.

There is good evidence that the fetus of a xanthinuric mother is not exposed to harmful levels of oxypurine such as might lead to brain damage, either on theoretical grounds or in the light of the number of normal children born to such mothers (Chalmers 1977; McKeran 1977).

A unique disorder was reported by Johnson and colleagues (1980) in a mentally subnormal female with serious neurological abnormalities, dislocated lens, and urinary xanthine stones. There was a combined deficiency of sulphite oxidase and xanthine oxidase activities due to primary molybdenum cofactor deficiency. A further case in a newborn male, distantly related to Johnson and colleagues' patient, suggests that the inheritance is probably autosomal recessive (Beemer 1981). A new case, in which prenatal diagnosis in a subsequent pregnancy of the mother yielded normal results, has recently been reported (Desjacques *et al.* 1985).

References

Auscher, C., Pasquier, C., de Gery, A., Weissenbach, R. and Delbarre, F. (1977). Xanthinuria: study of a large kindred with familial urolithiasis and gout. *Biomedicine* **27**, 57–9.

Beemer, F. A. (1981). Cited as a personal communication by V. A. McKusick in *Mendelian inheritance in man*, 6th edn. p. 831. Johns Hopkins University Press, Baltimore.

Boulieu, R., Bory, C., Baltassat, P. and Divry, P. (1984). Hypoxanthine and xanthine concentrations determined by high performance liquid chromatography in biological fluids from patients with xanthinuria. *Clin. Chim. Acta.* **142**, 83–9.

Bradford, M. J., Krakoff, I. H., Leeper, R. and Balis, M. E. (1968). Study of purine metabolism in a xanthinuric female. *J. Clin. Invest.* **47**, 1325–32.

Chalmers, R. A. (1977). Xanthinuria and pregnancy. *Lancet* **2**, 301.

——, Johnson, M., Pallis, C. and Watts, R. W. E. (1969). Xanthinuria with myopathy (with some observations on the renal handling of oxypurines in the disease). *Quart. J. Med.* **38**, 493–512.

Cifuentes Delatte, L. and Castro-Mendoza, H. J. (1967). Xanthinuria families. *Rev. Clin. Esp.* **107**, 244.

Dent, C. E. and Philpot, G. R. (1954). Xanthinuria, an inborn error (or deviation) of metabolism. *Lancet* **1**, 182–5.

Desjacques, P., Mousson, B., Vianey-Liaud, C., Boulieu, R., Bory, C., Baltassat, P., Divry, P., Zabot, M. T., Cotte, J., Lagier, P. and Philip, N. (1985). Combined deficiency of xanthine oxidase and sulphite oxidase: diagnosis of a new case followed by an antenatal diagnosis. *J. Inher. Metab. Dis.* **8**, Suppl. 2, 117–18.

Dickinson, C. J. and Smellie, J. M. (1959). Xanthinuria. *Br. Med. J.* **2**, 1217–21.

Engelman, K., Watts, R. W. E., Klinenberg, J. R., Sjoerdsma, A. and Seegmiller, J. E. (1964). Clinical, physiological and biochemical studies of a patient with xanthinuria and phaeochromocytoma. *Am. J. Med.* **37**, 839–61.

Johnson, J. L., Waud, W. R., Rajagopalan, K. V., Duran, M., Beemer, F. A. and Wadman, S. K. (1980). Inborn errors of molybdenum metabolism: combined deficiencies of sulfite oxidase and xanthine dehydrogenase in a patient lacking molybdenum cofactor. *Proc. Nat. Acad. Sci.* **77**, 3715–19.

McKeran, R. A. (1977). Xanthinuria and pregnancy. *Lancet* **2**, 86–7.

Sperling, O., Liberman, U. A., Frank, M. and De Vries, A. (1971). Xanthinuria: an additional case with demonstration of xanthine oxidase deficiency. *Am. J. Clin. Pathol.* **55**, 351–4.

Watts, R. W. E., Engelman, K., Klinenberg, J. R., Seegmiller, J. E. and Sjoerdsma, A. (1964a). Enzyme defect in a case of xanthinuria. *Nature* **201**, 395–6.

——, ——, ——, Sjoerdsma, A. and Seegmiller, J. E. (1964b). The enzyme defect in a case of xanthinuria. *Biochem. J.* **90**, 4P.
Wilson, D. M. and Tapia, H. K. (1974). Xanthinuria in a large kindred. In *Purine metabolism in man*, eds. Sperling, D., De Vries, A. and Wyngaarden, J. B. p. 343. Plenum, New York.
Wyngaarden, J. B. (1978). Xanthinuria. In *The metabolic basis of inherited disease*, 4th edn. eds. Stanbury, J. B., Wyngaarden, J. B. and Fredrickson, D. S. pp. 1037–44. McGraw-Hill, New York.

5.1.6. Hereditary orotic aciduria

This is a rare disorder of pyrimidine metabolism that occurs as two distinct but related enzymatic defects, types I and II, with similar clinical features of hypochromic megaloblastic anaemia.

Type I

Type I hereditary orotic aciduria was the first to be described (Huguley *et al.* 1959). It is characterized by megaloblastic anaemia which is not responsive to folic acid, vitamin B_{12} or other haematinics, and is associated with hypochromic, microcytic red cells. Large amounts of orotic acid are excreted and these may crystalize in the urine or within the urinary tract. The main findings in the earlier reports of type I are summarized in Table 5.1. The crystallization of orotic acid may result in ureteral or urethral obstruction (Huguley *et al.* 1959; Haggard and Lockhart 1965; Fox *et al.* 1969).

Treatment of the first reported case (J. R. in Table 5.1) with pyrimidine nucleotides led to haematological remission, a reduction of orotic aciduria, and weight gain. This suggested a block in pyrimidine biosynthesis at the orotic acid to uridine 5'-phosphate conversion step. This hypothesis was confirmed by the finding of reduced activity of the two enzymes involved, orotate phosphoribosyltransferase and orotidine 5'-phosphate decarboxylase, in the red cells of the patients and of two of three sibs (Smith *et al.* 1961). Deficient activity of these two enzymes was demonstrated in the second patient reported (D. G. in Table 5.1) by Smith *et al.* (1966) and has been confirmed in patients studied subsequently with this type of hereditary orotic aciduria in red and white blood cells, liver, and cultured fibroblasts (Krooth 1964). Red-cell activity is undetectable and that in fibroblasts only 2 to 5 per cent of normal.

Type II

Clinically this variant is indistinguishable from type I. The first reported case was a boy, probably born of an incestuous sib mating, diagnosed at

Table 5.1 *Patients with hereditary orotic aciduria type I*

Patient	Sex	Age at onset	Parental consanguinity	Hb at diagnosis	Urine	Urinary obstruction	Enzyme activity		References
							Patient	Parents	
J.R.	M	3 months	1st cousins once removed	6.7	Crystalluria	Ureteral and urethral	—	Reduced	Huguley et al. (1959) Smith et al. (1961) Fallon et al. (1963, 1964) Lotz et al. (1963)
D.G.	M	3 months	None	4.6	Crystalluria	—	Absent	Father reduced	Becroft et al. (1968, 1969) Smith et al. (1966) Smith and Gilmour (1975)
J.P.	M	7 months		4.8	Crystalluria	Ureteral	Absent	Reduced	Haggard and Lockhart (1965) Smith and Gilmour (1975)
T.H.	F	10 months		7.8	Crystalluria	—	Severely reduced	Reduced	Rogers et al. (1968) Beardmore et al. (1972) Worthy et al. (1974)
D.B.	F	$6\frac{1}{2}$ years		7.4	Crystalluria and haematuria	—	Severely reduced	Mother reduced	Tubergen et al. (1969) Beardmore et al. (1972)
C.P.	M	Birth		6.3	Crystalluria	Urethral	Severely reduced	Reduced	Fox et al. (1969) Beardmore et al. (1972)

$5\frac{1}{2}$ months of age from the finding of a megaloblastic anaemia and marked orotic acid crystalluria. As with type I patients he had a virtual absence of red-cell orotidine 5′-phosphate decarboxylase activity. However, his orotate phosphoribosyltransferase activity was initially elevated but fell following uridine therapy. Orotidine 5′-phosphate decarboxylase activity suggestive of the heterozygous state was obtained in his mother; urinary orotic acid excretion in the probable father also suggested heterozygosity. This child also showed mental retardation but as there is a family history of this it is not necessarily related to his metabolic defect (Fox *et al.* 1969, 1973).

The nature of the genetic defect remains obscure. There is some evidence that the two enzymes are in fact separate enzymes but may be associated in a single complex so that a mutation in one might affect the activity of both. Alternatively the two enzymes might share a common polypeptide chain which is involved in the mutation in type I, whereas a polypeptide unique to the decarboxylase might undergo mutation in type II. That a structural gene is involved in type I is supported by evidence of abnormal thermolability and electrophoretic mobility of the decarboxylase in heterozygotes (Worthy *et al.* 1974). The consistency of the finding of the double enzyme defect makes a double deletion of contiguous genes an unlikely explanation, as does the finding of improved enzyme activity under certain experimental cultural conditions. The enzyme studies on relatives undertaken by Fallon and colleagues (1963, 1964), in which obligate and presumed heterozygotes showed intermediate levels of decarboxylase activity, are entirely consistent with autosomal recessive inheritance. Rogers and colleagues (1968) obtained similar findings in further families of type I and so did Fox and coworkers (1973) in type II. Worthy and associates (1974) obtained evidence for differing defects in the two parents of their patient, suggesting that the later was a compound double heterozygote.

The incidence of the disorder is unknown. Rogers and Porter (1968) developed a screening test for heterozygotes and homozygotes. When applied in a survey of 1358 mentally subnormal individuals they detected two unrelated heterozygotes (Rogers *et al.* 1975). Nevertheless since unresponsive megaloblastic anaemia of infancy is rare then those cases due to orotic aciduria must also be very rare.

Heterozygote detection is complicated by the observation of increased orotic acid excretion following the administration of a variety of drugs and also in disorders other than hereditary orotic aciduria. Hence for clear identification of heterozygotes for type I estimation of urinary orotic acid excretion in the absence of any drug intake, assay of both enzymes and careful pedigree analysis are necessary (Kelley and Smith 1978).

208   *Urolithiasis and crystalluria*

References

Beardmore, T. D., Cashman, J. S. and Kelley, W. N. (1972). Mechanism of allopurinol mediated increase in enzyme activity in man. *J. Clin. Invest.* **51**, 1823–32.

Becroft, D. M. O. and Phillips, L. I. (1965). Hereditary orotic aciduria and megaloblastic anaemia: a second case, with response to uridine. *Br. Med. J.* **1**, 547–52.

——, —— and Simmonds, A. (1969). Hereditary orotic aciduria: long term therapy with uridine and trial of uracil. *J. Pediatr.* **75**, 885–91.

Fallon, H. J., Smith, L. H. Jr., Lotz, M., Graham, J. B. and Burnett, C. H. (1963). Hereditary orotic aciduria. *Trans. Assoc. Am. Phys.* **76**, 214–21.

——, ——, Grahams, J. B. and Burnett, C. H. (1964). A genetic study of hereditary orotic aciduria. *New Engl. J. Med.* **270**, 878–81.

Fox, R. M., O'Sullivan, W. J. and Firkin, B. G. (1969). Orotic aciduria. Differing enzyme patterns. *Am. J. Med.* **47**, 332–6.

——, Wood, M. H., Royse-Smith, D. and O'Sullivan, W. J. (1973). Hereditary orotic aciduria: Types I and II. *Am. J. Med.* **55**, 791–8.

Haggard, M. E. and Lockhart, L. H. (1965). Hereditary orotic aciduria, a disorder of pyrimidine metabolism responsive to uridine therapy (abs.). *J. Pediatr.* **67**, 906.

Huguley, C. M. Jr., Bain, J. A., Rivers, S. L. and Scoggins, R. B. (1959). Refractory megaloblastic anemia associated with excretion of orotic acid. *Blood* **14**, 615–34.

Kelley, W. N. and Smith, L. H. Jr. (1978). Hereditary orotic aciduria. Chapter 46 in *The metabolic basis of inherited disease*, 4th edn. eds. Stanbury, J. B., Wyngaarden, J. B. and Fredrickson, D. S. p. 1064. McGraw-Hill, New York.

Krooth, R. S. (1964). Properties of diploid cell strains developed from patients with an inherited abnormality of uridine biosynthesis. *Cold Spring Harbor Symp. Quart. Biol.* **29**, 189–212.

Lotz, M., Fallon, H. J. and Smith, L. H. Jr. (1963). Excretion of orotic acid and orotidine in heterozygotes of congenital orotic aciduria. *Nature* **197**, 194–5.

Rogers, L. E. and Porter, F. S. (1968). Hereditary orotic aciduria. II. A urinary screening test. *Pediatrics* **42**, 423–8.

——, Warford, L. R., Patterson, R. B. and Porter, F. S. (1968). Hereditary orotic aciduria. I. A new case with family studies. *Pediatrics* **42**, 415–22.

——, Nicolaisen, A. K. and Holt, J. G. (1975). Hereditary orotic aciduria: results of a screening survey. *J. Lab. Clin. Med.* **85**, 287–91.

Smith, L. H. Jr. and Gilmour, L. (1975). Determination of urinary carbamylaspartate and dihydro-orotate in normal subjects and in patients with hereditary orotic aciduria. *J. Lab. Clin. Med.* **86**, 1047–51.

——, Sullivan, M. and Huguley, C. M. (1961). Pyrimidine metabolism in man: IV. The enzymic defect of orotic aciduria. *J. Clin. Invest.* **40**, 656–64.

——, Huguley, C. M. and Bain, J. A. (1966). Hereditary orotic aciduria. In *The metabolic basis of inherited disease*, 2nd edn. eds. Stanbury, J. B., Wyngaarden, J. B. and Fredrickson, D. S. p. 739. McGraw-Hill, New York.

Tubergen, D. G., Krooth, R. S. and Heyn, R. M. (1969). Hereditary orotic aciduria with normal growth and development. *Am. J. Dis. Child.* **118**, 864–70.

Worthy, T. E., Grobner, W. and Kelley, W. N. (1974). Hereditary orotic aciduria: evidence for a structural gene mutation. *Proc. Nat. Acad. Sci.* **71**, 3031–5.

5.1.7. 2,8-dihydroxyadeninuria

This disorder is a rare cause of renal stones. It presents in childhood with crystalluria and radiolucent stones composed of 2,8-dihydroxyadenine. Adenine excretion is also increased, a defect correctable with allopurinol. 2,8-dihydroxyadenine also has a direct nephrotoxic action and patients may present in renal failure (Greenwood *et al.* 1982). There are no other clinical abnormalities and uric acid levels in blood and urine are normal (Cartier and Hamet 1974; Simmonds *et al.* 1976). About 20 per cent of subjects with this disorder are asymptomatic (Simmonds 1986).

2,8-dihydroxyadenine is formed by oxidation of adenine by xanthine oxidase and is less soluble in urine than uric acid or adenine. Adenine accumulates in these patients as a result of a block in the salvage pathway due to a complete deficiency in the activity of adenine phosphoribosyl-transferase (Cartier and Hamet 1974; Van Acker *et al.* 1977; Barratt *et al.* 1979). The disorder must be distinguished from the symptomless partial deficiency of the enzyme reported in other families as an auto-somal dominant trait. However, it is not known whether the complete deficiency represents the homozygous state for the partial defect or a different mutation. The fact that a heterozygote has been reported with urolithiasis would suggest the latter (Kuroda *et al.* 1980), and also that the inheritance is autosomal but incompletely recessive. Partial defi-ciency associated with urolithiasis has been reported in Japanese families (Fujimori *et al.* 1985). The same workers described a rapid diagnositic method for this variant of the disorder (Takeuchi *et al.* 1985).

Three recently reported families exhibited complete enzyme deficien-cies in the affected children with intermediate values in the parents in both families, and in an unaffected brother in one (Nakamoto *et al.* 1983; Witten *et al.* 1983).

The gene for adenine phosphoribosyltransferase has been assigned to the chromosome 16 long arm at position 16q 22 (Emmerson *et al.* 1975; Fox 1977). The heterozygote prevalence in a normal population has been found to be 0.42 per cent (Emmerson *et al.* 1977; Johnson *et al.* 1977). Recently Murray and colleagues (1984) have reported the cloning of the complete human adenine phosphoribosyltransferase gene.

References

Barratt, T. M., Simmonds, H. A., Cameron, J. S., Potter, C. F., Rose, G. A., Arkell, G. D. and Williams, D. I. (1979). Complete deficiency of adenine phos-phoribosyltransferase: a third case presenting as renal stones in a young child.

Arch. Dis. Child. **54**, 25–31.

Cartier, P. and Hamet, M. (1974). Une nouvelle maladie métabolique: le deficit complet en adenine phosphoribosyltransferase avec lithiase de 2,8-dihydroxyadenine. *C.R. Acad. Sci., Paris* **279**, Series D, 883.

Chevet, D., Le Pogamp, P., Gie, S., Gary, J., Daudon, M. and Hamet, M. (1984). 2,8-dihydroxyadenine (2,8-DHA) urolithiasis in an adult—complete adenine phosphoribosyltransferase deficiency—family study. *Kidney Int.* **26**, 226.

Emmerson, B. T., Gordon, R. B. and Thompson, L. (1975). Adenine phosphoribosyltransferase deficiency: its inheritance and occurrence in a female with gout and renal disease. *Aust. NZ. J. Med.* **5**, 440–6.

——, Johnson, L. A. and Gordon, R. B. (1977). Incidence of APRT deficiency. *Adv. Exp. Med. Biol.* **76A**, 293–4.

Fox, I. H. (1977). Purine enzyme abnormalities: a four year experience. *Adv. Exp. Med. Biol.* **76A**, 265–9.

Fujimori, S., Akooka, I., Sakamoto, K., Yamanaka, H., Nishioka, K. and Kamatani, N. (1985). Common characteristics of mutant adenine phosphoribosyltransferases from four separate Japanese families with 2,8-dihydroxyadenine urolithiasis associated with partial enzyme deficiencies. *Hum. Genet.* **71**, 171–6.

Greenwood, M. C., Dillon, M. J., Simmonds, H. A., Barratt, T. M., Pincott, J. R. and Metreneli, C. (1982). Renal failure due to 2,8-dihydroxyadenine urolithiasis. *Eur. J. Pediatr.* **138**, 346–9.

Johnson, L. A., Gordon, R. B. and Emmerson, B. T. (1977). Adenine phosphoribosyltransferase: a simple spectrophotometric assay and the incidence of mutation in the normal population. *Biochem. Genet.* **15**, 265–72.

Kuroda, M., Miki, T., Kiyohara, H., Usami, M., Nakamura, T., Kotake, T., Takemoto, M. and Sonoda, T. (1980). Urolithiasis composed of 2,8-dihydroxyadenine due to partial deficiency of adenine phosphoribosyltransferase. Report of a case. *Jap. J. Urol.* **71**, 283–8.

Murray, A. M., Drobetsky, E. and Arrand, J. E. (1984). Cloning the complete human adenine phosphoribosyltransferase gene. *Gene* **31**, 233–40.

Nakamoto, T., Nakatsu, H., Kishi, T., Sakura, N., Usui, T. and Nihira, H. (1983). Complete deficiency of adenine phosphoribosyltransferase: report of a new family. *J. Urol.* **130**, 580–2.

Simmonds, H. A. (1986). 2,8-dihydroxyadenine lithiasis. *Clin. Chim. Acta* **160**, 103–8.

——, Van Acker, K. J., Cameron, J. S. and Snedden, W. (1976). The identification of 2,8-dihydroxyadenine: a new component of urinary stones. *Biochemical J.* **157**, 485–7.

Takeuchi, F., Matsuta, K., Miyamoto, T., Enomoto, S., Fujimori, S., Akaoka, I., Kamatani, N. and Nishioka, K. (1985). Rapid method for the diagnosis of partial adenine phosphoribosyltransferase deficiencies causing 2,8-dihydroxyadenine urolithiasis. *Hum. Genet.* **71**, 167–70.

Van Acker, K. J., Simmonds, H. A., Potter, C. F. and Cameron, J. S. (1977). Complete deficiency of adenine phosphoribosyltransferase: report of a family. *New Engl. J. Med.* **297**, 127–32.

Witten, F. R., Morgan, J. W., Foster, J. G. and Glenn, J. F. (1983). 2,8-dihydroxyadenine urolithiasis: review of the literature and report of a case in the United States. *J. Urol.* **130**, 938–42.

5.1.8. Hypouricaemia, hypercalcinuria, and decreased bone density syndrome

A single family has been described in which two brothers and a sister, along with two grandchildren who are the products of a first-cousin marriage of obligate heterozygotes, are affected with this disorder. The features are low plasma uric acid associated with greatly increased renal clearance of uric acid, increased urinary calcium excretion and decreased bone density (Sperling *et al.* 1974). The disorder is presumably autosomal recessive.

Reference

Sperling, O., Weinberger, A., Oliver, I., Liberman, U. A. and De Vries, A. (1974). Hypouricemia, hypercalcinuria, and decreased bone density: a hereditary syndrome. *Ann. Intern. Med.* **80**, 482–7.

5.2. NON-SPECIFIC RENAL STONE FORMATION

5.2.1. Hypercalciuria

Goldwasser and colleagues (1986) have recently reviewed renal stone disease. Renal stones not associated with a known specific metabolic defect are mostly composed either of calcium oxalate (or phosphate) or of urate. Uric acid stones are discussed below. Here we are concerned with calcium oxalate or phosphate stones, especially when recurrent. Many authors have distinguished calcium stone formation associated with hypercalciuria from that in normocalciuric patients. Flocks (1940) found hypercalciuria in 66 per cent of patients with renal stones in the presence of normal serum calcium and phosphorus levels. Subsequent early workers confirmed these observations (Sutherland 1954; McGeown and Bull 1957; Boyce *et al.* 1958; Hodgkinson and Pyrah 1958). There has been considerable controversy as to the pathogenesis of both hypercalciuric and normocalciuric renal stone formation. Recent studies by Evans and colleagues (1984) appear to indicate that normocalciuric renal calcium stone formation is of similar aetiology to the hypercalciuric form, but with less marked changes. In particular they demonstrated that plasma calcium levels, although within the normal range in stone-formers who do not have primary hyperparathyroidism, are nevertheless higher than in controls. Furthermore this increase in plasma calcium, although greater in patients with hypercalciuria, is also present in those who are normocalciuric.

It was suggested by Dent and Watson (1965) that hypercalciuria could be due either to increased intestinal absorption of calcium or to renal tubular calcium loss. Several research groups have maintained that most patients have a renal tubular calcium leak with secondary hyperparathyroidism (Coe *et al.* 1973; Bordier *et al.* 1977; Muldowney *et al.* 1980), or that renal calcium loss is secondary to a primary renal loss of phosphate (Shen *et al.* 1977). Others have produced evidence that most hypercalciuric patients have a primary overabsorption of calcium (Pak *et al.* 1974, 1980; Broadus *et al.* 1978). Henneman and colleagues reported an apparently distinct form of idiopathic hypercalciuria with hypophosphataemia and a normal serum calcium (Albright *et al.* 1953; Henneman *et al.* 1958), and others observed similar patients (Harrison 1959; McGeown 1959; Maurice and Henneman 1961). The disorder was found only in males but a possible relationship to either pyelonephritis or hyperparathyroidism has not been excluded. McGeown certainly distinguished at least hyperparathyroidism from other causes of renal stone formation, finding this disorder in a fifth of her stone formers (McGeown and Morrison 1959). Nevertheless it remains doubtful if the disorder first described by Henneman and colleagues is distinct from other cases of idiopathic hypercalciuria.

A remarkable variety of further factors have been reported as playing a role in renal stone formation. The analysis of such factors has been difficult until recently because of the inability to assess independently the various physicochemical processes involved in renal stone formation. Bijvoet and his colleagues have developed a method for the independent assessment of solubility, crystal growth, and crystal agglomeration (Bijvoet *et al.* 1983; Blomen *et al.* 1983; Will *et al.* 1983). This group have recently demonstrated that in all seven members of a group of highly recurrent stone-formers their urine lacked the ability to inhibit the agglomeration of calcium oxalate monohydrate crystals, compared with the urine of 10 healthy subjects. This lack of inhibition of crystal agglomeration was associated in all seven stone-formers with hypocitraturia, and was corrected by normalization of the urine citrate concentration (Kok *et al.* 1986). Springmann and colleagues (1986), using different methods to those of Bijvoet's group, have confirmed deficient inhibition of crystal aggregation in calcium oxalate stone-formers. Although neither this factor, nor most of the other factors reported, appear to have been investigated from their genetic aspect, they are worth recording as areas of potential value for such analysis. Boyce and colleagues (Boyce and Garvey 1956; Boyce *et al.* 1954, 1955, 1956) promoted an earlier hypothesis that mucoproteins form an organic matrix on which minerals are deposited to form an insoluble complex. This theory received some experimental support from the observations of Hallson and Rose (1979) who obtained increased formation of calcium phosphate and oxalate, and clustering of the former, in the presence of uromucoids which are normal urinary constituents. It remains to be seen whether there are any differences in uromucoids between stone-formers and non-stone-formers, and whether or not individual variation is genetically determined. Nishio and associates (1985), and also Roberts and Resnick (1986) have analysed the glycosaminoglycan content of the matrix of renal stones, and found these to be mainly hyaluronic acid and heparan sulphate. Both groups suggest that these two glycosaminoglycans, in contrast to chondroitin sulphate, play a positive role in stone formation. Others have produced evidence that glycoproteins (Nakagawa *et al.* 1985), or glycosaminoglycans, especially chrondroitin sulphate, inhibit urinary stone formation (Robertson *et al.* 1973; Bowyer *et al.* 1979; Ryall *et al.* 1986). Ryall and colleagues further demonstrated that the inhibition of crystal aggregation by heparin and chondroitin sulphate is reduced in the presence of added monosodium urate. The description of an enzymatic method of measurement of urinary chondroitin sulphate content (Fellström *et al.* 1986) may lead to clarification of the apparently conflicting evidence of the studies mentioned above.

Other potential factors are the urine concentration of calcium or oxalate, and urine pH. Robertson and colleagues (1969) studied six male patients with idiopathic recurrent renal stones, and six controls. The stone-formers, on the same diet and fluid intake as the controls, had significantly higher calcium and oxalate concentrations in fresh urine and showed a greater increase on calcium or oxalate loading. When the urine was below pH 6.2 and was kept at 37 °C the stone-formers also showed the formation of larger crystals than controls. These were of calcium oxalate dihydrate and showed a tendency to aggregate not seen with the smaller calcium oxalate precipitates of the controls. Calcium phosphate crystalluria did not differ between the stone-formers and the controls. However, Vernon-Smith (1969) has suggested that their findings may be due to the presence of renal stones at the time of investigation.

Dent and Sutor (1971) produced evidence for a deficiency of a normal inhibitor of calcium oxalate crystal growth in stone-formers. Presence of the inhibitor was associated with the formation of calcium oxalate monohydrate, but in its absence the dihydrate was formed. The nature of the inhibitor was not identified and there do not appear to have been any genetic studies of this phenomenon.

It was originally claimed that apart from patients with hyperoxaluria, and occasional dietary oxaluria, oxalate excretion was not increased in renal stone patients. In addition to Robertson and colleagues' (1969) evidence of increased urinary oxalate concentration, other more recent studies confirm that oxalate, as well as calcium, shows both increased intestinal absorption (Hodgkinson 1978; Marangella *et al.* 1982) and increased urinary excretion (Robertson and Peacock 1980; Wallace *et al.* 1981; Baggio *et al.* 1983; Koide *et al.* 1985). Baggio and colleagues (1984b) suggest that this points to a defect in cellular transport of oxalate and produce evidence in support of this hypothesis. They have demonstrated increased flux of oxalate across the red blood cell membrane in patients with calcium oxalate stones. Although they were careful to exclude known primary causes of nephrolithiasis, they do not state whether or not their patients were hypercalciuric, but rather argue, with Robertson and Peacock (1980), that hypercalciuria is less important than hyperoxaluria in the determination of stone formation and crystalluria. They have demonstrated that the increased oxalate flux in red cells is restored to normal by inhibitors of the red-cell band 3 protein, which is an anion-transporting protein (Baggio *et al.* 1984a). Recently (Baggio *et al.* 1986), in a study of five families, they have demonstrated an autosomal dominant pattern of transmission of the increased oxalate flux in red cells, and its correction by diuretics.

Returning to the intestinal absorption–renal leak controversy it is recognized that the increased intestinal absorption, whether primary or secondary, helps to maintain calcium balance in hypercalciuria (Peacock and Nordin 1968; Nordin *et al.* 1972). There are those who maintain that the primary defect is the increased intestinal calcium absorption, probably due to increased 1,25-dihydroxy cholecalciferol (Martinez-Maldonado 1979; Pak 1979). In contrast Muldowney and coworkers (1980), in a comparison of idiopathic hypercalciuric patients' and controls' responses to an oral calcium load, found a similar increase in ionized calcium and concluded that there was no evidence for increased intestinal absorption but that a renal tubular calcium leak was clearly evident in the patients. Watts and his associates have shown in *in vitro* studies that in humans calcium flux across the jejunal brush border is a passive process in both patients and controls involving increased brush border permeability (Duncombe *et al.* 1980, 1984). This passive influx was found to be increased in most patients with hypercalciuria, but not in patients with renal stones without hypercalciuria. They were unable to distinguish between a primary increase in permeability and a secondary increase due to other factors; nor did they find any difference between the so-called 'absorptive' and 'renal' subtypes of hypercalciuria. Megevand and Faure (1984) produced evidence for distal tubular dysfunction, in the form of impaired hydrogen ion secretion and ammonium excretion after an ammonium chloride load, in stone-formers.

Recently Evans and colleagues (1984), on the basis of the observations mentioned earlier on plasma calcium levels and also of maximal increases in urinary calcium following oral loading in hypercalciurics with intermediate increases in normocalciuric stone-formers, have proposed the novel hypothesis of a primary parathyroid hyperactivity that falls short of hyperparathyroidism as usually defined.

How the various factors discussed above—renal calcium or oxalate leak, increased passive intestinal absorption of calcium, crystal growth promoters or inhibitors, and parathyroid overactivity—relate to one another remains obscure.

Despite the fact that genetic factors have long been suspected of playing a role in idiopathic renal stone formation, there have been remarkably few genetic studies. Early evidence comprises anecdotal reports of individual families such as those described by Clubbe (1874) and by Gram (1932). McGeown (1960) made the first genetic study of renal stone formation. She investigated the occurrence of renal stones among the first-degree relatives of 174 patients with idiopathic calcium stone formation, and those of matched controls, and found a significantly increased incidence among parents and sibs of the patients (see Table 5.2). A similar study by Resnick and colleagues (Pridgen *et al.* 1968; Resnick *et al.* 1968) on the parents and sibs of 106 patients and controls gave comparable results (see Table 5.2).

These two studies differed in several aspects apart from that of the different populations studied. McGeown used age- and sex-matched controls, Resnick and Pridgen used spouses as controls but denied that

Table 5.2 *Incidence of renal stones among relatives of calcium stone-formers*

| Study | Proportion affected (%) | | | |
| | Index families | | Control families | |
	Parents	Sibs	Parents	Sibs
Ireland McGeown (1960) (174 index patients with matched controls)	16/348(4.5)	15/708(2.1)	1/348(0.3)	4/732(0.5)
USA Resnick *et al.* (1968) (106 index patients with spouse controls)	28/212(13.2)	59/413(11.9)	8/197(4.1)	21/378(5.6)

this introduced any significant bias (Goodman *et al.* 1968), as was suggested by McGeown (1968). Resnick's cases were limited to patients with calcium oxalate stones whereas McGeown's may have included those with calcium phosphate stones, which could partially account for lower incidence in relatives (Thomas *et al.* 1966). McGeown's patients were drawn from a hospital renal stone clinic and the family history was obtained from a questionnaire completed by the proband. Resnick's group used patients, not necessarily hospitalized, whose renal stones had been sent to a stone analysis laboratory. Resnick's family histories were obtained from interviews with probands and their spouses, together with questionnaires completed by all their parents and sibs. His group estimate the prevalence of renal stones among all adult males at 2–4 per cent and among all adult females at about 1 per cent. These estimates greatly exceed those based on hospital surveys, as for example that of Boyce and colleagues (1956), for the same area as Resnick's study, of 0.14 per cent overall. Resnick's group also found a higher incidence of stones among the female relatives of both index cases and controls.

Resnick's estimate of prevalance among adult males agrees well with a more recent study in Leeds, Yorkshire, which found a 3.8 per cent prevalence (Robertson *et al.* 1983). The Leeds group found an increasing prevalence of renal stones, but not bladder stones, with social class, and a male:female ratio of 2:1. Among the relatives of their stone-formers there was a non-significant increase in stone-formers. This relatively low incidence among relatives, compared with the American study, is probably due to the family data being obtained only by questionnaire, as in McGeown's survey and in a more recent Swedish survey (Ljunghall 1979). The Swedish group have supplemented their earlier study with a more recent one in which they obtained family histories from 380 patients seen at a stone clinic (Ljunghall *et al.* 1985). In stark contrast to the Leeds study over half the patients had at least one first-degree relative with a history of renal stone formation, and an even higher proportion where the propositus had had recurrent renal stones, or was a female with incomplete renal tubular acidosis. They suggest that mild renal tubular acidosis may be a genetic factor in renal stone formation.

Both McGeown and Resnick's group postulate multifactorial inheritance. McGeown (1968) quotes an analysis of her data by Falconer (1965) giving a heritability of 46 ± 9 per cent. Resnick and colleagues estimate a life-risk for brothers of probands of about 50 per cent.

Recently Hymes and Warshaw (1985) have reported studies on the families of six children with idiopathic hypercalciuria. They divided the relatives into a group '1' with urolithiasis or unexplained haematuria and group '2' without signs or symptoms associated with hypercalciuria. The patients and their group 1 relatives showed an increased calciuria following an oral calcium load, and higher serum calcium and calcitriol levels, compared with the group 2 relatives. These authors propose that this evidence suggests a disturbance in the regulation of vitamin D metabolism, resulting in increased intestinal absorption.

Unfortunately, apart from the five studies discussed above, the genetic aspects of idiopathic renal stone formation have been largely ignored by research workers in this field. Neither the specific genetic factors involved, nor adequate family data for genetic counselling, have been established. Nevertheless there is plenty of scope for genetic studies in relation to any of the factors reputedly involved.

References

Albright, F., Henneman, P., Benedict, P. H. and Forbes, A. P. (1953). Idiopathic hypercalciuria. *Proc. R. Soc. Med.* **46**, 1077–81.

Baggio, B., Gambaro, G., Favaro, S. and Borsatti, A. (1983). Prevalence of hyperoxaluria in idiopathic calcium oxalate kidney stone disease. *Nephron* **35**, 11–14.

——, ——, Borsatti, A., Clari, G. and Moret, V. (1984a). Relation between band 3 red blood cell protein and transmembrane oxalate flux in stone formers. *Lancet* **2**, 223–4

——, ——, Marchini, F., Cicerelo, E. and Borsatti, A. (1984b). Raised transmembrane oxalate flux in red blood cells in idiopathic calcium oxalate nephrolithiasis. *Lancet* **2**, 12–13.

——, ——, ——, ——, Tenconi, R., Clementi, M. and Borsatti, A. (1986). An inheritable anomaly of red-cell oxalate transport in 'primary' calcium nephrolithiasis correctable with diuretics. *New Engl. J. Med.* **314**, 599–604.

Bijvoet, O. L. M., Blomen, L. J. M. J., Will, E. J. and vd Linden, H. J. (1983). Growth kinetics of calcium oxalate monohydrate III. *J. Crystal Growth* **64**, 316–25.

Blomen, L. J. M. J., Will, E. J., Bijvoet, O. L. M. and vd Linden, H. (1983). Growth kinetics of calcium oxalate monohydrate II. *J. Crystal Growth* **64**, 306–15.

Bordier, P., Ryckewart, A., Gueris, J. and Rasmussen, H. (1977). On the pathogenesis of so-called idiopathic hypercalciuria. *Am. J. Med.* **63**, 398–409.

Bowyer, R. C., Brockis, J. G. and McCulloch, R. K. (1979). Glycosaminoglycans as inhibitors of calcium oxalate crystal growth and aggregation. *Clin. Chim. Acta* **95**, 23–8.

Boyce, W. H. and Garvey, F. K. (1956). The amount and nature of the organic matrix in urinary calculi: a review. *J. Urol.* **76**, 213–27.

——, —— and Norfleet, C. M. (1954). The turbidity of urine in the normal and in patients with urinary calculi. *Exp. Med. Surg.* **12**, 450–9.

——, —— and —— (1955). The metal chelate compounds of urine. *Am. J. Med.* **19**, 87–95.

——, —— and Strawcutter, H. E. (1956). Incidence of urinary calculi among patients in general hospitals. *JAMA* **161**, 1437–42.

——, ——, Goven, C. E. and Winston-Salem, N. C. (1958). Abnormalities of calcium metabolism in patients with 'idiopathic' urinary calculi. *JAMA* **166**, 1577–83.

Broadus, A. E., Dominguez, M. and Bartter, F. C. (1978). Pathophysiological studies in idiopathic hypercalciuria: use of an oral calcium tolerance test to characterise distinctive hypercalciuric sub groups. *J. Clin. Endocr. Metab.* **47**, 751–60.

Clubbe, W. H. (1874). Notes, short comments and answers to correspondents: family disposition to urinary concretions. *Lancet* **2**, 823.

Coe, F. L., Canterbury, J. M., Firpo, J. J. and Reiss, E. (1973). Evidence for secondary hyperparathyroidism in idiopathic hypercalciuria. *J. Clin. Invest.* **52**, 134–42.

Dent, C. E. and Sutor, D. J. (1971). Presence or absence of inhibitor of calcium-oxalate crystal growth in urine of normals and of stone-formers. *Lancet* **2**, 775–8.

—— and Watson, L. (1965). Metabolic studies in a patient with idiopathic hyper-calciuria. *Br. Med. J.* **2**, 449–52.

Duncombe, V. M., Watts, R. W. E. and Peters, T. J. (1980). *In vitro* calcium uptake by jejunal biopsy specimens from patients with idiopathic hyper-calciuria. *Lancet* **2**, 1334–6.

——, —— and —— (1984). Studies on intestinal calcium absorption in patients with idiopathic hypercalciuria. *Quart. J. Med.* **53**, 69–79.

Evans, R. A., Hills, E., Wong, S. Y. P., Wyndham, L. E., Eade, Y. and Dunstan, C. R. (1984). The pathogenesis of idiopathic hypercalciuria: evidence for para-thyroid hyperfunction. *Quart. J. Med.* **53**, 41–53.

Falconer, D. S. (1965). The inheritance of liability to certain diseases, estimated from the incidence among relatives. *Ann. Hum. Genet.* **29**, 51–76.

Fellström, B., Danielson, B. G., Lind, E., Ljunghall, S. and Wikström, B. (1986). Enzymatic determination of urinary chrondroitin sulphate: applications in renal stone disease and acromegaly. *Eur. J. Clin. Invest.* **16**, 292–6.

Flocks, R.H. (1940). Calcium urolithiasis: role of calcium metabolism in patho-genesis and treatment of calcium urolithiasis. *J. Urol.* **43**, 214–33.

Goldwasser, B., Weinerth, J. L. and Carson, C. C. III (1986). Calcium stone disease: overview. *J. Urol.* **135**, 1–9.

Goodman, H. O., Resnick, M. and Pridgen, D. B. (1968). Inheritance of calcium renal stones. *Lancet* **1**, 1197.

Gram, H. C. (1932). Heredity of oxalic urinary calculi. *Acta Med. Scand.* **78**, 268–81.

Hallson, P. C. and Rose, G. A. (1979). Uromucoids and urinary stone formation. *Lancet* **1**, 1000–2.

Harrison, A. R. (1959). Some results of metabolic investigations in cases of renal stone. *Br. J. Urol.* **31**, 398–403.

Henneman, P. H., Benedict, P. H., Forbes, A. P. and Dudley, H. R. (1958). Idiopathic hypercalcuria. *New Engl. J. Med.* **259**, 802–7.

Hodgkinson, A. (1978). Evidence of increased oxalate absorption in patients with calcium-containing renal stones. *Clin. Sci.* **54**, 291–4.

—— and Pyrah, L. N. (1958). The urinary excretion of calcium and inorganic phosphate in 344 patients with calcium stone of renal origin. *Br. J. Surg.* **46**, 10–18.

Hymes, L. C. and Warshaw, B. L. (1985). Families of children with idiopathic hypercalciuria. Evidence for the hormonal basis of familial hypercalciuria. *Am. J. Dis. Child.* **139**, 621–4.

Koide, T., Bowyer, R. C. and Brockis, J. G. (1985). Comparison of urinary oxalate excretion in urolithiasis patients with and without hypercalciuria. *Br. J. Urol.* **57**, 505–9.

Kok, D. J., Papapoulos, S. E. and Bijvoet, O. L. M. (1986). Excessive crystal agglomeration with low citrate excretion in recurrent stone formers. *Lancet* **1**, 1056–8.

Ljunghall, S. (1979). Family history of renal stone in a population study of stone-formers and healthy subjects *Br. J. Urol.* **51**, 249–52.

——, Danielson, B. G., Fellstrom, B., Holmgren, K., Johansson, G. and Wikstrom, B. (1985). Family history of renal stones in recurrent stone patients. *Br. J. Urol.* **57**, 370–6.

McGeown, M. G. (1959). Hypercalciuria (letter). *Br. Med. J.* **1**, 857–8.

—— (1960). Heredity in renal stone disease. *Clin. Sci.* **19**, 465–71.

—— (1968). Inheritance of calcium renal stones. *Lancet* **1**, 866.

—— and Bull, G. M. (1957). The pathogenesis of urinary calculus formation. *Br. Med. Bull.* **13**, 53–6.

—— and Morrison, E. (1959). Hyperparathyroidism. *Postgrad. Med. J.* **35**, 330–7.

Marangella, M., Fruttero, B., Bruno, M. and Linari, F. (1982). Hyperoxaluria in idiopathic calcium stone disease: further evidence intestinal hyperabsorption of oxalate. *Clin. Sci.* **63**, 381–5.

Martinez-Maldonado, M. (1979). Continuing challenges to the understanding of the definition and pathophysiology of hypercalciuria. *Nephron* **24**, 209–11.

Maurice, P. F. and Henneman, P. H. (1961). Medical aspects of renal stones. *Medicine* **40**, 315–46.

Megevand, M. and Faure, H. (1984). Distal renal tubular dysfunction: a common feature in calcium stone formers. *Eur. J. Clin. Invest.* **14**, 456–61.

Muldowney, F. P., Freaney, R. and Ryan, J. G. (1980). The pathogenesis of idiopathic hypercalciuria: evidence for renal tubular calcium leak. *Quart. J. Med.* **49**, 87–94.

Nakagawa, Y., Abram, V., Parks, J. H., Lau, H. S.-H., Kawooya, J. K. and Coe, F. L. (1985). Urine glycoprotein crystal growth inhibitors. *J. Clin. Invest.* **76**, 1455–62.

Nishio, S., Abe, Y., Wakatsuki, A., Iwata, H., Ochi, K., Takeuchi, M. and Matsumoto, A. (1985). Matrix glycosaminoglycan in urinary stones. *J. Urol.* **134**, 503–5.

Nordin, B. E. C., Peacock, M. and Wilkinson, R. (1972). Hypercalciuria and calcium stone disease. *Clin. Endocr. Metab.* **1**, 169–83.

Pak, C. Y. C. (1979). Physiological basis for absorptive and renal hypercalciurias. *Am. J. Phyisol.* **237**(6), F415–23.

——, Ohata, M., Lawrence, E. C. and Snyder, W. (1974). The hypercalciurias: causes, parathyroid functions and diagnostic criteria. *J. Clin. Invest.* **54**, 387–400.

——, Britton, F. and Peterson, R. (1980). Ambulatory evaluation of nephrolithiasis. *Am. J. Med.* **69**, 19–30.

Peacock, M. and Nordin, B. E. C. (1968). Tubular reabsorption of calcium in normal and hypercalciuric subjects. *J. Clin. Pathol.* **21**, 353–8.

Pridgen, D. B., Resnick, M., Goodman, H. O. and Boyce, W. H. (1968). Inheritance of calcium renal stones. *Lancet* **1**, 537–8.

Resnick, M., Pridgen, D. B. and Goodman, H. O. (1968). Genetic predisposition to formation of calcium oxalate renal calculi. *New Engl. J. Med.* **278**, 1313–18.

Roberts, S. D. and Resnick, M. I. (1986). Glycosaminoglycans content of stone matrix. *J. Urol.* **135**, 1078–83.

Robertson, W. G. and Peacock, M. (1980). The cause of idiopathic stone disease: hypercalciuria or hyperoxaluria? *Nephron* **26**, 105–10.

——, —— and Nordin, B. E. C. (1969). Calcium crystalluria in recurrent renal-stone formers. *Lancet* **2**, 21–4.

——, —— and —— (1973). Inhibitors of the growth and aggregation of calcium oxalate crystals *in vitro*. *Clin. Chim. Acta* **43**, 31–7.

——, ——, Baker, M., Marshall, D. H., Pearlman, B., Speed, R., Sergeant, V. and Smith, A. (1983). Studies on the prevalance and epidemiology of urinary stone disease in men in Leeds. *Br. J. Urol.* **55**, 595–8.

Ryall, R. L., Harnett, R. M. and Marshall, V. R. (1986). Effect of monosodium urate on capacity of urine, chondroitin sulphate and heparin to inhibit calcium oxalate crystal growth and aggregation. *J. Urol.* **135**, 174–7.

Shen, F. H., Baylink, D. J., Nielsen, R. L., Sherrard, D. J., Ivey, J. L. and Haussler, M. R. (1977). Increased serum 1,25-dihydroxyvitamin D in idiopathic hypercalciuria. *J. Lab. Clin. Med.* **90**, 955–62.

Springmann, K. E., Drach, G. W., Gottung, B. and Randolph, A. D. (1986). Effects of human urine on aggregation of calcium oxalate crystals. *J. Urol.* **135**, 69–71.

Sutherland, J. W. (1954). Recurrence following operations for upper urinary tract stone. *Br. J. Urol.* **26**, 22–45.

Thomas, J., Berge, D., Brunschwig, J. F. and Aboulker, P. (1966). Caractéres sexuels et facteurs génétiques des trois grandes variété cliniques de lithiase rénale: urique, oxalique, phosphatique. *Rein et Foie* **18**, 147–50.

Vernon-Smith, M. J. (1969). Crystalluria and renal stones. *Lancet* **2**, 319–20.

Wallace, M. R., Mason, K. and Gray, J. (1981). Urine oxalate and calcium in idiopathic renal stone formers. *N.Z. Med. J.* **94**, 87–9.

Will, E. J., Bijroet, O. L. M., Blomen, L. J. M. J. and vd Linden, H. (1983). Growth kinetics of calcium oxalate monohydrate. I. *J. Crystal Growth* **64**, 287–305.

5.2.2. Hyperuricosuric nephrolithiasis

A number of families have been reported with uric acid lithiasis associated with an isolated defect in the renal tubular handling of urate (Praetorius and Kirk 1950; Khachadurian and Arslanian 1973; Benjamin *et al.* 1977; Sperling *et al.* 1977). Five of the reported families have been non-Ashkenazy Israeli Jews. A similar defect associated with hypercalciuria has also been described (Greene *et al.* 1972; Sperling *et al.* 1974; Frank *et al.* 1979). Renal handling of urate in humans is not fully understood but it has been proposed that it involves glomerular filtration, proximal reabsorption, secretion, and postsecretory reabsorption. It is also suggested that there is complete reabsorption of the filtered load by the presecretory mechanism so that urate excretion is regulated by the postsecretory reabsorption of the secreted urate (Rieselbach and Steele 1974). If this model of Rieselbach and Steele is correct then in theory excessive uric acid excretion could result from a failure of reabsorption at either the proximal or distal site, or at both. Studies of the effects of pyrazinamide, an inhibitor of uric acid secretion, not only support the model but suggest that hyperuricosuria shows genetic heterogeneity in that there is evidence for the occurrence of all three types of defective reabsorption. In normal subjects pyrazinamide almost completely suppresses uric acid excretion (Steele and Rieselbach 1967). In some cases of secondary renal hypouricaemia, with a high urate clearance, pyrazinamide also fully suppresses uric acid excretion (Bennett *et al.* 1972; Wilson and Goldstein 1973) and it is suggested that they have a defect of postsecretory reabsorption. In the cases of primary hyperuricosuria and hypercalciuria (Greene *et al.* 1972; Sperling *et al.* 1974; Frank *et al.* 1979) pyrazinamide reduced uric acid excretion but this remained abnormally high, suggesting a defect in presecretory reabsorption. In those patients with isolated primary hyperuricosia the uric acid clearance exceeded creatine clearance but equalled it following pyrazinamide administration, suggesting a defect of pre- and postsecretory reabsorption. A patient with a 48,XXYY karyotype has been reported with this defect, but his chromosomally normal brother was also affected (Nakajima *et al.* 1986).

Variation in uric acid reabsorption is presumably determined in a polygenic manner but there is very little evidence on this point. Whether hyperuricosuria in any of the families mentioned above is due to a single gene defect is unclear.

References

Bennett, J. S., Bond, J. and Singer, I. (1972). Hypouricemia in Hodgkin's disease. *Ann. Intern. Med.* **76**, 751–6.

Benjamin, D., Sperling, O., Weinberger, A., Pinkhas, J. and de Vries, A. (1977). Familial hypouricemia due to isolated renal tubular defect. Attenuated response of uric acid clearance to probenecid and pyrazinamide. *Nephron* **18**, 220–5.

Frank, M., Many, M. and Sperling, O. (1979). Familial renal hypouricaemia: two additional cases with uric acid lithiasis. *Br. J. Urol.* **51**, 88–91.

Greene, M. L., Marcus, R., Aurbach, G. D., Kazam, E. S. and Seegmiller, J. E. (1972). Hypouricemia due to isolated renal tubular defect. Dalmation dog mutation in man. *Am. J. Med.* **53**, 361–7.

Khachadurian, A. K. and Arslanian, M. J. (1973). Hypouricemia due to renal uricosuria. *Ann. Intern. Med.* **78**, 547–50.

Nakajima, H., Yajima, K., Nakajima, T., Iida, S., Sumi, S., Kono, N., Moriwaki, K., Nonaka, K. and Tarvi, S. (1986). Renal hypouricaemia in a patient with 48,XXYY syndrome. *Postgrad. Med. J.* **62**, 219–22.

Praetorius, E. and Kirk, J. E. (1950). Hypouricemia with evidence of tubular elimination of uric acid. *J. Lab. Clin. Med.* **35**, 865–8.

Reiselbach, R. E. and Steele, T. H. (1974). Influence of the kidney urate homeostasis in health and disease. *Am. J. Med.* **56**, 665–75.

Sperling, O., Weinberger, A., Oliver, I., Liberman, U. A. and de Vries, A. (1974). Hypouricemia, hypercalciuria and decreased bone density. A hereditary syndrome. *Ann. Intern. Med.* **80**, 482–7.

——, ——, Benjamin, D., Pinkhas, J. and de Vries, A. (1977). Hereditary renal hypouricemia: a comparative study of three families (abs.). *Hum. Hered.* **27**, 215.

Steele, T. H. and Rieselbach, R. E. (1967). The renal mechanism for urate homeostasis in normal man. *Am. J. Med.* **43**, 868–75.

Wilson, D. M. and Goldstein, N. P. (1973). Renal urate excretion in patients with Wilson's disease. *Kidney Int.* **4**, 331–6.

6. Renal tubular (transport) defects

There are now a variety of known defects involving specific renal tubular transport mechanisms for particular components of the glomerular filtrate. For most of these the defective mechanism has been localized to either the proximal or the distal convoluted tubule, and this provides the basis for a simple classification. Several are genetically heterogeneous. Hyperuricosuria has been discussed already in Chapter 5, on renal stones. The disorders described in this chapter are summarized in Tables 6.1 and 6.2. Calcium ions are reabsorbed in both proximal and distal tubules, about 99 per cent of the filtered load being reabsorbed. It is thought that the pathway involved is shared with magnesium ions. Parathormone increases reabsorption of calcium ions, whereas in familial hypocalciuric hypercalcaemia (listed arbitrarily in Table 6.1 for convenience) the increased reabsorption is parathormone independent, suggesting two separate transport mechanisms. Which of these is proximal tubular and which is distal tubular is unknown. The findings in the primary cystinurias are summarized in Table 6.3. The renal tubular acidoses, some of which are proximal and some of which are distal tubular, are summarized in Table 6.4. Renal tubular disorders are fully discussed in a recent text edited by Gonick and Buckalew (1985).

Reference

Gonick, C. and Buckalew, V. M. (eds.) (1985). *Renal tubular disorders: pathophysiology, diagnosis, and management. Kidney diseases, Vol. 5.* Marcel Dekker, New York.

Table 6.1 *Proximal renal tubular defects*

Disorder	Mechanism	Inheritance
1. Hypophosphataemia:		
(i) Familial hypophosphataemia	Renal phosphate leak due to loss of the parathormone inhibited mechanism of reabsorption	XD
(ii) Hypophosphataemic bone disease	Renal phosphate leak due to loss of the non-parathormone-inhibited mechanism of reabsorption	AD

223

Table 6.1—*Continued*

Disorder	Mechanism	Inheritance
(iii) Familial vitamin-D-dependent rickets, type I	Defective hydroxylation of 25,OH-vitamin D	AR
(iv) Familial vitamin-D-dependent rickets, type II	Dihydroxy vitamin D_3 receptor defect	?
(v) Hereditary hypophosphataemic rickets with hypercalciuria	?	Probably AR
2. Renal glycosuria (types A, B, and C)	Low threshold for glucose	Incomplete AR
3. Fanconi (or Fanconi renotubular) syndrome:		
(i) Type I, infantile	'Swan-neck' deformity of proximal tubule with generalized poor reabsorption	AR
(ii) Type II, adult	As above	AD or AR
4. Cystinuria:		
(i) Type I	Tubular and intestinal transport defect for a mechanism common to cystine and the dibasic amino acids	AR
(ii) Type II	Similar mechanism to type I	Incomplete AR
(iii) Type III (or I/II)	Tubular defect only, mainly for cystine	Incomplete AR
(iv) Hypercystinuria	Tubular defect in transport of cystine alone	AR
(v) Dibasic aminoaciduria	Tubular defect in transport of the dibasic amino acids but not cystine	AR
5. Glycinuria (iminoglycinuria)	Transport defect for a mechanism common to glycine and the imino acids proline and hydroxyproline:	
	heterozygotes: glycinuria and	AD
	homozygotes: glycinuria and iminoaciduria	AR

Table 6.1 — *Continued*

Disorder	Mechanism	Inheritance
6. Histidinuria	Renal tubular and intestinal transport defects for histidine	AR
7. Hartnup disease	Tubular and intestinal defect in transport of neutral α-amino acids	AR
8. Tubular acidosis, type II, proximal	Tubular defect in bicarbonate reabsorption with a low $T_{m_{HCO_3}}$ and marked bicarbonate urinary loss	?XR
9. Osteopetrosis with renal mixed tubular acidosis	Mixed tubular deficiency of carbonic anhydrase II as part of a general deficiency of this enzyme	AR
10. Familial hypocalciuric hypercalcaemia	Defect with increased calcium ion reabsorption; whether proximal or distal tubular is unknown	AD
11. Hypokalaemic alkalosis with proximal tubulopathy	Nature and site of defect not known	AR
12. Pseudohypoparathyroidism (Albright's hereditary osteodystrophy)	Tubular parathormone resistance, due to an N protein defect or other mechanisms	Most probably AD
13. Renal tubular insufficiency, cholestatic jaundice and multiple congenital abnormalities	?	Probably AR
14. Arthrogryposis multiplex congenita with renal and hepatic abnormality	?	Probably XR

Abbreviations: XD = X-linked dominant, XR = X-linked recessive, AD = Autosomal dominant, AR = Autosomal recessive.

Table 6.2 *Distal renal tubular defects*

Disorder	Mechanism	Inheritance
1. Renal diabetes insipidus (hereditary form)	Distal tubular and collecting duct vasopressin resistance; whether due to defective receptor affinity or to a failure of bound hormone to stimulate renal AMP cyclase synthesis is not known.	Incomplete XR
2. Tubular acidosis: Type I, classic or distal	Inability of distal tubule to produce the normal hydrogen ion gradient between the lumen and the peritubular blood	AD
Type III, dislocation (early and late onset forms)	Not known	AR
Renal tubular acidosis and nerve deafness	? Due to mutant form of carbonic anydrase B	AR
3. Bartler syndrome (familial renal hypoelectrolytaemia)	Hyperplasia of juxtaglomerular apparatus with hyperreninaemia and increased prostaglandin synthesis	AR
4. Pseudohypoaldosteronism	? Tubular aldosterone resistance	AR
5. Pseudohyperaldosteronism (Liddle's disease)	? Primary tubular membrane transport defect	AD
6. Systemic carnitine deficiency	Defect in tubular reabsorption of carnitine	AR
7. Blue-diaper syndrome	Intestinal tryptophan transport defect	AR

Abbreviations: XD=X-linked dominant, XR=X-linked recessive, AD=Autosomal dominant, AR=Autosomal recessive.

6.1. PROXIMAL TUBULAR DEFECTS

6.1.1. X-linked vitamin-D-resistant rickets (hypophosphataemia)

Albright and his associates first described a familial form of hypo-phosphataemia in vitamin-D-resistant rickets in 1937, which they termed renal osteodystrophy. Twenty years later Winters and colleagues showed that the common form of this disorder is inherited in an X-linked dominant manner (Winters *et al.* 1957, 1958, 1960; Graham *et al.* 1959). Earlier Christensen (1940/1941), had recorded a two-generation family without recognizing its X linkage. In 1942 it was suggested that the primary defect was a renal leak of phosphate (Robertson *et al.*), and in 1946 Albright and coworkers suggested that this might be due to resistance to vitamin D with secondary hyperparathyroidism (Albright *et al.* 1946), a view not subsequently confirmed. However, the concept of a renal phosphate leak did receive support from the work of both Dent (1952) and Fanconi and Girardet (1952). Fraser and associates (1957) showed that bone healing could be achieved by oral phosphate administration alone. Harrison and colleagues (1966) gave a detailed description of the clinical features, predominantly short stature with rickets in childhood and osteomalacia in the adult. Recently Polisson and associates (1985) have drawn attention to the frequent occurrence of calcification of tendons, ligaments, and joint capsules. In an analysis of the pedigrees of 24 cases—16 hereditary and 8 sporadic—Dents' group concluded that the key biochemical change is hypophosphataemia and that inheritance is X linked (Burnett *et al.* 1964). However, Briard-Guillemot and coworkers (1972) found that hypophosphataemia was an unreliable guide to affected individuals for genetic analysis. In an analysis of 23 families they found a pattern of inheritance compatible with incomplete X-linked dominance.

Condon and associates (1970) demonstrated reduced intestinal phosphate absorption, an observation confirmed by Short and colleagues (1973).

In a brilliant series of papers published between 1971 and the present time Scriver and his coworkers have elucidated the genetic defect in experimental studies on mice with an exact homologue of the human disease, and parallel clinical studies on patients with familial hypo-phosphataemia. Phosphate reabsorption in the proximal renal tubule depends on two separate transport mechanisms, one inhibited by para-thyroid hormone and the other independent of it (Tenenhouse *et al.* 1981). Glorieux and Scriver (1972) produced evidence from patients that it is the parathormone responsive mechanism only that is defective. Both in the human disease and in the mouse model, mice with the *Hyp* mutation, inheritance is X linked. The *Hyp*/Y mouse, like the human patient, has a low serum phosphate and reduced renal transport of phosphate. In the mouse the defect is localized to the renal tubular brush border membrane (Scriver *et al.* 1977; Tenenhouse and Scriver 1978, 1979; Tenenhouse *et al.* 1978), and this defect is not influenced by vitamin D therapy (Tenenhouse and Scriver 1981). Cole and Scriver (1984) found that sulphate reabsorption is not affected in either hypophosphataemic patients or *Hyp*/Y mice, and is not influenced by parathormone in normal subjects. They conclude that sulphate renal tubular transport is independent of that of phosphate. There is every reason to believe that the mechanism in the human patient is strictly comparable to that in the *Hyp* mouse, and that changes in intestinal absorption of phosphate are purely secondary to the primary renal defect (Eicher *et al.* 1976; Tenenhouse and Scriver 1978). The mechanism of the defect is illustrated in Fig. 6.1 where it is compared with that in the normal situation, in nutritional rickets, and in hypophosphataemic bone disease and vitamin-D-dependent rickets, discussed below.

References

Albright, F., Burnett, C. H., Parson, W., Reifenstein, E. C. and Roos, A. (1946). Osteomalacia and late rickets. *Medicine* **25**, 399–479.
——, Butler, A. M. and Bloomberg, E. (1937). Rickets resistant to vitamin D therapy. *Am. J. Dis. Child.* **54**, 529–47.
Briard-Guillemot, M.-L., Raverdy, E., Balsan, S., Rey, J. and Frezal, J. (1972). Etude critique de l'hypophosphatémie pour l'étude génétique du rachitisme vitamino-resistant hypophosphatémique familiel. *Arch. Fr. Pédiatr.* **29**, 1059–68.
Burnett, C. H., Dent, C. E., Harper, C. and Warland, B. J. (1964). Vitamin D-resistant rickets. Analysis of twenty-four pedigrees with hereditary and sporadic cases. *Am. J. Med.* **36**, 222–32.
Christensen, J. F. (1940/1941). Three familial cases of atypical late rickets. *Acta Paediatr. Scand.* **28**, 247–70.
Cole, D. E. C. and Scriver, C. R. (1984). The effects of mendelian mutation on renal sulfate and phosphate transport in man and mouse. *Pediatr. Res.* **18**, 25–9.
Condon, J. R., Nassim, J. R. and Rutter, A. (1970). Defective intestinal phosphate absorption in familial and non-familial hypophosphataemia. *Br. Med. J.* **3**, 138–41.
Dent, C. E. (1952). Rickets and osteomalacia from renal tubule defects. *J. Bone Jt. Surg.* **34B**, 266–74.
Eicher, E. M., Southard, J. L., Scriver, C. R. and Glorieux, F. H. (1976). Hypophosphatemia: mouse model for human familial hypophosphatemic (vitamin D-resistant) rickets. *Proc. Nat. Acad. Sci.* **73**, 4667–71.
Fanconi, G. and Girardet, P. (1952). Familiärer persistierender Phosphatdiabetes mit D-vitamin-resistenter Rachitis. *Helv. Paediatr. Acta* **7**, 14–41.

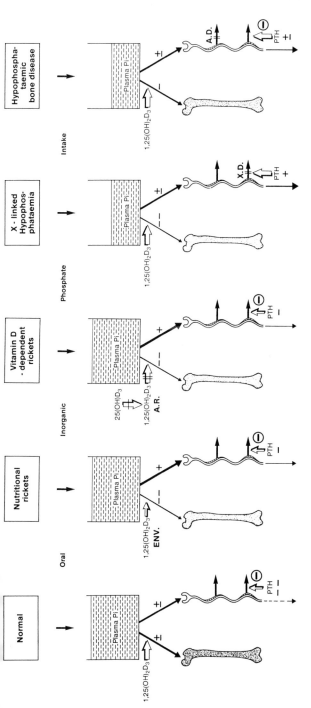

Fig. 6.1. Mechanism and aetiology of various forms of rickets, showing plasma phosphate level and phosphate excretion, transfer of phosphate to bone with consequent degree of mineralization, and site of origin of the defect.

Abbreviations and symbols: Pi = inorganic phosphate, $1,25(OH)_2D_3$ = 1,25-dihydroxy vitamin D_3, $25(OH)D_3$ = 25-hydroxy vitamin D_3, PTH = parathormone, ENV = environmental, AR = autosomal recessive, AD = autosomal dominant, XD = X-linked dominant, $\Leftrightarrow$ = stimulation, $\underline{\Leftrightarrow}$ = inhibition, $\nRightarrow$ = blocked stimulation.

Adapted from Tenenhouse *et al.* (1981) in *Transport and inherited disease*, eds. N. R. Belton and C. Toothill, with the permission of MTP Press, the Society for the Study of Inborn Errors of Metabolism, and Dr Toothill.

Fraser, D., Jaco, N. T., Yendt, E. K., Milne, J. D. and Lin, E. (1957). The induction of *in vitro* and *in vivo* calcification in bones of children suffering from vitamin D resistant rickets without recourse to large doses of vitamin D (abs.). *Am. J. Dis. Child.* **98**, 34.

Glorieux, F. and Scriver, C. R. (1972). Loss of parathyroid hormone-sensitive component of phosphate transport in X-linked hypophosphatemia. *Science* **175**, 997–1000.

Graham, J. B., McFalls, V. W. and Winters, R. W. (1959). Familial hypophosphatemia with vitamin D-resistant rickets. II. Three additional kindreds of sex-linked dominant type with a genetic analysis of four such families. *Am. J. Hum. Genet.* **11**, 311–32.

Harrison, H. E., Harrison, H. C., Lifshitz, F. and Johnson, A. D. (1966). Growth disturbance in hereditary hypophosphatemia. *Am. J. Dis. Child.* **112**, 290–7.

Polisson, R. P., Martinez, S., Khoury, M., Harrell, R. M., Lyles, K. W., Friedman, N., Harrelson, J. M., Reisner, E. and Drezner, M. K. (1985). Calcification of entheses associated with X-linked hypophosphataemic osteomalacia. *New Engl. J. Med.* **313**, 1–6.

Robertson, B. R., Harris, R. C. and McCune, D. J. (1942). Refractory rickets: mechanism of the genetic action of calciferol (abs.). *Am. J. Dis. Child.* **64**, 948–9.

Scriver, C. R., Stacey, T. E., Tenenhouse, H. S. and MacDonald, W. A. (1977). Transepithelial transport of phosphate anion in kidney. Potential mechanisms for hypophosphatemia. *Adv. Exp. Med. Biol.* **81**, 55–70.

Short, E. M., Binder, H. J. and Rosenberg, L. E. (1973). Familial hypophosphatemic rickets: defective transport of inorganic phosphate by intestinal mucosa. *Science* **179**, 700–2.

Tenenhouse, H. S. and Scriver, C. R. (1978). The defect in transcellular transport of phosphate in the nephron is located in brush-border membranes in X-linked hypophosphatemia (*Hyp* mouse model). *Can. J. Biochem.* **56**, 640–6.

—— and —— (1979). Renal adaptation to phosphate deprivation in the *Hyp* mouse with X-linked hypophosphatemia. *Can. J. Biochem.* **57**, 938–44.

—— and —— (1981). Effect of 1,25-dihydroxy vitamin D_3 on phosphate homeostasis in the X-linked hypophosphatemic (*Hyp*) mouse. *Endocrinology,* **109**, 658–60.

——, Cole, D. E. C. and Scriver, C. R. (1981). Mendelian hypophosphataemias as probes of phosphate and sulphate transport by mammalian kidney. In *Transport and inherited disease*, eds. Belton, N. R. and Toothill, C. pp. 231–62. MTP Press, Lancaster, Boston, The Hague.

——, Scriver, C. R., McInnes, R. R. and Glorieux, F. H. (1978). Renal handling of phosphate *in vivo* and *in vitro*, by the X-linked hypophosphatemic male mouse: evidence for a defect in the brush border membrane. *Kidney Int.* **14**, 236–44.

Winters, R. W., Graham, J. B., Williams, T. F., McFalls, V. W. and Burnett, C. H. (1957). A genetic study of familial hypophosphatemia and vitamin D-resistant rickets. *Trans. Assoc. Am. Phys.* **70**, 234–42.

——, ——, ——, ——, and —— (1958). A genetic study of familial hypophosphatemia and vitamin D resistant rickets with a review of the literature. *Medicine* **37**, 97–142.

——, McFalls, V. W. and Graham, J. B. (1960). 'Sporadic' hypophosphatemia and vitamin D-resistant rickets. *Pediatrics* **25**, 959–66.

Hypophosphataemic bone disease (see Fig. 6.1)

A relatively uncommon variant of familial hypophosphataemic bone disease was first reported by Harrison and colleagues as showing autosomal dominant inheritance (Harrison *et al.* 1966; Bianchine *et al.* 1971). Further reports of autosomal dominant inheritance followed shortly thereafter (Deluca 1969; Matsuda *et al.* 1969; Pak *et al.* 1972; Brickman *et al.* 1973). Scriver's group in their studies of X-linked hypophosphataemic rickets distinguished that disorder from this autosomal dominant form. The latter differs clinically in showing normal to slightly reduced stature with leg bowing and osteomalacia, but only rarely rickets. As in the X-linked form the renal threshold for phosphate ($T_{m_{P_i}}$) is reduced but in contrast the fractional excretion is briskly increased by parathyroid hormone, indicating that the defect lies in the parathormone-independent transport mechanism (Scriver *et al.* 1977).

References

Bianchine, J. W., Stambler, A. A. and Harrison, H. E. (1971). Familial hypophosphatemic rickets showing autosomal dominant inheritance. *The clinical delineation of birth defects. The endocrine system. Birth Defects Orig. Art. Series VII* (6), 287–94.

Brickman, A. S., Coburn, J. W., Kurokawa, K., Bethune, J. E., Harrison, H. E. and Norman, A. W. (1973). Actions of 1,25 dihydroxycholecalciferol in patients with hypophosphatemic, vitamin-D-resistant rickets. *New Engl. J. Med.* **289**, 495–8.

Deluca, H. F. (1969). Vitamin D. *New Engl. J. Med.* **281**, 1103–4.

Harrison, H. E., Harrison, H. C., Lifshitz, F. and Johnson, A. D. (1966). Growth disturbance in hereditary hypophosphatemia. *Am. J. Dis. Child.* **112**, 290–7.

Matsuda, J., Sugai, M. and Ohsawa, T. (1969). Laboratory findings in a child with pseudo-vitamin D deficiency rickets. *Helv. Paediatr. Acta* **24**, 329–36.

Pak, C. Y. C., Deluca, H. F., Bartter, F. C., Henneman, D. H., Frame, B., Simopoulos, A. and Delea, C. S. (1972). Treatment of vitamin-D-resistant rickets with 25-hydroxycholecalciferol. *Arch. Intern. Med.* **129**, 894–9.

Scriver, C. R., MacDonald, W., Reade, T., Glorieux, F. H. and Nogrady, B. (1977). Hypophosphatemic nonrachitic bone disease: an entity distinct from X-linked hypophosphatemia in the renal defect, bone involvement, and inheritance. *Am. J. Med. Genet.* **1**, 101–17.

Familial vitamin-D-dependent rickets, type I (see Fig. 6.1)

This disorder, also known as pseudo-vitamin-D-deficient rickets, clinically mimics nutritional rickets. It was possibly first recognized by Fraser and Salter (1958), as their type IIIB. A detailed description was given by Prader and colleagues (1961) who noted a low plasma calcium but normal plasma phosphate. They also observed that the phosphaturia was corrected by administration of vitamin D. They initially suggested that the inheritance was autosomal dominant but later accepted that it was recessive (Fanconi and Prader 1969; Prader *et al.* 1976). Recessive inheritance was established by reports from several groups (Stoop *et al.* 1967; Dent *et al.* 1968; Scriver 1970).

The disorder is not in fact a renal tubular transport defect but is described here in order to distinguish it from X-linked and autosomal dominant hypophosphatemia. It has been shown to be an inborn error of metabolism involving defective hydroxylation of 25-hydroxy vitamin D_3 to 1α, 25-dihydroxy vitamin D_3 (Fraser *et al.* 1973). The dihydroxy vitamin is the active promotor of phosphate incorporation into bone— hence the similarity to nutritional rickets in which there is a dietary vitamin deficiency. Prader and colleagues (1976) demonstrated a specific response to the dihydroxy vitamin but not the the 25-hydroxy vitamin, which supports the concept of a specific deficiency of the 1α-hydroxylase in the mitochondria of renal cells.

References

Dent, C. E., Friedman, M. and Watson, L. (1968). Hereditary pseudo-vitamin-D deficiency rickets (Hereditare Pseudo-Mangelrachitis). *J. Bone Jt. Surg.* **50B**, 708–19.

Fanconi, A. and Prader, A. (1969). Pseudo-vitamin D-deficiency rickets. In *Mineral metabolism in pediatrics,* eds. Burland, W. L. and Barltrop, D. p. 19. Blackwell Scientific, Oxford.

Fraser, D. and Salter, R. B. (1958). The diagnosis and management of the various types of rickets. *Pediatr. Clin. North Am.* **5**, 417–41.

——, Kooh, S. W., Kind, H. P., Holick, M. F., Tanaka, Y. and De Luca, H. F. (1973). Pathogenesis of hereditary vitamin-D-dependent rickets. An inborn error of vitamin D metabolism involving defective conversion of 25-hydroxy vitamin D to 1α, 25-dihydroxy-vitamin D. *New Engl. J. Med.* **289**, 817–22.

Prader, A., Illig, R. and Heierli, E. (1961). Eine besondere Form der primaren vitamin-D-resistenten Rachitis mit Hypocalcamie und autosomal-dominantem Erbgang: die hereditare Pseudo-mangelrachitis. *Helv. Paediatr. Acta.* **16**, 452–68.

——, Kind, H. P and De Luca, H. F. (1976). Pseudovitamin D deficiency (vitamin D dependency). In *Inborn errors of calcium and bone metabolism,* eds. Bickel, H. and Stein, J. pp. 115–23. University Park Press, Baltimore.

Scriver, C. R. (1970). Vitamin D dependency (editorial). *Pediatrics* **45**, 361–3.

Stoop, J. W., Schraagen, M. J. C. and Tiddens, H. A. W. M. (1967). Pseudo vitamin D-deficiency rickets: report of four new cases. *Acta Paediatr. Scand.* **56**, 607–16.

In a variant of this disorder, type II, there appears to be a defect in receptors for the dihydroxy vitamin D_3 and no response to this vitamin (Brooks *et al.* 1978; Kudoh *et al.* 1981). Failure of dihydroxy vitamin D_3

to reduce the incorporation of (^{14}C) thymidine in phytohaemaglutinin stimulated lymphocytes is claimed to provide a rapid diagnostic test of this disorder (Takeda *et al.* 1986). Evidence of genetic heterogeneity has also been reported (Liberman *et al.* 1986).

References

Brooks, M. H., Bell, N. H., Love, L., Stern, P. H., Orfei, E., Queener, S. F., Hamstra, A. J. and De Luca, H. F. (1978). Vitamin-D-dependent rickets type II: resistance of target organs to 1,25-dihydroxy-vitamin D. *New Engl. J. Med.* **298**, 996–9.

Kudoh, T., Kumagai, T., Uetsuji, N., Tsugawa, S., Oyanagi, K., Chiba, Y., Minami, R. and Nakao, T. (1981). Vitamin D dependent rickets: decreased sensitivity to 1,25-dihydroxy vitamin D. *Eur. J. Pediatr.* **137**, 307–11.

Liberman, V. A., Eil, C. and Marx, S. J. (1986). Receptor-positive hereditary resistance of 1,25-dihydroxyvitamin D: chromatography of hormone-receptor complexes on deoxyribonucleic acid-cellulose shows two classes of mutation. *J. Clin. Endocrinol. Metab.* **62**, 122–6.

Takeda, E., Kuroda, Y., Saijo, T., Toshiwa, K., Naito, E., Kobashi, H., Iwakumi, Y. and Miyao, M. (1986). Rapid diagnosis of vitamin-D dependent rickets type II by one of phytohemagglutinin-stimulated lymphocytes. *Clin. Chim. Acta* **155**, 245–50.

Hereditary hypophosphataemic rickets with hypercalciuria

Tieder and colleagues (1985) have recently described a new disorder in an inbred Bedouin tribe, to which they give the above name. Onset is in childhood with rickets, short stature, and increased renal phosphate clearance. There is hypercalciuria with normal serum calcium and increased intestinal absorption of calcium and phosphorus. Serum 1,25-dihydroxy vitamin D is markedly elevated and parathyroid function suppressed. Apart from a bladder stone in one patient out of six studied, there was no evidence of urolithiasis or nephrocalcinosis. The authors suggest that the disorder is due to renal phosphate leak with secondary increase in 1,25-dihydroxy vitamin D, but this is difficult to reconcile with the evidence for involvement of the parathormone-inhibited and independent mechanisms of phosphate reabsorption in X-linked hypophosphatemia and hypophosphataemic bone disease respectively. At present the primary defect must be accepted as being unknown. Inheritance appears to be autosomal recessive.

Reference

Tieder, M., Modai, D., Samuel, R., Arie, R., Halabe, A., Bab, I., Gabizon, D. and Liberman, U. A. (1985). Hereditary hypophosphatemic rickets with hyper-calciuria. *New Engl. J. Med.* **312**, 611–17.

6.1.2. Renal glycosuria

This benign condition was first recognized in the early part of this century as one that needed to be distinguished from diabetes (Hjärne 1927; Parkes Weber 1931; Lawrence 1934; Brown and Poleschuck 1935). These authors, and others, reported families with apparently typical autosomal dominant inheritance. The condition is diagnosed on the finding of an isolated glycosuria in the presence of a normal blood glucose. Early studies of heritability relied on oral glucose tolerance tests (Hjärne 1927; Brown and Poleshuck 1935; Houston and Merivale 1949). Later studies revealed complications to this simple genetic interpretation of the findings in that the severity of glycosuria varied within families (Froesch *et al.* 1957), that severe glycosuria was less common than milder degrees (Lawrence 1947; Marble 1952; Harkness 1962), and that mild glycosuria was seen in consanguineous parents of children with more severe glycosuria (Khachadurian and Khachadurian 1964). In the most severe form there may be no reabsorption of glucose at all. Analysis of the renal threshold for glucose and of maximal glucose reabsorptive capacity (T_{m_G}) defined two types of renal glycosuria: type A characterized by low threshold and T_{m_G}, thought to be due to a reduced number of carrier sites; and type B characterized by low threshold with a widened splay and normal T_{m_G}, thought to be due to a lowered affinity of the carrier for glucose (Reubi 1954; Khachadurian and Khachadurian 1964; Monasterio *et al.* 1964). Elsas and Rosenberg (1969) showed inheritance of the type A defect in a fully autosomal recessive manner in one family, and the occurrence of mild and severe type A and type B glycosuria all within another family. They also showed normal intestinal glucose transport in one family. In a further study (Elsas *et al.* 1971) they demonstrated severe type A renal glycosuria in a boy and mild type A in both of his parents and in one grandparent on each side of the family. The findings in this latter family are similar to those in the families studied by the Khachadurians. Thus mild type A is inherited in a dominant and severe type A in a recessive manner, or put another way type A glycosuria is incompletely recessive. The inheritance of type B is less clear but is probably dominant, mutations for both types probably having been present in Elsas and Rosenberg's second family. Reubi (1962) has estimated that 0.5 to 1.0 per cent of the population have either type A or B renal glycosuria.

A third type of renal glycosuria, type C, with autosomal dominant inheritance has been described, in which proximal tubular reabsorption fatigues rapidly at high filtered loads (Govaerts and Lambert 1949; Chaptal *et al.* 1954).

Further light is thrown on the mechanisms of glucose transport by studies of the autosomal recessive glucose–galactose malabsorption syndrome in which there is severe neonatal diarrhoea (Calcagno and Hollerman 1975). Elsas and colleagues (1970) showed grossly impaired glucose transport by the jejunum, and a partial defect of renal glucose reabsorption in an affected child. The asymptomatic parents had a less marked impairment of intestinal transport. Scriver and colleagues (1976) suggested that there are two mechanisms of hexose transport, G_1 and G_2. G_1 is a carrier for both glucose and galactose and its function is defective in glucose–galactose syndrome with both intestine and renal tubule involved. Scriver and coworkers proposed that G_1 accounts for only 30 per cent of renal tubular reabsorption of glucose, resulting in only mild glycosuria. The G_2 mechanism functions only in the kidney, and accounting for 70 per cent of the transport, its mutations result in the isolated but more severe glycosuria of the various recognized types.

References

Brown, M. S. and Poleshuck, R. (1935). Familial renal glycosuria. *J. Lab. Clin. Med.* **20**, 605–8.

Calcagno, P. L. and Hollerman, A. (1975). Hereditary renal disease, including certain renal tubular disorders. In *Pediatric nephrology,* eds. Rubin, M. I. and Barratt, T. p. 668. Williams & Wilkins, Baltimore.

Chaptal, J., Benezech, C., Jean, R., Campo, C. and Dejeanne, M. G. (1954). Etude sur le diabete renal chez l'enfant: exploration biologique de deux cas, discussion nosologique. *Arch. Fr. Pédiatr.* **11**, 273–80.

Elsas, L. J. and Rosenberg, L. E. (1969). Familial renal glycosuria: a genetic reappraisal of hexose transport by kidney and intestine. *J. Clin. Invest.* **48**, 1845–54.

——, Hillman, R. E., Patterson, J. H. and Rosenberg, L. (1970). Renal and intestinal hexose transport in familial glucose–galactose malabsorption. *J. Clin. Invest.* **49**, 576–85.

——, Busse, D. and Rosenberg, L. E. (1971). Autosomal recessive inheritance of renal glycosuria. *Metabolism* **20**, 968–75.

Froesch, E. R., Winegrad, A. I. and Renold, A. E. (1957). Die tubulare Nierenfunktion bei verschiedenen Formen des renalen Diabetes mellitus. *Helv. Med. Acta.* **24**, 548–55.

Govaerts, P. and Lambert, P. P. (1949). Pathogénie du diabét renal. *Acta Clin. Belg.* **4**, 341–70.

Harkness, J. (1962). Prevalence of glycosuria and diabetes mellitus. *Br. Med. J.* **1**, 1503–7.

Hjärne, U. (1927). A study of orthoglycaemic glycosuria with particular reference to its hereditability. *Acta Med. Scand.* **67**, 422–94.

Houston, J. C. and Merivale, W. H. H. (1949). Renal glycosuria in a family. *Guy's Hosp. Rep.* **98**, 233–40.

Khachadurian, A. K. and Khachadurian, L. A. (1964). The inheritance of renal glycosuria. *Am. J. Hum. Genet.* **16**, 189–94.

Lawrence, R. D. (1934). Heredity in diabetes mellitus and renal glycosuria. In *Chances of morbid inheritance*, ed. Blacker, C. P. pp. 346–8. H. K. Lewis, London.

—— (1947). Symptomless glycosurias: differentiation by sugar tolerance tests. *Med. Clin. N. Amer.* **31**, 289–97.

Marble, A. (1952). Non-diabetic mellituria. In *The treatment of diabetes mellitus*, eds. Joslin, E. P., Root, H. F., White, P. and Marble, A. p. 699. Lea & Febiger, Philadelphia.

Monasterio, G., Oliver, J., Muiesan, G., Pordelli, G., Marinozzi, V. and McDowell, M. (1964). Renal diabetes as a congenital tubular dysplasia. *Am. J. Med.* **37**, 44–61.

Parkes Weber, F. (1931). A glycosuric family without hyperglycaemia. *Lancet* **2**, 71–2.

Reubi, F. C. (1954). Glucose titration in renal glycosuria. In *Ciba foundation symposium on the kidney*, eds. Lewis, A. A. G. and Wolstenholme, G. E. W. p. 96. Little Brown, Boston.

—— (1962). In *Erbliche Stoffwechsoelkronkheiten*, ed. Linneweb, F. Urban und Schwarzenberg, München.

Scriver, C. R., Chesney, R. W. and McInnes, R. R. (1976). Genetic aspects of renal tubular transport: diversity and topology of carriers. *Kidney Int.* **9**, 149–71.

6.1.3. Fanconi syndrome (renal phospho-gluco-aminoaciduria, Fanconi renotubular syndrome)

This syndrome is highly heterogeneous in origin, being a non-specific renal tubular disorder resulting in rickets in childhood and osteomalacia in adult life (Fanconi 1936). It may be inherited or acquired. The acquired forms include those due to a variety of toxins and drugs, and those secondary to myeloma, hypokalaemia and several forms of metabolic bone disease. It may also occur secondary to a number of inherited diseases including cystinosis, galactosaemia, Wilson's disease, Lowe's syndrome, Von Gierke's disease, tyrosinosis, oxalosis, and hereditary fructose intolerance.

The primary or idiopathic form of the disorder is a generalized defect in renal tubular reabsorption involving glucose, amino acids, phosphate, potassium, water, and bicarbonate. There may also be a tubular acidosis (Dent 1952). Early reports recognized childhood (Bickel *et al.* 1952a) and adult (Milne *et al.* 1952) forms of the disorder. In the former many of the patients show deposition of cystine in tissues. This childhood form came to be termed Lignac–Fanconi disease (Bickel *et al.* 1952a and b), or type I Fanconi syndrome, and is inherited in an autosomal recessive manner with affected sibs and parental consanguinity (Bickel and Harris 1952). The childhood cases with cystinosis are now recognized as being due to primary cystinosis, which is discussed elsewhere in this volume.

There remains a rare recessive childhood form without cystinosis (Klajman and Arber 1967).

Primary, adult, idiopathic, or type II Fanconi syndrome without cystinosis is also rare. Hunt and colleagues (1966) could identify only six adult cases. In the families reported by Hunt and associates (1966) and by others (Sheldon *et al.* 1961; Ben-Ishay *et al.* 1961), inheritance appeared to be autosomal dominant, although in other families autosomal recessive inheritance seemed more likely (Illig and Prader 1961). This primary form of the disease, although variable in expression especially in the dominant form, has a relatively good prognosis in contrast to the cystinotic form (Dent and Harris 1956; Brenton *et al.* 1981); it does, however, share with it the pathological lesion of 'swan neck' deformity of the junction of the proximal renal tubule with the glomerulus (Clay *et al.* 1953; Darmady 1954). Recurrence of primary Fanconi syndrome following renal transplantation, suggesting a continuing pathogenetic mechanism, has been reported (Briggs *et al.* 1972).

References

Ben-Ishay, D., Dreyfuss, F. and Ullman, T. D. (1961). Fanconi syndrome with hypouricemia in an adult: family study. *Am. J. Med.* **31**, 793–800.

Bickel, H. and Harris, H. (1952). Cystine storage disease with aminoaciduria and dwarfism (Lignac–Fanconi disease). Part 2: The genetics of Lignac-Fanconi disease. *Acta Paediatr.* **42**, Suppl. 90, 22–6.

——, Smallwood, W. C., Smellie, J. H., Baar, H. S. and Hickmans, E. M. (1952a). Cystine storage disease with aminoaciduria and dwarfism (Lignac–Fanconi disease). Part I: Introduction. *Acta Paediatr.* **42**, Suppl. 90: 9–21.

——, ——, —— and Hickmans, E. M. (1952b). Cystine storage disease with aminoaciduria and dwarfism (Lignac–Fanconi Disease). Part 3: Clinical description, factual analysis, prognosis and treatment of Lignac–Fanconi disease. *Acta Paediatr.* **42**, Suppl. 90: 27–78.

Brenton, D. P., Isenberg, D. A., Cusworth, D. C., Garrod, P., Krywawych, S. and Stamp, T. C. B. (1981). The adult presenting idiopathic Fanconi Syndrome. *J. Inherit. Metab. Dis.* **4**, 211–15.

Briggs, W. A., Kominami, N., Wilson, R. E. and Merril, J. P. (1972). Kidney transplantation in Fanconi syndrome. *New Engl. J. Med.* **286**, 25.

Clay, R. D., Darmady, E. M. and Hawkins, M. (1953). The nature of the renal lesion in Fanconi syndrome. *J. Pathol. Bact.* **65**, 551–8.

Darmady, E. M. (1954). Renal lesion in amino-aciduria and water diuresis. *Ciba Foundation Symposium on the Kidney.* Churchill, Livingstone, London.

Dent, C. E. (1952). Rickets and osteomalacia from renal tubule defects. *J. Bone Jt. Surg.* **34B**, 266–74.

—— and Harris, H. (1956). Hereditary forms of rickets and osteomalacia. *J. Bone Jt. Surg.* **38B**, 204–26.

Fanconi, G. (1936). Der Frühinfantile nephrotisch–glykosurische Zwergwuchs mit hypophosphatamischer Rachitis. *Jahrb. Kinderheilk.* **147**, 299–338.

Hunt, D. D., Stearns, G., McKinley, J. B., Froning, E., Hicks, P. and Bonfiglio, M. (1966). Long-term study of family with Fanconi syndrome without cystinosis (De Toni–Debre–Fanconi syndrome). *Am. J. Med.* **40**, 492–510.

Illig, R. and Prader, A. (1961). Primary tubulopathies. II. A case of idiopathic gluco-amino-phosphate diabetes (De Toni–Debre–Fanconi syndrome). *Helv. Paediatr. Acta.* **16**, 622–46.

Klajman, A. and Arber, I. (1967). Familial glycosuria and amino-aciduria associated with low serum alkaline phosphatase. *Israel J. Med. Sci.* **3**, 392–6.

Milne, M. D., Stanbury, S. W. and Thomson, A. E. (1952). Observations on the Fanconi syndrome and renal hyperchloraemic acidosis in the adult. *Quart. J. Med.* **21**, 61–82.

Sheldon, W., Linder, J. and Webb, B. (1961). A familial tubular reabsorption defect of glucose and amino acids. *Arch. Dis. Child.* **36**, 90–5.

6.1.4. Cystinuria, hypercystinuria, and dibasic aminoaciduria

Cystine stones were first recognized as early as 1810 by Wollaston, and cystinuria was discussed by Garrod (1908). The disorder is one in which there is impaired amino acid transport by the proximal renal tubular and gastrointestinal epithelial cells. Clinically patients are liable to form cystine renal stones, which may present with renal colic and lead on to complicating infection or renal failure; as a group they are slightly below average in height (Coliss *et al.* 1963). A number of associated clinical abnormalities have been reported, many probably fortuitous, and others, such as Lowe's syndrome (Bailey *et al.* 1976) and hereditary pancreatitis, in which the cystinuria is secondary (Gross *et al.* 1964). An association with mental subnormality remains of uncertain significance. Several groups have undertaken amino acid chromatography of retarded patients and found an apparent excess of cystinuria (Visakorpi and Hyrske 1960; Berry 1962; Carson and Neil 1962; Efron 1965; Scriver *et al.* 1970; Wadman and van Sprang 1971; Hill and Zaleski 1972; Cavanagh *et al.* 1974). At least some of the apparent excess of cystinurics in these surveys is likely to be due to the detection of heterozygotes (Smith and Procopis 1975) for the incompletely recessive form of the disorder, as well as of homozygotes. The doubtful significance of these earlier reports is born out by the findings of Gold and colleagues (1977) who could not detect any increase in the incidence of mental subnormality among a group of cystinurics.

Amongst a variety of other neurological associations are a few families with muscular dystrophy or hypotonia. Clara and Lowenthal (1966) reported a family in which four out of five sibs had severe congenital hypotonia, dwarfism, and excess excretion of cystine and the diabasic amino acids. Hurwitz and colleagues (1967) described a family with incompletely recessive cystinuria and a muscular dystrophy of the facio-scapulo-humeral type. The present author investigated a family, under the care of Dr J. M. Littlewood, in which the eldest and youngest of a family of three children had cystinuria of the fully recessive type. The parents were first cousins. The affected children, both girls, but not their unaffected brother, also had a marked hypotonia and joint hyper-extensability, premature dental caries, eyelid cysts, persistent loose stools, and speech delay. The only abnormality observed on muscle biopsy in the younger child was variation in fibre calibre. Since the clinical picture in these different families with cystinuria and myopathy varies there is no firm evidence of a causal relationship in any of them, although one or more may eventually prove to be true associations in rare genetically distinct variants.

Yeh and colleagues (1947) were the first to observe that cystinuric patients excrete excess amounts of the dibasic amino acids lysine and arginine in addition to cystine. This was confirmed by Dent and Rose (1951) and by Stein (1951) who also demonstrated high urinary concentrations of the third dibasic amino acid, ornithine. Harris and Dent and their colleagues found that the high urinary concentrations of these amino acids were associated with normal or low plasma levels, thus demonstrating that the defect must be one of renal tubular reabsorption (Fowler *et al.* 1952; Dent *et al.* 1954; Arrow and Westall 1958; Lester and Cusworth 1973; Kato 1977). Robson and Rose (1957), and subsequently Lester and Cusworth (1973) and Kato (1977), showed that in normal subjects intravenous infusion of lysine resulted in increased excretion of the other dibasic amino acids. These amino acids must, therefore, share a common step in reabsorption, as postulated by Dent and Rose (1951). Arginine inhibition of cystine uptake in microperfusion studies on rat proximal tubules adds further evidence for a common pathway (Silbernagl and Deetjen, 1972). Some cystinuric patients actually have a renal clearance of cystine that exceeds the glomerular filtration rate, implying secretion (Frimpter *et al.* 1962; Crawhall *et al.* 1967; Morin *et al.* 1971; Lester and Cusworth 1973), an observation that so far remains unexplained. A similar apparent secretion of cystine occurs on lysine infusion in the normal (Webber *et al.* 1961) and cystinuric dog (Segal and Bovee 1979). Dent and Rose's original postulate of a single mechanism of reabsorption of cystine and the dibasic amino acids has had to be modified in the light of lysine infusion experiments in cystinuric subjects which indicate two lysine transport systems: a low capacity system active at low substrate concentration, defective in cystinuria, and a high capacity system effective at high lysine concentration, which is unaffected (Lester and Cusworth 1973; Kata 1977). Further evidence for dual transport systems comes from the observations of patients with either isolated cystinuria without dibasic aminoaciduria, termed hypercystinuria (Brodehl *et al.* 1966, 1967), or cystinuria with only minimal dibasic aminoaciduria (Stephens and Perrett 1967), or with hyperdibasic aminoaciduria alone (Whelan and Scriver 1968; Oyanagi *et al.* 1970). Hyperdibasic aminoaciduria is associated with increased excretion of all three dibasic amino acids along with a similar intestinal transport defect. Several types have been described: type I with growth retardation and malabsorption syndrome, and type II or lysinuric protein intolerance, with mental retardation, but neither with renal stones. Inheritance, although presumably autosomal, is uncertain though probably incompletely recessive (Scriver *et al.* 1976). A further type, hyperlysinuria with hyperammonaemia, with mental retardation has been reported (Brown *et al.* 1972). These clinical observations suggest that the dibasic amino acids share a common pathway of tubular reabsorption for which cystine does not compete. This suggestion is confirmed by experiments on rat (Rosenberg *et al.* 1962; Segal *et al.* 1967; Segal and Crawhall 1968) and human (Fox *et al.* 1964) renal cortex slices. This mechanism of dibasic amino acid transport is impaired in cystinuria whereas cystine uptake by cystinuric renal slices is not (Fox *et al.* 1964), nor is that of cysteine (Segal and Crawhall 1967). Furthermore *in vitro* lysine transport is mediated by similar high affinity, low capacity and low affinity, high capacity carrier systems, to those defined *in vivo*. The former only, as in the *in vivo* studies, shows impaired capacity in cystinuric kidney (Rosenberg *et al.* 1967a). Cysteine uptake, although showing a dual transport mechanism in human kidney slices (Segal and Crawhall 1967), also shows no mutual inhibition with the dibasic amino acids (Schwartzman *et al.* 1966). More recently the study of rat tubule fragments (Foreman *et al.* 1980) and brush border membrane vesicles (Segal *et al.* 1977; Foreman *et al.* 1981; McNamara *et al.* 1981) has clarified the transport mechanisms for these amino acids in the proximal renal tubule. In the rat at least there are two transport systems for cystine, a high affinity, low K_m and a low affinity, high K_m system, the former being inhibited by the dibasic amino acids and, it is concluded, shared with them. Thus there are three systems for cystine and the dibasic amino acids: one shared with a high affinity for both cystine and lysine, one low affinity system for cystine alone, and a similar one for the dibasic amino acids. The shared system is sodium ion and oxygenation dependent. The cystine systems transport this sulphur amino acid across the brush border in unreduced form and it is only within the renal epithelial cell that it is reduced to cysteine (Crawhall and Segal 1967). Some of the past confusion over *in vitro* findings arises from the fact that using kidney slices only the high K_m system of cystine transport is revealed. The brush border vesicle and tubule fragment

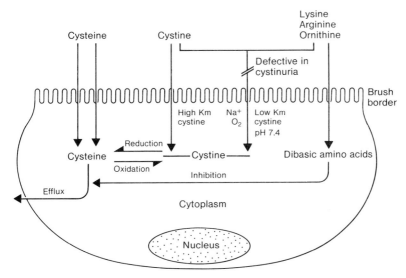

Fig. 6.2. Sulphur and dibasic amino acid transport defects in a proximal renal tubular epithelial cell in cystinuria (for references see text).

studies thus confirm the original theory of Dent and Rose (1951) that cystinuria results from a defect in a common transport system. It can be postulated that the unshared high K_m system of cystine transport is defective in isolated hypercystinuria and the unshared high K_m system of lysine transport is defective in hyperdibasic aminoaciduria (Fig. 6.2).

Milne and colleagues demonstrated *in vivo* that, in addition to the renal defect, cystinuric patients have a defect in the intestinal uptake of both cystine and all of the dibasic amino acids which compete for a common mechanism of absorption (Milne *et al.* 1961; Asatoor *et al.* 1962). Others using *in vitro* methods have confirmed this absorptive defect (McCarthy *et al.* 1964; Thier *et al.* 1964, 1965; Rosenberg *et al.* 1965, 1966a, 1967b). Segal and colleagues (1968) demonstrated that lysine uptake by intestinal mucosa, unlike that in the kidney, is wholly sodium ion and oxygen dependent, indicating that only one transport mechanism, that shared with cystine, is present (Fig. 6.3). Cysteine absorption is not impaired in cystinuria (Foley and London 1965). Overall dibasic amino acid absorption is maintained through normal oligopeptide absorption (Asatoor *et al.* 1972). Rosenberg and his coworkers (1966a) described three types of cystinuria on the basis of *in vivo* and *in vitro* studies of the intestinal transport defect. In type I, which corresponds to the fully recessive type of Harris and colleagues (1954a), there is no demonstrable active transport of cystine or any of the dibasic amino acids in jejunal biopsies, and no rise in plasma cystine level

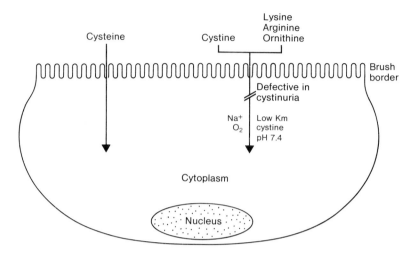

Fig. 6.3. Sulphur and dibasic amino acid transport defect in a jejunal epithelial cell in cystinuria (for references see text).

following an oral load. Types II and III correspond to the incompletely recessive form of cystinuria of Harris and colleagues (1954a, 1955b). In type II there is a minor degree of transport of cystine but no transport of lysine on jejunal biopsy, and no rise in plasma cystine after an oral load. In type III there is active but reduced transport of cystine, lysine and arginine on biopsy, and a reduced rise in plasma cystine after an oral load. The transport defect in the intestine has been localized to the luminal brush border membrane (Coicaden *et al.* 1980). Morin and colleagues (1971) confirmed the existence of types I and II but concluded that individuals with findings suggestive of type III were double heterozygotes for I and II.

A classification of cystinuria combining the renal and intestinal transport defects is outlined in Table 6.1.

The earliest proper genetic studies of cystinuria were those of Harris and his colleagues in the 1950s (Harris and Warren 1953; Harris *et al.* 1954a and b, 1955a and b; Harris and Robson 1955, 1957). On the basis of urinary amino acid excretion patterns in patients with cystine stones, and their relatives, they recognized fully and incompletely recessive forms of cystinuria. Their heterozygotes for the incompletely recessive form did not form stones and they suggested that this type might be under polygenic influence. Like Harris and colleagues the group at St Bartholomews Hospital also found marked variation in the amounts of the different amino acids excreted by both homozygotes and heterozygotes (Crawhall *et al.* 1969) (Table 6.3). They supported the idea that

Table 6.3 *A classification of primary cystinuria*

Types of cystinuria	Cystine and dibasic amino acid transport							
	Renal excretion (μmol/g creatinine)				Intestinal absorption (Distribution ratios: 1.0 = no transport, and plasma rise (μg/ml)			
	Cystine	Lysine	Arginine	Ornithine	Cystine	Lysine	Arginine	Rise in plasma cystine after oral load
Type 1: Homozygote	1250–3790	2350–17 300	273–19 200	390–4440	1.1	1.0	0.9	None
Heterozygote	11–754	45–3900	5–129	3–694	—	—	—	Normal
Type II: Homozygote	1260–4940	2400–21 400	215–19 300	476–19 300	2.4	1.0	—	None
Heterozygote	63–755	390–2990	4–234	22–401	—	—	—	Normal
Type I/II: Double Heterozygote	Increased	Increased	Increased	Increased	Normal to reduced	Variably reduced	Variably reduced	4–9 in 2 hours
Controls: Excretion ± 2 SD in μmol/g creatinine	8–89	40–490	0–177	10–153				8–13 in 1 hour
Absorption: Distribution ratios and plasma rise (μg/ml)					7	11	28	

Based on date of Rosenberg *et al.* (1966), especially for absorption, Crawhall *et al.* (1969) for excretion in types I and II, and Morin *et al.* (1971).

this variation may be due to polygenic influences. Studies of intestinal absorption enabled Rosenberg and his coworkers to subdivide the incompletely recessive cases into two types, types II and III, with the fully recessive form termed type I (Rosenberg *et al.* 1966b, 1967). They considered that their type III individuals were distinct from their single or double heterozygotes for their types I and II and that their three types were therefore allelic (Rosenberg 1966, 1967; Rosenberg *et al.* 1966b). Hershko and colleagues (1965) also obtained evidence for types I and II being allelic. Others have tried to refine the diagnosis of heterozygotes for the different types on the basis of amino acid excretion patterns (Kelly and Copeland 1968; Crawhall *et al.* 1969; Morin *et al.* 1971) or by cystine loading (Minami *et al.* 1975). As previously mentioned Morin and colleagues could not distinguish more than two allelic forms and considered Rosenberg's type III to be wholly compatible with double heterozygosity for types I and II. The resolution of this question of the number of allelic forms will probably await studies of the molecular level.

Various estimates of incidence or prevalence have been attempted on the basis of urine amino acid excretion but these have not all distinguished the patterns produced by homozygotes from those of heterozygotes. Estimates of homozygote prevalence in Caucasian populations vary from the low value of 1 in 100 000 in Sweden (Boström and Hambraeus 1964), through values in the 1 in 10 000–1 in 20 000 range for England, Germany, and Australia (Crawhall *et al.* 1966; Crawhall and Watts 1968; Crawhall *et al.* 1969; Turner and Brown 1970; Thalhammer *et al.* 1975), to the high value of 1 in 2500 among Israeli Jews of Libyan origin (Weinberger *et al.* 1974). Milne (1967) puts the frequency of type I at twice that of types II and III (or I/II) combined. Newborn screening programmes have given higher estimates for birth frequency. Woolf (1967) obtained a figure of 1 in 2000 in England, Turner and Brown (1972) found 1 in 4000, and Levy and colleagues (1971) 1 in 15 000 in the United States. Levy (1973) in a review of these results estimated a birth incidence for Caucasians of 1 in 7000, making cystinuria a relatively common disorder. Estimates of heterozygote prevalence on adult populations vary even more widely than those for homozygotes, from about 1 in 500 to 1 in 2000 (Dent and Harris 1951; Boström and Tottie 1959; Crawhall *et al.* 1966; Crawhall and Watts 1968; Turner and Brown 1970), but on the basis of homozygote frequencies quoted above would all appear to be low. It has been suggested that heterozygosity for cystinuria may predispose to recurrent calcium oxalate stone formation. Surveys of such patients have given conflicting results. In the United States 8 to 14 per cent of recurrent stone-formers are cystinuric heterozygotes (Resnick *et al.* 1979; Thomas *et al.* 1981) and in Brazil 4 per cent (Giugliani and Ferrari 1980), whereas in the Netherlands the figure is only 2.8 per cent (Carpentier *et al.* 1983). Nevertheless, Carpentier and colleagues also found that heterozygosity for cystinuria was confined to their recurrent stone-formers, and was not found among patients with non-recurring calcium oxalate stones. A further observation is that in an inbred population with a high incidence of cystinuria there is also a high prevalence of calcium oxalate stone formation (Caldwell *et al.* 1978), lending support to the hypothesis that cystinuric heterozygosity may be a significant factor in recurrent stone formation. Giugliani and colleagues (1985) found that the cystinuric heterozygotes among their stone formers were heterozygous for types II and III but not type I.

References

Arrow, V. K. and Westall, R. G. (1958). Amino acid clearances in cystinuria. *J. Physiol. (Lond.)* **142**, 141–6.

Asatoor, A. M., Lacey, B. W., London, D. R. and Milne, M. D. (1962). Amino acid metabolism in cystinuria. *Clin. Sci.* **23**, 285–304.

——, Harrison, B. D. W., Milne, M. D. and Prosser, D. I. (1972). Intestinal absorption of an arginine-containing peptide in cystinuria. *Gut* **13**, 95–8.

Bailey, R. R., Carrell, R. W. and Shannon, F. T. (1976). Homozygous cystinuria and oculo-cerebro-renal dystrophy of Lowe in the same family. *Arch. Dis. Child.* **51**, 558–62.

Berry, H. K. (1962). Detection of metabolic disorders among mentally retarded children by means of paper spot tests. *Am. J. Ment. Defic.* **66**, 555–60.

Boström, H. and Hambraeus, L. (1964). Cystinuria in Sweden. VII. Clinical histopathological and medico-social aspects of the disease. *Acta Med. Scand.* Suppl. **411**, 1–128.

—— and Tottie, K. (1959). Cystinuria in Sweden. II. The incidence of homozygous cystinuria in Swedish school children. *Acta Paediatr.* **48**, 345–52.

Brodehl, J., Gellissen, K. and Kowalewski, S. (1966). Isolated cystinuria (without lysine, ornithine-argininuria) in a family with hypocalcaemic tetany. *Proc. 3rd Int. Congr. on Nephrology,* Washington, 1966.

——, Gellissen, K. and Kowalewski, S. (1967). Isolated cystinuria (without lysine–ornithine–argininuria) in a family with hypocalcaemic tetany. *Klin. Wschr.* **45**, 38–40.

Brown, J. H., Fabre, L. F., Farrell, G. L. and Adams, E. D. (1972). Hyperlysinuria with hyperammonemia. *Am. J. Dis. Child.* **124**, 127–32.

Caldwell, R. J., Townsend, J. I. and Smith, M. J. V. (1978). Genetics of cystinuria in an inbred population. *J. Urol.* **119**, 531–3.

Carpentier, P. J., Kurth, K. H., Blom, W. and Huijmans, J. G. M. (1983). Heterozygous cystinuria and calcium oxalate urolithiasis. *J. Urol.* **130**, 302–4.

Carson, N. A. J. and Neill, D. W. (1962). Metabolic abnormalities detected in a survey of mentally backward individuals in Northern Ireland. *Arch. Dis. Child.* **37**, 505–13.

Cavanagh, N. P. C., Bicknell, J. and Howard, F. (1974). Cystinuria with mental retardation and paroxysmal dyskinesia in two brothers. *Arch. Dis. Child.* **49**, 662–4.

Clara, R. and Lowenthal, A. (1966). Familial and congenital lysine-cystinuria with benign myopathy and dwarfism. *J. Neurol. Sci.* **3**, 433–4.

Coicadan, L., Heyman, M., Grasset, E. and Desjeux, J. F. (1980). Cystinuria: reduced lysine permeability of the brush border of intestinal membrane cells. *Pediatr. Res.* **14**, 109–12.

Colliss, J. E., Levi, A. J. and Milne, M. D. (1963). Stature and nutrition in cystinuria and Hartnup disease. *Br. Med. J.* **1**, 590–2.

Crawhall, J. C. and Segal, S. (1967). The intracellular ratio of cysteine and cystine in various tissues. *Biochem. J.* **105**, 891–6.

—— and Watts, R. W. E. (1968). Cystinuria. *Am. J. Med.* **45**, 736–55.

——, Saunders, E. P. and Thompson, C. J. (1966). Heterozygotes for cystinuria. *Ann. Hum. Genet.* **29**, 257–69.

——, Scowen, E. F., Thompson, C. J. and Watts, R. W. E. (1967). The renal clearance of amino acids in cystinuria. *J. Clin. Invest.* **46**, 1162–71.

——, Purkiss, P., Watts, R. W. E. and Young, E. P. (1969). The excretion of amino acids by cystinuric patients and their relatives. *Ann. Hum. Genet.* **33**, 149–69.

Dent, C. E. and Harris, H. (1951). The genetics of 'cystinuria'. *Ann. Eug.* **16**, 60–87.

—— and Rose, G. A. (1951). Aminoacid metabolism in cystinuria. *Quart. J. Med.* **20**, 205–19.

——, Senior, B. and Walshe, J. M. (1954). The pathogenesis of cystinuria. 2. Polarographic studies of the metabolism of sulphur containing amino acids. *J. Clin. Invest.* **33**, 1216–26.

Efron, M. L. (1965). Aminoaciduria. *New Engl. J. Med.* **272**, 1058–67 and 1107–13.

Foley, T. H. and London, D. R. (1965). Cysteine metabolism in cystinuria. *Clin. Sci.* **29**, 549–54.

Foreman, J. W., Hwang, S.-M. and Segal, S. (1980). Transport interactions of cystine and dibasic amino acids in isolated rat renal tubules. *Metabolism* **29**, 53–61.

——, McNamara, P. D. and Segal, S. (1981). Renal transport of cystine by isolated renal tubules and brush border membrane vesicles. In *Transport and inherited disease*, eds. Belton, N. R. and Toothill, C. pp. 263–75. MTP Press, Lancaster.

Fowler, D. I., Harris, H. and Warren, F. L. (1952). Plasma-cystine levels in cystinuria. *Lancet* **1**, 544.

Fox, M., Thier, S., Rosenberg, L., Kiser, W. and Segal, S. (1964). Evidence against a single renal transport defect in cystinuria. *New Engl. J. Med.* **270**, 556–61.

Frimpter, G. W., Horwith, M., Furth, E., Fellows, R. E. and Thompson, D. D. (1962). Inulin and endogenous amino acid renal clearances in cystinuria: evidence for tubular secretion. *J. Clin. Invest.* **41**, 281–8.

Garrod, A. E. (1908). Inborn errors of metabolism (1908 Croonian Lectures). *Lancet* **21**, 1, 73, 142, and 214.

Giugliani, R. and Ferrari, I. (1980). Metabolic factors in urolithiasis: a study in Brazil. *J. Urol.* **124**, 503–7.

Gold, R. J. M., Dobrinski, M. J. and Gold, D. P. (1977). Cystinuria and mental deficiency. *Clin. Genet.* **12**, 329–32.

Gross, J. B., Ulrich, J. A. and Jones, J. D. (1964). Urinary excretion of amino acids in a kindred with hereditary pancreatitis and aminoaciduria. *Gastroenterology,* **47**, 41–8.

Giugliani, R., Ferrari, I. and Greene, L. J. (1985). Heterozygous cystinuria and urinary lithiasis. *Am. J. Med. Genet.* **22**, 703–15.

Harris, H. and Robson, E. B. (1955). Variation in homozygous cystinuria. *Acta Genet.* **5**, 381–90.

—— and —— (1957). Cystinuria. *Am. J. Med.* **22**, 774–83.

—— and Warren, F. L. (1953). Quantitative studies on the urinary cystine in patients with cystine stone formation and their relatives. *Ann. Eug.* **18**, 125–71.

——, Mittwoch, U., Robson, E. B. and Warren, F. L. (1954a). Genetical studies on urinary cystine, lysine and arginine excretion in man. *Caryologia,* Vol. 6 (Suppl.), 1188–9.

——, ——, —— and —— (1954b). Excretion of amino acids in cystinurics. *Biochem. J.* **57**, 33.

——, ——, —— and —— (1955a). The pattern of amino-acid excretion in cystinuria. *Ann. Hum. Genet.* **19**, 196–208.

——, ——, —— and —— (1955b). Phenotypes and genotypes in cystinuria. *Ann. Hum. Genet.* **20**, 57–91.

Hershko, C., Ben-Ami, E., Paciorkovski, J. and Levin, N. (1965). Allelomorphism in cystinuria. *Proc. Tel-Hashomer Hosp.* **4**, 21–3.

Hill, A. and Zaleski, W. A. (1972). Screening for metabolic disorders associated with mental retardation. *Clin. Biochem.* **5**, 33–45.

Hurwitz, L. F., Carson, N. A. J., Allen, I. V., Fannin, T. F., Lyttle, J. A. and Neill, D. W. (1967). Clinical, biochemical and histopathological findings in a family with muscular dystrophy. *Brain* **90**, 799–816.

Kato, T. (1977). Renal handling of dibasic amino acids and cystine in cystinuria. *Clin. Sci. Mol. Med.* **53**, 9–15.

Kelly, S. and Copeland, W. (1968). Amino acid patterns in cystinuric families. *J. Med. Genet.* **5**, 281–5.

Lester, F. T. and Cusworth, D. C. (1973). Lysine infusion in cystinuria: theoretical renal thresholds for lysine. *Clin. Sci.* **44**, 99–111.

Levy, H. L. (1973). Genetic screening. In *Advances in human genetics,* Vol. 4, eds. Harris, H. and Hirschhorn, K. p. 1. Plenum, New York.

——, Madigan, P. M. and Shih, V. E. (1972). Massachusetts metabolic disorders screening program. I. Technics and results of urine screening. *Pediatrics* **49**, 825–36.

McCarthy, C. F., Borland, J. L., Lynch, H. J., Owen, E. E. and Tyor, M. P. (1964). Defective uptake of basic amino acids and L-cystine by intestinal mucosa of patients with cystinuria. *J. Clin. Invest.* **43**, 1518–24.

McNamara, P. D., Pepe, L. M. and Segal, S. (1981). Cystine uptake by renal brush border vesicles. *Biochem. J.* **194**, 443–9.

Milne, M. D. (1967). Cystinuria 1810–1965. In *The scientific basis of medicine annual reviews 1967.* The Athlone Press, London.

——, Asatoor, A. M., Edwards, K. D. G. and Loughridge, L. W. (1961). The intestinal absorption defect in cystinuria. *Gut* **2**, 323–37.

Minami, R., Olek, K. and Wardenbach, P. (1975). Cystinuric heterozygotes and cystine loading. *Humangenetik.* **29**, 145–9.

Morin, C. L., Thompson, M. W., Jackson, S. H. and Sass-Kortsak, A. (1971). Biochemical and genetic studies in cystinuria: observations on double hetero-zygotes of genotype I/II. *J. Clin. Invest.* **50**, 1961–76.

Oyanagi, K., Miura, R. and Yamanoughi, T. (1970). Congenital lysinuria: a new inherited disorder of dibasic amino acids. *J. Pediatr.* **77**, 259–66.

Resnick, M. I., Goodman, H. O. and Boyce, W. H. (1979). Heterozygous cystinuria and calcium oxalate urolithiasis. *J. Urol.* **122**, 52–4.

Robson, E. B. and Rose, G. A. (1957). The effect of intravenous lysine on the renal clearances of cystine, arginine and ornithine in normal subjects, in patients with cystinuria and Fanconi syndrome and in their relatives. *Clin. Sci.* **16**, 75–93.

Rosenberg, L. E. (1966). Cystinuria. Genetic heterogeneity and allelism. *Science* **154**, 1341–3.

—— (1967). *Amino acid metabolism and genetic variation.* ed. Nyhan, W. L. p. 341. McGraw-Hill, New York.

——, Downing, S. J. and Segal, S. (1962). Competitive inhibition of dibasic amino acid transport in rat kidney. *J. Biol. Chem.* **237**, 2265–70.

——, Durant, J. L. and Holland, J. M. (1965). Intestinal absorption and renal excretion of cystine and cysteine in cystinuria. *New Engl. J. Med.* **273**, 1239–45.

——, Downing, S., Durant, J. L. and Segal, S. (1966a). Cystinuria: biochemical evidence for three genetically distinct diseases. *J. Clin. Invest.* **45**, 365–71.

——, Durant, J. L. and Albrecht, I. (1966b). Genetic heterogeneity in cystinuria: evidence for allelism. *Trans. Assoc. Am. Phys.* **79**, 284–96.

——, Albrecht, I. and Segal, S. (1967a). Lysine transport in human kidney: evidence for two systems. *Science* **155**, 1426–8.

——, Crawhall, J. C. and Segal, S. (1967b). Intestinal transport of cystine and cysteine in man: evidence for separate mechanisms. *J. Clin. Invest.* **46**, 30–4.

Schwartzman, L., Blair, A. and Segal, S. A. (1966). A common renal transport system for lysine, ornithine, arginine and cystine. BBRC **23**, 220–6.

Scriver, C. R., Whelan, D. T., Clow, C. L. and Dallaire, L. (1970). Cystinuria: increased prevalence in patients with mental disease. *New Engl. J. Med.* **283**, 783–6.

——, Chesney, R. W. and McInnes, R. R. (1976). Genetic aspects of renal tubular transport: diversity and topology of carriers. *Kidney Int.* **9**, 149–71.

Segal, S. and Bovee, K. (1979). Canine models of human renal transport disorders. In *Models for the study of inborn errors of metabolism,* ed. Hommes, F. A. pp. 19–30. Elsevier-North Holland, Amsterdam.

—— and Crawhall, J. C. (1967). Transport of cysteine by human kidney cortex *in vitro. Biochem. Med.* **1**, 141.

—— and —— (1968). The characteristics of cystine and cysteine transport in rat kidney cortex slices. *Proc. Nat. Acad. Sci.* **59**, 231–37.

——, Schwartzman, L., Blair, A. and Bertoli, D. (1967). Dibasic amino acid transport in rat kidney cortex slices. *Biochim. Biophys. Acta.* **135**, 127–35.

——, Lowenstein, L. M. and Wallace, A. (1968). Comparison of the transport characteristics by rat intestine and kidney cortex. *Gastroenterology* **55**, 386–91.

——, McNamara, P. D. and Pepe, L. M. (1977). Transport interaction of cystine and dibasic amino acids in renal brush border vesicles. *Science* **197**, 169–71.

Silbernagal, S. and Deetjen, P. (1972). The tubular reabsorption of L-cystine and L-cysteine: a common transport system with L-arginine or not? *Pflügers Arch.* **337**, 277–84.

Smith, A. and Procopis, P. G. (1975). Cystinuria and its relationship to mental retardation. *Med. J. Aust.* **2**, 932–3.

Stein, W. H. (1951). Excretion of amino acids in cystinuria. *Proc. Soc. Exp. Biol., NY,* **78**, 705–8.

Stephens, A. D. and Perrett, D. (1976). Cystinuria: a new genetic variant. *Clin. Sci. Mol. Med.* **51**, 27–32.

Thalhammer, O., *et al.* (1975). Frequency of inborn errors of metabolism especially PKU, in some representative newborn screening centers around the world. A collaborative study. *Humangenetik.* **30**, 273–86.

Thier, S., Fox, M., Segal, S. and Rosenberg, L. E. (1964). Cystinuria: *in vitro* demonstration of an intestinal transport defect. *Science* **143**, 482–4.

——, Segal, S., Fox, M., Blair, A. and Rosenberg, L. E. (1965). Cystinuria: defective intestinal transport of dibasic amino-acids and cystine. *J. Clin. Invest.* **44**, 442–8.

Thomas, W. C., Malagodi, M. H. and Rennert, O. M. (1981). Amino acids in urine and blood of calculous patients. *Invest. Urol.* **19**, 115–22.

Turner, B. and Brown, D. A. (1970). Amino acid excretion in infancy and early childhood. A survey of 100 000 infants. *Med. J. Aust.* **1**, 11–14.

—— and —— (1972). Amino acid excretion in infancy and early childhood: a survey of 200 000 infants. *Med. J. Aust.* **1**, 62–5.

Visakorpi, J. K. and Hyrske, I. (1960). Urinary amino-acids in mentally retarded patients. *Ann. Paediatr. Fenn.* **6**, 112–18.

Wadman, S. K. and Van Sprang, F. J. (1971). Frequency of mental retardation and neurological disturbances in patients with cystinuria. In *Inherited disorders of sulphur metabolism, 8th Symposium Society for Study of Inborn Errors of Metabolism,* eds. Carson, N. A. J. and Raine, D. M. pp. 81–4. Churchill Livingstone, London.

Webber, W. A., Brown, J. L. and Pitts, R. F. (1961). Interactions of amino acids in renal tubular transport. *Am. J. Physiol.* **200**, 380–6.

Weinberger, A., Sperling, O., Rabinowvitz, M., Brosh, S., Adam, A. and DeVries, A. (1974). High frequency of cystinuria among Jews of Libyan origin. *Hum. Hered.* **24**, 568–72.

Whelan, D. T. and Scriver, C. R. (1968). Hyperdibasic aminoaciduria: an inherited disorder of amino acid transport. *Pediatr. Res.* **2**, 525–34.

Wollaston, W. H. (1810). On cystic oxide: a new species of urinary calculus. *(Phil.) Trans. R. Soc. Lond.* **100**, 223.

Woolf, L. I. (1967). Large-scale screening for metabolic disease in the newborn in Great Britain. In *Phenylketonuria and allied metabolic disorders,* eds. Anderson, J. A. and Swaiman, K. F. pp. 50–9. US Dept. of Health, Education and Welfare (Childrens' Bureau), Washington.

Yeh, H. L., Frankl, W., Dunn, M. S., Parker, P., Hughes, B. and György, P. (1947). The urinary excretion of amino acids by a cystinuric subject. *Am. J. Med. Sci.* **214**, 507–12.

6.1.5. Familial glycinuria (iminoglycinuria)

Glycine and the imino acids, proline and hydroxyproline, are normally excreted by the human infant up to about 6 months of age. Persistent iminoglycinuria beyond this age may be secondary to generalized aminoaciduria as in Fanconi syndrome or hyperprolinaemia and hyper-hydroxyprolinaemia. It also occurs as a specific inherited defect of proximal renal tubular transport—familial (renal) glycinuria or imino-glycinuria.

Excessive excretion of glycine in the presence of normal plasma levels was reported by De Vries and coworkers (1957) in association with renal stones. The following year Joseph and colleagues (1958) described familial iminoglycinuria in association with convulsions. Scriver (1983) quotes a similar family described to him in 1962 by Jonxis in Holland. Reports of familial iminoglycinuria and mental retardation appeared from Japan (Tada *et al.* 1965; Morikama *et al.* 1966), France (Mardens *et al.* 1968), Israel (Statter *et al.* 1976). The first report of familial imino-glycinuria without any clinical abnormality was that of Scriver and Wilson (1967) in a North American Ashkenazic Jewish family. Many subsequent reports have appeared (Goodman *et al.* 1967; Bank *et al.* 1972; Blehova *et al.* 1973; Greene *et al.* 1973) in all of which the imino-glycinuria was a coincidental finding. It thus appears that this transport defect is benign (Fraser *et al.* 1968; Rosenberg, *et al.* 1968; Whelan and Scriver 1968). This view is confirmed by findings in newborn-screening programmes (Procopis and Turner 1971; Levy 1973).

Renal clearance studies of amino acids in iminoglycinuric families (Tada *et al.* 1967; Hoefnagal and Pomeroy 1968/1969; Rosenberg *et al.* 1968; Scriver 1968) show that only the imino acids and glycine have increased clearance and reduced tubular reabsorption. This defect in reabsorption is not absolute in homozygotes showing some net absorption, and even normal proline excretion at low plasma levels. Proline or hydroxyproline infusion results in saturation of imino acid transport and normal plasma concentrations in homozygotes; and a T_m intermediate between the values of normals and homozygotes in hetero-zygotes, with normal reabsorption below that T_m (Scriver and Wilson 1967; Rosenberg *et al.* 1968; Scriver 1968). The effect is for homo-zygotes to present with iminoglycinuria but some heterozygotes with hyperglycinuria alone (Rosenberg *et al.* 1968; Whelan and Scriver 1968).

Genetic heterogeneity is suggested by the observation of Greene and colleagues (1973) that in their case there was a mutation that impaired the affinity of the transport system for imino acids and glycine rather than its loss. In the homozygote the normal competitive inhibition of glycine reabsorption by proline and hydroxyproline is lost, suggesting that the residual glycine transport involves a non-shared pathway (Scriver and Wilson 1967; Scriver 1968). On the other hand competitive inhibition between the two imino acids is retained in the homozygote (Scriver 1968). Scriver and colleagues (1976) have suggested that there are at least four alleles on the basis of interfamilial variation. Renal tubular brush border membrane vesicles studies by two groups in rat or rabbit kidney confirms that there is a common pathway for proline, hydroxyproline, and glycine, which is sodium ion dependent and of high capacity, and other low capacity sites selective for either glycine or the imino acids (McNamara *et al.* 1976; Hammerman and Sacktor 1977; Slack *et al.* 1977; McNamara *et al.* 1979). A further genetic variant is suggested by the family of Käser and associates (1962) with gluco-glycinuria.

Studies of intestinal transport also bear out the genetic heterogeneity suggested by the renal studies. Some homozygotes have impaired intestinal absorption and plasma uptake (Morikawa *et al.* 1966; Goodman *et al.* 1967), whereas others show no defect in intestinal transport (Rosenberg *et al.* 1968; Scriver 1968; Tancredi *et al.* 1970).

The autosomal recessive inheritance of iminoglycinuria is established by the frequent occurrence of homozygous sibs, the identification of heterozygosity in parents and children of homozygotes, and the observation of parental consanguinity (Tada *et al.* 1965; Fraser *et al.* 1968).

References

Bank, H., Crispin, M., Ehrlich, D. and Szeinberg, A. (1972). Iminoglycinuria: a defect of renal tubular transport. *Israel J. Med. Sci.* **8**, 606–12.

Blehovà, B., Pazoutová, N., Hyánek, J. and Jirásek, J. (1973). Iminoglycinuria in a child in Czechoslovakia. *Humangenetic* **19**, 207–10.

DeVries, A., Kochwa, S., Lazebnik, J., Frank, M. and Djaldetti, M. (1957). Glycinuria, a hereditary disorder associated with nephrolithiasis. *Am. J. Med.* **23**, 408–15.

Fraser, G. R., Friedmann, A. I., Patton, V. M., Wade, D. N. and Woolf, L. I. (1968). Iminoglycinuria—a 'harmless' inborn error of metabolism? *Humangenetik* **6**, 362–7.

Goodman, S. I., McIntyre, C. A. Jr., and O'Brien, D. (1967). Impaired intestinal transport of proline in a patient with familial iminoaciduria. *J. Pediatr.* **71**, 246–9.

Greene, M. L., Lietman, P. S., Rosenberg, L. E. and Seegmiller, J. E. (1973). Familial hyperglycinuria: new defect in renal tubular transport of glycine and iminoacids. *Am. J. Med.* **54**, 265–71.

Hammerman, M. R. and Sacktor, B. (1977). Transport of amino acids in renal brush border membrane vesicles. Uptake of L-proline. *J. Biol. Chem.* **252**, 591–5.

Hoefnagel, D. and Pomeroy, J. (1968/1969). Cited as personal communications by Scriver, C. R. (1983). Familial iminoglycinuria, Chapter 81 in *The metabolic basis of inherited disease,* 5th edn., eds. Stanbury, J. B., Wyngaarden, J. B., Frederickson, D. S., Goldstein, J. L. and Brown, M. S. p. 1393. McGraw-Hill, New York.

Joseph, R., Ribierre, M., Job, J. C. and Girault, M. (1958). Maladie familiale associate des convulsions a début trés précoce, une hyperalbumino-rachie et une hyperaminoacidurie. *Arch. Fr. Pédiatr.* **15**, 374–87.

Käser, H., Cottier, P. and Antener, I. (1962). Glucoglycinuria, a new familial syndrome. *J. Pediatr.* **61**, 386–94.

Levy, H. L. (1973). Genetic screening. In *Advances in human genetics,* Vol. 4, eds. Harris, H. and Herschhorn, K. p. 1. Plenum, New York.

McNamara, P. D., Ozegovic, B., Pepe, L. M. and Segal, S. (1976). Proline and glycine uptake by renal brush border membrane vesicles. *Proc. Nat. Acad. Sci.* **73**, 4521–5.

——, Pepe, L. M. and Segal, S. (1979). Sodium gradient dependence of proline and glycine uptake in renal brush-border membrane vesicles. *Biochim. Biophys. Acta* **556**, 151–60.

Mardens, Y., Andriaenssens, K. and Van Sande, M. (1968). Glycinurie et imino-acidurie rénales associés à une oligophrenie: étude clinique et biochimique. *J. Neurol. Sci.* **6**, 333–46.

Morikawa, T., Tada, K., Ando, T., Yoshida, T., Yokoyama, Y. and Arakowa, T. (1966). Prolinuria: defect in intestinal absorption of imino acids and glycine. *Tohoku J. Exp. Med.* **90**, 105–16.

Procopis, P. G. and Turner, B. (1971). Iminoaciduria: a benign renal tubular defect. *J. Pediatr.* **79**, 419–22.

Rosenberg, L. E., Durant, J. L. and Elsas, L. J. II. (1968). Familial imino-glycinuria: an inborn error of renal tubular transport. *New Engl. J. Med.* **278**, 1407–13.

Scriver, C. R. (1968). Renal tubular transport of proline, hydroxyproline and glycine. III. Genetic basis for more than one mode of transport in human kidney. *J. Clin. Invest.* **47**, 823–35.

—— (1983). Familial iminoglycinuria, Chapter 81 in *The metabolic basis of inherited disease,* 5th edn. eds. Stanbury, J. B., Wyngaarden, J. B., Fredrickson, D. S., Goldstein, J. L. and Brown, M. S. p. 1793. McGraw-Hill, New York.

—— and Wilson, O. H. (1967). Amino acid transport in human kidney: evidence for genetic control of two types in human kidney. *Science* **155**, 1428–30.

——, Chesney, R. W. and McInnes, R. R. (1976). Genetic aspects of renal tubular transport: diversity and topology of carriers. *Kidney Int.* **9**, 149–71.

Slack, E. N., Lian, C.-C. T. and Sacktor, B. (1977). Transport of L-proline and D-glucose in luminal (brush border) and contraluminal (basal-lateral) membrane vesicles from the renal cortex. *Biochem. Biophys. Res. Commun.* **77**, 891–7.

Statter, M., Ben-Zvi, A., Shina, A., Schein, R. and Russell, A. (1976). Familial iminoglycinuria with normal intestinal absorption of glycine and imino acids in association with profound mental retardation, a possibel cerebral phenotype. *Helv. Paediatr. Acta* **31**, 173–82.

Tada, K., Morikawa, T., Ando, T., Yoshida, T. and Miragawa, A. (1965). Prolinuria: a new renal tubular defect in transport of proline and glycine. *Tohoku J. Exp. Med.* **87**, 133–43.

Tancredi, F., Guazzi, G. and Aurichio, S. (1970). Renal iminoglycinuria without intestinal malabsorption of glycine and imino acids. *J. Pediatr.* **76**, 386–92.
Whelan, D. T. and Scriver, C. R. (1968). Cystathioninuria and renal iminoglycinuria in a pedigree: a perspective on counselling. *New Engl. J. Med.* **278**, 924–7.

6.1.6. Histidinuria

Holmgren and colleagues (1974) described a patient with renal histidinuria, normal plasma histidine levels, and myoclonic seizures. A similar patient was reported by Kamoun and associates (1981). The possibility of genetic heterogeneity is raised by a family in which two mentally retarded brothers, aged 9 and 11 years, had renal histidinuria and impaired intestinal histidine absorption (Sabater *et al.* 1976). Parents showed impaired intestinal absorption of intermediate degree, thereby confirming autosomal recessive inheritance. It is not known whether the patients in the other two reports also had an intestinal absorption defect. This renal tubular disorder is to be distinguished from histidinaemia.

References

Holmgren, G., Hambraeus, L. and Chateau, P. (1974). Histidinemia and normo-histidinemic histidinuria. *Acta Paediatr. Scand.* **63**, 220–4.
Kamoun, P. P., Parvy, P., Cathelineau, L. and Meyer, B. (1981). Renal histidinuria. *J. Inher. Metab. Dis.* **4**, 217–19.
Sabater, J., Ferre, C., Puliol, M. and Maya, A. (1976). Histidinuria: a renal and intestinal histidine transport deficiency found in two mentally retarded children. *Clin. Genet.* **9**, 117–24.

6.1.7. Hartnup disease

This disease was first described by Charles Dent's group and takes its name from that of their family (Baron *et al.* 1956). The family comprised eight children of first-cousin parents. Four of the children were affected with a light-sensitive skin rash in which the skin becomes rough and reddened and in the more severe instances becomes typically pellagra like. The rash was exacerbated by infection and poor nutrition and the worst attacks were accompanied by a transient cerebellar ataxia. The older affected sibs were mentally retarded but subsequent reports have shown this to be an inconsistent feature and probably not specific. For example all of 12 children with Hartnup disease detected in a neonatal-screening programme in New South Wales and followed up for 8 years showed normal mental development (Wilcken *et al.* 1977). The light sensitivity results in symptoms appearing predominantly during the summer months and sometimes being totally absent in winter (Borrie and Lewis 1962).

Dent's group observed an aminoaciduria in their patients unlike anything observed hitherto. There was increased excretion of several neutral α-amino acids but not of the imino acids, nor of the basic or acidic amino acids. In addition there was excess indican and indolylacetic acid in the urine. Jepson (1956) demonstrated excretion of further indole derivatives. Milne and colleagues (1960) studied two of Dent's patients and confirmed that the aminoaciduria was renal in origin and found that this was a more constant abnormality than the indicanuria. They also demonstrated that intestinal absorption of tryptophan following an oral load was delayed and incomplete. The unabsorbed tryptophan was converted to indole and other products of bacterial tryptophan metabolism in the colon. They concluded that there is defective transport of tryptophan across the jejunal mucosa and the proximal renal tubule in Hartnup disease, and suggested that the attacks of cerebellar ataxia are due to indolic acid intoxication. Others have confirmed that the disorder is one of transport of a group of neutral amino acids, presumably sharing a common pathway, as in cystinuria. Scriver (1965) who also carried out further studies on a Hartnup family found that indole-3-pyruvic acid is normally absorbed from the gut and subsequently metabolized, unlike its α-amino analogue, in Hartnup disease, thereby confirming that the defect is one of transport rather than subsequent metabolism of tryptophan and other neutral amino acids. Shih and coworkers (1971) confirmed the defective intestinal transport of tryptophan, and of methionine, with a minimal reduction in transport of lysine and glycine, correlated with modest increases of these latter amino acids in urine.

The numerous reports of affected sibs and parental consanguinity from Dent's family leave no doubt that inheritance is autosomal recessive. There is some evidence for minor biochemical deviation in heterozygotes, at least in childhood, from the finding of modest increases in urinary tryptophan and indole derivatives, and in one case even skin sensitivity to sunlight, among the children of affected homozygotes (Pomeroy *et al.* 1968). The karyotype shows no abnormality (Lopez *et al.* 1969). Evidence for genetic heterogeneity comes from the observation of families with the urinary defect but either only partial impairment of intestinal transport (Seakins and Ersser 1967) or no such impairment (Srikantia *et al.* 1964).

The symptoms of Hartnup disease appear to be mainly attributable to the impaired intestinal absorption of tryptophan, which reduces the amount of this amino acid available for conversion to nicotinamide, and also results in the conversion of residual gut tryptophan to indole derivatives. Under conditions of good nutrition, as prevail in Australia and North America, expression is minimal. Estimates of the incidence of the disorder at birth vary between about 1 in 30 000 (Wilcken *et al.* 1977) in New South Wales and 1 in 15 000 (Levy *et al.* 1972) in Massachusetts.

References

Baron, D. N., Dent, C. E., Harris, H., Hart, E. W. and Jepson, J. B. (1956). Hereditary pellagra-like skin rash with temporary cerebellar ataxia, constant renal amino-aciduria and other bizarre biochemical features. *Lancet* **2**, 421–33.

Borrie, P. F. and Lewis, C. A. (1962). Hartnup disease. *Proc. R. Soc. Med.* **58**, 231–2.

Jepson, J. B. (1956). Indolylacetyl–glutamine and other indole metabolites in Hartnup disease. *Biochem. J.* **64**, 14p.

Levy, H. L., Madigan, P. M. and Shih, V. E. (1972). Massachusetts metabolic screening program. I. Technique and results of urine screening. *Pediatrics* **49**, 825–36.

Lopez, G. F., Velez, A. H. and Toro, G. G. (1969). Hartnup disease in two Colombian siblings. *Neurology* **19**, 71–6.

Milne, M. D., Crawford, M. A., Girao, C. B. and Loughridge, L. W. (1960). The metabolic disorder in Hartnup disease. *Quart. J. Med.* **29**, 407–21.

Pomeroy, I., Efron, M. L., Dayman, J. and Hoefnagel, B. (1968). Hartnup disorder in a New England family. *New Engl. J. Med.* **278**, 1214–16.

Scriver, C. R. (1965). Hartnup disease. A genetic modification of intestinal and renal transport of certain neutral alpha amino acids. *New Engl. J. Med.* **273**, 530–2.

Seakins, J. W. T. and Ersser, R. S. (1967). Effects of amino acid loads on a healthy infant with the biochemical features of Hartnup disease. *Arch. Dis. Child* **42**, 682–8.

Shih, V. E., Bixby, E. M., Alpers, D. H., Bartsocas, C. S. and Thier, S. O. (1971). Studies of intestinal transport defect in Hartnup disease. *Gastroenterology* **61**, 445–53.

Srikantia, S. G., Venkatachalam, P. S. and Reddy, V. (1964). Clinical and biochemical features of a case of Hartnup disease. *Br. Med. J.* **1**, 282–5.

Wilcken, B., Yu, J. S. and Brown, D. A. (1977). Natural history of Hartnup disease. *Arch. Dis. Child.* **52**, 38–40.

6.1.8. Renal tubular acidosis, type II, proximal or bicarbonate wasting type

Morris has proposed a classification of renal tubular acidosis into types I, II, III, and IV (Morris 1969; McSherry *et al.* 1972). These are discussed more fully in the next section as most forms, including the commonest, classic or type I, involve a defect of the distal tube. Type II is discussed here since in this form the lesion is in the proximal tubule. This type of renal tubular acidosis is associated with a reduction of reabsorption of bicarbonate, and to a less extent of potassium (Sebastian *et al.* 1971). It may occur as part of a Fanconi syndrome in a wide range of disorders including cystinosis, Wilson's disease, tyrosinaemia, hereditary fructose intolerance (Morris 1968), metachromatic leucodystrophy, Lowe's syndrome (Lamy *et al.* 1962), Leigh's syndrome, vitamin-D-deficient rickets, nephrotic syndrome, renal amyloidosis, chronic renal failure, myeloma, and intoxication including the administration of a carbonic anhydrase inhibitor. The genetically determined among those quoted are discussed elsewhere in this monograph.

Isolated proximal renal tubular acidosis may occur as a transient abnormality in infancy (Latner and Burnard 1950). This genetically determined form was more fully described in 1967 by Rodriguez-Soriano, Edelmann, and their associates. They described a syndrome of renal tubular acidosis occuring in boys in which they demonstrated a low bicarbonate threshold. This was associated with a low serum bicarbonate, and gave rise to a hyperchloraemicacidosis with an acid urine, as low as a pH of 5.0. They also showed that administration of acetazolamide further reduced reabsorption of bicarbonate. They interpreted these observations as being due to a depressed proximal tubular reabsorption of bicarbonate with either a lowered $T_{m_{HCO_3^-}}$ or a widened splay, and as not being due to any inhibitor of carbonic anhydrase. Apart from a possible slight glomerular hypercellularity they detected no histological changes (Rodriguez-Soriano *et al.* 1967a and b; Rodriguez-Soriano and Edelmann 1969).

Further families have been reported since and it has become clear that two forms exist, both apparently showing X-linked recessive inheritance. The first is the transient form already described, of which further instances have been reported by Edelmann (1970), and by Nash and coworkers (1972) in association with growth retardation. A form in which the bicarbonate wasting tubular acidosis persists into adult life with a consequent short stature has been described by Brenes and colleagues (1977). They observed nine members of a family to be· affected and suggested that the pattern of inheritance was autosomal dominant. However, there was no male-to-male transmission and there were three apparently unaffected gene transmitters. The pattern is at least as well explained on an X-linked basis. Winsnes and others (1979) reported two brothers with a severe persistent renal tubular acidosis and with bicarbonate reabsorption only about half that of normal. Associated abnormalities included both growth and mental retardation; nystagmus, cataract, and corneal opacities; enamel defects of the permanent teeth and increased red-cell osmotic resistance. Acetazolamide induced further reduction of bicarbonate reabsorption indicating the presence of carbonic anhydrase. The younger brother died at the age of $4\frac{1}{2}$ years. Histologically the renal tubule cells were swollen with vacuoles but the glomeruli appeared normal.

References

Brenes, L. G., Brenes, J. N. and Hernandez, M. M. (1977). Familial renal tubular acidosis: a distinct clinical entity. *Am. J. Med.* **63**, 244–52.

Edelmann, C. M. Jr. (1970). Cited by McKusick, V. A. (1978) in *Mendelian inheritance in man*, 5th edn. p. 796. Johns Hopkins University Press, Baltimore.

Lamy, M., Freza, J., Rey, J. and Larsen, C. (1962). Etude metabolique du syndrome de Lowe. *Rev. Fr. Étude. Clin. Biol.* **7**, 271–83.

Latner, A. L. and Burnard, E. D. (1950). Idiopathic hyperchloraemic renal acidosis of infants (nephrocalcinosis infantum): observations on the site and nature of the lesion. *Quart. J. Med.* **19**, 285–301.

McSherry, E., Sebastian, A. and Morris, R. C. Jr. (1972). Renal tubular acidosis in infants: the several kinds, including bicarbonate wasting, classic renal tubular acidosis. *J. Clin. Invest.* **51**, 499–514.

Morris, R. C. (1968). An experimental renal acidification defect in patients with hereditary fructase intolerance. II. Its distinction from classic renal acidification defect associated with the Fanconi syndrome of children with cystinosis. *J. Clin. Invest.* **47**, 1648–63.

—— (1969). Renal tubular acidosis. Mechanisms, classification and implications. *New Engl. J. Med.* **281**, 1405–13.

Nash, M. A., Torrado, A. D., Griefer, I., Spitzer, A. and Edelmann, C. M. (1972). Renal tubular acidosis in infants and children. *J. Pediatr.* **80**, 738–48.

Rodriguez-Soriano, J. and Edelmann, C. M. (1969). Renal tubular acidosis. *Ann. Rev. Med.* **20**, 363–82.

——, Boichis, H. and Edelmann, C. M. Jr. (1967a). Bicarbonate reabsorption and hydrogen ion excretion in children with renal tubular acidosis. *J. Pediatr.* **71**, 802–13.

——, ——, Stark, H. and Edelmann, C. M. Jr. (1967b). Proximal renal tubular acidosis. A defect in bicarbonate reabsorption with normal urinary acidification. *Pediatr. Res.* **1**, 81–98.

Sebastian, A., McSherry, E. and Morris, R. C. Jr. (1971). On the mechanism of renal potassium wasting in renal tubular acidosis associated with the Fanconi syndrome (type 2 RTA). *J. Clin. Invest.* **50**, 231–43.

Winsnes, A., Monn, E., Stokke, O. and Feyling, T. (1979). Congenital persistent proximal type renal tubular acidosis in two brothers. *Acta Paediatr. Scand.* **68**, 861–8.

6.1.9. Osteopetrosis with renal tubular acidosis (marble brain disease)

In 1972 three groups independently reported a familial form of osteopetrosis distinct from the better-known benign autosomal dominant and lethal autosomal recessive forms of the disease (Guibaud *et al.* 1972; Sly *et al.* 1972; Vainsel *et al.* 1972). The new type was associated with renal tubular acidosis, short stature, dull mentality, dental malocclusion, and optic nerve compression leading to visual impairment. Onset is typically at about 2 years of age with fractures, and there is a mild anaemia in infancy which improves with age. The disease is compatible with long survival. A full report of the family described by Sly and associates appeared 8 years later, by which time two of their three affected sisters had developed basal ganglion calcification and renal tubular acidosis, reported as type I (Whyte *et al.* 1980).

Also in 1980, Ohlsson and colleagues described three Saudi Arabian families with parental consanguinity, cerebral calcification and strikingly similar facies. They coined the name 'marble brain disease' for this disorder. They have subsequently shown that the cerebral calcification may be present even in childhood (Cumming and Ohlsson 1985), and have reported two further Saudi Arabian families with parental consanguinity in one of them (Ohlsson *et al.* 1986). Guibaud and colleagues' (1972) family, with two affected brothers, also involved parental consanguinity. A further family involved two Kuwaiti Bedouin sibs with basal ganglion calcification in one (Bourke *et al.* 1981).

A further study by Sly's group has demonstrated that activity of the soluble isozyme of carbonic anhydrase, carbonic anhydrase II, which is found in the cystosol of the proximal renal tubule cells and also in brain, erythrocytes and many other tissues, is absent in erythrocytes of their patients (Sly *et al.* 1983). On both high pressure liquid chromatography and fluorescein diacetate staining of starch gels of haemolysates for esterase activity the affected sisters showed no activity, whereas their parents and an unaffected sister showed about half-normal activities. Protein staining of the gels, and ouchterlony immunodiffusion plates using an antiserum to carbonic anhydrase II, showed complete absence of the enzyme protein in the haemolysates of the affected individuals, and on the gels reduced amounts of protein in the presumed carriers. By all of these methods carbonic anhydrase I was normal. The same group have recently confirmed these findings in 18 patients from 11 further families, and in their obligate heterozygote parents (Sly *et al.* 1985b). They have demonstrated a positive renal response to intravenous acetazolamide (Sly *et al.* 1985a). They have also described a simplified enzyme assay method based on selective inhibition of carbonic anhydrase I (Sundaram *et al.* 1986). A similar method has been described by Conroy and Maren (1985). Ohlsson's group have also demonstrated a 50 per cent reduction in carbonic anhydrase II activity in the father of one of their patients (Ohlsson *et al.* 1986).

Carbonic anhydrase II, which is known to be present in the cytosol of tubule cells, is believed to hydrate carbon dioxide to carbonic acid, which after dissociation into hydrogen and bicarbonate permits transport of the latter into the interstitial fluid or the peritubular capillary. This is not to be confused with the membrane-bound isozyme of carbonic anhydrase in the brush border of the proximal tubule cell, which catalyses the breakdown of luminal carbonic acid into water and carbon dioxide allowing the carbon dioxide to diffuse into the tubule cell to become available to the type II isozyme. The finding of a distal tubular, as well as a proximal, component of the tubular acidosis in these patients (Whyte *et al.* 1980; Bourke *et al.* 1981) may be a consequence of the more intense reaction of the distal tubules to an immunohistochemical stain for carbon anhydrase II than the proximal tubules (Spicer *et al.* 1982). Inheritance is almost certainly autosomal recessive.

References

Bourke, E., Delaney, V. B., Mosawi, M., Reavey, P. and Weston, M. (1981). Renal tubular acidosis and osteopetrosis in siblings. *Nephron* **28**, 268–72.

Conroy, C. W. and Maren, T. H. (1985). The determination of osteopetrotic phenotypes by selective inactivation of red cell carbonic anhydrase phenotypes. *Clin. Chim. Acta* **152**, 347–54.

Cumming, W. A. and Ohlsson, A. (1985). Intracranial calcification in children with osteopetrosis caused by carbonic anhydrase II deficiency. *Radiology* **157**, 325–7.

Guibaud, P., Larbre, F., Freycon, M. T. and Genoud, J. (1972). Osteopetrose et acidose renale tubulaire. Deux cas de cette association dans une fratrie. *Arch. Fr. Pédiatr.* **29**, 269–86.

Ohlsson, A., Stark, G. and Sakati, N. (1980). Marble brain disease: recessive osteopetrosis, renal tubular acidosis and cerebral calcification in three Saudi Arabian families. *Develop. Med. Child. Neurol.* **22**, 72–84.

——, Cumming, W. A., Paul, A. and Sly, W. S. (1986). Carbonic anhydrase II deficiency syndrome: recessive osteopetrosis with renal tubular acidosis and cerebral calcification. *Pediatrics* **77**, 371–81.

Sly, W. S., Lang, R., Avioli, L., Haddad, J., Lubowitz, H. and McAlister, W. (1972). Recessive osteopetrosis: a new clinical phenotype (abs.). *Am. J. Hum. Genet.* **24**, 34.

——, Hewett-Emmett, D., Whyte, M. P., Yu, Y-S. L. and Tashian, R. E. (1983). Carbonic anhydrase II deficiency identified as the primary defect in the autosomal recessive syndrome of osteopetrosis with renal tubular acidosis and cerebral calcification. *Proc. Nat. Acad. Sci.* **80**, 2752–6.

——, Whyte, M. P., Krupin, T. and Sundaram, V. (1985a). Positive renal response to intravenous acetazolamide in patients with carbonic anhydrase II deficiency. *Pediatr. Res.* **19**, 1033–6.

——, ——, Sundaram, V., Tashian, R. E., Hewett-Emmett, D., Guibaud, P., Vainsel, M., Baluarte, H. J., Gruskin, A., Al-Mosawi, M., Sakati, N. and

Ohlsson, A. (1985b). Carbonic anhydrase II deficiency in 12 families with the autosomal recessive syndrome of osteopetrosis with renal tubular acidosis and cerebral calcification. *New. Engl. J. Med.* **313**, 139–45.

Spicer, S. S., Sens, M. A. and Tashian, R. E. (1982). Imunocytochemical demonstration of carbonic anhydrase in human epithelial cells. *J. Histochem. Cytochem.* **30**, 864–73.

Sundaram, V., Rumbolo, P., Grubb, J., Strisciuglio, P. and Sly, W. S. (1986). Carbonic anhydrase II deficiency: diagnosis and carrier detection using differential enzyme inhibition and activation. *Am. J. Hum. Genet.* **38**, 125–36.

Vainsel, M., Fondu, P., Cadranel, S., Rocmans, C. L. and Gepts, W. (1972). Osteopetrosis associated with proximal and distal tubular acidosis. *Acta Paediatr. Scand.* **61**, 429–34.

Whyte, M. P., Murphy, W. A., Fallon, W. S., Teitelbaum, S. L., McAlister, W. H. and Avioli, L. V. (1980). Osteopetrosis, renal tubular acidosis and basal ganglia calcification in three sisters. *Am. J. Med.* **69**, 64–74.

6.1.10. Familial hypocalciuric hypercalcaemia (familial benign hypercalcaemia)

The clinical importance of this benign condition, first described in 1972 as familial benign hypercalcaemia (Foley *et al.* 1972), arises from the fact that it is frequently misdiagnosed as primary hyperparathyroidism, resulting in unnecessary and ineffective parathyroidectomy. Although hypercalcaemia is a feature of both disorders only familial hypocalciuric hypercalcaemia is usually familial or associated with low urinary calcium excretion as evidenced by a low, less than 0.01, calcium to creatinine clearance ratio (Marx *et al.* 1978, 1980).

The disorder has been defined in a series of papers by Marx and his colleagues who introduced the term familial hypocalciuric hyper-calcaemia. In a study of the families of 25 index patients with a diagnosis of primary parathyroid hyperplasia they identified two inherited disorders: type 1 multiple endocrine adenomatosis and the present disorder in two families (Marx *et al.* 1977). In a detailed study of these two families plus one further family they showed that there was increased tubular reabsorption of magnesium as well as calcium and that the resultant hypermagnesaemia closely correlated with the hyper-calcaemia (Marx *et al.* 1978, 1981). Marx (1980) reviewed 66 reported cases and showed that the age of onset of hypercalcaemia was less than 10 years, that peptic ulcer and renal stones were uncommon among affected individuals, but that fatigue, muscle weakness, pancreatitis, and chondrocalcinosis (Marx *et al.* 1980, 1981) were occasional complications. This group confirmed that the underlying defect is of increased tubular reabsorption of calcium, which is independent of parathormone (Attie *et al.* 1980), and that it is associated with increased urinary excretion of cyclic AMP, related to the glomerular filtration rate, in more than a third of patients (see also Heath and Purnell 1980).

Law and colleagues (1984) studied 32 adult patients from 12 families. They found normal levels of immunoreactive parathyroid hormone and of 25-hydroxy vitamin D but lower levels of 1,25-dihydroxy vitamin D in the serum or plasma of their patients than in normal controls or patients with hyperparathyroidism.

A curious, ill-understood affect of the disorder is that the newborn infants of affected parents may have a severe neonatal primary hyperparathyroidism (Marx *et al.* 1980, 1981, 1982). This effect is not due purely to maternal influence, as in the three families reported by Marx and coworkers (1982) it was the father who had familial hypocalciuric hypercalcaemia. In one of these three families the mother was also affected, and in each of them there were also children with hypocalciuric hypercalcaemia as well as those with severe neonatal primary hyperparathyroidism.

An autosomal dominant mode of inheritance was suggested by the earliest report in which there were 12 affected members of a family over four generations, but there was no male-to-male transmission (Foley *et al.* 1972). The several families studied by Marx and coworkers (Marx *et al.* 1978, 1980, 1981, 1982, 1985; Attie *et al.* 1980) confirm this hypothesis and demonstrate virtually full penetrance. Further large families consistent with autosomal dominance have been reported by Paterson and Gunn (1981) and Menko and colleagues (1983). For example, in the family reported by Menko's group there are five instances of male-to-male transmission and both affected and unaffected daughters of affected fathers. This group also confirm that the hypercalcaemia is entirely due to increased renal tubular reabsorption of calcium and that changes in phosphate transport are secondary to the increased filtered load of calcium. They were not able to confirm any alteration in urinary excretion of cyclic AMP so that the mechanism of increased reabsorption remains unknown; as does the site of the defect, proximal or distal tubular. Menko and colleagues (1984) have also reported a linkage study with negative results. The subject has been reviewed in a *Lancet* editorial in 1982. That there may be genetic heterogeneity is evidenced by the observation of Marx and colleagues (1985) of a family in which the hypercalcaemia in heterozygotes is milder than in their other families and intermittent, and in which neonatal severe primary hyperparathyroidism occurred in homozygotes. Homozygosity may also be the cause of neonatal severe primary hyperparathyroidism in at least some cases in other families. A curious family in which some members had benign hypercalcaemia and others had benign hypocalcaemia has been reported (Bannister *et al.* 1986).

References

Attie, M. F., Gill, J. R., Stock, J. L., Spiegel, A. M., Downs, R. W., Levine, M. A. and Marx, S. J. (1980). Parathyroid hormone (PTH) independent abnormality of renal tubular transport of calcium in familial hypocalciuric hypercalcaemia. *Clin. Res.* **28**, 384A (abs.).

Bannister, P., Sheridan, P., Dibble, J. and Payne, R. B. (1986). Benign hypercalcaemia and benign hypocalcaemia in the same family. *Ann. Intern. Med.* **105**, 217–19.

Foley, T. P., Harrison, H. C., Arnaud, C. D. and Harrison, H. E. (1972). Familial benign hypercalcaemia. *J. Pediatr.* **81**, 1060–7.

Heath, H. and Purnell, D. C. (1980). Urinary cyclic 3′,5′-adenosine monophosphate responses to exogenous and endogenous parathyroid hormone in familial hypercalcaemia and primary hyperparathyroidism. *J. Lab. Clin. Med.* **96**, 974–84.

Lancet (1982). Familial hypocalciuric hypercalcaemia. *Lancet* **1**, 488–9.

Law, W. M., Bollman, S., Kumar, R. and Heath, H. (1984). Vitamin D metabolism in familial benign hypercalcaemia (hypocalciuric hypercalcaemia) differs from that in primary hyperparathyroidism. *J. Clin. Endocrinol. Metab.* **58**, 744–7.

Marx, S. J. (1980). Familial hypocalciuric hypercalcaemia (editorial). *New Engl. J. Med.* **303**, 810–11.

——, Spiegel, A. M., Brown, E. M. and Aurbach, G. D. (1977). Family studies in patients with primary parathyroid hyperplasia. *Am. J. Med.* **62**, 698–706.

——, ——, ——, Koehler, J. O., Gardner, D. G., Brennan, M. F. and Aurbach, G. D. (1978). Divalent cation metabolism. Familial hypocalciuric hypercalcaemia versus typical primary hyperparathyroidism. *Am. J. Med.* **65**, 235–42.

——, Stock, J. L., Attie, M. F., Downs, R. W., Gardner, D. G., Brown, E. M., Spiegel, A. M., Doppman, J. L. and Brennan, M. F. (1980). Familial hypocalciuric hypercalcaemia: recognition among patients referred after unsuccessful parathyroid exploration. *Ann. Intern. Med.* **92**, 351–6.

——, Attie, M. F., Levine, M. A., Spiegel, A. M., Downs, R. W. and Lasker, R. D. (1981). The hypocalciuric or benign variant of familial hypercalcaemia: clinical and biochemical features in fifteen kindreds. *Medicine* **60**, 397–412.

——, ——, Spiegel, A. M., Levine, M. A., Lasker, R. D. and Fox, M. (1982). An association between neonatal severe hyperparathyroidism and familial hypocalciuric hypercalcaemia in three kindreds. *New Engl. J. Med.* **306**, 257–64.

——, Fraser, D. and Rapoport, A. (1965). Familial hypocalciuric hypercalcaemia: mild expression of the gene in heterozygote and severe expression in homozygotes. *Am. J. Med.* **78**, 15–22.

Menko, F. H., Bijvoet, O. L. M., Fronen, J. L. H. H., Sandler, L. M., Adami, S., O'Riordan, J. L. H. and Schopman, W. (1983). Familial benign hypercalcaemia. Study of a large family. *Quart. J. Med.* **52**, 120–40.

——, ——, Meera Khan, P., Nijenhuis, L. E., v. Loghem, E., Schreuder, I., Bernini, L. F., Pronk, J. C., Madan, K. and Went, L. N. (1984). Familial benign hypercalcaemia (FBH; McK. No. 14598, 1983): Linkage studies in a large Dutch family. *Hum. Genet.* **67**, 452–4.

Paterson, C. R. and Gunn, A. (1981). Familial benign hypercalcaemia. *Lancet* **2**, 61–3.

6.1.11. Hypokalaemic alkalosis hypomagnesaemia and renal proximal tubulopathy

A new syndrome, with similarities to Bartter's syndrome, has recently been described in three out of four sibs, two girls and a boy (Güllner *et al.* 1979a and b, 1981, 1983). The main clinical and biochemical features are growth retardation, a hypokalaemic alkalosis, hyperreninaemia, normal plasma aldosterone levels, increased urinary excretion of prostaglandin E_2, and normal blood pressure with resistance of blood pressure to angiotensin II. These features are all found in Bartter's syndrome which is associated with hyperplasia of the juxtaglomerular apparatus and a defect in chloride reabsorption in the loop of Henle. However, histopathology of renal biopsies of Güllner and coworkers' patients showed a normal appearance of the glomeruli and the juxtaglomerular apparatus, intense staining of the proximal renal tubular cells with methylene blue/basic fuchsin, and a marked hypertrophy of the proximal tubular basement membranes. On electron microscopy the tubular cells showed a dense cytoplasm with pyknotic nuclei and compact mitochondria. In addition chloride reabsorption in the thick ascending limb of the loop of Henle was shown to be normal, as was the distal delivery of proximal tubular solute.

The three affected sibs showed identical HLA-A and -B haplotypes, whereas an unaffected sib showed a complementary haplotype. On the reasonable assumption of autosomal recessive inheritance this finding gave a maximum lod score of 1.322 with odds of 21:1 in favour of linkage of the gene for the disease to the gene complex for the HLA system on chromosome 6.

Whether or not the basic defect in this disorder is a proximal tubular one remains uncertain. Histological changes were confirmed to the proximal tubule but the delivery of solute to the distal nephron was normal and potassium reabsorption in the proximal tubule is known to be linked with that for sodium, which was not disturbed. The authors suggest that there may be an increased secretion of potassium by the distal convoluted tubule and collecting duct.

It is possible, but by no means certain, that the two brothers reported earlier by Potter and colleagues (1974) had the same disorder.

References

Güllner, H.-G., Gill, J. R., Bartter, F. C., Chan, J. C. M. and Dickman, P. S. (1979a). A familial disorder with hypokalemic alkalosis, hyperreninemia, aldosteronism, high urinary prostaglandins and normal blood pressure that is not 'Bartter's syndrome'. *Trans. Assoc. Am. Phys.* **92**, 175–88.

——, Terasaki, P. I., Bartter, F. C., Gill, J. R. and Tiwari, J. (1979b). Linkage between histocompatibility antigens (HLA) and familial hypokalemia. Quoted by McKusick, V. A. (1983) in *Mendelian inheritance in man,* 6th edn. p. 778. Johns Hopkins University Press, Baltimore.

——, Bartter, F. C., Gill, J. R., Dickman, P. S., Wilson, C. B. and Tiwari, J. L. (1983). A sibship with hypokalemic alkalosis and renal proximal tubulopathy. *Arch. Intern. Med.* **143**, 1534–40.

——, Gill, J. R. and Bartter, F. C. (1981). Correction of hypokalemia by magnesium repletion in familial hypokalemic alkalosis with tubulopathy. *Am. J. Med.* **71**, 578–82.

Potter, W. Z., Trygstad, C. W., Helmer, O. M., Nance, W. E. and Judson, W. E. (1974). Familial hypokalemia associated with renal interstitial fibrosis. *Am. J. Med.* **57**, 971–77.

6.1.12. Pseudohypoparathyroidism (Albright's hereditary osteodystrophy)

This disorder was first described by Albright and his associates (Albright *et al.* 1942, 1952; Elrich *et al.* 1950). The disorder is a familial one resembling true hypoparathyroidism but with normal or hyperplastic parathyroid glands. Clinically patients are typically round faced with a depressed nasal bridge, and are of short stature with skeletal deformities, including brachydactyly with short metacarpals that may lead to the mis-diagnosis of Turner's syndrome (Miller *et al.* 1965) or of type E brachy-dactyly in which there are similar dermatoglyphic patterns (Forbes 1964). There may also be vertebral disc calcification or dislocation of the hips (Kelly 1968), or even rickets or the bone changes of hyperpara-thyroidism (McArthur *et al.* 1979; Kidd *et al.* 1980). Subcutaneous calcification or even bone formation, and more seriously basal ganglia calcification (Palubinskas and Davies 1959), may also occur. The latter may be the basis of the epileptic convulsions which occur in 60 per cent of patients. Mental retardation is a common feature (Farfel and Friedman 1986), as is also an olfactory defect (Henkin 1968). Psychotic symptoms or tetany may be features associated with hypocalcaemia. Bronsky and coworkers (1958) found a 35 per cent incidence of cataracts of the ocular lenses. Several authors have reviewed the skeletal and radiological changes (Arnstein *et al.* 1966; Steinbach and Young 1966; Spranger 1969). In addition to short phalanges, metacarpals, and metatarsals the skeletal changes include curvature of the radius (Werder *et al.* 1975) and cubitus valgus, coxa vara and valga and genu varum or valgum. Enamel hypoplasia and other dental defects are also common.

In classical pseudohypoparathyroidism there is hypocalcaemia and hyperphosphataemia. Serum levels of parathyroid hormone are typically elevated rather than low in patients not on vitamin D therapy (Lee *et al.*

1968; Chase *et al.* 1969; Drezner *et al.* 1976). Growth hormone secretion and sulphation factor activity are normal (Urdanivia *et al.* 1975). Hypothyroidism has recently been reported as an unusual presentation in sibs (Levine *et al.* 1985).

In Albright's second paper (1952) on the disorder, he described a patient with all the physical signs but with normal serum calcium and phosphate. He termed this form of the disease pseudo-pseudohypoparathyroidism. It has since been observed that both hypocalcaemic and normocalcaemic patients may occur in the same family (Mann *et al.* 1962; Chase *et al.* 1969; Williams *et al.* 1977), and that the two forms may even be observed in the same patient at different stages of the disease (Mautalen *et al.* 1967; Logan and Miller 1979).

The underlying defect in pseudohypoparathyroidism appears to be a target organ resistance to parathormone. Evidence for the mechanism of this resistance came from the observation of Chase and Aurbach that the normal response to parathormone administration of increased urinary excretion of cAMP was absent in patients with this disease (Chase and Aurbach 1968; Chase *et al.* 1969). However, they observed that in patients with pseudo-pseudohypoparathyroidism the cyclic AMP excretory response to parathormone was normal and that there was a high basal excretion of cAMP. They also demonstrated that parathormone and vasopressin act separately on adenyl cyclase in the cortex and medulla respectively, suggesting that in pseudohypoparathyroidism there may be a defective parathormone receptor in the renal tubule. This end-organ resistance results in a failure of renal phosphate excretion in response to parathormone with consequent phosphate retention (Coulson and Moses 1975; Nagant de Deuxchaisnes and Krane 1978). As a secondary effect there is renal calcium loss, malabsorption of calcium, and impaired flow of calcium from bone to the extracellular fluid. The main site of hormone-dependent phosphate reabsorption is the proximal tubule, and there is evidence that distal tubular calcium reabsorption is normal (Nagant de Deuxchaisnes and Krane 1978).

More recent studies have indicated heterogeneity in the mechanism of parathormone resistance, with at least three types being recognized: types 1A and 1B, and type 2. In type 1 there is a normal phosphate diuresis on administration of dibutyryl cAMP indicating a normal renal response to cyclic AMP (Bell *et al.* 1972). The synthesis of cAMP is catalysed by adenylate cyclase, the activation of which is in turn stimulated by parathormone binding to a receptor in the proximal tubular cell membrane. This activation involves a complex hormone–receptor–enzyme system which incorporates a nucleotide regulatory protein, N protein, in an intermediary step (Maguire *et al.* 1977). Studies on plasma membrane from the renal cortex of patients with pseudohypoparathyroidism type 1 have produced evidence for defective action of this N protein. There was no evidence for any defect of either the receptor or cyclase ends of the chain (Marcus *et al.* 1971; Drezner and Burch 1978a and b). In those patients designated type 1A, who show the full Albright syndrome, there is 50 per cent reduction of N protein activity in red cells (Farfel and Bourne 1980; Farfel *et al.* 1980, 1981; Levine *et al.* 1980; Akita *et al.* 1985). Type 1B patients in contrast have normal N protein activity, and usually show normal somatic features, but the nature of their defect remains obscure. Recently Bourne and colleagues (1981) have confirmed these observations for type 1A patients in fibroblast membranes. The presumption must be that the N protein defect of red-cell and fibroblast membranes is also the defect determining resistance of adenylate cyclase complex to parathormone in the kidney. There is some evidence that the action of other hormones may also be affected: excessive thyrotrophin response to thyrotrophin-releasing hormone (Werder *et al.* 1975), and decreased prolactin secretion in response to thyrotrophin-releasing hormone (Carlson *et al.* 1977). Despite these new insights into the underlying defect in type 1 pseudohypoparathyroidism the mechanism of hypocalcaemia is not fully understood. One factor may be an associated resistance to parathormone of renal $25(OH)_D-1\alpha$-hydroxylase. Evidence supporting this hypothesis comes from the observation of reduced basal levels of serum $1,25(OH)_2$ vitamin D in type 1 patients and a failure of administered parathormone to raise the level, as it does in normal subjects (Drezner *et al.* 1976; Metz *et al.* 1977; Aksnes and Aarskog 1980; Lambert *et al.* 1980; Mason *et al.* 1980).

Type 2 pseudohypoparathyroidism was first defined in an infant with retarded stature, mental subnormality, and the typical biochemical findings of pseudohypoparathyroidism. However, urinary cAMP excretion was raised and increased further in a normal manner after parathormone injection without a concommitant increase in phosphate excretion. This excluded classical pseudohypoparathyroidism (Drezner *et al.* 1973). Drezner and colleagues postulated that the parathormone–receptor–adenyl cyclase complex was normal in the red-cell membrane but that intracellular cAMP hormone-related activity in the kidney was defective. They termed this form of the disease type 2. Several reports of similar cases have been subsequently published, such as those of Rodriguez and colleagues (1974), Stogmann and Fischer (1975), and Matsuda and others (1979). These patients generally lack the skeletal anomalies of typical Albright's hereditary osteodystrophy seen in type 1, and have been consistently sporadic in occurrence. As would be expected N protein activity is normal (Farfel *et al.* 1980).

The genetic analysis of type 1 pseudohypoparathyroidism has

presented considerable problems. It was for a long time regarded as being an X-linked dominant disorder (Mann *et al.* 1962; Aurbach and Potts 1964) since the female:male ratio of cases is about 2:1 and male-to-male transmission was not seen in most families. However, the severity of the disorder in affected females is as severe as in affected males, contrary to expectation for an X-linked dominant disorder. A more serious objection to X linkage is the observation of unaffected daughters of affected males (Weinberg and Stone 1971; Levine *et al.* 1981). Drezner and Neelon (1983) have analysed the published adequate pedigrees and have found that this ratio is confirmed, 50 affected females to 32 affected males, but that among the affected sibs of index cases there were 15 males to 9 females. This suggests that affected females are more likely to be diagnosed than males and certainly excludes X-linked inheritance.

A number of individual pedigrees have suggested other modes of inheritance than X linkage. As early as 1963 Minozzi and colleagues suggested autosomal dominance in their family, and Hermans and others (1964) reported a family in which there was definite male-to-male transmission. Similar families indicative of autosomal dominance have been reported by Goeminne (1965) and by Weinberg and Stone (1971). Drezner and Neelon's (1983) analysis of published pedigrees gives a ratio of affected to unaffected sibs of 22:20, which is consistent with autosomal dominant inheritance, and if X linkage is excluded the frequent occurrence of the disease in a parent and child further supports this mode of inheritance. The finding of about half the normal levels of N protein in affected individuals for type 1A suggests autosomal dominance for that type. This is confirmed by the observations of Van Dop and coworkers (1984) of reduced red-cell N protein activity in a man with typical type Ia pseudohypoparathyroidism, and in his son and daughter who both had partial expression of the disorder.

Nevertheless several families with normal parents and more than one affected offspring have suggested autosomal recessive inheritance (Fanconi *et al.* 1964; Spranger and Rohwedder 1965; Cederbaum and Lippe 1973; Farfel *et al.* 1981). Farfel and colleagues reinvestigated the family of Cederbaum and Lippe. These observations suggest genetic heterogeneity. An alternative possibility is that proposed by Johnson (1980) who suggests that inheritance is autosomal with both types of homozygote being normal but the heterozygote being abnormal due to interaction between the two alleles.

There are as yet insufficient fully investigated families to resolve these different possibilities, nor does the recent report of the disease in both of a pair of 19-year-old identical twin girls (Janke 1985) indicate the mode of inheritance.

References

Akita, Y., Saito, T., Yajima, Y. and Sakuma, S. (1985). The stimulatory and inhibitory guanine nucleotide-binding proteins of adenylate cyclase in erthrocytes from patients with pseudohypoparathyroidism type I. *J. Clin. Endocrinol. Metab.* **61**, 1012–17.

Aksnes, L. and Aarskog, D. (1980). Effect of parathyroid hormone on 1,25-dihydroxyvitamin D formation in type 1 pseudohypoparathyroidism. *J. Clin. Endocrinol. Metab.* **51**, 1223–6.

Albright, F., Burnett, C. H., Smith, P. H., Parson, W. (1942). Pseudohypoparathyroidism—an example of the 'Seabright–Bantam syndrome': report of three cases. *Endocrinology* **30**, 922–32.

——, Forbes, A. P. and Henneman, P. H. (1952). Pseudo-pseudohypoparathyroidism. *Trans. Assoc. Am. Physicians* **65**, 337–50.

Arnstein, A. R., Frame, B., Frost, H. M. and Block, M. A. (1966). Albright's hereditary osteodystrophy: report of a family with studies of bone remodelling. *Ann. Intern. Med.* **64**, 996–1008.

Aurbach, G. D. and Potts, J. T. Jr. (1964). The parathyroids. In *Advances in metabolic disorders*, eds. Levine, R. and Luft, R. Vol. 1. p. 45. Academic Press, New York.

Bell, N. H., Avery, S., Sinha, T., Clark, C. M., Allen, D. O. and Johnston, C. (1972). Effects of dibutyryl cyclic adenosine 3′,5′-monophosphate and parathyroid extract on calcium and phosphorus metabolism in hypoparathyroidism and pseudohypoparathyroidism. *J. Clin. Invest.* **51**, 816–23.

Bourne, H. R., Kaslow, H. R., Brickman, A. S. and Farfel, Z. (1981). Fibroblast defect in pseudohypoparathyroidism, type 1: reduced activity of receptor cyclase coupling protein. *J. Clin. Endocrinol. Metab.* **53**, 636–40.

Bronsky, D., Kushner, D. S., Dubin, A. and Snapper, I. (1958). Idiopathic hypoparathyroidism and pseudohypoparathyroidism: case reports and review of the literature. *Medicine (Baltimore)*, **37**, 317–52.

Carlson, H. E., Brickman, A. S. and Bottazzo, G. F. (1977). Prolactin deficiency in pseudohypoparathyroidism. *New Engl. J. Med.* **296**, 140–4.

Cederbaum, S. D. and Lippe, B. M. (1973). Probable autosomal recessive inheritance in a family with Albright's hereditary osteodystrophy and evaluation of the genetics of the disorder. *Am. J. Hum. Genet.* **25**, 638–45.

Chase, L. R. and Aurbach, G. D. (1968). Renal adenyl cyclase: anatomically separate sites for parathyroid hormone and vasopressin. *Science* **159**, 545–7.

——, Melson, G. L. and Aurbach, (1969). Pseudohypoparathyroidism: defective excretion of 3′-5′-AMP in response to parathyroid hormone. *J. Clin. Invest.* **48**, 1832–44.

Coulson, R. and Moses, A. M. (1975). Effect of chlorpropamide on renal response to parathyroid hormone in normal subjects and in patients with hypoparathyroidism and pseudohypoparathyroidism. *J. Pharmacol. Exp. Ther.* **194**, 603–13.

Drezner, M. K. and Burch, W. M. Jr. (1978a). Pseudohypoparathyroidism (PsH): a disorder due to an abnormal adenylate cyclase enzyme (abs.). *Clin. Res.* **26**, 413A.

—— and —— (1978b). Altered activity of the nucleotide regulatory site in the parathyroid hormone-sensitive adenylate cyclase from the renal cortex of a patient with pseudohypoparathyroidism *J. Clin. Invest.* **62**, 1222–7.

—— and Neelon, F. A. (1983). Pseudohypoparathyroidism. Chapter 69 in *The metabolic basis of inherited disease,* 5th edn. eds. Stanbury, J. B., Wyngaarden, J. B., Frederickson, D. S., Goldstein, J. L. and Brown, M. S. pp. 1508–27. McGraw-Hill, New York.

——, —— and Lebovitz, H. E. (1973). Pseudohypoparathyroidism type II: a possible defect in the reception of the cyclic AMP signal. *New Engl. J. Med.* **289**, 1056–60.

——, ——, Haussler, M., McPherson, H. T. and Lebovitz, H. E. (1976). 1,25-dihydro-cholecalciferol deficiency: the probable cause of hypocalcemia and metabolic bone disease in pseudohypoparathyroidism. *J. Clin. Endocrinol.* **42**, 621–8.

Elrich, H., Albright, F., Bartter, F. C., Forbes, A. P. and Reeves, J. D. (1950). Further studies on pseudohypoparathyroidism: report of four new cases. *Acta Endocrinol.* **5**, 199–225.

Fanconi, A., Heinrich, H. G. and Prader, A. (1964). Klinischer und biochemischer Hypoparathyreoidismus mit radiologischem Hyperparathyriodismus. *Helv. Paediatr. Acta* **19**, 181–206.

Farfel, Z. and Bourne, H. R. (1980). Deficient activity of receptor-cyclase coupling protein in platelets of patients with pseudohypoparathyroidism. *J. Clin. Endocrinol. Metab.* **51**, 1202–4.

—— and Friedman, F. (1986). Mental deficiency in pseudohypoparathyroidism type I is associated with Ns-protein deficiency. *Ann. Intern. Med.* **105**, 197–9.

——, Brickman, A. S., Kaslow, H. R., Brothers, V. M. and Bourne, H. R. (1980). Defect of receptor-cyclase coupling protein in pseudohypoparathyroidism. *New Engl. J. Med.* **303**, 237–42.

——, Brothers, V. M., Brickman, A. S., Conte, F., Neer, R. and Bourne, H. R. (1981). Pseudohypoparathyroidism: inheritance of deficient receptor-cyclase coupling activity. *Proc. Nat. Acad. Sci.* **78**, 3098–102.

Forbes, A. P. (1964). Fingerprints and palm prints (dermatoglyphics) and palmar flexion creases in gonadal dysgenesis, pseudohypoparathyroidism and Klinefelter's syndrome. *New Engl. J. Med.* **270**, 1268–77.

Goeminne, L. (1965). Albright's hereditary poly-osteochondrodystrophy (pseudo-pseudo-hypoparathyroidism with diabetes, hypertension, artentis and polyarthrosis). *Acta Genet. Med. Gemollol.* **14**, 226–81.

Henkin, R. I. (1968). Impairment of olfaction and of the tastes of sour and bitter in pseudohypoparathyroidism. *J. Clin. Endocrinol.* **28**, 624–8.

Hermans, P. E., Gorman, C. A., Martin, W. J. and Kelly, P. J. (1964). Pseudopseudohypoparathyroidism (Albright's hereditary osteodystrophy). A family study. *Mayo Clin. Proc.* **39**, 81–91.

Janke, P. G. (1985). A case of pseudohypoparathyroidism in identical twins. *Br. Med. J.* **290**, 1628.

Johnson, W. G. (1980). Metabolic interference and the +− heterozygote. A hypothetical form of single inheritance which is neither dominant nor recessive. *Am. J. Hum. Genet.* **32**, 374–86.

Kelly, J. J. (1968). Albright's hereditary osteodystrophy associated with disc calcification and bilateral dislocation of the hips. *Br. J. Clin. Pract.* **22**, 399–403.

Kidd, G. S., Schaaf, M., Adler, R. A., Lassman, M. N. and Wray, H. L. (1980).

Skeletal responsiveness in pseudohypoparathyroidism: a spectrum of clinical disease. *Am. J. Med.* **68**, 772–81.

Lambert, P. W., Hollis, B. W., Bell, N. H. and Epstein, S. (1980). Demonstration of a lack of change in serum 1α,25-dihydroxy vitamin D in response to parathyroid extract in pseudohypoparathyroidism. *J. Clin. Invest.* **66**, 782–91.

Lee, J. B., Tashjian, A. H. Jr., Streeto, J. M. and Frantz, A. G. (1968). Familial pseudohypoparathyroidism. Role of parathyroid hormone and thyrocalcitonin. *New Engl. J. Med.* **279**, 1179–84.

Levine, M. A., Downs, R. W., Singer, M., Marx, S. J., Aurbach, G. D. and Spiegel, A. M. (1980). Deficient activity of guanine nucleotide regulatory protein in erythrocytes from patients with pseudohypoparathyroidism. *Biochem. Biophys. Res. Commun.* **94**, 1319–24.

——, ——, Marx, S. J., Lasker, R. D., Aurbach, G. D. and Spiegel, A. M. (1981) Clinical and biochemical features of pseudohypoparathyroidism. *Proc. VI Parathyroid Conf. Excerpta Medica*, pp. 95–101. Elsevier, Amsterdam.

——, Jap, T.-S. and Hung, W. (1985). Infantile hypothyroidism in two sibs: an unusual presentation of pseudohypoparathyroidism type Ia. *J. Pediatr.* **107**, 919–22.

Logan, K. R. and Miller, J. H. D. (1979). Pseudo-pseudohypoparathyroidism developing pseudohypoparathyroidism. *Irish J. Med. Sci.* **148**, 194.

McArthur, R. G., Hayles, A. B. and Lambert, P. W. (1979). Albright's syndrome with rickets. *Mayo Clin. Proc.* **54**, 313–20.

Maguire, M. E., Ross, E. M. and Gilman, A. G. (1977). Beta-adrenergic receptor: ligand binding properties and the interaction with adenyl cyclase. *Adv. Cycl. Nuc. Res.* **8**, 1–83.

Mann, J. B., Alterman, S. and Hills, A. G. (1962). Albright's hereditary osteodystrophy comprising pseudohypoparathyroidism and pseudo-pseudohypoparathyroidism, with a report of two cases representing the complete syndrome occurring in two successive generations. *Ann. Intern. Med.* **56**, 315–42.

Marcus, R., Wilber, J. F. and Aurbach, G. D. (1971). Parathyroid hormone-sensitive adenyl cyclase from the renal cortex of a patient with pseudohypoparathyroidism. *J. Clin. Endocrinol.* **33**, 537–41.

Mason, R. S., Lissner, D. and Posen, S. (1980). Parathyroid hormone effect on 1,25-dihydroxy vitamin D in hypoparathyroidism. *Ann. Intern. Med.* **92**, 260.

Matsuda, I., Takekoshi, Y., Tanaka, M., Matsuura, N., Nagai, B. and Seino, Y. (1979). Pseudohypoparathyroidism type II and anticonvulsant rickets. *Eur. J. Pediatr.* **132**, 303–8.

Mautalen, C. A., Dymling, J.-F. and Horwith, M. (1967). Pseudohypoparathyroidism 1942–1966. A negative progress report. *Am. J. Med.* **42**, 977–85.

Metz, S. A., Baylink, D. J., Hughes, M. R., Haussler, M. R. and Robertson, R. P. (1977). Selective deficiency of 1,25-dihydrocholecalciferol: a cause of isolated skeletal resistance to parathyroid hormone. *New Engl. J. Med.* **297**, 1084–90.

Miller, J. Q., Rostafinski, M. J. and Hyde, M. S. (1965). Gonadal dysgenesis and brachymetacarpal dwarfism (pseudo-pseudohypoparathyroidism). *Arch. Intern. Med.* **116**, 940–3.

Minozzi, M., Faggiano, M., Bianio, A., Brizzi, G. and Coligianni, A. (1963). Su un caso di osteodistrofia ereditaria de Albright varieta normocalcemia con documentata transmissione da maschio a maschio. *Folio Endocrinol. (Roma)* **16**, 166–88.

Nagant de Deuxchaisnes, C. and Krane, S. M. (1978). Hypoparathyroidism. In *Metabolic bone disease*, eds. Avioli, L. V. and Krane, S. M. p. 218. Academic Press, New York.

Palubinskas, A. J. and Davies, H. (1959). Calcification of the basal ganglia of the brain. *Am. J. Roentgenol.* **82**, 806–22.

Rodriguez, H. J., Villarreal, H. Jr., Klahr, S. and Slatopolsky, E. (1974). Pseudo-hypoparathyroidism type II: restoration of normal renal responsiveness to parathyroid hormone by calcium administration. *J. Clin. Endocrinol.* **39**, 693–701.

Spranger, J. W. (1969). Skeletal dysplasias and the eye: Albright's hereditary osteodystrophy. *Birth Defects Orig. Art. Series No. 4*, 122–8.

—— and Rohwedder, J. (1965). Zur Genetik der Osteodystrophia hereditaria Albright. *Med. Welt.* **41**, 2308–12.

Steinbach, H. L. and Young, D. A. (1966). The roentgen appearance of pseudo-hypoparathyroidism and pseudo-pseudohypoparathyroidism. *Am. J. Roentgenol. Radium. Ther. Nucl. Med.* **97**, 49–66.

Stogmann, W. and Fischer, J. A. (1975). Pseudohypoparathyroidism: disappearance of the resistance to parathyroid extract during treatment with vitamin D. *Am. J. Med.* **59**, 140–4.

Urdanivia, E., Mataverde, A. and Cohen, M. P. (1975). Growth hormone secretion and sulfation factor activity in pseudohypoparathyroidism. *J. Lab. Clin. Med.* **86**, 772–6.

Van Dop, C., Bourne, H. R. and Neer, R. M. (1984). Father to son transmission of decreased Ns activity in pseudohypoparathyroidism type Ia. *J. Clin. Endocrinol. Metab.* **59**, 825–8.

Weinberg, A. G. and Stone, R. T. (1971). Autosomal dominant inheritance in Albright's hereditary osteodystrophy. *J. Pediatr.* **79**, 996–9.

Werder, E. A., Illig, R., Bernaconi, S., Kind, H., Prader, A., Fischer, J. A. and Fanconi, A. (1975). Excessive thyrotropin response to thyrotropin-releasing hormone in pseudohypoparathyroidism. *Pediatr. Res.* **9**, 12–16.

Williams, A. J., Wilkinson, J. L. and Taylor, W. H. (1977). Pseudohypoparathyroidism: variable manifestations within a family. *Arch. Dis. Child.* **52**, 798–800.

6.1.13. Biliary malformation with renal tubular insufficiency

There was a report in 1973 of two brothers, with second-cousin parents, both affected by a syndrome leading to infantile death. They had biliary hyperplasia and a generalized renal tubular failure with non-specific aminoaciduria, proteinuria, glycosuria, and metabolic acidosis. It is likely that both proximal and distal tubules were involved (Lutz-Richner and Landolt 1973). A second pair of brothers, also born to second-cousin parents, has appeared recently (Mikati *et al.* 1984). The latter group emphasize the association of odd facies, club foot and hypotonia in their own and in Lutz–Richner and Landolt's cases. Although they observed occasional calcification of distal tubules histologically they regard the defect as a proximal tubular one. These two reports leave little doubt that this is an autosomal recessive disorder.

References

Lutz-Richner, A. R. and Landolt, R. F. (1973). Familiaere Gallengang miss-bildungen mit tubularer Niereninsuffizienz. *Helv. Paediatr. Acta* **28**, 1–12.
Mikati, M. A., Barakat, A. Y., Sulh, H. B. and Der Kaloustian, V. M. (1984). Renal tubular insufficiency cholestatic jaundice, and multiple congenital anomalies—a new multisystem syndrome. *Helv. Paediatr. Acta* **39**, 463–71.

6.1.14. Arthrogryposis multiplex congenita with renal and hepatic abnormality

The disorder described by Nezeloff and colleagues (1979) is probably distinct from biliary malformation with renal tubular insufficiency. Nezeloff and colleagues described a family in which four brothers out of a family of seven of North African descent had arthrogryposis multiplex congenita with jaundice and renal dysfunction. Death occurred at 2 months, 12 days, and 42 weeks. At autopsy there was rarefaction of the anterior horns of the spinal cord, pigmentary deposits in the liver, and renal tubular degeneration with nephrocalcinosis.

In their mother's family eight other males had died at birth or in early infancy, suggesting that this disorder is probably one with X-linked recessive inheritance.

Reference

Nezeloff, C., Dupart, M. C., Jaubert, F. and Eliachar, E. (1979). A lethal familial syndrome associating arthrogryposis multiplex congenita, renal dysfunction, and a cholestatic and pigmentary liver disease. *J. Pediatr.* **94**, 258–80.

6.2. DISTAL TUBULAR DISEASES

6.2.1. Renal (or nephrogenic) diabetes insipidus (hereditary form)

Renal diabetes insipidus can occur secondary to intoxication, systemic disease or urinary tract obstruction. We are here concerned solely with the familial form.

Familial diabetes insipidus or 'water babies' have been recognized since the 19th century (LaCombe 1841; Weil 1884; McIlraith 1892). McIlraith reported severely affected males, with extreme thirst, in three generations of a family and slightly affected females who transmitted the disorder to their children. Neither McIlraith, nor deLange (1935) who reported a four-generation family, observed male-to-male transmission. DeLange distinguished the disorder from pituitary diabetes insipidus through the observation that injection of posterior pituitary lobe extract did not reduce the urine volume nor increase the urinary specific gravity in his patients. He also observed that the male patients may or may not be mentally retarded.

The clinical picture was defined in the 1940s with onset, shortly after birth, of polyuria and polydipsia not responding to pitressin, and if free availability of fluid is withheld, as in the non-breast-fed baby, this may lead to dehydration with fever, vomiting, failure to thrive, and convulsions (Forssman 1942, 1945; Waring *et al.* 1945; Williams and Henry 1947; Dancis *et al.* 1948). All of these workers recognized the insensitivity of this form of diabetes insipidus to pitressin. Forssman (1945) noted that affected adults may have daily urine volumes in excess of four litres and urinary specific gravity after water deprivation of no more than 1.003 to 1.008. Like McIlraith he recognized partial defects in carrier females with excess thirst and nocturnal water consumption. Williams and Henry introduced the term nephrogenic diabetes insipidus. Forssman, Williams and Henry, and Dancis and colleagues all confirmed McIlraith's observation that affected males may or may not be mentally retarded. Dancis and colleagues observed normal plasma levels of vasopressin on bioassay. The mental defect observed in some patients is due to organic brain damage secondary to the hypernatraemia associated with early dehydration (Reuss and Rosenthal 1963), and does not develop if severe dehydration is prevented. Another more recently recognized feature is radiological evidence of urinary tract dilatation, even to the extent of hydronephrosis and hydroureter (Ten Bensel and Peters 1970). It is postulated that this may be due to urinary flow rates exceeding the normal emptying capacity of the bladder (Shapiro *et al.* 1978).

The basic defect is still not fully understood. Morphologically Abelson (1968) reported an abnormal mitrochondrial structure throughout the nephron on electron microscopy, and on microdissection the proximal convoluted tubule was found to measure only about half the length observed in controls (Darmady *et al.* 1964). The morphological observations are difficult to reconcile with the physiological abnormalities that have been repeatedly observed. In particular the observation of short proximal tubules is based on only two cases with the range of measured lengths overlapping those in controls. DeLange's observation of pitressin resistance, which affects the distal convoluted tubule, thick ascending limb of Henle's loop, and the collecting ducts, remains the principle observed physiological defect. It has been confirmed by numerous authors (Forssman 1942, 1945; Waring *et al.* 1945; Williams and Henry

1947; Dancis *et al.* 1948; Crawford and Kennedy 1959; Robinson and Kaplan 1960). Since Dancis and coworkers' observation of normal plasma vasopressin levels on bioassay others have confirmed normal or even increased levels by both sensitive radioimmunoassay (Robertson 1974) and bioassay (Andreoli and Schafer 1978). Robertson (1974) demonstrated that in both normal subjects and patients with nephrogenic diabetes insipidus serum osmolalities greater than 280 mosmol/kg were associated with near-linear increments in serum arginine vasopressin concentration, whereas in pituitary diabetes insipidus plasma arginine vasopressin concentration was not influenced by osmotic challenge. He also found that in normal subjects and patients with pituitary diabetes insipidus or primary polydipsia there was a near-linear relationship of urine osmolality and plasma arginine vasopressin concentration, whereas patients with nephrogenic diabetes insipidus excreted a consistently hypotonic urine despite an up to 15-fold variation in plasma arginine vasopressin concentration.

Normally binding of vasopressin by the distal nephron stimulates adenyl cyclase synthesis, which in turn catalyses the synthesis of cAMP, which leads to increased permeability to water of the duct or tubule luminal membrane. The vasopressin resistance of the distal nephron could be due to a variety of abnormalities. Darmady and associates suggested that it was secondary to large dilute urine volume, owing to the short proximal tubule presenting to the distal nephron and overwhelming the reabsorptive mechanism. This is inconsistent with Robertson's observation of a linear relationship between plasma osmolality and vasopressin concentration, and subsequent studies on cAMP excretion discussed below. Another possibility is a defect in the counter-current urine-concentrating mechanism. This may contribute in those cases with secondary urinary tract dilatation but is unlikely to be involved in the primary pathogenesis. Primary vasopressin resistance could be due to a vasopressin receptor defect in the distal nephron epithelial cells, to a defect in adenyl cyclase or to a defect beyond cAMP production. Evidence in support of a vasopressin receptor defect comes from the observation that the synthetic vasopressin analogue DDAVP fails to elicit the normal factor VIII response in patients with nephrogenic diabetes insipidus, and that a half normal response is obtained with carriers of the gene (Kobrinsky *et al.* 1985). There is some evidence that more than one of these possibilities may apply in different families, and Zimmerman and Green (1975) termed patients with evidence of a receptor defect type I and those with a defect beyond the receptor type II. A mouse model, with impaired stimulation of renal medullary adenyl cyclase by vasopressin in the presence of normal affinity, is probably not relevant to the human disease as it is not X linked (Jackson *et al.* 1980).

The early reports of familial occurrence of nephrogenic diabetes insipidus, with severely affected males, mildly affected females, and an absence of male-to-male transmission, strongly suggested X-linked recessive inheritance with variable partial expression in female heterozygotes (McIlraith 1892; deLange 1935; Forssman 1942, 1945; Williams and Henry 1947). Cannon (1955) claimed that there was male-to-male transmission in his family and suggested autosomal dominant inheritance. However, later studies on this family (Bode and Crawford 1969; Ten Bensel and Peters 1970) found that Cannon's information on this point was incorrect and that the family is consistent with X-linked inheritance. Nevertheless some authors have observed families apparently consistent with autosomal dominant inheritance and with females as severely affected as males (Dancis *et al.* 1948; Weller *et al.* 1950; Levinger and Escamilla 1955; Childs and Sidbury 1957; Crawford and Kennedy 1959; Robinson and Kaplan 1960). An exceptionally rare autosomal form cannot be altogether excluded but a reanalysis of some of these families by Allen (1972) led him to reject the autosomal hypothesis and to favour X linkage even for these families. Nevertheless the family reported by Ohzeki and colleagues (1984), suffering from nephrogenic diabetes insipidus type II, showed clear autosomal dominant inheritance with male-to-male transmission. The disease has been mainly reported in Caucasian populations but has also been reported in others, for example in American Blacks (Feigin *et al.* 1970), in Japanese (Ohzeki *et al.* 1978, 1984) and in a Samoan family (Nakano 1969). Bode and Crawford (1969) traced the origins of several North American families back to Ulster Scots who emigrated to Nova Scotia in 1761 on the ship 'Hopewell'.

Further evidence for X linkage comes from studies on heterozygous females. West and Kramer (1955) reported obligate heterozygous sisters with low morning urine specific gravity and little response of urine concentration to vasopressin. Carter and Simpkiss (1956) used a 12-hour water deprivation test to detect such heterozygotes, and found that they could not concentrate their urine beyond a specific gravity of 1.018. Others have confirmed defective urine concentration in a proportion of female relatives of male patients (Schoen 1960; Andreoli and Schafer 1978), but Schoen was unable to demonstrate such a defect in all obligate female heterozygotes. Yet others have claimed a partial responsiveness of female heterozygotes to vasopressin (Childs and Sidbury 1957) although this method does not seem to have been properly assessed as a method of carrier detection. Kobrinsky and colleagues (1985) suggest that the reduced factor VIII response to DDAVP observed by them in carriers might be used for carrier detection.

Bode and Miettinen (1970) were unable to detect close genetic linkage to the X-linked blood group system, Xg, which excludes assignment of the gene to the tip of the short arm.

Several studies suggest genetic heterogeneity, on the basis of varying response of cAMP excretion to administered vasopressin. In some patients there is no increase in urinary cAMP excretion when vasopressin is administered in doses which do lead to such an increase in normal subjects or patients with pituitary diabetes insipidus (Fichman and Brooker 1972; Bell *et al.* 1974; Ohzeki *et al.* 1978), These are the families regarded by Zimmerman and Green (1975) as probably having a receptor defect and which they designate type I. In contrast other studies have reported children with nephrogenic diabetes insipidus in whom both basal and vasopressin-stimulated urinary cAMP excretion exceeds that in normals (Zimmerman and Green 1975; Monn *et al.* 1976; Usberti *et al.* 1980), who constitute type II. The family of this type described by Ohzeki and colleagues (1984) has been mentioned above as a clear example of autosomal dominant inheritance. Uttley and Thistlethwaite (1972) were unable to demonstrate changes in cAMP excretion after vasopressin any different from those in normal subjects in whom they could only demonstrate a two- to three-fold increase. However, the more recent studies have used more sensitive assays and probably do represent valid distinctions. In summary current evidence indicates at least two X-linked forms, with a probable receptor defect and a postreceptor defect respectively, and an autosomal form with a postreceptor defect.

References

Abelson, H. (1968). Nephrogenic diabetes insipidus. *Pediatr. Res.* **2**, 271–82.

Allen, G. (1972). Quoted by J. Orloff and M. B. Burg in *The metabolic basis of inherited disease*, 3rd edn. eds. Stanbury, J. B., Wyngaarden, J. B. and Fredrickson, D. S. p. 1576. McGraw-Hill, New York.

Andreoli, T. E. and Schafer, J. A. (1978). Nephrogenic diabetes insipidus. In *Metabolic basis of inherited disease*, 4th edn. eds. Stanbury, J. B., Wyngaarden, J. B. and Fredrickson, D. S. pp. 1634–59. McGraw-Hill, New York.

Bell, N. H., Clark, C. M., Avery, S., Sinha, T., Trygstad, C. W. and Allen, D. O. (1974). Demonstration of a defect in the function of adenosine 3′,5′monophosphate in vasopressin-resistant diabetes insipidus. *Pediatr. Res.* **8**, 223–30.

Bode, H. H. and Crawford, J. D. (1969). Nephrogenic diabetes insipidus in North America—the *Hopewell* hypothesis. *New Engl. J. Med.* **280**, 750–4.

—— and Miettinen, O. S. (1970). Nephrogenic diabetes insipidus: absence of close linkage with Xg. *Am. J. Hum. Genet.* **22**, 221–7.

Cannon, J. F. (1955). Diabetes insipidus: Clinical and experimental studies with consideration of genetic relationships. *Arch. Intern. Med.* **96**, 215–72.

Carter, C. and Simpkiss, M. J. (1956). The 'carrier' state in nephrogenic diabetes insipidus. *Lancet* **2**, 1069–73.

Childs, B. and Sidbury, J. B. (1957). A survey of genetics as it applies to problems in medicine. *Pediatrics* **20**, 177–218.

Crawford, J. D. and Kennedy, G. C. (1959). Chlorthiazide in diabetes insipidus. *Nature* **183**, 891–2.

Dancis, J., Birmingham, J. R. and Leslie, S. H. (1948). Congenital diabetes insipidus resistant to treatment with pitressin. *Am. J. Dis. Child.* **75**, 316–28.

Darmady, E. M., Offer, J., Prince, J. and Stranack, F. (1964). The proximal convoluted tubule in the renal handling of water. *Lancet* **2**, 1254–7.

deLange, C. (1935). Uber erblichen Diabetes insipidus. *Jahrb. f. Kindesheilk.* **145**, 1.

Feigin, R. D., Rimoin, D. L. and Kaufman, R. L. (1970). Nephrogenic diabetes insipidus in a Negro kindred. *Am. J. Dis. Child.* **120**, 64–8.

Fichman, M. P. and Brooker, G. (1972). Deficient renal cyclic adenosine 3'-5' monophosphate production in nephrogenic diabetes insipidus. *J. Clin. Endocrinol. Metab.* **35**, 35–47.

Forssman, H. H. (1942). Om ärftlighetsgangen vid diabetes insipidus. *Nord. Med.* **16**, 3211.

—— (1945). On hereditary diabetes insipidus: with special regard to a sex-linked form. *Acta Med. Scand.* **121** Suppl. 159, 1–196.

Jackson, B. A., Edwards, R. M., Valton, H. and Dousa, T. P. (1980). Cellular action of vasopressin in medullary tubules of mice with hereditary nephrogenic diabetes insipidus. *J. Clin. Invest.* **66**, 110–22.

Kobrinsky, N. L., Doyle, J. J., Israels, E. D., Winter, J. S. D., Cheang, M. S., Walker, R. D. and Bishop, A. J. (1985). Absent factor VIII response to synthetic vasopressin analogue (DDAVP) in nephrogenic diabetes insipidus. *Lancet* **1**, 1293–4.

LaCombe, L. U. (1841). De la polydipsie. L'Expérience. *J. Med. Chir.* **7**, 305.

Levinger, E. L. and Escamilla, R. F. (1955). Hereditary diabetes insipidus: report of 20 cases in seven generations. *J. Clin. Endocrinol.* **15**, 547–52.

McIlraith, C. H. (1892). Notes on some cases of diabetes insipidus with marked family and hereditary tendencies. *Lancet* **2**, 767.

Monn, E., Osnes, J. B. and Oye, I. (1976). Basal and hormone-induced urinary cyclic AMP in children with renal disorders. *Acta Pediatr. Scand.* **65**, 739–45.

Nakano, K. K. (1969). Familial nephrogenic diabetes insipidus. *Hawaii Med. J.* **28**, 205–8.

Ohzeki, T., Egi, S., Takehiro, A. and Igarashi, Y. (1978). Urinary cyclic AMP excretion in vasopressin sensitive and nephrogenic diabetes insipidus. *Proc. Ann. Meet. of the Eastern Division of the Japan Endocrine Soc.* (in Japanese), Maebashi, Japan.

——, Igarashi, T. and Okamoto, A. (1984). Familial cases of congenital nephrogenic diabetes insipidus type II: remarkable increment of urinary adenosine 3',5'-monophosphate in response to antidiuretic hormone. *J. Pediatr.* **104**, 593–5.

Reuss, A. L. and Rosenthal, I. M. (1963). Intelligence in nephrogenic diabetes insipidus. *Am. J. Dis. Child.* **105**, 358–63.

Robertson, G. L. (1974). Vasopressin in osmotic regulation in man. *Ann. Rev. Med.* **25**, 315–22.

Robinson, M. G. and Kaplan, S. A. (1960). The inheritance of vasopressin-resistant ('nephrogenic') diabetes insipidus. *Am. J. Dis. Child.* **99**, 164–74.

Schoen, E. J. (1960). Renal diabetes insipidus. *Pediatrics* **26**, 808–16.

Shapiro, S. R., Woener, S., Adelman, R. D. and Palmer, J. M. (1978). Diabetes insipidus and hydronephrosis. *J. Urol.* **119**, 715–19.

Ten Bensel, R. W. and Peters, E. R. (1970). Progressive hydronephrosis, hydroureter, and dilatation of the bladder in siblings with congenital nephrogenic diabetes insipidus. *J. Pediatr.* **77**, 439–43.

Usberti, M., Dechaux, M., Guillot, M., Seligmann, R., Pavlovitch, H., Loirat, C., Sachs C. and Broyer, M. (1980). Renal prostaglandin E^2 in nephrogenic diabetes insipidus: effects of inhibition of prostaglandin synthesis by indomethacin. *J. Paediatr.* **97**, 476–8.

Uttley, W. S. and Thistlethwaite, D. (1972). Failure to detect the carrier in congenital nephrogenic diabetes insipidus. *Arch. Dis. Child.* **47**, 137–9.

Waring, A. J., Kajdi, L. and Tappan, V. (1945). A congenital defect of water metabolism. *Am. J. Dis. Child.* **69**, 323–4.

Weil, A. (1884). Uber die hereditäre Form des Diabetes insipidus. *Arch. J. Pathol. Anat.* **95**, 70.

Weller, C. G., Elliott, W. and Gusman, A. R. (1950). Hereditary diabetes insipidus: unusual urinary tract changes. *J. Urol.* **64**, 716–21.

West, J. R. and Kramer, J. G. (1955). Nephrogenic diabetes insipidus. *Pediatrics* **15**, 424–32.

Williams, R. H. and Henry, C. (1947). Nephrogenic diabetes insipidus: transmitted by females and appearing during infancy in males. *Ann. Intern. Med.* **27**, 84–95.

Zimmerman, D. and Green, O. C. (1975). Nephrogenic diabetes insipidus type II: defect distal to the adenylate-cyclase step (abs.). *Pediatr. Res.* **9**, 381.

6.2.2. Renal tubular acidosis

Introduction

Hereditary renal tubular acidosis is a heterogeneous disorder including several distinct entities. The proximal tubular and mixed proximal and distal forms have already been discussed in the previous section and all the main types are summarized in Table 6.4. Albright is usually credited with the first description of renal tubular acidosis (Albright *et al.* 1946) and the disorder has sometimes been called Albright's syndrome. However, Baines and coworkers (1945), and later Govan (1950), reported a family in which a man had renal stones and his daughter had renal tubular acidosis. Huth and colleagues (1960) distinguished primary and secondary forms of the disease.

The hereditary forms must not be confused with the sporadic transient infantile renal acidosis which was recognized in the 1930s to 1950s as a relatively common disorder (Lightwood 1935; Doxiadis 1952; Carré *et al.* 1954), but which subsequently declined in incidence (Lightwood and Butler 1963). Nor must they be confused with the many primary disorders, hereditary and acquired, which may be complicated by a secondary renal tubular acidosis, of type I, II, or IV (Morris and Sebastian 1983).

Table 6.4 *Inherited renal tubular acidosis*

Type	Sub-type	Site of defect	Primary defect	Onset	HCO₃⁻ Wasting	Urine Ca	Nephro-calcinosis	Hypo-citraturia	Osteo-malacia	T_{mHCO_3}	Inheritance
Classic, gradient or distal type (Type I)	San Francisco	Distal tubules and collecting ducts	Acidification (?H+ secretion)	Childh.	+	↑	+	+	+	N	AD
	Philadelphia		Acidification (?H+ secretion)	Childh.	+	↑	+	±	+	N	AD
	Atlanta		Hypercalciuria	Childh. (acidosis adult)	± to ±	↑↑	+	–	+	N	AD
	Oklahoma City		Hypercalciuria (absorptive)	Adult	± to ±	↑↑	–	–	+	N	AD
Proximal, bicarbonate wasting type (Type II)		Proximal tubule	HCO₃⁻ reabsorption	Childh.	++	N	–	–	–	↓↓	Prob. XR
Dislocation type (Type III)	Early onset	Distal tubule	Unknown	Childh.	+	N	–	–	–	N	Prob. AR
	Late onset			Adult	+	N	–	–	–	N	?
Renal tubular acidosis and nerve deafness		Distal tubule	Unknown	Childh.	± to +	↑	+	–	+	↓	AR
Renal tubular acidosis and osteopetrosis		Proximal and distal tubules	Carbonic anhydrase II deficiency	Childh.	+	N	–	–	–	↓	AR
Renal tubular magnesium transport defect		Distal tubule and intestine	Tubular transport of magnesium	Childh.	±	↑	+	+	–	?	Prob. AR.

Abbreviations: N=normal, ±=equivocal, +=represent, ++=marked, ↑=increased, ↑↑=markedly increased, ↓=decreased, ↓↓=markedly decreased, –=absent, AD=autosomal dominant, AR=autosomal recessive, XR=X-linked recessive, HCO₃⁻=bicarbonate, Ca=calcium, T_{mHCO_3}=maximal tubular reabsorption of bicarbonate.

Several workers have attempted classifications of renal tubular acidosis. Morris (1969) recognized three main types: type I, the common classic, gradient, or distal type in which the bicarbonate threshold is normal, the defect is in the distal tubule, and inheritance is autosomal dominant; type II, with a low bicarbonate threshold due to a proximal tubular defect and recessive inheritance, now thought to be probably X linked; and a very rare type III or dislocation type also recessively inherited. He subsequently recognized a hybrid type I–II, incomplete forms of types I and II, and a type IV. Muldowney (1979) proposed a modified classification based on the definability of bicarbonate threshold and the severity of bicarbonate wasting at a plasma level of 25 mEq/l. He suggested that this basis of classification was therapeutically useful. His classification is set out in Table 6.5 in comparison with the updated Morris classification.

The splay, or type IV, renal tubular acidosis has not been reported as a primary hereditary disorder, but has always been secondary to some other disorder, either hereditary or acquired. Type IV is usually secondary to chronic renal disease, especially interstitial nephritis, and diabetic nephropathy. It is associated with hyperkalaemia, caused by alderosterone deficiency or renal resistance to mineral ocorticoid steroids. It is in many ways similar to type II pseudohypoaldosteronism, which is discussed later, but in that disorder aldosterone production is normal and there is no resistance to mineralocorticoids. A good example of type IV (hyperkalaemic) renal acidosis in an inherited disorder is that recently described in salt-losing congenital adrenal hyperplasia (Rodriguez-Soriano *et al.* 1986). A brief review of renal acidosis and its relationship to renal stone formation is given by Pohlman and colleagues (1984).

More recently the hereditary type I disorder has been further subdivided into the San Francisco and Philadelphia syndromes with

Table 6.5 *Muldowney's and Morris' renal tubular acidosis classifications*

Muldowney		Morris type
Renal bicarbonate threshold	Severity of bicarbonate wasting at a plasma level of 25 mEq/l	
Not definable	Minimal (1–3 mEq/kg/day)	I
	Moderate (4–7 mEq/kg/day)	III
	Severe (10 or more mEq/kg/day)	Hybrid I–II
Definable	Minimal	Splay type IV
	Moderate	} Type II
	Severe	

secondary nephrocalcinosis, and the Atlanta and Oklahoma City syndromes with primary nephrocalcinosis (Morris and Sebastian, 1983). These are all autosomal dominant in inheritance. In addition a type-I-like tubular acidosis is seen in three autosomal recessive syndromes, in association with sensorineural deafness in one, with osteopetrosis in another, and with hypomagnesemia in the third.

Familial type I renal tubular acidosis

Since Albright's original report numerous families have been reported with type I renal tubular acidosis. The principal feature is a renal acidification defect such that the urine pH will not fall below a fixed minimal value, usually about pH 5.0, on challenge with ammonium chloride administration. This is usually of sufficient severity to produce a hyperchloraemic acidosis with a low serum bicarbonate and hypocalcaemia. The commonest form of the disease presents in infancy and responds to alkali therapy (McSherry and Morris 1978). In the majority of families hypercalciuria and nephrocalcinosis, with or without renal calculi, are seen in at least some of the affected members (Musgrave *et al.* 1972), and osteomalacia may also be found. However the precise status of these early families, in terms of current classification, is unclear. Some early reports seemed to establish the autosomal dominant pattern of inheritance of familial type I tubular acidosis (Schreiner *et al.* 1953; Foss *et al.* 1956; Wilansky and Schneiderman 1957; Wilansky and Schucher 1960; Seedat 1964, 1967, 1968, 1972; Kolb 1967; Gyory and Edwards 1968; Musgrave *et al.* 1972). Male-to-male transmission occurs in several of these families. Other groups report affected sibs (Cooke and Kleeman 1950; Engel 1951; Mozziconacci *et al.* 1958; Dedmon and Wrong 1962; Richardson 1962; Kuhlencordt *et al.* 1967), or twins (Rendle-Short 1953), but in several of these parents were not available for study so they do not provide convincing evidence for a recessive type. This is even the case for the concordantly affected identical twins with first-cousin parents reported by Kuhlencordt and colleagues.

A family reported by Pitts and coworkers (1955) has been extensively studied by further workers (Randall and Targgart 1961; Randall 1967; Musgrave *et al.* 1972). The designation of the San Francisco type of renal tubular acidosis I is based on this family. It is characterized by the frequent occurrence of hypercalciuria and hypocitraturia with consequent nephrocalcinosis. However, in both this family and other similar families alkali therapy instituted before the age of 4 years corrects the hypercalciuria and hypocitraturia, preventing the development of nephrocalcinosis (Morris and Sebastian 1983). Incomplete forms of distal renal tubular acidosis with nephrocalcinosis and a renal acidification defect, but without actual acidosis, have been reported (Wrong and

Davies 1959; Wrong and Feest 1980). Nevertheless families are also seen in which some affected members are acidotic and others are not (Richards and Wrong 1972).

In another form of type I renal tubular acidosis, the Philadelphia syndrome, the course of the disease is progressive with a non-acidotic phase preceding the onset of the complete syndrome, with acidosis coinciding with the development of nephrocalcinosis (Elkinton *et al.* 1967). This form is of later onset than the San Francisco type with one family showing onset of incomplete renal tubular acidosis at an age of about 15 years, and the complete form with nephrocalcinosis at about 24 years (Norman *et al.* 1978). These workers showed a similar age-related difference in other families with presumably the same syndrome. Buckalew and coworkers (1968) have also described the development of progressive acidosis in a patient with renal tubular acidosis in association with nephrocalcinosis and stone formation. The studies of Coe and Parks (1980) suggest that, at least in this type, hypocitraturia, as well as the acidification defect, may be a primary metabolic defect leading to nephrocalcinosis and stone formation.

A third variant of renal tubular acidosis I is the Atlanta syndrome, studied by Buckalew and colleagues, in which hypercalciuria seems to be the primary defect leading to a progressive nephrocalcinosis, renal acidification defect, and acidosis (Buckalew *et al.* 1974). In their family there were patients with nephrocalcinosis and hypercalciuria but without an acidification defect. Other features present in the more severely affected members of this family suggest that the proximal as well as the distal tubule may be involved. The family appears to be unique.

A fourth variant is the Oklahoma City syndrome in which there is autosomal dominant inheritance of hypercalciuria. As in the Atlanta syndrome, renal tubular acidosis develops as a consequence of nephrocalcinosis and distal tubular damage in some older members of the family (Hamed *et al.* 1979).

A metabolic renal tubular acidosis resembling type I has been described in the autosomal recessive Schwachman's syndrome, often associated with glycosuria or aminoaciduria (Agget *et al.* 1980; Marra *et al.* 1986).

References

Agget, P. J., Cavanagh, N. P. C., Matten, D. J., Pincott, J. R., Sutcliff, J. and Harries, J. T. (1980). Schwachman's syndrome: a review of 21 cases. *Arch. Dis. Child.* **55**, 331–47.

Albright, F., Burnett, C. H., Parson, W., Reifenstein, E. C. Jr. and Roos, A. (1946). Osteomalacia and late rickets: the various etiologies met in the United States with emphasis on that resulting in a specific form of renal acidosis, and therapeutic indications for etiological sub-groups, and the relationship between osteomalacia and Milkman's syndrome. *Medicine (Baltimore)* **25**, 399–479.

Baines, G. H., Barclay, J. A. and Cook, W. T. (1945). Nephrocalcinosis associated with hyperchloraemia and low plasma bicarbonate. *Quart. J. Med.* **14**, 113–23.

Buckalew, V. M., McCurdy, K. D., Ludwig, G. D., Chaykin, L. B. and Elkinton, J. R. (1968). The syndrome of incomplete renal tubular acidosis: physiologic studies in three patients with a defect in lowering urine pH. *Am. J. Med.* **45**, 32–42.

——, Purvis, M. L., Shulman, M. G., Herndon, C. N. and Rudman, D. (1974). Hereditary renal tubular acidosis. Report of a 64 number kindred with variable expression including idiopathic hypercalcinuria. *Medicine* **53**, 229–54.

Carré, I. J., Wood, B. S. B. and Smallwood, W. C. (1954). Idiopathic renal acidosis in infancy. *Arch. Dis. Child.* **29**, 326–33.

Coe, F. L. and Parks, J. H. (1980). Stone disease in hereditary distal renal tubular acidosis. *Ann. Intern. Med.* **93**, 60–1.

Cooke, R. E. and Kleeman, C. R. (1950). Distal tubular function with renal calcification. *Yale J. Biol. Med.* **23**, 199.

Dedmon, R. E. and Wrong, O. (1962). The excretion of organic anion in renal tubular acidosis with particular reference to citrate. *Clin. Sci.* **22**, 19–32.

Doxiadis, S. A. (1952). Idiopathic renal acidosis in infancy. *Arch. Dis. Child.* **27**, 409–27.

Elkinton, J. R., McCurdy, D. K. and Buckalew, V. M. Jr. (1967). Hydrogen ion and the kidney. In *Renal Disease*, 2nd edn. ed. Black, D. A. K. p. 110. Davis, Philadelphia.

Engel, W. J. (1951). Nephrocalcinosis. *JAMA* **145**, 288–94.

Foss, G. L., Perry, C. B. and Wood, F. J. Y. (1956). Renal tubular acidosis. *Quart. J. Med.* **25**, 185–99.

Govan, A. D. T. (1950). Nephrocalcinosis associated with hyperchloraemia and low plasma bicarbonate. *Quart. J. Med.* **19**, 277–83.

Gyory, A. Z. and Edwards, K. D. G. (1968). Renal tubular acidosis. A family with an autosomal dominant genetic defect, in renal hydrogen ion transport with proximal tubular and collecting duct dysfunction and increased metabolism of citrate and ammonia. *Am. J. Med.* **45**, 43–62.

Hamed, I. A., Czerwinski, A. W., Coats, B., Kaufman, C. and Altmiller, D. H. (1979). Familial absorptive hypercalcinuria and renal tubular acidosis. *Am. J. Med.* **67**, 385–91.

Huth, E. J., Webster, G. D. Jr. and Elkinton, J. R. (1960). The renal excretion of hydrogen ions in renal tubular acidosis. III. An attempt to detect latent cases in a family: comments on nosology, genetics, and etiology of the primary disease. *Am. J. Med.* **29**, 586–98.

Kolb, F. O. (1967). Cited by McKusick, V. A. in *Mendelian inheritance in man*, 5th edn. (1978) p. 340.

Kuhlencordt, F., Lenz, W., Seeman, N. and Zukschwert, L. (1967). Renal tubular acidosis and bilateral nephrocalcinosis in uniovular twins. *Germ. Med. Monthly* **12**, 565–70.

Lightwood, R. (1935). Calcium infarction of the kidneys in infants. *Arch. Dis. Child.* **10**, 205–6.

—— and Butler, N. (1963). Decline in primary infantile renal acidosis, aetiological implications. *Br. Med. J.* **1**, 855–7.

McSherry, E. and Morris, R. C. (1978). Attainment and maintenance of normal stature with alkali therapy in infants and children with classic renal tubular acidosis. *J. Clin. Invest.* **61**, 509–27.

Marra, G., Appiani, A. C., Romeo, L., Marzorati, D., Valade, A., Goj, V. and Assael, B. M. (1986). Renal tubular acidosis in a case of Schwachman's syndrome. *Acta Paediatr. Scand.* **75**, 682–4.

Morris, R. C. (1969). Renal tubular acidosis. Mechanisms, classification and implications. *New Engl. J. Med.* **281**, 1405–13.

—— and Sebastian, A. (1983). Renal tubular acidosis and Fanconi syndrome. Chapter 84 in *The metabolic basis of inherited disease*, 5th edn. eds. Stanbury, J. B., Wyngaarden, J. B., Fredrickson, D. S., Goldstein, J. L. and Brown, M. S. pp. 1808–43. McGraw-Hill, New York.

Mozziconacci, P., Lestradet, H., Attal, C., Girard, H. and Pham-Huu-Trung (1958). Acidose rénale hyperchlorémique avec nephrocalcinose familiale, rétinité albescente et hypocalciurie. *Sem. Hôp. Paris.* **2**, 3167–72P.

Muldowney, F. P. (1979). Renal acidosis. Chapter 19 in *Renal disease*, 4th edn. eds. Black, D. and Jones, N. F. pp. 587–614. Blackwell Scientific, Oxford, London, Edinburgh and Shelbourne.

Musgrave, J. E., Bennett, W. M., Campbell, R. A. and Eisenberg, C. S. (1972). Renal tubular acidosis (letter). *Lancet* **2**, 1364.

Norman, M. E., Feldman, N. I., Cohn, R. M., Roth, K. S. and McCurdy, D. K. (1978). Urinary citrate excretion in the diagnosis of distal renal tubular acidosis. *J. Pediatr.* **92**, 394–400.

Pitts, H. H., Schulte, J. W. and Smith, D. R. (1955). Nephrocalcinosis in a father and three children. *J. Urol.* **73**, 208–11.

Pohlman, T., Hruska, K. A. and Menon, M. (1984). Renal tubular acidosis. *J. Urol.* **132**, 431–6.

Randall, R. E. Jr. (1967). Familial renal tubular acidosis revisited (letter). *Ann. Intern. Med.* **66**, 1024–5.

—— and Targgart, W. H. (1961). Familial renal tubular acidosis. *Ann. Intern. Med.* **54**, 1108–16.

Rendle-Short, J. (1953). Idiopathic renal acidosis in twins. Alkalosis resulting from overdosage of a citrate mixture. *Arch. Dis. Child.* **28**, 55–6.

Richards, P. and Wrong, O. M. (1972). Dominant inheritance in a family with familial renal tubular acidosis. *Lancet* **2**, 998–9.

Richardson, R. E. (1962). Nephrocalcinosis with special reference to its occurrence in renal tubular acidosis. *Clin. Radiol.* **13**, 224–30.

Rodriguez-Soriano, J., Vallo, A., Castillo, G., Oliveros, R. and Fernandez-Garnica, J. M. (1986). Hyperkalemic distal renal tubular acidosis in salt-losing congenital adrenal hyperplasia. *Acta Paediatr. Scand.* **75**, 425–32.

Schreiner, G. E., Smith, L. H. and Kyle, L. H. (1953). Renal hyperchlorenic acidosis. Familial occurrence of nephrocalcinosis with hyperchloremia and low serum bicarbonate. *Am. J. Med.* **15**, 122–9.

Seedat, Y. K. (1964). Some observations of renal tubular acidosis—a family study. *S. Afr. Med. J.* **38**, 606–10.

—— (1967). Renal tubular acidosis. *S. Afr. Med. J.* **41**, 1007–12.

—— (1968). Familial renal tubular acidosis (letter). *Ann. Intern. Med.* **69**, 1329.

—— (1972). Renal tubular acidosis (letter). *Lancet* **2**, 1364.

Wilansky, D. L. and Schneiderman, C. (1957). Renal tubular acidosis with recurrent nephrolithiasis and nephrocalcinosis. *New Engl. J. Med.* **257**, 399–403.

—— and Schucher, R. (1960). Familial acidosis of renal tubular origin. *Can. Med. Assoc. J.* **83**, 308–12.

Wrong, O. and Davies, H. E. F. (1959). The excretion of acid in renal disease. *Quart. J. Med.* **28**, 259–313.

—— and Feest, T. G. (1980). The natural history of distal renal tubular acidosis. *Contr. Nephrol.* **21**, 137–44.

Type III renal tubular acidosis

This exceedingly rare type of distal tubular acidosis, also known as the 'dislocation type', is characterized by a moderate degree of bicarbonate wasting. There appear to be two forms. In one onset begins in infancy or early childhood (Huth *et al.* 1960; Morris *et al.* 1969; McSherry *et al.* 1972). Huth and colleagues (1960) described affected sibs with normal parents, and in two cases first-cousin parents. Morris and colleagues (1969) reported two sporadic cases. Whilst this form is probably autosomal recessive the genetic status of a late onset form (Wilson *et al.* 1967) is unknown.

References

Huth, E. J., Webster, G. D. Jr. and Elkinton, J. R. (1960). The renal excretion of hydrogen ion in renal tubular acidosis. III. An attempt to detect latent cases in a family: comments on nosology, genetics and etiology of the primary disease. *Am. J. Med.* **29**, 586–98.

McSherry, E., Sebastian, A. and Morris, R. C. (1972). Renal tubular acidosis in infants: the several kinds, including bicarbonate-wasting, classic and tubular acidosis. *J. Clin. Invest.* **51**, 499–514.

Morris, E., Sebastian, A., Kranhold, J. and Morris, R. C. (1969). Infantile renal tubular acidosis (RTA), a distinct type (abs.). *Clin. Res.* **17**, 441.

Wilson, I. D., Williams, R. C. Jr. and Tobian, L. Jr. (1967). Renal tubular acidosis: three cases with immunoglobulin abnormalities in the patients and their kindreds. *Am. J. Med.* **43**, 356–70.

Renal tubular acidosis with nerve deafness

This type was first described by Konigsmark in 1966, in a 17-year-old girl with bilateral renal calculi, renal tubular acidosis, and progressive nerve deafness. She had a 20-year-old brother who was similarly affected, but her unrelated parents and another brother were normal. Further reports of similar cases followed (Royer and Broyer 1967; Nance 1970; Nance and Sweeney 1971; Walker *et al.* 1974; Donckerwolcke *et al.* 1976; Cremers *et al.* 1980) in several of which there were affected sibs and in one instance cousin parents, confirming an autosomal recessive pattern of inheritance. Dunger and colleagues (1980) considered the renal defect to be a distal tubular one similar to that in the classic type I tubular acidosis. Cohen and coworkers (1973) studied two families, each with affected sibs and parental consanguinity, in which both the renal lesion and the hearing defect were more severe than in other such families. It is probable that their families have a disorder due to a different gene rather than an allelic mutation because in one of their families Shapira and associates (1974) detected an inactive red-cell carbonic anhydrase I (or B) with an additional lysine residue. This observation is difficult to interpret in the light of the report of complete red-cell carbonic anhydrase I deficiency without renal tubular acidosis (Kendall and Tashian 1977), and the evidence that carbonic anhydrase II (or C) is the only soluble isoenzyme present in kidney (Wistrand 1980; Dobyan and Bulger 1982, Spicer *et al.* 1982). Similar difficulties arise over the two unrelated boys with renal tubular acidosis, but without mention of deafness, reported by Kondo and coworkers (1978). They found an inactive red-cell carbonic anhydrase I in both cases which differed from that found by Shapira and associates in being stable to high temperature and to 8M urea. The apparent contradiction in these cases has yet to be resolved.

References

Cohen, T., Brand-Auraban, A., Karshai, C., Jacob, A., Gay, I., Tsitsianov, J., Shapiro, T., Jatziv, S. and Ashkenazi, A. (1973). Familial infantile renal tubular acidosis and congenital nerve deafness: an autosomal recessive syndrome. *Clin. Genet.* **4**, 275–8.

Cremers, C. W. R. J., Monnens, L. A. H. and Marres, E. H. M. A. (1980). Renal tubular acidosis and sensorineural deafness: an autosomal recessive syndrome. *Arch. Otolaryngol.* **106**, 287–9.

Dobyan, D. C. and Bulger, R. E. (1982). Renal carbonic anhydrase. *Am. J. Physiol.* **243**, F311–F324.

Donckerwolcke, R. A., van Biervliet, J. P., Koorevar, G., Kuijten, R. H. and van Stekelenburg, G. J. (1976). The syndrome of renal tubular acidosis with nerve deafness. *Acta Paediatr. Scand.* **65**, 100–4.

Dunger, D. B., Brenton, D. P. and Cain, A. R. (1980). Renal tubular acidosis and nerve deafness. *Arch. Dis. Child.* **55**, 221–5.

Kendall, A. G. and Tashian, R. E. (1977). Erythrocyte carbonic anhydrase I: inherited deficiency in humans. *Science* **197**, 471–2.

Kondo, T., Taniguchi, N., Taniguchi, K., Matsuda, I. and Murao, M. (1978). Inactive form of erythrocyte carbonic anhydrase B in patients with primary renal tubular acidosis. *J. Clin. Invest.* **62**, 610–17.

Konigsmark, B. W. (1966). Cited by McKusick, V. A. (1978) in *Mendelian inheritance in man*, 5th edn. pp. 658–9.

Nance, W. E. (1970). Cited by McKusick, V. A. (1978) in *Mendelian inheritance in man*, 5th edn. pp. 658–9.

—— and Sweeny, A. (1971). Evidence for autosomal recessive inheritance of the syndrome of renal tubular acidosis with deafness. *Clin. Delineation Birth Defects. IX. Ear. Birth Defects Orig. Art. Series VII* (4), 70–2.

Royer, P. and Broyer, M. (1967). L'Acidose rénale an cours des tubulopathies congénitales. *Actualites Néphrologiques de l'hopital Necker.* p. 73. Flammarion, Paris.

Shapira, E., Ben-Yoseph, Y., Eyal, G. and Russell, A. (1974). Enzymatically inactive red cell carbonic anhydrase B in a family with renal tubular acidosis. *J. Clin. Invest.* **53**, 59–63.

Spicer, S. S., Sens, M. A. and Tashian, R. E. (1982). Immunocytochemical demonstration of carbonic anhydrase in human epithelial cells. *J. Histochem. Cytochem.* **30**, 864–73.

Walker, W. G., Ozer, F. L. and Whelton, A. (1974). Syndrome of perceptive deafness and renal tubular acidosis. *Birth Defects Orig. Art. Series* **10**, 163.

Wistrand, P. J. (1980). Human renal cytoplasmic carbonic anhydrase. *Acta Physiol. Scand.* **109**, 239–48.

Renal tubular defect in magnesium transport

Renal tubular magnesium wasting may occur secondary to the administration of drugs, such as diuretics, gentamicin, or mercurials; to renal transplantation; to urinary tract obstruction; or to the diuretic phase of acute renal failure or to intestinal malabsorption of magnesium. It is associated with an incomplete distal renal tubular acidosis (Passer 1975). Several groups have reported a familial form with affected sibs, including brother and sister, or sister and sister, sib pairs (Michelis *et al.* 1972; Manz *et al.* 1978; Evans *et al.* 1981). The clinical and investigative picture is one of polyuria with excretion of urine of low specific gravity, hypomagnesaemia with increased urinary excretion of magnesium, low citrate excretion, mild bicarbonate wasting and nephrocalcinosis.

Inheritance is probably autosomal recessive.

This disorder should not be confused with the primary hypomagnesaemia reported by Friedman and others (1967). Urinary magnesium excretion was low in this patient and they attributed the defect to a primary intestinal specific malabsorption of magnesium. The parents of their patient were first cousins.

References

Evans, R. A., Carter, J. N., George, C. R. P., Walls, R. S., Newland, R. C., McDonnell, G. D. and Lawrence, J. R. (1981). The congenital magnesium-losing kidney: report of two patients. *Quart. J. Med.* **197**, 39–52.

Friedman, M., Hatcher, G. and Watson, L. (1967). Primary hypomagnesaemia with secondary hypocalcaemia in an infant. *Lancet* **1**, 203–5.

Manz, F., Scharer, K., Janka, P. and Lombeck, J. (1978). Renal magnesium wasting, incomplete tubular acidosis, hypercalcinuria and nephrocalcinosis in siblings. *Eur. J. Pediatr.* **128**, 67–79.

Michelis, M. F., Drash, A. L., Linarelli, L. G., De Rubertis, F. R. and Davis, B. B.

(1972). Decreased bicarbonate threshold and renal magnesium wasting in a sibship with distal tubular acidosis. *Metabolism* **21**, 905–20.

Passer, J. (1975). Incomplete distal renal tubular acidosis in hypomagnesemia-dependent hypocalcemia. *Arch. Intern. Med.* **136**, 462–5.

6.2.3. Bartter's syndrome (familial renal hypoelectrolytaemia) and familial hypokalaemic alkalosis with tubulopathy

The syndrome of hypokalaemic alkalosis with hypochloraemia and hyponatraemia was first described by Bartter and his colleagues (Pronove *et al.* 1960; Bartter *et al.* 1962). Onset is usually shortly after birth with failure to thrive with polyuria and polydipsia but no oedema, salt craving, and muscle weakness or even tetany. James and coworkers (1975) described atypical facies. Blood pressure remains normal despite usually high blood levels of aldosterone, and of renin and angiotensin. However, hyperaldosteronism is not invariable (Saruta *et al.* 1984). Subsequent growth retardation during childhood is a common and mental retardation a more variable finding, although these features may be absent (Tarm *et al.* 1973). Persistent hypercalciuria, although unusual, has been reported (Girardin *et al.* 1986). Gout has also been reported as a complication of Bartter's syndrome (Meyer *et al.* 1975). Erkelens and van Eps (1973) suggested that both renin and erythropoietin are produced in the juxtaglomerular apparatus on the basis of observing erythrocytosis in their patient.

Histologically changes in the kidney point to the renal location of the lesion. The juxtaglomerular apparatus is hyperplastic, and the macula densa is enlarged with a p-aminosalicylic acid (PAS)-positive membrane separating the macula densa from the juxtaglomerular apparatus (Bartter *et al.* 1962; Cannon *et al.* 1968; Arant *et al.* 1970). More recently hyperplasia of the interstitial cells of the renal medulla, the site of renal prostaglandin synthesis, has been demonstrated (Verberckmoes *et al.* 1976).

There has been considerable controversy, still unresolved, regarding the pathogenesis of the disorder. Some of the earlier hypotheses were reviewed by Calcagno and Hollerman (1975). Gill and Bartter (1964) suggested that there was a primary vascular resistance to the pressor effect of angiotensin with other effects secondary to this. However, there is resistance to other pressors, and this resistance is not specific to Bartter's syndrome. Laragh and Cannon, in a series of papers, have postulated defective proximal tubular reabsorption of sodium (Laragh and Kelly 1964; Laragh *et al.* 1964; Cannon *et al.* 1968). Gardner and others (1970) claimed to find evidence for generalized disturbance of membrane sodium transport. There is undoubtedly a defect in renal handling of sodium with a consequent natriuresis (White 1972; Gill and Bartter 1978; Delany *et al.* 1981). However, Gill and Bartter (1978) proposed that this was due to a defect in chloride reabsorption in the thick ascending limb of the loop of Henle, a view supported by Baehler and associates (1980). Gill and colleagues (1976) observed increased urinary excretion of prostaglandin E and demonstrated that the hyper-reninaemia of the syndrome was dependent on prostaglandin synthesis. However, prostaglandins are known to decrease chloride reabsorption in the ascending limb of Henle's loop (Stokes and Kokko 1977), and normalization of urinary prostaglandin E excretion with drug administration does not always correct the hypokalaemia (Bourke and Delaney 1977; Gill 1980; Delaney *et al.* 1981). It has been suggested that sodium, rather than chloride, is actively transported in the ascending limb of the loop of Henle and that in Bartter's syndrome a defect in this mechanism results in impaired sodium reabsorption, with hypokalaemia resulting from increased potassium secretion distally as a consequence of the increased sodium load (Westenfelder and Kurtzman 1981). Bargette and Stein (1978) and Costello and Bourke (1983) have resurrected the hypothesis of a primary potassium-losing distal tubular defect to meet objections to the salt-wasting hypothesis. Furthermore Korff and colleagues (1984), in a study of nine patients with Bartter's syndrome, have recently confirmed that red-cell intracellular sodium is increased, and that the ouabain-sensitive and furosemide-sensitive sodium effluxes are also increased, but were all restored to normal when the hypokalaemia was corrected. Their observations provide direct evidence that the sodium disturbances are secondary to hypokalaemia but still leave the mechanism of hypokalaemia unknown. Very high plasma levels of atrial natriuretic peptide, quite inappropriate for a disorder with low blood volume, have recently been reported in Bartter's syndrome (Tunny and Gordon 1986; Yamada *et al.* 1986).

Following Bartter's original description further reports followed. Campbell and coworkers (1966) and Sutherland and associates (1970) reported affected twins, with the latter group also reporting an affected child of an incestuous mating. Others have described families with affected sibs (Bailey *et al.* 1963; Trygstad *et al.* 1967; Arant *et al.* 1970; Sutherland *et al.* 1970; Dillon *et al.* 1979; Delaney *et al.* 1981). These reports taken together establish an autosomal recessive pattern of inheritance. The disorder appears to occur with relatively high frequency among people of African origin, over three-quarters of affected families in the United States being Black (Hall 1971; Mace *et al.* 1971). No association with any histocompatibility antigen has been established (Watson *et al.* 1982).

A number of atypical families have been described that may or may not represent mutations at different loci. De Jong and others (1980) described sibs with a Bartter-like syndrome but with hypertension. The early report of familial Bartter's syndrome of Arant and coworkers (1970) mentioned above was atypical in that both of the affected brothers had severe uraemia at the time of onset, and one had renal osteodystrophy. On renal biopsy there was glomerulonephritis as well as mild hyperplasia of the juxtaglomerular apparatus. The defective platelet aggregation observed in one family (Stoff *et al.* 1980) does not necessarily imply a separate disorder, but may be just another side effect of increased prostaglandin synthesis. Kurtz and colleagues (1981) described five sibs with a Bartter-like syndrome with hypercalciuria and nephrocalcinosis. In another variant a partial resistance to vasopressin produced a Bartter-like syndrome with diabetes insipidus (Robertson and Scheidler 1981).

Neither heterozygote detection nor prenatal diagnosis have been described.

A disorder very similar to Bartter's syndrome has been described earlier (p. 263). It differs in lacking hyperplasia of the juxtaglomerular apparatus and was described in 1974 in two brothers (Potter *et al.* 1974). Gullner and colleagues studied another family with three affected sibs, two girls and a boy (Güllner *et al.* 1979a and b, 1981). They demonstrated that the distal fractional reabsorption of chloride, which is low in Bartter's syndrome, was normal. They obtained evidence of possible linkage to the HLA locus and suggested that the defect was a specific tubulopathy involving magnesium and introduced the term 'familial hypokalaemic alkalosis with tubulopathy'.

Yet another similar but possibly separate disorder, with congenital hypokalaemia and hypercalcinuria but normal tubular chloride reabsorption was described in 5 patients by Seyberth and colleagues from Heidelberg. These workers considered that this is a distinct disorder due to increased production of prostaglandin E_2 (Seyberth *et al.* 1985), which they term 'hyperprostaglandin E syndrome'.

References

Arant, B. S., Brackett, N. C. Jr., Young, R. B. and Still, W. J. S. (1970). Case studies of siblings with juxtaglomerular hyperplasia and secondary aldosteronism associated with severe azotemia and renal rickets—Bartter's syndrome or disease? *Pediatrics* **46**, 344–61.

Baehler, R. W., Work, J., Kotchen, T. A., McMorrow, G. and Guthrie, G. (1980). Studies on the pathogenesis of Bartter's syndrome. *Am. J. Med.* **69**, 933–8.

Bailey, J. E., Sutherland, L. E. and Hartroft, P. M. (1963). Familial electrolyte-losing nephropathy. *Can. Med. Assoc. J.* **88**, 252.

Bargette, J. J. and Stein, J. H. (1978). In *Contemporary issues in nephrology: acid, base and potassium handling*, eds. Brenner, B. M. and Stein, J. H. pp. 269–88. Churchill Livingstone, New York.

Bartter, F. C., Pronove, P., Gill, J. R. Jr. and MacCardle, R. C. (1962). Hyperplasia of the juxtaglomerular complex with hyperaldosteronism and hypokalemic alkalosis. A new syndrome. *Am. J. Med.* **33**, 811–28.

Bourke, E. and Delaney, V. B. (1977). Pathogenesis of Bartter's syndrome: a family study. *Kidney Int.* **12**, 447.

Calcagno, P. L. and Hollerman, C. E. (1975). Hereditary renal disease and certain renal tubular disorders. Chapter 30 in *Pediatric nephrology*, eds. Rubin, M. I. and Barratt, T. M. pp. 672–3. Williams & Wilkins, Baltimore.

Campbell, R. A., Blair, H. R., Klevit, H. D. and Goodnight, S. H. (1966). Hypokalemic alkalosis and normopoiesis with elevated aldosterone excretion in an 8-year old girl twin. (Abs.). p. 111. Soc. Pediat. Res., Atlantic City.

Cannon, P. J., Leeming, J. M., Sommers, S. C., Winters, R. W. and Laragh, J. H. (1968). Juxtaglomerular cell hyperplasia and secondary hyperaldosteronism (Bartter's syndrome): a re-evaluation of the pathophysiology. *Medicine* **47**, 107–31.

Costello, J. and Bourke, E. (1983). Bartter's syndrome—the case for a primary potassium-losing tubulopathy: discussion paper. *J. R. Soc. Med.* **76**, 53–65.

De Jong, P. E., Donker, A. J. M., van der Wall, E., Erkelens, D. W., van der Hem, G. K. and Doorenbos, H. (1980). Effects of indomethacin in two siblings with a renin-dependent hypertension, hyperaldosteronism and hypokalaemia. *Nephron* **25**, 47–52.

Delaney, V. B., Oliver, J. F., Simms, M., Costello, J. and Bourke, E. (1981). Bartter's syndrome: physiological and pharmacological studies. *Quart. J. Med.* **50**, 213–32.

Dillon, M. J., Shah, V. and Mitchell, M. D. (1979). Bartter's syndrome: 10 cases in childhood: results of long-term indomethacin therapy. *Quart. J. Med.* **48**, 429–46.

Erkelens, D. W. and van Eps, L. W. S. (1973). Bartter's syndrome and erythrocytosis. *Am. J. Med.* **55**, 711–19.

Gardner, J., Lapey, A., Simopoulos, A. and Bravo, E. (1970). Evidence for a primary disturbance of membrane transport in Bartter's syndrome and Liddle's syndrome. (abs.). *J. Clin. Invest.* **49**, 32A.

Gill, J. R. (1980). Bartter's syndrome. *Ann. Rev. Med.* **31**, 405–19.

—— and Bartter, F. C. (1964). In *West European Symposia on Clinical Chemistry*, Vol. 3. *Water and electrolyte metabolism II,* eds. de Graeff, J. and Leijnse, B. pp. 119–24. Elsevier.

—— and —— (1978). Evidence for a prostaglandin-independent defect in chloride reabsorption in the Loop of Henle as a proximal cause of Bartter's syndrome. *Am. J. Med.* **65**, 766–72.

——, Frölich, J. C., Bowden, R. E., Taylor, A. A., Keiser, H. R., Seyberth, H. W., Oates, J. A. and Bartter, F. C. (1976). Bartter's syndrome: a disorder characterized by high urinary prostaglandins and a dependence of hyperreninemia on prostaglandin synthesis. *Am. J. Med.* **61**, 43–51.

Girardin, E., Favre, L., Valloton, M. B. and Paunier, L. (1986). Familial Bartter's syndrome: report of a case with early manifestations and persistent hypercalciuria. *Helv. Paediatr. Acta.* **41**, 221–8.

Güllner, H.-G., Gill, J. R., Bartter, F. C., Chan, J.-C. M. and Dickman, P. S. (1979a). A familial disorder with hypokalemic alkalosis, hyperreninemia, aldosteronism, high urinary prostaglandins and normal blood pressure that is not 'Barter's Syndrome'. *Trans. Assoc. Am. Phys.* **71**, 578–82.

——, Terasaki, P. I., Bartter, F. C., Gill, J. R. and Tiwari, J. (1979b). Linkage between histocompatibility antigens (HLA) and familial hypokalemia. Quoted by McKusick, V. A. (1983) in *Mendelian inheritance in man*, 6th edn. p. 778. Johns Hopkins University Press, Baltimore.

——, Gill, J. R. and Bartter, F. C. (1981). Correction of hypokalemia by magnesium repletion in familial hypokalemia alkalosis with tubulopathy. *Am. J. Med.* **71**, 578–82.

Hall, B. D. (1971). Preponderance of Bartter syndrome among Blacks (letter). *New Engl. J. Med.* **285**, 581.

James, T., Holland, N. H. and Preston, D. (1975). Bartter syndrome: typical facies and normal plasma volume. *Am. J. Dis. Child.* **129**, 1205–7.

Korff, J. M., Siebens, A. W. and Gill, J. R. Jr. (1984). Correction of hypokalemia corrects abnormalities in erhthrocyte sodium transport in Bartter's syndrome. *J. Clin. Invest.* **74**, 1724–9.

Kurtz, I., Maheer, T., Jones, J. W., Sutton, J. M., Schambelan, M., Hulter, H. N., Rector, F. C., Morris, R. C. and Sebastian, A. (1981). Familial chloride-resistant renal alkalosis and hypokalemia with fasting hypercalciuria and medullary nephrocalcinosis: a unique variant of Bartter's syndrome without impaired renal diluting ability (abs.). *Clin. Res.* **29**, 555A.

Laragh, J. H. and Kelly, W. G. (1964). Aldosterone: its biochemistry and physiology. *Adv. Metab. Dis.* **1**, 217–62.

——, Cannon, P. J. and Ames, R. P. (1964). Interaction between aldosterone secretion, sodium, and potassium balance, and angiotensin activity in man: studies in hypertension and cirrhosis. *Can. Med. Assoc. J.* **90**, 248–56.

Mace, J., Hambridge, K. M., Gotlin, R. and Dubois, R. (1971). Bartter's syndrome in Blacks (letter). *New Engl. J. Med.* **285**, 1488.

Meyer, W. J. III, Gill, J. R. Jr. and Bartter, F. C. (1975). Gout as a complication of Bartter's syndrome. A possible role of alkalosis in the decreased clearance of uric acid. *Ann. Intern. Med.* **83**, 56–9.

Potter, W. Z., Trygstad, C. W., Helmes, O. M., Nance, W. E. and Judson, W. E. (1974). Familial hypokalemia associated with renal interstitial fibrosis. *Am. J. Med.* **57**, 971–7.

Pronove, P., MacCardle, R. C. and Bartter, F. C. (1960). Aldosteronism, hypokalaemia and a unique renal lesion in a five year old boy. *Acta Endocrinol.* (Suppl.) **51**, 167.

Robertson, G. L. and Scheidler, J. A. (1981). A newly recognized variant of familial nephrogenic diabetes insipidus distinguished by partial resistance to vasopressin (type 2). (abs.). *Clin. Res.* **29**, 555A.

Saruta, T., Fujimaki, M., Senba, S., Saito, I. and Konishi, K. (1984). Aldosterone and other mineral corticoids in Bartter's syndrome. *J. Lab. Clin. Med.* **103**, 848–53.

Seyberth, H. W., Rascher, W., Schweer, H., Kuhl, P. G., Mehls, O. and Scharer, K. (1985). Congenital hypokalemia with hypercalciuria in preterm infants: a hyperprostaglandinuric tubular syndrome different from Bartter syndrome. *J. Pediatr.* **107**, 694–701.

Stoff, J. S., Stemerman, M., Steer, M., Salzman, E. and Brown, R. S. (1980). A defect in platelet aggregation in Bartter's syndrome. *Am. J. Med.* **68**, 171–80.

Stokes, J. B. and Kokko, J. P. (1977). Inhibition of sodium transport by prostaglandin E_2 across the isolated, perfused rabbit collecting tubule. *J. Clin. Invest.* **59**, 1099–104.

Sutherland, L. E., Hartroft, P., Balis, J. U., Bailey, J. D. and Lynch, M. J. (1970). Bartter's syndrome. A report of four cases, including three in one sibship, with comparative histologic evaluation of the juxtaglomerular apparatuses and glomeruli. *Acta Paediatr. Scand.* **59**, (Suppl. 201): 1–24.

Tarm, F., Juncos, L. L., Anderson, C. F. and Donadio, J. V. Jr. (1973). Bartter's syndrome: an unusual presentation. *Mayo. Clin. Proc.* **48**, 280–3.

Trygstad, C. W., Mangos, J. A., Hansen, M. F. and Lobeck, C. C. (1967). Familial hypokalemic alkalosis with growth failure (abs.). p. 66. Am. Pediatr. Soc., Atlantic City.

Tunny, T. J. and Gordon, R. D. (1986). Plasma atrial natriuretic peptide in primary aldosteronism (before and after treatment) and in Bartter's and Gordon's syndromes. *Lancet* **1**, 272–3.

Verberckmoes, R., van Damme, B., Clement, J., Amery, A. and Michielsen, P. (1976). Bartter's syndrome with hyperplasia of renomedullary cells: successful treatment with indomethacin. *Kidney Int.* **9**, 302–7.

Watson, A., Bourke, E., Delaney, V. B., Pollock, M. S. and Dupont, B. (1982). HLA typing in Bartter's syndrome (B.S.). *Kidney Int.* **21**, 160A.

Westenfelder, C. and Kurtzman, N. A. (1981). Bartter's syndrome: a disorder of active sodium and/or passive chloride transport in the thick ascending limb of Henle's loop. *Min. Electrol. Metab.* **5**, 135–43.

White, M. G. (1972). Bartter's syndrome: a manifestation of renal tubular defects. *Arch. Intern. Med.* **129**, 41–7.

Yamada, K., Tajima, K., Moriwaki, K., Tarui, S., Miyata, A., Kangawa, K. and Matsuo, H. (1986). Atrial natriuretic peptide in Bartter's syndrome. *Lancet* **1**, 273.

6.2.4. Pseudohypoaldosteronism

This disorder appears to be a heterogeneous one, there being two types, known as types I and II, but with uncertainty regarding their genetic determination and at least the possibility of heterogeneity within them.

The classic, or type I, pseudohypoaldosteronism was first described as a renal salt-wasting disorder of infancy with failure to thrive, dehydration and hyponatraemia, hyperkalaemia, and renal acidosis of type 4 (Cheek and Perry 1958). Plasma renin activity and aldosterone were increased. Further reports followed over the next few years establishing a renal tubular insensitivity to mineralocorticoids (Donnell *et al.* 1959; Lelong *et al.* 1960; Raine and Roy 1962; Royer *et al.* 1963; Trung *et al.* 1970; Levine 1973). One curious feature that may have initially obscured the pattern of inheritance is a lessening of the severity of the salt-wasting disturbance after the infantile period (Postel-Vinay *et al.* 1974). The underlying pathogenesis of the defect is unknown.

The majority of reported cases have been sporadic but a proportion are familial. Some of the familial cases suggest autosomal recessive inheritance, in particular that reported in seven Persian–Jewish children by Rösler *et al.* (1973). Their patients, four boys and three girls, came from five families and in six of the seven there was parental consanguinity. Other possibly recessive families include those of Raine and Roy (1962) in which a boy and possibly his sister were affected, and of Bonnici (1977). However, the majority of reported instances of familial occurrence are suggestive of autosomal dominant inheritance, especially when plasma renin and aldosterone levels of older relatives have been estimated (LeLong *et al.* 1960; Roy 1977; Hanukoglu *et al.* 1978; Lauras *et al.* 1978; Limal *et al.* 1978).

A rare type II pseudohypoaldosteronism, with renal acidosis and renal hyperkalaemia but without salt wasting, has also been described (Schambelan *et al.* 1981). The genetic basis, if any, of this type is uncertain although Licht and colleagues (1985) have described a patient with affected relatives, indicative of autosomal dominant inheritance.

References

Bonnici, F. (1977). Pseudohypoaldosteronisme familial à transmission autosomique recessive. *Arch. Fr. Pédiatr.* **34**, 915–16.

Cheek, D. B. and Perry, J. W. (1958). A salt wasting syndrome in infancy. *Arch. Dis. Child.* **33**, 252–6.

Dillon, M. J., Leonard, J. V., Buckler, J. M., Ogilvie, D., Lillystone, D., Honour, J. W. and Shackleton, C. H. L. (1980). Pseudohypoaldosteronism. *Arch. Dis. Child.* **55**, 427–34.

Donnell, G. N., Litman, N. and Roldan, M. (1959). Pseudohypoadrenalcorticism: renal sodium loss, hyponatremia and hyperkalemia due to a renal tubular insensitivity to mineralo-corticoids. *Am. J. Dis. Child.* **97**, 813–28.

Hanukoglu, A., Fried, D. and Gotlieb, A. (1978). Inheritance of pseudo-hypoaldosteronism. *Lancet* **1**, 1359.

Lauras, B., Ravussin, J.-J., David, M., Freycon, F. and Jeune, M. (1978). Pseudo-hypoaldosteronism chez l'enfant: apropos de quatre observations dont deux concernant des freres. *Pédiatrie* **33**, 119–35.

LeLong, M., Alagille, D., Phillipe, A., Gentil, C. and Gabilan, J. C. (1960). Diabete salin par insensibilite congénitale du tubule à l'aldosterone: pseudo-hypoadrenocortisme. *Rev. Fr. Études Clin. Biol.* **5**, 558–65.

Levine, S. (1973). Personal communication quoted by Rösler *et al.* (1973). *Lancet* **1**, 959–62.

Licht, J. H., Amundson, D., Hsueh, W. A. and Lombardo, J. V. (1985). Familiar hyperkalaemic acidosis. *Quart. J. Med.* **54**, 161–76.

Limal, J. M., Rappaport, R., Dechaux, M., Riffaud, C. and Morin, C. (1978). Familial dominant pseudohypoaldosteronism. *Lancet* **1**, 51.

Postel-Vinay, M.-C., Alberti, G. M., Ricour, C., Limal, J.-M., Rappaport, R. and

Royer, P. (1974). Pseudohypoaldosteronism: persistence of hyperaldosteronism and evidence for renal tubular and intestinal responsiveness to endogenous aldosterone. *J. Clin. Endocrinol. Metab.* **39**, 1038–44.

Raine, D. N. and Roy, J. (1962). A salt losing syndrome in infancy: pseudo-hypoaldocorticalism. *Arch. Dis. Child.* **37**, 548–56.

Rösler, A., Theodor, R., Gazit, E., Biochis, H. and Rabinowitz, D. (1973). Salt-wastage, raised plasma-renin activity, and normal or high plasma-aldosterone: a form of pseudohypoaldosteronism. *Lancet* **1**, 959–62.

Roy, C. (1977). Pseudohypoaldosteronisme familial (á propos de 5 cas). *Arch. Fr. Pédiatr.* **34**, 37–54.

Royer, P., Bonnette, J., Mathieu, H., Gabilan, J.-C., Klutchko, G. and Ziltoun, R. (1963). Pseudohypoaldosteronisme. *Ann. Pédiatr. (Paris)* **10**, 596–605.

Schambelan, M., Sebastian, A. and Rector, F. C. (1981). Mineralocorticoid-resistant renal hyperkalemia without salt wasting (type II pseudohypoaldoster-onism): role of increased renal chloride reabsorption. *Kidney Int.* **19**, 716–27.

Trung, P. H., Piussan, C., Rodary, C., Legrand, S., Attal, C. and Mozziconacci, P. (1970). Etude du taux de secretion de l'aldosterone et de l'activité de la renine plasmatique d'un cas de pseudo-hypoaldosteronism. *Arch. Fr. Pédiatr.* **27**, 603–15.

6.2.5. Pseudohyperaldosteronism (Liddle's syndrome)

Liddle and coworkers (1963, 1964) reported a family of six sibs and members of two further generations with a syndrome of hypertension and hypokalaemic alkalosis resembling hyperaldosteronism. However, aldosterone secretion was low and renin and angiotensin were also decreased. They attributed the disorder to a renal tubular abnormality. Although there was no male-to-male transmission the pattern of inheritance in their family suggested an autosomal dominant trans-mission.

This suggestion regarding the pattern of inheritance was supported but not confirmed by studies in a further family (Gardner *et al.* 1970). These workers demonstrated a low red blood cell sodium content and increased total fractional sodium efflux. They suggested that the primary defect was in distal tubular membrane transport. Further isolated case reports such as the recent one by Mutoh and colleagues (1986) do not contribute to our understanding of the genetics of this syndrome.

References

Gardner, J., Lapey, A., Simopoulos, A. and Bravo, E. (1970). Evidence for a primary disturbance of membrane transport in Bartter's syndrome and Liddle's syndrome (abs.). *J. Clin. Invest.* **49**, 32A.

Liddle, G. W., Bledsoe, T. and Coppage, W. S. Jr. (1963). A familial renal disorder simulating primary aldosteronism but with negligible aldosterone secretion. *Trans. Assoc. Am. Phys.* **76**, 199–213.

——, —— and —— (1964). In *Aldosterone*, eds. Baulieu, E. E. and Robel, P. p. 352. Blackwell Scientific, Oxford.

Mutoh, S., Hirayama, H., Ueda, S., Tsuruta, K., Imafuji, M. and Ikegami, K. (1986). Pseudohyperaldosteronism (Liddle's syndrome): a case report. *J. Urol.* **135**, 557–8.

6.2.6. Systemic carnitine deficiency

This disorder, which is distinct from myopathic carnitine deficiency, is characterized by muscle weakness, cardiomegaly, and hypoglycaemic attacks without ketosis, presenting in infancy (Karpati *et al.* 1975). Chapoy and coworkers (1980) demonstrated low levels of carnitine in plasma, liver, and muscle in their case, and a favourable response to oral carnitine. It has subsequently been shown that carnitine biosynthesis is normal (Rebouche and Engel 1981), and that there is evidence for a renal tubular defect in carnitine reabsorption (Engel *et al.* 1981; Waber *et al.* 1981, 1982).

Several groups have recorded the occurrence of this disorder in sibs (Tripp *et al.* 1981; Waber *et al.* 1981), which is indicative of autosomal recessive inheritance.

References

Chapoy, P. R., Angelini, C., Brown, W. J., Stiff, J. E., Shug, A. and Cederbaum, S. D. (1980). Systemic carnitine deficiency—a treatable inherited lipid-storage disease presenting as Reye's syndrome. *New Engl. J. Med.* **303**, 1389–94.

Engel, A. G., Rebouche, C. J., Wilson, D. M., Glasgow, A. M., Romshe, C. A. and Cruse, R. P. (1981). Primary systemic carnitine deficiency. II. Renal handling of carnitine. *Neurology* **31**, 819–25.

Karpati, G., Carpenter, S., Engel, A. G., Watters, G. V., Allen, J., Rothman, S., Klassen, G. and Mamer, O. A. (1975). The syndrome of systemic carnitine deficiency: clinical morphologic, biochemical, and pathophysiologic features. *Neurology* **25**, 16–24.

Rebouche, C. J. and Engel, A. G. (1981). Primary systemic carnitine deficiency. I. Carnitine biosynthesis. *Neurology* **31**, 813–18.

Tripp, M. E., Katcher, M. L., Peters, H. A., Gilbert, E. F., Arya, S., Hodach, R. J. and Shug, A. L. (1981). Systemic carnitine deficiency presenting as familial endocardial fibroelastosis. *New Engl. J. Med.* **305**, 385–90.

Waber, L., Valle, D., Neill, C. and Shug, A. (1981). Systemic carnitine deficiency: a treatable cause of familial cardiomyopathy (abs.). *Am. J. Hum. Genet.* **33**, 58A.

——,——, ——, Dimauro, S. and Shug, A. (1982). Carnitine deficiency presenting as familial cardiomyopathy: a treatable defect in carnitine transport. *J. Pediatr.* **101**, 700–5.

6.2.7. Blue-diaper syndrome

This disorder is not known to be a renal tubular transport defect, but is rather a defect in intestinal transport of tryptophan. Bacterial degradation of the tryptophan within the intestine results in the production of excessive amounts of indole. The indole is absorbed and is metabolized to indican with a consequent indicanuria, detected in the newborn infant as blue staining of the nappy or diaper.

The syndrome is only mentioned here because it has been reported in two brothers with an associated hypercalcaemia and nephrocalcinosis of unknown pathogenesis (Drummond *et al.* 1964). It is probably inherited in an autosomal recessive manner.

Reference

Drummond, K. N., Michael, A. F., Ulstrom, R. A. and Good, R. A. (1964). The blue diaper syndrome: familial hypercalcemia with nephrocalcinosis and indicanuria. A new familial disease, with definition of the metabolic abnormality. *Am. J. Med.* **37**, 928–48.

7. Primary hereditary nephropathies

7.1. PRIMARY GLOMERULONEPHRITIS

The term 'typical primary non-familial glomerulonephritis' designates a common group of renal disorders of varied histopathological appearance generally thought to reflect varying immune responses to different stimuli. Associations of several glomerulonephritides with specific HLA antigens have been observed suggesting some degree of genetic acid predisposition or perhaps determination of pattern of response. Associations of minimal change disease with HLA-B12 (Trompeter *et al.* 1980), B8 (O'Regan *et al.* 1980; Rashid *et al.* 1983), and DR7 or DRW7 (Alfiler *et al.* 1980; de Mouzon-Cambon *et al.* 1983) have been reported. That with DR7 is particularly strong, especially in children with atopy. Associations of idiopathic membranous nephropathy with HLA-DR3 and B8 or B18 have also been reported (Klouda *et al.* 1979; Müller *et al.* 1981; Rashid *et al.* 1983). Short and coworkers (1983) have identified a haplotype HLA-B18, DR3, properdin factor B phenotype BfF1, in membranous nephropathy which carries a worse prognosis than is seen in patients without this haplotype.

Wank and colleagues (1984) in a study of 59 patients with various forms of primary glomerulonephritis have found an association with a rare allele at the HLA-linked C4B locus. This allele, C4B*2.9, was found in a quarter of the patients compared with 2 per cent of the normal population. The association was strongest for membranoproliferative glomerulonephritis, being found in seven out of 11 patients. Regueiro and Arnaiz-Villena (1984) observed that the non-HLA-linked complement component C3 shows an association of the common C3^F allele with chronic renal failure in Spaniards. Twenty patients, all on haemodialysis awaiting renal transplantation and suffering from a variety of renal diseases leading to renal failure, gave C3^F and C3^S gene frequencies of 0.425 and 0.575 respectively compared with frequencies of 0.225 and 0.775 respectively among 196 controls ($P<0.025$). However, because of the heterogeneity of their patient group this observation is difficult to interpret.

McLean and colleagues (1980) have reported arthritis and glomerulonephritis in a patient with the rare hypomorphic C3 allele, C3*f. More recently the same group have described a new hypomorphic C3 variant, of slow electrophoretic mobility, C3*s, in a 4-year-old boy with hypocomplementaemia and haematuria (McLean *et al.* 1985). They clearly demonstrated its maternal inheritance.

Apart from the hypomorphic variants of C3 discussed above a number of inherited complement component deficiencies may be associated with renal disease, with varying frequency. The renal disease seen in patients with such complement deficiencies may be one of the immune glomerulonephritides or may be lupus nephritis occurring as a complication of systemic lupus erythematosus. In one instance the haemolytic uraemic syndrome has been reported in a patient with a deficiency of factor H (Ross and Densen 1984). The inherited complement component abnormalities have recently been reviewed by Schur (1986) and Table 7.1, summarizing the complement component deficiencies reported as occuring in association with renal disease, is largely based on data from his review. The evidence regarding C2 deficiency is conflicting. Some workers have found renal disease to be uncommon in C2 deficiency (Agnello 1978), and in one case a patient developed severe lupus nephritis after a blood transfusion, suggesting that C2 deficiency may even prevent the development of immune-complex-mediated glomerular nephritis (Roberts *et al.* 1978). In contrast Sobel and others (1979) have described the occurrence of a non-specific glomerulonephritis in association with inherited C2 deficiency.

Table 7.1 *Complement component deficiencies associated with renal disease*

Complement component	Associated disease	
Classical pathway:		
Clq	LN	GN
Clr	LN	GN
C4	LN	MPGN
Alternative pathway:		
C3	GN	
Final pathway:		
C7	(LN)	GN
C8	(LN)	
Complement receptor:		
CR1	LN	
Properdin factor:		
BF1	MGN	

Abbreviations: LN = Lupus nephritis, GN = glomerulonephritis, MGN = membranous glomerulonephritis, MPGM = membranoproliferative glomerulonephritis. Designations in brackets indicate occasional reports only. Based on data largely from Schur (1986).

Recently Short and colleagues (1984) have reported familial membranous nephropathy presenting as adult onset nephrotic syndrome in three separate pairs of brothers. One pair were monozygotic twins and therefore HLA identical.

Julian and associates (1985) have reported a remakable observation of a striking familial aggregation of IgA nephropathy in several interrelated Kentucky families. There was no HLA antigen or haplotype common to the affected members of these families, nor did the pattern of occurrence in their pedigrees suggest Mendelian inheritance. Cederholm and others (1986) have demonstrated circulating IgA anti-basement membrane antibodies, reacting with structures common to collagens, I, II, and IV, in patients with IgA nephropathy.

The Goodpasture syndrome (see p. 437) of glomerulonephritis with anti-glomerular basement membrane antibodies and lung disease is usually of sporadic occurrence, but familial cases have been reported (Maddock *et al.* 1967; Gossain *et al.* 1972; D'Apice *et al.* 1978). This disease shows a strong association with HLA-DRW2 (Rees *et al.* 1978, 1984).

References

Agnello, V. (1978). Complement deficiency states. *Medicine* **57**, 1–24.

Alfiler, C. A., Roy, L. P., Doran, T., Sheldon, A. and Bashir, H. (1980). HLA-DRw7 and steroid responsive nephrotic syndrome of childhood. *Clin. Nephrol.* **14**, 71–4.

Cederholm, B., Wieslander, J., Bygren, P. and Heinegärd, D. (1986). Patients with IgA nephropathy have circulating anti-basement membrane antibodies reacting with structures common to collagen I, II and IV. *Proc. Nat. Acad. Sci.* 6151–5.

D'Apice, A. J. F., Kincaid-Smith, P., Becker, G. J., Loughhead, M. G., Freeman, J. W. and Sands, J. M. (1978). Goodpasture's syndrome in identical twins. *Ann. Intern. Med.* **88**, 61–2.

Gossain, V. V., Gerstein, A. R. and Janes, A. W. (1972). Goodpasture's syndrome: a familial occurrence. *Am. Rev. Resp. Dis.* **105**, 621–4.

Julian, B. A., Quiggins, P. A., Thompson, J. S., Woodford, S. Y., Gleason, K. and Wyatt, R. J. (1985). Familial Iga nephropathy. *New Engl. J. Med.* **312**, 202–8.

Klouda, P. T., Manos, J., Acheson, E. J., Dyer, P. A., Goldby, F. S., Harris, R., Lawler, W., Mallick, N. P. and Williams, G. (1979). Strong association between idiopathic membranous nephropathy and HLA-DR3. *Lancet* **2**, 770–1.

McLean, R. H., Weinstein, A., Damjanov, I. and Rothfield, N. (1980). Hypomorphic variant of C3 arthritis and glomerulonephritis. *J. Pediatr.* **93**, 937–43.

——, Bryan, R. K. and Winkelstein, J. (1985). Hypomorphic variant of the slow allele of C3 associated with hypocomplementemia and hematuria. *Am. J. Med.* **78**, 865–8.

Maddock, R. K., Stevens, L. E., Reemtsma, K. and Bloomer, H. A. (1967). Goodpasture's syndrome: cessation of pulmonary hemorrhage after bilateral nephrectomy. *Ann. Intern. Med.* **67**, 1259–64.

de Mouzon-Cambon, A., Ohayon, E., Bouissou, F. and Barthe, P. (1980). HLA-DR typing in children with glomerular diseases. *Lancet* **2**, 868.

Müller, G. A., Müller, C., Liebau, G., Kömpf, J., Ising, H. and Wernet, P. (1981). Strong association of idiopathic membranous nephropathy (IMN) with HLA-DR3 and MT-2 without involvement of HLA-B18 and no association to BfF1. *Tissue Antigens* **17**, 332–7.

O'Regan, D., O'Callaghan, U., Dundon, S. and Reen, D. J. (1980). HLA antigens and steroid responsive nephrotic syndrome of childhood. *Tissue Antigens* **16**, 147–51.

Rashid, H. U., Papiha, S. A., Agroyannis, B., Morley, A. R., Ward, M. K., Roberts, D. F. and Kerr, D. N. S. (1983). The associations of HLA and other genetic markers with glomerulonephritis. *Hum. Genet.* **63**, 38–44.

Rees, A. J., Peters, D. K., Compston, D. A. S. and Batchelor, J. R. (1978). Strong association between HLA-DRW2 and antibody-mediated Goodpasture's syndrome. *Lancet* **1**, 966–8.

——,——, Amos, N., Welsh, K. I. and Batchelor, J. R. (1984). The influence of HLA-linked genes on the severity of anti-GBM antibody-mediated nephritis. *Kidney Int.* **26**, 445–50.

Regueiro, J. R. and Arnaiz-Villena, A. (1984). C3 polymorphism, HLA and chronic renal failure in Spaniards. *Hum. Genet.* **67**, 437–40.

Roberts, J. L., Schwartz, M. M. and Lewis, E. J. (1978). Hereditary C2 deficiency and systemic lupus erythematosus associated with severe glomerulonephritis. *Clin. Exp. Immunol.* **31**, 328–38.

Ross, S. C. and Densen, P. (1984). Complement deficiency states and infection: epidemiology, pathogenesis and consequences of Neisserial and other infections in an immune deficiency. *Medicine* **163**, 243–73.

Schur, P. H. (1986). Inherited complement component abnormalities. *Ann. Rev. Med.* **37**, 333–46.

Short, C. D., Dyer, P. A., Cairns, S. A., Manos, J., Walton, C., Harris, R. and Malick, N. P. (1983). A major histocompatibility system haplotype associated with poor prognosis in idiopathic membranous nephropathy. *Disease Markers* **1**, 189–96.

——, Feehaly, J., Gokal, R. and Mallick, N. P. (1984). Familial membranous nephropathy. *Br. Med. J.* **289**, 1500.

Sobel, A. T., Moisy, G. and Hirbec, G. (1979). Hereditary C2 deficiency associated with non-systemic glomerulonephritis. *Clin. Nephrol.* **12**, 132–6.

Trompeter, R. S., Barratt, T. M., Kay, R., Turner, M. W. and Soothill, J. F. (1980). HLA, atopy and cyclophosphamide in steroid responsive childhood nephrotic syndrome. *Kidney Int.* **17**, 113–17.

Wank, R., Schendl, D. J., O'Neill, G. J., Rietmüller, G., Held, E. and Feucht, H. E. (1984). Rare variant of complement C4 is seen in high frequency in patients with primary glomerulonephritis *Lancet* **1**, 872–4.

7.2. BENIGN FAMILIAL HAEMATURIA

Persistent or recurrent haematuria is a common clinical finding in otherwise healthy children, or occasionally adults. As early as 1926, Baehr recognized that after the exclusion of recognizable serious renal or lower urinary tract disease, such haematuria has a benign prognosis. However, recent studies have shown that Alport's disease and IgA nephropathy are the most common individual causes of recurrent haematuria in childhood (Miller *et al.* 1985; White 1986). The terms benign, essential, or idiopathic have all been applied to this condition whose harmless nature has been amply confirmed (Wyllie 1955; Livaditis and Ericsson 1962; Travis *et al.* 1962). However, families have been reported in which haematuria has been asymptomatic in younger affected members for many years, but older members have eventually developed chronic nephritis (Atlee 1901; Russell and Smith 1959; Habib *et al.* 1982). Similar families with hereditary nephritis, in which only asymptomatic affected individuals have been detected, may have been included among those families reported as having benign familial haematuria. More recent studies on asymptomatic haemtauria, described below, have identified varying pathological changes on renal biopsy, especially of glomerular basement membranes. As yet the prognosis for patients with benign haematuria has not been determined in relation to renal biopsy appearance. Hence caution should be exercised in giving a clinical prognosis, even when the patient has had a renal biopsy, unless an adequate investigation of renal function in all close relatives has been undertaken, and there has been a reasonable period of follow-up (Miller *et al.* 1985).

The clinical picture of benign haematuria varies from a gross macro-scopic haematuria, often at the height of a febrile illness, with associated red-cell casts and proteinuria, to a symptomless microscopic haematuria with no associated provocative episode or other urinary abnormality. The essential feature, apart from the haematuria, is that renal function is unimpaired. If renal biopsy is performed a mild focal or diffuse nephritis with mild hypercellularity of the mesangium on light microscopy has been described. In many of these cases there are mesangial deposits of IgA (Berger and Hinglais 1968; Berger 1969). In such patients the haematuria is probably due to an immunological reaction to antigens of an infective agent, and must be distinguished from the cases described below with basement membrane thinning or other structural defects.

The disorder may be familial, especially in the milder, microscopic form without significant proteinuria and with normal light microscopy on renal biopsy. There is considerable disparity in the literature as to the proportion of cases that are familial. Ayoub and Vernier (1965), in the first clearly documented report of benign familial haematuria, found a high frequency of familial occurrence among children with idiopathic haematuria. In an earlier report of what was probably benign familial haematuria Aitken (1909) described a family in which 10 of 17 members had haematuria. He likened his family to that of Guthrie (1902) who gave the earliest published account of Alport's much studied family. However, the clinical course in Aitken's family was benign apart from one child who died from an acute nephritic episode, which was possibly coincidental. Several other groups have also found a high proportion of familial cases (McConville *et al.* 1966; Johnston and Shuler 1969; Cotton *et al.* 1975). However, familial occurrence was considered rare by further groups (Arneil *et al.* 1969; Glasgow *et al.* 1970).

The lack of changes suggestive of nephritis on light microscopy was confirmed by McConville and colleagues (1966), but Rogers and coworkers (1973) described changes on electron microscopy of renal biopsies from the affected members of their family. These consisted of focal thinning of the glomerular basement membrane, especially of the lamina densa. Similar observations were made by Cotton and associates (1975), and by Yoshikawa and others (1982), but it has also been claimed that this is a non-specific finding (Hill *et al.* 1974), and Yoshikawa and colleagues (1984) in an extensive Japanese study of renal biopsies observed non-specific glomerular basement membrane thinning in 10 sporadic cases of persistent microscopic haematuria, as well as in a further 10 familial cases. Furthermore, Dische and colleagues (1984) reported similar glomerular basement membrane thinning in 14 patients, 13 of whom had haematuria, including 10 with proteinuria as well, with or without hypertension or impaired renal function. Kohaut and colleagues (1976), in an ultrastructural study of heriditary nephritis, used patients with benign recurrent haematuria as one group of controls. They did not give details of their benign recurrent haematuria patients, nor did they state the proportion if any that were familial. However, the appearance of the glomerular basement membrane in this group did not suffer from that of normal controls.

In contrast to the above reports of normal glomerular basement membrane ultrastructural appearance, or of focal thinning, whether regarded as characteristic or non-specific, Yum and Bergstein (1983) claimed to be able to separate their patients into three groups. They examined renal biopsies by electron microscopy from 19 patients with asymptomatic haematuria, normal-looking glomeruli on light microscopy, and negative immunofluorescence. They classified four patients as belonging to their type I with thickening and lamellation of the basement membrane. As will be seen in sections 7.3 and 7.4 this appearance is typical of that reported by others in hereditary nephritis with or without deafness. One may speculate that despite the asymptomatic nature of their haematuria these patients nevertheless belong in that category. Indeed one patient in their type I category had a mother and an elder brother with microscopic haematuria, and progressively increasing proteinuria in the brother suggestive of an hereditary nephritis. Yum and Bergstein's type II was represented by seven patients who showed extensive attenuation of the basement membranes with only occasional small areas of lamellation or fragmentation. This probably corresponds to the thinning observed by earlier workers in benign familial haematuria, for which they had evidence from relatives in one case. However, in one other case of type II the mother of the patient developed renal failure at the age of 44 years and was found to have sensorineural deafness. Although eight of the 11 patients with types I and II nephropathy had a family history of renal disease this could not be defined in most cases. Relatives of the patients without a family history were not investigated. Eight patients with type III changes exhibited only moderate variation in basement membrane thickness, and possibly correspond to the benign recurrent haematuria subjects used as controls by Kohaut and colleagues (1976) discussed above. Clearly groups studied in this way will need to be followed over many years to determine the natural history of patients with different renal biopsy pictures, and will also need to be correlated with the findings in relatives.

In all of the above reports of benign familial haematuria and in other large families (Argianas *et al.* 1975; Eisenstein *et al.* 1979) the pattern of incidence and transmission has been consistent with autosomal dominant inheritance, although Eisenstein and colleagues in particular produced evidence of incomplete penetrance and variable expressivity. They did observe several instances of male-to-male transmission. Their paper describes the only systematic study published to date, with examination of the first-degree relatives of 130 children seen for asymptomatic persistent or recurrent haematuria over a 7-year period in Tel Aviv. In 34 cases haematuria was found in other family members. In 23 of these this was considered to be due to benign familial haematuria (18 per cent of all benign haemtauria), and in 11 instances to other causes. Of these 23 families 18 were non-Ashkenazi (8 being Iraqui) and 5 were Ashkenazi, compared to a non-Ashkenazi:Ashkenazi ratio of 2:1 for all children admitted to their hospital.

On the present limited information genetic heterogeneity of the familial form of benign haematuria is not excluded and the true incidence in populations outside Israel remains uncertain. Such heterogeneity is suggested by the exceptional family of Marks and Drummond (1969) in which seven out of eight sibs in one family were observed to have persistent microscopic and recurrent macroscopic haematuria over periods of up to 8 years, whereas the parents and several other close relatives had normal urine analyses.

References

Aitken, J. (1909). Congenital, hereditary and family haematuria. *Lancet* **2**, 444–6.
Argianas, E., Melissinos, K. and Belimezis, A. (1975). Hereditary recurrent haematuria. *Lancet* **2**, 715.

Arneil, G. C., Lam, C. N., McDonald, A. M. and McDonald M. (1969). Recurrent haematuria in 17 children. *Br. Med. J.* **2**, 233–5.

Atlee, W. H. W. (1901). Three cases of recurrent haemturia occurring in one family. *St Bart. Hosp. J.* **9**, 41–2.

Ayoub, E. M. and Vernier, R. L. (1965). Benign recurrent hematuria. *Am. J. Dis. Child.* **109**, 217–23.

Baehr, G. (1926). Benign and curable form of hemorrhagic nephritis. *JAMA* **86**, 1001–4.

Berger, J. (1969). IgA glomerular deposits in renal disease. *Transplant. Proc.* **1**, 939–44.

—— and Hinglais, N. (1968). Les Dépots intercapillaires d'IgA–IgG. *J. Urol. Nephrol.* **47**, 694–5.

Cotton, J. R., Schwartz, M. M., Antonovych, T. T. and Hunsicker, L. K. (1975). Benign familial hematuria (BFH): frequency studies in 12 families (abs.). *Kidney Int.* **8**, 408.

Dische, F. E., Weston, M. J. and Parsons, V. (1984). Abnormally thin glomerular basement membranes associated with hematuria, proteinuria, or renal failure in adults. *Am. J. Nephrol.* (in press). Quoted in leading article, *Lancet* (1984) **1**, 1450.

Eisenstein, B., Stark, H. and Goodman, R. M. (1979). Benign familial haematuria in children from the Jewish communities of Israel: clinical and genetic studies. *J. Med. Genet.* **16**, 369–72.

Glasgow, E. F., Moncrieff, M. W. and White, R. H. R. (1970). Symptomless haematuria in childhood. *Br. Med. J.* **2**, 687–92.

Guthrie, L. G. (1902). 'Idiopathic' or congenital, hereditary and family haematuria. *Lancet* **1**, 1243–6.

Habib, R., Gubler, M., Hinglais, N., Noel, L.-H., Droz, D., Levy, M., Mahieu, P., Fordart, J. M., Perrin, D., Bois, E. and Grünfeld, J.-P. (1982). Alport's syndrome: experience at Hospital Necker. *Kidney Int.* **21**, (Suppl. 11), S20–S28.

Hill, G. S., Jenis, E. H. and Goodloe, S. J. (1974). The non-specificity of the ultrastructural alterations in hereditary nephritis, with additional observations on benign familial hematuria. *Lab. Invest.* **31**, 516–32.

Johnston, C. and Shuler, S. (1969). Recurrent haematuria in childhood: a five year follow-up. *Arch. Dis. Child.* **44**, 483–6.

Kohaut, E. C., Singer, D. B., Nevels, B. K. and Hill, L. L. (1976). The specificity of split renal membranes in hereditary nephritis. *Arch. Pathol.* **100**, 475–9.

Livaditis, A. and Ericsson, N. O. (1962). Essential hematuria in children—prognostic aspects. *Acta Paediatr.* **51**, 630–4.

McConville, J. M., West, C. D. and McAdams, A. J. (1966). Familial and non-familial benign hematuria. *J. Pediatr.* **69**, 207–14.

Marks, M. I. and Drummond, K. N. (1969). Benign familial hematuria. *Pediatrics* **44**, 590–3.

Miller, P. F. W., Spiers, N. I., Aparvio, S. R., Lendon, M., Savage, J. M., Postlethwaite, R. J., Brocklebank, J. T., Houston, I. B. and Meadow, S. R. (1985). Long term prognosis of recurrent haematuria. *Arch. Dis. Child.* **60**, 420–5.

Reyersbach, G. C. and Butler, A. M. (1954). Congenital hereditary hematuria. *New Engl. J. Med.* **251**, 377–80.

Rogers, P. M., Kurtzmann, N. A., Bunn, S. N. and White, M. G. (1973). Familial, benign essential hematuria. *Arch. Intern. Med.* **131**, 257–62.

Russell, E. P. and Smith, N. J. (1959). Hereditary hematuria. *Am. J. Dis. Child.* **98**, 353–8.

Travis, L. B., Daeschner, C. W., Dodge, W. F., Hopps, H. C. and Rosenberg, H. S. (1962). 'Idiopathic' hematuria. *J. Pediatr.* **60**, 24–32.

White, R. H. R. (1986). Asymptomatic microscopical haematuria. *Lancet* **1**, 1599.

Wyllie, G. C. (1955). Haematuria in children. *Proc. Roy. Soc. Med.* **48**, 1113–17.

Yoshikawa, N., White, R. H. R. and Cameron, A. H. (1982). Familial haematuria: clinicopathological correlations. *Clin. Nephrol.* **17**, 172–82.

——, Hashimoto, H., Katayama, Y., Yamada, Y., Matsuo, T. and Okada, S. (1984). The thin glomerular basement membrane in children with haematuria. *J. Pathol.* **142**, 253–7.

Yum, M. and Bergstein, J. M. (1983). Basement membrane nephropathy: a new classification for Alport's syndrome and asymptomatic hematuria based on ultrastructural findings. *Hum. Pathol.* **14**, 996–1003.

7.3. UNCOMPLICATED (PURE) HEREDITARY NEPHRITIS

There have been many reports of hereditary or familial nephritis uncomplicated by deafness, ocular, or other non-renal abnormalities. A review of the literature reveals no consistent clinical, pathological, or genetic picture, the reported families clearly being highly heterogeneous. The majority of families show dominant inheritance, although even this is not invariable, but a clearly autosomal or X-linked dominant pattern is only present in a minority.

Many reports appeared before the association with deafness in Alport's disease had been recognized, and even in most of the more recent studies audiometry was not performed, or is not reported, so that Alport's disease can often not be excluded. Unfortunately several very recent studies of ultrastructural changes, and of tissue binding of anti-glomerular basement membrane antisera, in hereditary nephritis also fail to distinguish between families with and without an associated perceptive deafness. Some authors add to the confusion by referring to a specific ultrastructural abnormality of the glomerular basement membrane, seen in Alport's disease but also in some cases of pure hereditary nephritis, as 'Alport-like' (Jenis *et al.* 1981).

The earliest reported families were those of Samelsohn (1874) and of Dickinson (1875). Samelsohn described two brothers in their fifties and the 19-year-old son of the younger, all with proteinuria and chronic nephritis. Dickinson reported a family in which 12 out of 16 members, over three generations, had proteinuria and there had been several early deaths from Bright's disease. There was a single instance of male-to-male transmission.

These and other similar early reports (Tyson 1881; Kidd 1882; Meigs 1883; Guthrie 1897; Eichhorst 1899; Pel 1899; Atlee 1901; Frölich 1906; Mitchell 1930; Morin *et al.* 1958; Marie *et al.* 1960, families 5–7; Whalen *et al.* 1961, Case B; Hobolth 1963, family I; Bodalski and Margolis 1966, family I; Urbanczyk 1969) support an autosomal dominant mode of inheritance in most such families. Pel's two families in particular have several clear instances of male-to-male transmission, and also of unaffected daughters of affected fathers, as do Bodalski and Margolis' and Urbanczyk's single families. However, several of these reports are equally compatible with X-linked dominant inheritance (Morin *et al.* 1958; Marie *et al.* 1960; Whalen *et al.* 1961, Case B; Hobolth 1963), a situation that echoes that in relation to the inheritance of Alport's disease. A minority of families are suggestive of autosomal recessive inheritance. Rinkoff and associates (1939) reported familial glomerulonephritis in three out of four brothers who each died in their twenties after a brief period of renal failure with a histological picture of glomerulonephritis. Repeated investigation of the parents and a surviving brother and sister showed no renal abnormality. Joshi (1968) described three brothers, including a twin pair, with a mixed glomerulo-, pyelo-, and interstital nephritis. Two of the brothers died in renal failure aged 30 and 24 years. None of the three were deaf but no audiometry was undertaken. Another family with possible autosomal recessive inheritance is that of Albert and coworkers (1969) who described two sisters and a brother with nephritis, one of whom developed nephrotic syndrome. The parents were apparently normal and unrelated, but two otherwise unaffected brothers had congenital cataracts. As with Rinkoff's and Joshis' families none of the family were deaf. Clark (1951) described two families in which several sibs had pyelonephritis but there was no evidence to support a genetic basis for the familial occurrence. Extensive bibliographies of these and other early reports are given by Antonovych and colleagues (1969), and by Royer and others (1970).

More recent studies, whilst providing data on the results of new methods of investigation, have done little to clarify the pathogenesis and genetics of hereditary nephritis, which remain as confused as those of Alport's disease. Indeed it is not even clear whether or not the continued separation of Alport's disease and pure hereditary nephritis remains valid. However, this is an empirically useful distinction for the time being and will be maintained in this monograph. The degree of heterogeneity, or common aetiology, of the hereditary nephritides will become clear only when they have been elucidated at the molecular level. For the present a working classification of pure hereditary nephritis is presented in Table 7.2.

Although the presenting symptom in most cases of Alport's disease is haematuria the picture in pure hereditary nephritis is more variable with

Table 7.2 *A provisional classification of pure hereditary nephritis*

Syndrome	GBM Ultrastructure	Inheritance	References
A. Glomerulo- or mixed nephritis of			
1. Acute or insidious onset[1]:	(a) ABN	AD	Gaboardi et al. (1974) families 9 and 13
	(b) ABN	AD or XD[2]	Gaboardi et al. (1974) families 7 and 15–18.
	(c) ABN	XD	O'Neill et al. (1978) family C.
	(d) N	AD	Grünefeld et al. (1973) family 9.
	(e) N	AD or XD	Grünefeld et al. (1973) families 7, 8, and 10–13.
	(f) ?	AD	Furhmann (1959); Wasserman et al. (1965); Ben-Ishay et al. (1967).
	(g) ?	AR	Rinkoff et al. (1939); Bohrer et al. (1964).
	(h) ?	AD or XD	Russel and Smith (1959); Whalen et al. (1961). Case B; Bruno and Ober (1964); Walker (1966/1974).
	(i) ?	XD	Hashimoto et al. (1970).
2. Acute onset with evidence of an immune defect:	?	AR	Teisberg et al. (1973); Sobel et al. (1979).

B. Chronic interstital nephritis[3]:	(a) ABN	AD or XD	Grünefeld et al. (1973) family 3.
	(b) ?	AD	Richmond (1981).
	(c) ?	AD or XD	Glaser (1918).
	(d) ?	AR	Barber (1913); Taylor (1920).
C. Infantile haematuria progressing to early chronic nephritis and death	?	AD or XD	Dockhorn (1967).
D. Microscopic haematuria with occassionally impaired renal function	?	AD	Hooft et al. (1962).
E. Chronic glomerulonephritis with development of the GBM lesion late in the course of the disease	ABN	AD	Beathard and Granholm (1977).

Abbreviations: GBM = glomerular basement membrane, ABN = presence of the characteristic lesion of membrane thickening and splitting, N = lacking the characteristic lesion, ? = basement membrane ultrastructure not known, AD = autosomal dominant, XD =X-linked dominant, AR = autosomal recessive.

[1] This and other categories refer to hereditary, not the more common sporadic forms. In this category both acute and insidious onset have been described in different families and this further distinction overlaps with the subcategories listed, creating further heterogeneity.

[2] The abbreviation AD or XD means that in the families described it is not possible to state which of these two modes of inheritance applies.

[3] Although this is listed as a separate category its subcategories are not necessarily distinct from the equivalent ones in category A.

proteinuria, haematuria, both together, or established chronic nephritis as the initial picture. There is also a greater variation in age of onset and severity than in typical Alport's disease, especially in males, sometimes within a single family (Ben-Ishay *et al.* 1967). Nevertheless, as in Alport's disease the nephropathy tends to be more severe in males than in females. One form of presentation is with the relatively acute onset of marked proteinuria, which may progress to chronic nephritis (Ben-Ishay *et al.* 1967; Teisburg *et al.* 1973; Grottum *et al.* 1975) or to nephrotic syndrome (Bohrer *et al.* 1964; Churg and Sherman 1973; Kobierska-Szezepanska *et al.* 1974). Only Teisberg's group excluded deafness by audiometry. They also produced evidence of *in vivo* and *in vitro* activation of the third component of complement and suggested an immune defect as the cause. A similar immune deficiency mechanism was proposed by Sobel and coworkers (1979) for a family with hereditary C2 deficiency associated with glomerulonephritis. Ben-Ishay's family shows a pattern of segregation suggestive of autosomal dominant inheritance with incomplete penetrance. Recessive inheritance is suggested by the families of Teisberg, who studied three affected sibs, and of Bohrer with two pairs of identical twins. In one family reported by Gagnon and colleagues (1963) chromosomal mosaicism was detected in several affected members. Since this study predates the techniques for chromosome banding it is difficult to interpret.

Another presentation is with chronic nephritis with more or less rapid progression to renal failure (Rinkoff *et al.* 1939; Fuhrmann, 1959; Russell and Smith 1959; Bohrer *et al.* 1964; Bruno and Ober 1964; Wasserman *et al.* 1965, families L and D; Walker 1966/1974; Hashimoto *et al.* 1970; Churg and Sherman 1973; Grünefeld *et al.* 1973, cases 7–13; Gaboardi *et al.* 1974, families 7, 9, 13, and 15–18; O'Neil *et al.* 1978). This form may also occasionally progress to nephrotic syndrome (Bruno and Ober 1964; Knepshield *et al.* 1968). Audiometry was undertaken in Fuhrmann's family but is not reported in most of the other cases. Wasserman and colleagues (1965) demonstrated that in their families, with either Alport's disease or pure hereditary nephritis, there was no activation of serum complement, in contrast to patients with postinfectious glomerulonephritis and the group of patients with hereditary nephritis of acute onset discussed above. Male-to-male transmission and the presence of unaffected daughters of affected fathers confirm autosomal dominant inheritance in Fuhrmann's family, and also in family D of Wasserman and colleagues, family 9 of Grünefeld and associates, and families 9 and 13 of Gaboardi and coworkers. In contrast, in the family reported by Hashimoto and colleagues (1970) the pattern of transmission strongly suggests X-linked dominant inheritance, as is also the case for family C of O'Neill and colleagues (1978). The pattern in the remaining families is compatible with either autosomal or X-linked dominant inheritance.

Whether chronic interstitial nephritis occurring in families is distinct from hereditary glomerular nephritis is debatable. There have been several reports of interstitial nephritis affecting sibs with normal parents, suggesting autosomal recessive inheritance (Brill and Libman 1899; Barber 1913; Taylor 1920). However, this type of hereditary nephritis is not necessarily recessive. As early as 1918 Glaser described interstitial chronic nephritis in a mother and her two daughters. Case 3 of Grünefeld and colleagues (1973) demonstrates dominant, either autosomal or X-linked, inheritance. Richmond and associates (1981) recently described a family in which several affected individuals presented in adult life with hypertension, proteinuria, and a renal biopsy picture of interstitial nephritis with secondary glomerular atrophy. Men and women were equally severely affected and inheritance appeared to be autosomal dominant. The family of Hellendall (1897) is more difficult to interpret. He described two sisters, out of a family of eight children, who died aged 2 years and 6 months respectively with chronic interstitial nephritis, established at autopsy. Their mother was investigated at the age of 36 years for recurring episodes of oedema, especially during pregnancy, and found to have proteinuria, urinary casts, and epithelial cells, and was diagnosed as having chronic nephritis.

An exceptional family is that of Dockhorn (1967) in which the presenting feature, in infancy, was haematuria which progressed to early death from chronic nephritis. Audiometry excluded deafness. A further group presenting with haematuria and difficult to distinguish from benign familial haematuria comprises families in which affected members have haematuria for the most part with normal renal function, but one or a few show some impairment of function. An example is the family reported by Hooft and colleagues (1962) in which a girl, her father, and two other close paternal relatives had microscopic haematuria, but her brother had gross haematuria with some impairment of renal function.

Another example, which is difficult to classify, is the family described by Rome and coworkers (1966) in which 17 members in three generations had haematuria, with or without proteinuria. Renal biopsies showed minimal changes on light microscopy but irregular thickening of the lamina densa of the glomerular basement membrane on electron microscopy. There was no hearing loss on audiometry apart from one subject with an acquired unilateral loss. There were, however, lens opacities in four affected females. The pedigree does not permit distinction between autosomal and X-linked dominant inheritance. The authors suggest that this family have Alport's disease but the evidence presented does not bear this out.

A further family which cannot be readily classified is that of Wallace and Jones (1960). They reported a family in which two brothers and a sister died with glomerulonephritis. All three sibs, along with two other brothers and both parents all without nephritis, also had a generalized aminoaciduria. There was no mention of hearing defect. The authors propose that an inherited defect producing the aminoaciduria also pre-disposes to glomerulonephritis, but there is no further evidence to support this hypothesis.

Several groups have undertaken ultrastructural studies of patients from families with hereditary nephritis, with or without deafness. They have demonstrated the presence of thickening and splitting of the glomerular basement membrane in kidneys from some patients with pure hereditary nephritis similar to those seen in Alport's disease, but not in others. Grünefeld and colleagues (1973) observed such changes in five Alport's disease and one pure hereditary nephritis family, but no such changes in seven further such families. Churg and Sherman (1973) likewise were unable to detect the characteristic basement membrane splitting of Alport's disease in eight patients from families lacking deafness. Gaboardi and coworkers (1974) on the other hand found specific glomerular basement membrane abnormalities in all of four Alport's disease and four pure hereditary nephritic families. Similar changes were reported by O'Neill and associates (1978) in one very large family with Alport's disease, the original Utah family of Stephens and Perkoff, and also in a new large family with pure hereditary nephritis (their family C). Their genetic analysis of both of these families indicates dominant inheritance and is strongly suggestive of X linkage. All of these groups of workers agree that the ultrastructural glomerular changes are consistent within any one family.

An unusual family with pure hereditary nephritis was reported by Beathard and Granholm (1977) in which the basement membrane lesion developed late in the course of the disease, and only in some affected members. Inheritance was autosomal dominant with male-to-male transmission.

It is clear from these studies that glomerular basement membrane splitting is not specific to a single gene defect. It remains an open question as to whether or not patients with apparently pure hereditary nephritis and glomerular basement membrane splitting may in fact have Alport's disease without expression of deafness in them or their affected relatives. Families in which there is hereditary nephritis, but perceptive deafness only in relatives without nephropathy, also present a diagnostic problem.

The overall incidence of uncomplicated hereditary nephritis is difficult to assess. Some earlier workers, such as Osman (1927) who found a history of nephritis among relatives of index patients in over 25 per cent of his families, may have been observing multiple occurrence of non-hereditary glomerulonephritis within families. This was indeed subsequently reported, often with evidence of streptococcal infection, by several groups (Eason *et al.* 1924; Ernstene and Robb 1931; Ellenberg and Martin 1940; Tudor 1943; Goldsmith *et al.* 1958; Dodge *et al.* 1967). Dodge and colleagues (1967) in a study of 20 children with acute glomerulonephritis, proved on renal biopsy, found proved or suspected acute nephritis in 19 out of 91 sib contacts. Whilst this may well suggest familial predisposition, it is certainly not hereditary nephritis.

References

Albert, M. S., Leeming, J. M. and Wigger, H. J. (1969). Familial nephritis associated with the nephrotic syndrome in a family with severe involvement in females. *Am. J. Dis. Child.* **117**, 153–5.

Antonovych, T. T., Deasy, P. F., Tina, L. U., D'Albora, J. B., Hollerman, C. E. and Calcagno, P. L. (1969). Hereditary nephritis: early clinical, functional, and morphological studies. *Pediatr. Res.* **3**, 545–56.

Atlee, W. H. W. (1901). Three cases of recurrent haematuria occurring in one family. *St Bart. Hosp. J.* **9**, 41–2.

Barber, H. (1913). Chronic interstitial nephritis in children: a brother and sister affected. *Br. Med. J.* **2**, 1204–5.

Beathard, G. A. and Granholm, N. A. (1977). Development of the characteristic ultrastructural lesion of hereditary nephritis during the course of the disease. *Am. J. Med.* **62**, 751–6.

Ben-Ishay, D., Biran, S. and Ullmann, T. D. (1967). Familial nephritis. *Israel J. Med. Sci.* **3**, 106–12.

Bodalski, J. and Margolis, A. (1966). Nefropatia rodzinna. *Ped. Pol.* **41**, 836–41.

Bohrer, N., Churg, J. and Gribetz, D. (1964). Glomerulonephritis in two sets of twins. *Am. J. Med.* **36**, 787–94.

Brill, N. E. and Libman, E. (1899). A contribution to the subjects of chronic interstitial nephritis and arteritis in the young and family nephritis; with a note on calcification in the liver. *J. Exp. Med.* **4**, 541–57.

Bruno, M. S. and Ober, W. B. (eds.) (1964). Clinicopathologic Conference. Proteinuria and haematuria in an adolescent. *NY State J. Med.* **64**, 2783–9.

Churg, J. and Sherman, R. L. (1973). Pathologic characteristics of hereditary nephritis. *Arch. Pathol.* **95**, 374–9.

Clark, N. S. (1951). Familial renal insufficiency. *Arch. Dis. Child.* **26**, 351–7.

Dickinson, W. H. (1875). *Disease of the kidney and urinary derangements.* Part 2. p. 379. Longmans Green, London.

Dockhorn, R. J. (1967). Hereditary nephropathy without deafness. *Am. J. Dis. Child.* **114**, 135–8.

Dodge, W. F., Spargo, B. H. and Travis, L. B. (1967). Occurrence of acute glomerulonephritis in sibling contacts of children with sporadic acute glomerulonephritis. *Pediatrics* **40**, 1028–30.

Eason, J., Smith, G. L. M. and Buchanan, G. (1924). Hereditary and familial nephritis. *Lancet* 2, 639–46.

Eichhorst, (1899). Cited by Senator, H. Erkrankungen der Nieren, in *Specielle Pathologie und Therapie*, Vol. 19, ed. Nothnagel, H. p. 249. Holder, Vienna.

Ellenberg, S. L. and Martin, A. T. (1940). Acute nephritis simultaneously affecting three siblings. *Arch. Pediatr.* 57, 38–42.

Ernstene, A. C. and Robb, G. P. (1931). Familial epidemic of acute diffuse glomerulonephritis. *JAMA* 97, 1382–3.

Frölich, T. (1906). Zwei Fälle von hereditärer, familiärer, kongenitaler (?) nephritis. *Jahrb. f. Kinderheilk.* 64, 244.

Fuhrmann, W. (1959). Ein erbliches Nieron leiden mit dem Leitsymptom der Hämaturie. *Z. Kinderheilk.* 82, 514–25.

Gaboardi, F., Edefonti, A., Imbasciati, E., Tarantino, A., Mihatsch, M. J. and Zollinger, H. U. (1974). Alport's syndrome (progressive hereditary nephritis). *Clin. Nephrol.* 2, 143–56.

Gagnon, J., Archambault, L., Ducharme, J. R. and Katyk-Longtin, N. (1963). Résultats préliminaires sur une étude cytogénétique d'une famille affecté de néphropathie. *Rev. Canad. Biol.* 22, 133–6.

Glaser, F. (1918). Uber juvenile primäre Schrumpfniere. *Jahrb. f. Kinderheilk.* 87, 95–108.

Goldsmith, H. J., Cowan, M. A. and Gooder, E. (1958). Familial outbreak of acute glomerulonephritis due to Griffith type 1 steptococcus. *Lancet* 2, 674–5.

Grottum, K. A., Flatmark, A., Myhre, E., Jansen, H., Teisberg, P., Oystese, B., Husby, G. and Hovin, T. (1975). Immunological hereditary nephropathy. *Acta Med. Scand.* 197, Suppl. 571, 28.

Grünefeld, J.-P., Bois, E. P. and Hinglais, N. (1973). Progressive and non-progressive hereditary chronic nephritis. *Kidney Int.* 4, 216–28.

Guthrie, L. G. (1897). Chronic interstitial nephritis in childhood. *Lancet* 1, 585, 728.

Hashimoto, Y., Mori, M., Kanazawa, I., Ishikawa, T., Tanaka, T., Dofuku, R., Kinugasa, K. and Sekiguti, T. (1970). Hereditary familial nephritis (complete sex-linked dominant inheritance) the first report: the genetic study (in Japanese). *J. Jap. Soc. Int. Med.* 59, 41–6.

Hellendall, H. (1897). Hereditäre Schrumpfniere in frühen Kindesalter. *Arch. f. Kinderheilk.* 22, 61–74.

Hobolth, N. (1963). Hereditary nephropathy with haematuria. *Acta Paediatr. (Stockh.)* 52, 581–7.

Hooft, C., van Acker, K. and Verbeek, J. (1962). Familiale hematurie. *Maandschrift voor Kindergeneeskunde* 30, 357–68.

Jenis, E. H., Valeski, J. E. and Calcagno, P. L. (1981). Variability of anti-GBM findings in hereditary nephritis. *Clin. Nephrol.* 15, 111–14.

Joshi, V. V. (1968). Pathology of hereditary nephritis. *J. Clin. Pathol.* 21, 744–7.

Kidd, J. (1882). The inheritance of Bright's disease of the kidney. *Practitioner* 29, 104–14.

Knepshield, J. H., Roberts, P. L., Davis, C. J. and Moser, R. H. (1968). Hereditary chronic nephritis complicated by nephrotic syndrome. *Arch. Intern. Med.* 122, 156–8.

Kobierska-Szezepanska, A., Jonczyk, K. and Dziuba, P. (1974). Nefropatia rodzinna na podstawie przypadkow obserwowanych w I Klinice Pediatric w Zabrzu. *Pol. Tyg. Lek.* 29, 233–4.

Marie, J., Royer, P., Habib, R., Mathieu, H. and Reveillaud, R.-J. (1960). La néphropathie hématurique héréditaire avec surdité. *Ann. de Pédiatrie* **36**, 84–103.

Meigs, A. V. (1883). Clinical observations on albuminuria, based upon study of 62 cases seen in private practice. *Tr. Coll. Physicians, Philadelphia.* **6**, 163–79.

Mitchell, A. G. (1930). Nephrosclerosis (chronic interstitial nephritis) in childhood, with special reference to renal rickets. *Am. J. Dis. Child.* **40**, 101–45, 345–88.

Morin, M., Graveleau, J., Schimmel, H., Gremy, F. and Testard, R. (1958). Néphropathie hématuirique familiale. *Sem. Hôp. Paris.* **34**, 907–15.

O'Neill, W. M., Atkin, C. L. and Bloomer, H. A. (1978). Hereditary nephritis: a re-examination of its clinical and genetic features. *Ann. Intern. Med.* **88**, 176–82.

Osman, A. A. (1972). The constitutional factor in disease. *Br. Med. J.* **1**, 938.

Pel, P. K. (1899). Die Erblichkeit der chronischen Nephritis. *Z. Klin. Med.* **38**, 127–39.

Richmond, J. M., Whitworth, J. A. and Kincaid-Smith, P. S. (1981). Familial interstitial nephritis. *Clin. Nephrol.* **16**, 109–13.

Rinkoff, S. S., Stern, A. and Schumer, H. (1939). Familial nephritis. Report of cases and review of literature. *JAMA* **113**, 661–4.

Rome, L., Cuppage, F. E., Vertes, V. (1966). Familial hematuric nephritis. *Pediatrics* **38**, 808–18.

Royer, P., Frezal, J., Bois, E. and Feingold, J. (1970). Les néphropathies héréditaires. *Arch. Fr. Pédiatr.* **27**, 293–317.

Russell, E. P. and Smith, N. J. (1959). Hereditary hematuria. *Am. J. Dis. Child.* **98**, 353–8.

Samelsohn, F. (1874). Über hereditäre Nephritis und über den Hereditätsbegriff im Allgemeinen. *Virchow's Arch. f. Pathol. Anatom.* **59**, 257–69.

Sobel, A. T., Moisy, G., Hirbec, G. (1979). Hereditary C2 deficiency associated with non-systemic glomerulonephritis. *Clin. Nephrol.* **12**, 132–6.

Taylor, R. (1920). Chronic interstitial nephritis in children. *Minnesota Med.* **3**, 481–5.

Teisberg, P., Grottum, K. A., Myhre, E. and Flatmark, A. (1973). *In vivo* activation of complement in hereditary nephropathy. *Lancet* **2**, 356–8.

Tudor, R. B. (1943). Acute glomerulonephritis occurring in three children in the same family. *Am. J. Dis. Child.* **66**, 528–30.

Tyson, J. (1881). *A treatise of Bright's disease and diabetes.* p. 166. Lindsay & Blakiston, Philadelphia.

Urbanczyk, J. (1969). Rodzinne, dziedzicne zapalenie nerek. *Wiad. Lek.* **22**, 1881–4.

Walker, W. G. (1966/74). Personal communications quoted by McKusick, V. A. (1978). *Mendelian inheritance in man*, 5th edn. pp. 20, 272. Johns Hopkins University Press.

Wallace, I. R. and Jones, J. H. (1960). Familial glomerulonephritis and aminoaciduria. *Lancet* **1**, 941–4.

Wasserman, E., Schwarz, F., Wachstein, M. and Lange, K. (1965). Diagnostic value of serum complement determination in hereditary glomerulonephritis. *J. Lab. Clin. Med.* **65**, 589–99.

Whalen, R. E., Huang, S., Peschel, E. and McIntosh, H. D. (1961). Hereditary nephropathy, deafness and renal foam cells. *Am. J. Med.* **31**, 171–86.

7.4. HEREDITARY NEPHRITIS WITH DEAFNESS (ALPORT'S DISEASE)

7.4.1. Introduction

In 1927 A. C. Alport gave the first clear description of the disease that now bears his name. It is of historical interest that in his paper he acknowledged the assistance of A. E. Garrod for urine investigations and of Alexander Fleming for bacteriological studies on his family. This family had been the subject of several earlier papers (Guthrie 1902; Kendall and Hertz 1912; Hurst 1923; Eason *et al.* 1924). Guthrie did not comment on the presence of deafness and, at the time of his observations, did not observe symptoms more serious than haematuria. By the time Kendall and Hertz studied the family a decade later the nephritic nature of the disorder was apparent. When Hurtz, who had by then anglicized his name to Hurst, gave a further report on the family, after the passage of another decade, a third generation had become involved and there had been further deaths. He noted on his pedigree that three of the patients were deaf but makes no further comment on this point. Eason and coworkers (1924) provided further details of the third generation, and drew attention to the severe course of the disease with early death in males and its relatively benign course in females. Alport, who at the time of writing was first assistant at the Medical Unit, St Mary's Hospital, London and shortly after became the first holder of the chair of medicine at Cairo University, made the important contribution of recognizing that the nerve deafness from which several affected members suffered was an integral part of the disease. Like Hurst he also recognized its hereditary nature. It is an indication of the lethality of the disorder in males that a reinvestigation of the family 40 years later revealed no new cases (Crawfurd and Toghill 1968).

Following Alport's paper there were no new case reports until Perkoff and Stephens and their colleagues published a detailed study of a large Mormon family from Utah (Perkoff *et al.* 1951; Stephens *et al.* 1951; Perkoff *et al.* 1958). Taking their two studies reported in 1951 and 1958 together 90 members of their family had had renal disease, typically a chronic interstitial nephritis or pyelonephritis, or carried the trait. Of 44 of those examined by the authors in their earlier study, seven out of 15 males had died of the disease but none of 29 females. The predominant urinary findings were proteinuria, haematuria, pyuria, and casts. Eighty-six members of the family had audiograms, and 15 of the affected members, all but one male, had progressive perceptive high tone hearing loss. In addition five apparently unaffected males were also deaf. Post-mortem renal pathology showed contracted kidneys with lymphocytic infiltration of the interstitial connective tissue, and the presence of an excess of foam cells. The pattern of inheritance suggested dominance but few of the affected males had affected fathers and most of the daughters of affected fathers were themselves affected. Perkoff and colleagues interpreted this as evidence for the hitherto purely hypothetical mechanism of partially sex-linked dominant inheritance with crossing-over between X and Y chromosomes, an interpretation that has subsequently been disputed, and was the first of many controversial hypotheses regarding the genetics of this disease. Their family although much larger than Alport's shows essentially similar features. Following their report there has been a steady flow of papers on Alport's disease over the last 30 years, now covering about 200 families, from which a detailed picture of the clinical features and pathology has built up, although the genetics of the disorder has remained controversial. Recent studies have begun to give an insight into the likely pathogenesis of the disorder, and have provided convincing evidence of genetic hetero-geneity. Detailed investigation of this heterogeneity will doubtless be undertaken, in the not too distant future, using recombinant DNA methodology.

7.4.2. Clinical features

The picture presented by the families of Alport, and Perkoff and colleagues, has been confirmed with only minor modifications by subsequent reports. This is essentially of a presentation with haematuria, which may be intermittent and is mostly microscopic but may be macroscopic, proteinuria, and red-cell casts, more severe in males than females. In males the renal disorder progresses to renal failure and death typically in the late teens to early twenties, whereas in females renal failure is postponed to middle life or later. Occasionally patients may first present with renal failure.

A proportion of patients develop a progressive perceptive hearing loss, again more noticeable in males than females, with the severity of hearing loss correlated with that of nephropathy. Subclinical hearing loss may be demonstrated by audiometry, but nevertheless some affected family members with nephropathy, especially females, never develop clinical or audiometric hearing loss. Many families contain some members with hearing loss but no nephropathy, and it is often unclear as to whether such members have the disease or not. This variable penetrance of hearing loss raises the question as to whether in some smaller families apparently pure hereditary nephritis may in fact be due to the Alport gene. Although Alport's disease and pure hereditary nephritis are discussed separately here it remains possible that at least some families of each disorder may be due to identical, or to allelic, mutant genes.

Perkoff and colleagues emphasized the proteinuria, pyuria and casts found in many of their patients and regarded the disease as a familial chronic pyelonephritis. Pyelonephritis, which may or may not be present, has subsequently been regarded as a complication due to secondary infection, although some have suggested that the disease increases susceptibility to infection, especially streptococcal (Poli 1953, 1955; Chappel and Kelsey 1960). A few other authors have emphasized the proteinuria as a presenting or diagnostic sign (Hamburger 1956), but many have given equal emphasis to proteinuria and haematuria (Gobin *et al.* 1958; Ohlsson 1963), and others have laid emphasis on haematuria as being a more specific sign (Reyersbach and Butler 1954; Sturtz and Burke 1956, 1958; Nichol and Miller 1965; Wood and Knight 1966; Maurer *et al.* 1968; Tishler and Rosner 1974; O'Neill *et al.* 1978; Evans *et al.* 1980; Gubler *et al.* 1981). O'Neill and associates (1978) in particular have shown that haematuria, and to a less extent in males red-cell casts, are more reliable indicators of affected individuals in families under investigation than is proteinuria. Proteinuria when present was invariably associated with haematuria. They found pyuria to be a quite unreliable indicator.

However, since microscopic haematuria may be intermittent, especially in females, several tests for haematuria may be necessary before a particular individual can be accepted as not manifesting the disease (Mulrow *et al.* 1963; Pashayan *et al.* 1971; O'Neill *et al.* 1978). Ferguson and Rance (1972) reckoned that affected females in their seven families developed haematuria by the age of 20 years. Nevertheless even with repeated testing there remain some individuals who have transmitted the gene to children but who have given consistently negative results for haematuria or other manifestations of the disease, that is, they remain asymptomatic obligatory heterozygotes. Such failures of penetrance are seen only rarely in males (Poli 1953; Chappel and Kelsy 1960; Shaw and Glover 1961; Cohen *et al.* 1961; Mulrow *et al.* 1963; Ohlsson 1963), but are comparatively common among female hetero-zygotes. Tishler (1979) in a survey of the literature estimated the overall proportion of non-manifesting female heterozygotes at 12.1 per cent, and the proportion did not vary according to either age or the severity of the disease in their affected male relatives. A survey of the literature presented in Table 7.4, for non-ocular families, gives a similar figure of 13.2 per cent, with little variation as between three subgroups for I auto-somal dominant, II X linked dominant and III uncertain inheritance (e.g. I 11.9 per cent, II 13.3 per cent, III 14.6 per cent). The frequency of asymptomatic female heterozygotes is slightly higher for the ocular group of families at 18.6 per cent (Table 7.3), and shows greater variation between subgroups (A 30 per cent, C 7.1 per cent). The existence of such asymptomatic affected females has important genetic implications, both for counselling and for genetic analysis as will be discussed below. Proteinuria remains a useful prognostic sign in known patients as it tends to increase sharply before the onset of renal failure (Gubler *et al.* 1981).

In most patients the predominant protein excreted is albumin but in advanced cases higher molecular weight proteins such as IgG and transferrin may appear in the urine (Hobday and Jones 1969). Protein-uria may exceptionally become sufficiently severe to produce nephrotic syndrome (Kinoshita *et al.* 1969; Zavala *et al.* 1969; Felts 1970; Chazan *et al.* 1971; Schneegans *et al.* 1971; Hinglais *et al.* 1972; Churg and Sherman 1973; Gaboardi *et al.* 1974). There have been several families reported with a more specific aminoaciduria, hyperprolinaemia, and Alport's disease. These are discussed in a later section of this chapter.

A non-specific aminoaciduria may also be observed (Onisawa *et al.* 1965).

Several authors have reported the results of renal function tests in patients (Nieth 1959; Chappel and Kelsey 1960; Rosencranz 1963; White *et al.* 1964; Cassady *et al.* 1965; Onisawa *et al.* 1965; Antonovych *et al.* 1969; Spear *et al.* 1970; Hinglais *et al.* 1972; Grunefeld *et al.* 1973; Kryzmanski *et al.* 1973; Beathard and Granholm 1977). Nieth (1959) reported the results of clearance studies, T_m estimates, phenolsulphtha-lein (PSP) excretion and urine concentration. Rosenkrantz (1963) recorded urine concentration, PSP excretion, inulin and creatine clearance, and urine pH. Cassady and colleagues (1965) reported detailed biochemical studies on blood, creatinine clearance, PSP excretion, urine concentration and constituents, and intravenous pyelography. The other authors mentioned above have described similar combinations of renal function findings. In general clearance rates and PSP excretion have been impaired only in patients in advanced renal failure, often with marked uraemia. Some such patients have also have marked proteinuria but by no means all. Impaired urine-concentrating ability and acidification may precede reduced renal clearance values. Patients with renal failure may also show angiographic changes (Chuang and Reuter 1974).

Since Alport (1927) drew attention to the significance of sensorineural hearing loss in the family studied by him subsequent authors have paid greater or less attention to this aspect. Some papers report the results of audiometric studies. Stephens and colleagues (1951) studied two small groups in their Utah family and found high tone loss or at least a dip in the audiogram at 4096 cycles per second (c.p.s). The milder changes were observed in the younger members of the family and hearing defect was limited to males. Onset of hearing loss is invariably insidious. Their

Table 7.3 *Published pedigrees of families with Alport's disease with lenticular and/or macular ocular lesions*

Ocular lesions present and mode of inheritance	Proportion of affected subjects with ocular lesions	Proportion of affected subjects with hearing loss	Mean age of death of affected males (range)	Proportion of asymptomatic obligate female heterozygotes	Ratio of affected males to females	Offspring of affected parents								References
						Fathers				Mothers				
						AS	US	AD	UD	AS	US	AD	UD	
Autosomal dominant (A)														
Cataracts	2/83	5/38	—	4/12 (2/2)[1]	12:26	2	3	1	3	8	10	25	18	Shaw and Glover (1961).
Lens opacities	2/5[2]	3/5[2]	27	0/2	3:2	2	0	0	0	0	0	1	2	Junod (1963) and Perrin (1964) [fam. Tr]
Lens abnormality	1/7	6/7	—	0/0	8:5	3	1	1	1	2	0	2	1	Symboulidis et al. (1968) [fam. 4]
Macular change	4/26	11/26	20 (11–24)	1/4	14:12	1	5	2	5	2	8	1	7	Purriel et al. (1970) [fam. 1]
Macular change	1/8	1/8	—	1/1 (1/3)	6:2[3]	5	6	1	12	0	0	0	0	Purriel et al. (1970) [fam. 2]
Macular change	3/20	8/20	20 (15–23)	2/7	8:12	1	3	1	2	8	5	0	9	Purriel et al. (1970) [fam. 4]
Unspecified	3/39	5/39	43[14] (37–48)	1/4	18:21	9	23	16	12	2	23	4	14	Goldman and Haberfelde (1959); Kenya et al. (1977) [fam. C]
Totals	16/143	39/143		9/30	69:80	23	41	22	35	22	46	33	51	
Probable X-linked dominant (B)														
Stellate cataract	1/6	6/6	26 (23–30)	0/1	3:3	0	1	2	0	3	0	0	0	Lachhein et al. (1969)

Autosomal or X-linked dominant (C)

	4/22	14/22	18 (13–29)	0/9	16:10	0	2	0	0	14	4	6	8	
Cataracts														Reyersbach and Butler (1954) [fam. M] Case Records Massachussetts General Hospital (1957) Robin *et al.* (1957) [fam. 1]
Spherophakia and posterior cataract	4/8	7/8	23 (22–24)	0/1	6:2	0	0	0	0	4	0	1	2	Sohar (1954, 1956)
Anterior cortical cataract	1/4	2/4	7½ (5–10)	0/1	3:1	0	0	0	0	3	0	0	0	Goldbloom *et al.* (1957)
Keratoconus	1/6	4/6	28 (17–36)	0/1	4:2	0	0	0	0	4	9	2	6	Nieth (1959)
Cataracts, posterior	1/2	1/2	21	–	2:0	–	–	–	–	–	–	–	–	Whalen *et al.* (1961) [fam. A]
Anterior lenticonus	2/3	3/3	25 (24–26)	–	3:0	–	–	–	–	–	–	–	–	Mettier (1961) [fam. 1]
Anterior lenticonus	2/5	2/5	28 (23–33)	0/1	3:2	0	0	0	0	0	0	1	0	Mettier (1961) [fam. 2]
Anterior lenticonus	4/23	11/23	–	–	–	–	–	–	–	–	–	–	–	Howe and Smythe (1962)
Anterior lenticonus	2/4	3/4	21 (17–25)	0/1	1:3	0	0	0	0	1	0	2	0	Junod (1963) [fam. Ab] Perrin (1964)
Anterior and posterior lenticonus	2/2	1/2	–	0/1	1:1	0	0	0	0	1	0	0	1	Junod (1963) [fam. Bon]

Table 7.3.—*Continued*

Ocular lesions present and mode of inheritance	Proportion of affected subjects with ocular lesions	Proportion of affected subjects with hearing loss	Mean age of death of affected males (range)	Proportion of asymptomatic obligate female heterozygotes	Ratio of affected males to females	Offspring of affected parents								References
						Fathers				Mothers				
						AS	US	AD	UD	AS	US	AD	UD	
Right lens rupture and left anterior cataract	1/1	1/1	17	0/0	1:0	0	0	0	0	0	0	0	0	McKennan Hospital Clinical-Pathological Conference (1963) Greg and Becker (1963)
Anterior and posterior lenticonus and anterior subcapsular catacacts or opacities	6/7	3/7	19	1/1^5	4:3	0	0	0	0	4	1	2	2	Brownell and Wolter (1964)
Bilateral anterior and left posterior lenticonus	1/1	1/1	—	—	1:0	0	0	0	0	0	0	0	0	Asperti (1964)
Anterior or posterior lenticonus	3/8	6/8	19½ (18–22)	1/3	6:2	0	0	0	0	6	6	1	3	Arnott *et al.* (1966)
Anterior lenticonus or cataract	2/8	4/8	—	0/2	5:3	0	0	0	0	5	3	2	2	Symboulidis *et al.* (1968) [fam. 1]

Eye abnormality														Reference
Cataract	1/3	3/3	0/0	—[4]	1:2	0	0	0	0	0	1	1	0	1	Symboulidis *et al.* (1968) [fam. 3]
Cataract	2/4	1/4	0/1	57	3:1	0	0	0	0	1	2	2	0	0	Symboulidis *et al.* (1968) [fam. 6]
Lenticonus and cataract	1/3	2/3	0/1	—	1:2	0	0	0	0	1	0	0	2	1	Symboulidis *et al.* (1968) [fam. 7]
Cataracts	2/16	4/16	0/4	19	5:11	0	0	0	0	5	7	7	10	7	Grace *et al.* (1970)
Lens opacities and macular changes	2/2	2/2	0/0	—	1:1	0	0	0	0	0	0	0	0	0	Hinglais *et al.* (1972) [Cases 7 & 8]
Anterior lenticonus	2/2	2/2	0/0	—	0:2	0	0	0	0	0	0	0	0	0	Grunefeld *et al.* (1973) [fam. 6]
Cataract and macular changes	1/3	1/7	0/1	—	1:2	0	0	0	0	1	0	1	1	0	Polak and Hogewind (1977) [fam. 1]
Total	47/141	78/141	2/28		68:50	0	2	0	0	51	33	33	30	33	
Grand total	64/290	123/290	11/59		140:133	27	44	24	35	76	79	63	84		

Abbreviations; AS = affected son, US = unaffected son, AD = affected daughter, UD = unaffected daughter, — = information not given.

[1] Figures in brackets = proportion of asymptomatic obligate male heterozygotes
[2] Excluding three uncertainly affected males
[3] Including one asymptomatic male and one male with deafness but without nephropathy
[4] Indicates the presence of surviving affected males over the age of 30 years
[5] A female with lens defect only

report highlights one of the problems in studying deafness in Alport's disease families, namely the occurrence of deafness unrelated to the disease, in that otosclerosis was segregating independently within the family. Sohar (1956) published an audiogram on one of four affected brothers, said to be typical of all four, showing hearing loss in air and bone maximal at 2000–8000 c.p.s. with a loss in that range of 70–80 decibels (dB). Other authors have published audiograms showing similar medium to high tone loss, mostly as in the study of Stephens and colleagues maximal around 4000 c.p.s., and with a loss frequently of the order of 70–80 dB or more (Bouchet and Paquelin 1956; Flower 1964; Tiliakos *et al.* 1964; Chaptal *et al.* 1965; Johnson and Hagan 1965; Nichol and Miller 1965; Winter *et al.* 1968). Although most of these reports concern affected males some do show similar medium to high tone hearing loss in females (Flower 1964; Nichol and Miller 1965). Yet others have reported similar audiometric findings without actually publishing audiograms (Sturtz and Burke 1956; Cassady *et al.* 1965; Crawfurd and Toghill 1968; Chazan *et al.* 1971; Hinglais *et al.* 1972).

Cassady and colleagues found audiometric evidence of hearing defect in just over half of their patients with renal disease. Progressive deterioration of hearing on audiometry in individual male patients has also been reported (Klotz 1959; Gregg and Becker, 1963; McKennan Hospital Clinical–Pathological Conference 1963; Beaudoing *et al.* 1970). Typically hearing loss has an onset in the second decade in males and later in females, but there is considerable variation and its detection in infancy has been reported (Mamou 1966). Temporal bone pathology has been examined postmortem from patients with sensorineural hearing loss. In one case involving a 22-year-old male with at least 10 years hearing loss the principal changes were a reduction in the spiral ganglion cells of the basal turn of about a half, some degeneration of spiral nerves supplying the basal turns, and vesicle formation in the spiral ligament of each basal turn and under each utricular macule. The tectorial membrane, organ of Corti, and Reissner's membrane were all normal (Winter *et al.* 1968). Similar changes including atrophy of spiral ganglion cells in the basal turns had been previously described in two affected brothers (Minder *et al.* 1965). Other authors have reported more drastic changes including degeneration of hair cells and of the stria vascularis, with absence of the tectorial membrane (Gregg and Becker 1963; McKennan Hospital Clinical–Pathological Conference, 1963), or even absence or atrophy of the organ of Corti with collapse or Reisnner's membrane (Crawfurd and Toghill 1968; Lachhein *et al.* 1969). It is unclear as to whether these more severe changes reflect the true pathology of the inner ear lesion or are artefactual. Turner (1970) reported audiometric screening on 92 members of three Alport's disease families, aged 5 to over 50 years, with more detailed audiometric examination of 54 of these subjects (22 males and 32 females). He observed a drop in sensitivity at 6000 c.p.s., probably significant for females over the age of 15 years. The reason for this rather higher peak of hearing loss than obtained in earlier studies is unclear. An analysis of 147 published families (Tables 7.3 and 7.4) shows that deafness, assessed by clinical history or audiometry, was present in 35 per cent (495 out of 1419) of family members with renal disease. Among families with male-to-male transmission the proportion is 30 per cent (229/753), and among those strongly suggestive of X-linked dominance only 22 per cent (57/255). Among the families that could be either autosomal or X-linked dominant as many as 51 per cent (209/407) were deaf. These figures are very crude and not too much should be read into these differences.

Another important clinical abnormality found in some affected members of a minority of families is an ocular defect. Earlier observations were of lens defects, most characteristically anterior (Goldbloom *et al.* 1957; Mettier 1961; Howe and Smythe 1962; Gregg and Becker 1963; Junod 1963, Fam. Ab.; Arnott *et al.* 1966; Hinglais *et al.* 1972; Grunefeld *et al.* 1973; Nielsen 1978; Farboody *et al.* 1979, families 11 and 15; Perrin *et al.* 1980; Gubler *et al.* 1981; Habib *et al.* 1982), or less commonly anterior and posterior lenticonus (Junod 1963, family Bon; Asperti 1964; Brownell and Wolter 1964; Perrin 1964). Other lens abnormalities described include cataracts, especially anterior or posterior subcapsular cataracts (Reyersbach and Butler 1954; Goldbloom *et al.* 1957; Robin *et al.* 1957; Shaw and Glover 1961; Whalen *et al.* 1961, family A; Junod 1963, family Tr; Brownell and Wolter 1964; Symboulidis *et al.* 1968; Lachhein *et al.* 1969; Felts 1970; Grace *et al.* 1970; Purriel 1970; Hinglais *et al.* 1972; Farboody *et al.* 1979, family 22), spherophakia (Sohar 1954, 1956; Goldbloom *et al.* 1957; Farboody *et al.* 1979, family 10), and keratoconus (Nieth 1959). In the patient reported by Gregg and Becker (1963), and also in the McKennan Hospital Clinical–Pathological Conference (1963), the lens lesion was associated with a rupture of the capsule on the right and extrusion of the lens contents. Farboody and colleagues (1979), reporting on 23 families with hereditary nephritis, recorded hearing loss in 17 of these families. Lens defects were present in four of these 17 families, lenticonus in two families, spherophakia in one, and cataracts in the fourth. Arnott and colleagues (1966) reviewed the literature on anterior lenticonus and found that it almost invariably occurs in males, only three cases in a female having been reported, and that, out of 30 cases previously reported, other than those recognized as being associated with Alport's disease, five were in patients with nephritis (Jaworski 1910; Kienecker 1929; Tsukahara 1930; Ehrlich 1946; Unger 1957). A further example

Table 7.4 *Published pedigrees of families with Alport's disease without lenticular or macular lesions*

Mode of inheritance	Mean age at death of affected subjects with (range) – male	Mean age at death – female	Proportion of affected subjects with hearing loss	Proportion of asymptomatic obligate female heterozygotes	Ratio of affected males to females	Offspring of affected parents – Fathers AS	US	AD	UD	Mothers AS	US	AD	UD	References
Autosomal dominant (1)														
	—	—	3/28	3/18 (1/17)[1]	17:18	5	5	3	5	12	9	8	10	Poli (1953, 1955)
	—	17 (15–21)	—	0/1	11:6	3	3	5	4	3	3	1	0	Robin et al. (1957) [fam. 2]
	—	—	1/11	0/1 (1/1)[1]	4:7	1	0	0	0	3	7	6	0	Chappel and Kelsey (1960) [fam. 1]
	—	—	12/46	0/13	20:26	1	2	4	1	18	9	15	12	Cohen et al. (1961) [fam. 2] Cassady et al. (1965) [fam. M]
	—	—	18/43	0/15 (3/9)[1]	15:28	3	7	6	3	5	9	14	12	Cohen et al. (1961) [fam. 3] Cassady et al. (1965) [fam. H]
	—	—	7/23	1/11	8:15	1	3	2	3	5	12	7	3	Cohen et al. (1961) [fam. 4] Cassady et al. (1965) [fam. C]
	—	—	26/88	4/26 (3/22)[1]	37:51	12	28	19	16	17	32	22	23	Cohen et al. (1961) [fam. 5] Cassady et al. (1965) [fam. K]
	39.5 (26–50)	—	5/32	3/6 (1/7)[1]	13:19	1	7	13	6	11	4	6	3	Mulrow et al. (1963)
	29	—	3/8	0/3	4:4	1	1	1	0	3	2	1	1	Giacomelli (1963)
	—	—	4/6	0/1	2:4	1	0	2	2	0	0	0	2	Ellis and Yaffe (1964)
	36 (13–55)	36 (11–52)	7/9	0/3	4:5	1	1	0	2	2	7	5	3	Tiliakos (1964) [fam. A]
	—	27[2] (21–35)	4/14	0/3	5:9	1	6	2	6	4	0	6	2	Tiliakos et al. (1964) [fam. B]
	—	—[2]	4/15	4/5	9:6	1	3	1[3]	2	7	3	4	4	Flower (1964) [fam. M]
	—	—[2]	3/7	0/1	3:4	1	0	2	1	2	2	1	2	Nichol and Miller (1965)
	—	—[2]	2/2	0/0	2:0	1	0	0	0	0	0	0	0	Chaptal et al. (1965) [fam. 1]
	—	—	4/4	0/0	3:1	2	1	1	0	0	0	0	0	Chaptal et al. (1965) [fam. 2]
	35 (35–40)	—	4/9	0/1	1:1	0	0	0	0	1	0	0	0	Maurer et al. (1968)

Reference									M:F			Age	Age
Crawford and Toghill (1968) [fam. G]	5	6	1	4	0	0	0	0	8:1	0/1	5/7	—	25.5[2] (24-27)
Westley (1970)	1	4	2	7	9	4	7	6	10:10	0/5 (1/2)[1]	8/20	—	15 (11-21)
Turner (1970) [fam. 1]	2	10	7	3	12	17	16	12	17:26	0/12	10/43	—	—
Turner (1970) [fam. 2]	1	3	3	2	5	6	11	4	8:16	1/11	4/24	—	—
Turner (1970) [fam. 3]	1	2	4	1	20	8	14	13	23:21	0/12	11/44	—	—
Chazan et al. (1970, 1971) [fam. A]	1	4	7	2	6	3	4	2	7:12	0/6	6/19	42 (25-58)	32[2] (26-35)
Chiricosta et al. (1970)	1	14	6	3	6	3	2	7	13:9	1/4	4/22	—	22 (20-25)
Felts (1970) [fam. E]	1	3	3	4	5	3	6	3	7:11	3/6	5/18	48	34 (21-60)
Miller et al. (1970) [fam. 1]	3	0	0	0	0	0	0	0	4:0	—	2/4	—	—
Miller et al. (1970) [fam. 2]	3	1	3	0	2	0	1	0	6:7	0/2	8/13	—	18
Chazan et al. (1971) [fam. G]	4	3	6	2	5	4	4	2	9:11	0/6	11/20	—	—[2]
Chavis and Groshong (1973)	2	1	1	1	0	0	0	0	3:1	0/0	3/4	18	—
Gaboardi et al. (1974) [fam. 12]	2	0	0	0	0	0	0	0	3:2	0/1	1/5	—	—
Kenya et al. (1977) [fam. B]	3	6	5	8	7	7	1	6	11:7	1/2	3/18	—	—
Evans et al. (1980) [fam. N]	2	0	0	0	1	1	0	1	3:1	0/1	2/4	—	—
Totals	68	124	109	87	171	155	162	133	290:339	21/177	190/610		
Probable X linked dominant (II)													
Stephens et al. (1951); Perkoff et al. (1951, 1958); O'Neill et al. (1978); Hasstedt and Atkin (1983)	0	22	31	3	36	48	22	40[4]	38:64	2/39 (1/14)[1]	17/88	31 (22-37)	
Ohlsson (1963)	2	2	3	0	6	0	3	2	6:7	0/4 (1/2)[1]	3/13	—[2]	
Peters (1964)	0	2	1	1	9	5	4	9	10:8	3/6	3/18	25 (17-37)	
White et al. (1964)	0	4	1[1]	1	2	0	0	2	3:1	1/1	2/4	39	
Hobday and Jones (1969)	0	2	4	0	6	6	4	7	6:9	0/8	5/15	17 (2-32)	
Patton (1970)	0	8	4	5	7	3	4	2	8:11	3/7	5/19	—	
Chazan et al. (1971) [fam. L]	0	3	2	0	6	1	6	2	6:9	0/2	7/15	27[2]	

Table 7.4.—*Continued*

Mode of inheritance	Mean age at death of affected subjects with (range)		Proportion of affected subjects with hearing loss	Proportion of asymptomatic obligate female heterozygotes	Ratio of affected males to females	Offspring of affected parents								References
						Fathers				Mothers				
	male	female				AS	US	AD	UD	AS	US	AD	UD	
	27^2 (17–35)	42	3/52	1/14	26:26	0	5	4	1	18	11	20	15	Preus and Fraser (1971) Pashayan et al. (1971)
	—	—	2/9	0/2	6:3	0	1	1	0	6	1	2	3	Gaboardi et al. (1974) [fam. 1]
	—	—	3/13	2/4	5:8	0	1	3	0	3	1	3	0	Gaboardi et al. (1974) [fam. 2]
	—	—	1/7	0/3	2:5	0	1	1	0	2	0	3	3	Gaboardi et al. (1974) [fam. 3]
	—	—	—	10/75	23:75	0^s	22	18	11	22	59	60	43	Evans et al. (1980) [Grand Rapids fam. 1].
Total			51/253	22/165	139:226	0	73	76	22	123	135	131	128	
Autosomal or X linked dominant (III)	$14\frac{1}{2}$ (4–24)	$54\frac{1}{2}$ (19–90)	9/10	0/10	7:10	0	0	0	0	7	4	10	6	Guthrie (1902) Kendall and Hertz (1912) Hurst (1923) Eason et al. (1924) Alport (1927) Crawfurd and Toghill (1968)
	—	—	2/2	0/0	2:0	0	0	0	0	0	0	0	0	Reyersbach and Butler (1954) [fam. S]
	18	—	4/13	0/3	7:6	0	0	0	0	7	3	5	3	Hamburger (1956) Naffah (1956) Marie et al. (1960)
	$8\frac{1}{2}$ (18–19)	—	4/13	0/3	7:5	0	0	0	0	7	3	4	4	Bouchet and Paquelin (1956) Lemoyne and Fleury (1962)
	24 (19–28)	53 (30–75)	9/16	4/8	8:8	0	0	0	0	8	7	5	7	Sturtz and Burke (1956, 1958) [fam. A]
	—	—	5/14	—	—	—	—	—	—	—	—	—	—	Gobin et al. (1958) [fam. T]
	<20	—	4/10	—	—	—	—	—	—	—	—	—	—	Gobin et al. (1958) [fam. L]

Reference												
Sturtz and Burke (1958) [fam. B]	3	3	1	1	0	0	0	1:4	1/2	1/5	26	—
Klotz (1959)	0	5	0	3	0	0	0	3:5	0/4	3/6	20½	58
Chappel and Kelsey (1960) [fam. 2]	7	10	9	7	0	1	0	7:12	0/7	8/19	24	45 (25–65)
Whalen et al. (1961) [St. J. fam.] Felts (1970) [fam. F]												
Cohen et al. (1961) [fam. 1] Cassady et al. (1965) [fam. D]	4	3	4	4	0	0	0	4:4	0/3	7/8	—	—
Williamson (1961) [fam. A]	1	1	0	4	0	0	0	4:2	0/2	3/6	13	—
Williamson (1961) [fam. B]	0	0	0	3	0	0	0	3:1	0/1	2/4	—	—
Williamson (1961) [fam. C]	0	2	0	0	0	0	0	1:3	0/1	2/4	29	—
Opitz (1962)	8	7	14	5	0	0	0	5:10	2/8	6/10	19	—
Rosenkranz (1963) [fam. 2]	1	2	1	4	0	0	0	4:2	2/2	4/6	(17–21)	—
Holbolth (1963) [fam. II]	6	6	1	6	0	1	1	6:7	1/5	2/13	25½	—
Schneider (1963)	11	10	4	8	0	1	1	8:12	2/9	6/20	(14–60)	78
Wasserman et al. (1963, 1965) [fam. G–M]	2	1	0	1	3	1	1	3:2	1/2	2/5	50	—
Wasserman et al. (1963, 1965) [fam. G]	0	0	1	3	0	0	0	3:2	0/1	2/5	21½ (17–26)	26
Flower (1964) [fam. B]	0	3[2]	0	3	2	0	0	3:4	1/3	4/7	—	—
Flower (1964) [fam. S]	0	3	0	5	2	0	0	5:4	0/2	4/9	—	—
Flower (1964) [fam. K]	2	5	4	5	4	0	0	5:6	2/5	6/11	—	—
Johnson and Hagan (1965)	1	1	2	2	0	0	0	2:2	0/2	3/4	17	32
Goetz et al. (1965)	2	1	0	2	0	0	0	3:1	0/0	4/4	—	—
Onisawa et al. (1966)	0	0	0	2	0	1	0	3:1	0/1	1/4	—	—
Burguet et al. (1966	1	2	1	2	0	0	0	5:4	0/4	6/9	22	—
Wood and Knight (1966)	0	0	0	0	0	0	0	2:2	0/0	2/4	25 (18–24)	—
Winter et al. (1968)	0	0	0	1	0	0	0	2:2	0/1	1/4	19	—
Crawfurd and Toghill (1968) [fam. S]	0	0	0	1	0	0	0	1:1	0/1	2/2	(14–23)	—

Table 7.4.—*Continued*

Mode of inheritance	Mean age at death of affected subjects with (range)		Proportion of affected subjects with hearing loss	Proportion of asymptomatic obligate female heterozygotes	Ratio of affected males to females	Offspring of affected parents								References
						Fathers				Mothers				
	male	female				AS	US	AD	UD	AS	US	AD	UD	
	36	—	10/11	0/1	6:5	0	0	0	1	7	2	4	1	Symboulidis et al. (1968) [fam. 2]
	16	—	2/8	0/1	3:5	0	0	0	0	3	0	4	3	Cohen-Solal et al. (1970) [fam. M]
	—	—	1/3	0/1	2:1	0	0	0	0	2	0	0	0	Cohen-Solal et al. (1970) [fam. S. G.]
	16	—	3/8	0/2	2:6	0	0	0	0	2	0	4	0	Beaudoing et al. (1970)
	—	—	3/4	0/2	1:3	0	0	0	0	1	1	2	1	Spear et al. (1970) [fam. 1]
	—	—	1/4	0/1	3:1	0	0	0	0	2	1	0	1	Spear et al. (1970) [fam. 2]
	—	—	2/5	0/2	2:3	0	0	0	0	2	1	2	2	Spear et al. (1970) [fam. 3]
	—	—	1/2	0/1	1:1	0	0	0	0	1	0	2	0	Spear et al. (1970) [fam. 4]
	—	—	1/2	0/1	6:1	0	0	0	0	1	1	0	2	Spear et al. (1970) [fam. 5]
	—	—	3/3	0/1	2:1	0	0	0	0	2	0	0	0	Felts (1970) [fam. C]
	—	34	4/5	—	—	0	0	0	0	0	0	0	0	Felts (1970) [fam. D]
	35 (16–53)	31	3/5	0/2	3:2	0	0	1	0	2	2	1	1	Jain et al. (1970)
	—	—	2/3	1/2	1:2	0	0	0	0	1	0	1	0	Miller et al. (1970) [fam. 3]
	15	—	—	—	—	0	0	0	0	0	0	0	0	Miller et al. (1970) [fam. 4]
	11	—	1/6	1/3	3:3	0	0	0	0	3	0	2	1	Schneegans et al. (1971)
	—	—	3/6	0/5	3:5	0	0	0	0	4	4	3	2	Feingold and Bois (1971) [fam. 1]
	—	—	5/8	0/3	2:5	0	0	0	0	2	5	5	2	Feingold and Bois (1971) [fam. 2]
	—	—	2/3	0/1	3:4	0	0	1	0	1	0	0	2	Feingold and Bois (1971) [fam. 3]
	—	—	2/2	0/3	4:4	0	0	0	0	3	0	2	2	Feingold and Bois (1971) [fam. 4]

Reference											
Feingold and Bois (1971) [fam. 5]	0	0	1	2	0	0	2:1	0/1	2/2	—	—
Feingold and Bois (1971) [fam. 6]	3	5	0	5	0	0	5:6	1/4	2/2	—	—
Feingold and Bois (1971) [fam. 7]	3	5	5	6	1	0	6:6	0/3	3/3	—	—
Feingold and Bois (1971) [fam. 8]	0	0	0	2	0	0	3:3	0/1	1/2	—	—
Feingold and Bois (1971) [fam. 9]	0	0	0	0	0	0	2:0	0/0	2/2	—	—
Feingold and Bois (1971) [fam. 10]	2	0	0	1	0	0	1:1	0/1	1/2	—	—
Chazan et al. (1971) [fam. P]	4	10	6	3	0	0	3:11	0/7	7/14	34	19½ (17–22)
Chazan et al. (1971) [fam. W]	3	3	2	4	0	0	4:4	0/2	3/8	—	18
Acecka and Dowbor (1972)	3	0	1	4	0	0	4:1	0/0	2/5	47	24 (19–27)
Hinglais et al. (1971) [Case 1. fam. 1]	4	3	1	1	0	0	1:5	0/1	1/6	—	—
Grunefeld et al. (1973) [fam. 1]	0	0	1	3	0	0	3:1	0/1	2/4	24	—
Hinglais et al. (1972) [Case 2. fam 2] Grunefeld et al. (1973) [fam. 2]	0	1	0	2	0	1	3:2	0/1	1/5	27	—
Hinglais et al. (1972) [Case 6. fam 5] Grunefeld et al. (1973) [fam. 4]	3	0	0	0	1	0	2:0	0/0	2/2	—	—
Hinglais et al. (1972) [cases 9 and 10. fam. 7]	0	0	0	—	—	—	—	0/1	—	—	—
Grunefeld et al. (1973) [fam. 5]	0	1	0	1	0	0	1:2	0/1	1/1	—	—
Gaboardi et al. (1974) [fam. 4]	0	4	0	2	0	0	2:8	1/4	1/9	—	—
Gaboardi et al. (1974) [fam. 5]	1	1	1	3	0	0	3:2	2/2	3/5	—	—
Gaboardi et al. (1974) [fam. 6]	0	1	2	1	0	0	1:2	0/2	1/3	—	—
Gaboardi et al. (1974) [fam. 8]	0	0	0	0	0	0	2:0	—	2/2	—	—
Gaboardi et al. (1974) [fam. 10]	2	0	0	1	0	0	1:1	0/1	2/2	—	—

Table 7.4.—*Continued*

Mode of inheritance	Mean age at death of affected subjects with (range)		Proportion of affected subjects with hearing loss	Proportion of asymptomatic obligate female heterozygotes	Ratio of affected males to females	Offspring of affected parents								References
	male	female				Fathers				Mothers				
						AS	US	AD	UD	AS	US	AD	UD	
	—	—	1/4	0/1	0:4	0	0	0	0	0	0	2	0	Gaboardi *et al.* (1974) [fam. 11]
	—	—	1/2	0/1	1:1	0	0	0	0	1	0	0	0	Gaboardi *et al.* (1974) [fam. 14]
	—	—	2/2	—	1:1	0	0	0	0	0	0	0	0	Gaboardi *et al.* (1974) [fam. 19]
	16	—	2/4	1/2	2:2	0	0	0	0	2	1	2	5	Sherman *et al.* (1974)
	34 (31–40)	—	3/5	0/1	4:1	0	0	0	0	3	0	0	1	Miyoshi *et al.* (1975) [fam. K]
	—	—	1/1	0/0	1:0	0	0	0	0	0	0	0	0	Miyoshi *et al.* (1975) [fam. X]
Totals			131/266	23/158	208:239	0	6	6	12	186	96	157	121	
Grand Totals			372/1129	66/500	637:804	68	203	191	121	480	386	450	382	

Abbreviations: AS = affected son, US = unaffected son, AD = affected daughter, UD = unaffected daughter.

1 Figures in brackets are proportion of asymptomatic obligate male heterozygotes.

2 Indicates the presence of surviving affected males over the age of 30 years.

3 Including one asymptomatic obligate female heterozygote.

4 The figures for this family are taken from O'Neill *et al.* (1978), apart from those for the proportion with perceptive deafness and for age at death of affected males, both of which were obtained from Perkoff *et al.* (1951).

5 This zero figure excludes four doubtful cases: two boys with hearing defect only and two young boys with occasional haematuria. If any of these four boys were proved to be affected this family would have to be reclassified as autosomal dominant.

was in a human embryo whose mother had nephritis (Rones 1934). These findings strongly suggest that a high proportion of all cases of anterior lenticonus are associated with Alport's disease. Any patient presenting with this lenticular lesion should be fully investigated for haematuria or nephritis. Several non-lenticular ocular lesions have been reported in single families and are probably just chance associations. These include retinal detachment (Williamson 1961), arcus juvenilis (Tsukahara 1930; Arnott *et al.* 1966; Chavis and Groshong 1973), severe myopia (Holbolth 1963; Ohlsson 1963), optic nerve atrophy (Bodalski and Margolis 1966), posterior corneal opacities (Chaptal *et al.* 1965), a scleral defect (Symboulidis *et al.* 1968, 1972, familiy S), and a combination of strabismus, heterophoria, and nystagmus (Tiliakos 1964). A more significant abnormality is the frequent observation of a macular lesion, occuring either alone or in association with anterior lenticonus or lens opacities. Purriel and colleagues (1970) found in their series of 230 patients that eye defects were present in 22 (9.5 per cent), 19 being in male patients. These included 20 with macular lesions, 16 without nephropathy. The macular lesion was mainly pigmentary, usually a fine but occasionally a more course pigmentation, sometimes associated with adjoining whitish depigmented areas. Hinglais and associates (1972) observed similar macular lesions in association with lens opacities in one patient. Polak and Hogewind (1977) performed detailed ophthalmological studies in three families and observed whitish lesions in the macular area in association with cataracts in the index cases in each of their families. Fluorescin angiography in their case 1 was normal. Similar macular changes occurring in association with anterior lenticonus were described by Nielsen (1978) in four out of his six cases. Perrin and colleagues (1980), at the Hospital Necker in Paris, reported on 79 patients with Alport's disease studied ophthalmologically. In 29 of these (24 male) from 23 families similar whitish or yellowish dense granulations were observed surrounding the fovea. Fluorescein angiography was normal in eight patients in which it was undertaken. All 29 patients had neural hearing loss and 26 had anterior lenticonus. In contrast, none of 50 patients without macular changes had lenticonus. This study would appear to confirm the suggestion from the earlier studies that macular changes are a specific component of the ocular abnormalities in this disease and are frequently associated with lenticular defects, especially anterior lenticonus. Further support for this view comes from more recent reports from the Paris group including that of Gubler and associates (1981), who reported on 58 patients, of whom 18 had anterior lenticonus and/or macular lesions; and of Habib and colleagues (1982) who studied 41 affected children of whom 10 boys had anterior lenticonus and macular changes, and six boys and two girls had macular changes without lens defect. The data on the 30 families with lenticular or macular ocular lesions listed in Table 7.1 provide some evidence for genetic heterogeneity within this group. None of these families provide unequivocal evidence of X linkage (group B), the most likely candidate being the family of Lachhein and colleagues (1969) in which the finding of a stellate cataract may not in fact be associated with the Alport's disease present. Only seven families show male-to-male transmission indicative of autosomal dominance (group A) (Shaw and Glover 1961; Junod 1963, family Tr; Perrin 1964, family Tr; Symboulidis *et al.* 1968, family 4; Purriel *et al.* 1970, families 1, 2, and 4; Kenya *et al.* 1977). Among these seven, family Tr, and families 1 and 4 of Purriel and colleagues show typical early death of affected males. The family originally reported by Goldman and Haberfelde (1959) showed no convincing deafness at that time but when reinvestigated by Kenya and colleagues (1977) did so. Unfortunately the eye defect present in three members is not specified. This family is unusual in the advanced age of the affected males. Shaw and Glover's family is also atypical in that not only are four out of 12 obligatory heterozygous females asymptomatic but so also are the only two transmitting males. Thus even among these seven autosomal dominant families there appears to be heterogeneity. In the remaining families (group C) it is impossible to say whether inheritance is autosomal dominant or X-linked dominant as there are too few offspring of affected males, in fact only two in the one family of Reyersbach and Butler's (1954) (family S) out of 22 families. In those families, within this subgroup C, where affected males have died this has mostly been at an early age, that is, under 30 years. The only exceptions are family 3 of Symboulidis and colleagues (1968) where there was an affected male surviving at 45 years, and their family 6 with death of an affected male at 57 years. Hence there would again appear to be at least a few atypical families among this subgroup. Comparison of the data from the 30 families in groups A, B, and C with one another, and with the 117 families without ocular lesions in the comparable groups I, II, and III in Table 7.4 shows up further differences. The ratio of families with ocular lesions to those without, 30 to 117, is similar to that in the series of Farboody and colleagues (1979), 4 to 13, that is, both about 1 to 4. The relevant comparisons, derived from the data in Tables 7.3 and 7.4, are set out in Table 7.5.

Within the ocular group the incidence of ocular lesions and of perceptive deafness is lower in group A than group C, and in the case of the ocular lesions is not attributable to the higher proportion of cases with macular lesions only in group C. There is a modest deficit of affected offspring of affected mothers in group A, compared with an excess of affected sons in group C. However, the striking difference in both the ocular and non-ocular groups among offspring is the extreme dearth of children born to affected fathers in groups C and III, of uncertain inheritance. This gross deficit is associatd with a low mean age of death of affected males in most of the families in these two groups and would appear to demarcate sharply most of these large groups of families from those with more clear-cut patterns of inheritance.

The remarkable overlap of clinical and pathological features between different forms of hereditary nephritis is illustrated by the family of Zavala and colleagues (1969) in which an Alport's syndrome-like combination of hereditary nephritis and perceptive deafness with hyper-prolinaemia, an association discussed in a later section of this chapter, is associated with anterior lenticonus and cataracts, demonstrating that anterior lenticonus is not confined to pure Alport's disease.

Arnott and colleagues (1966) noted that deafness was more common among affected members of families with lens defects (0.62) than among those without such defects (0.44). The present data indicate a lower overall incidence in both groups but do not support the earlier excess in the ocular families when comparing groups A with I, B with II, and C with III. Similarly, Arnott and colleagues (1966) found the sex ratio for affected members of the ocular families to be double that for the non-ocular (2.3 to 1.04), whereas those calculated from the present data, excluding the X-linked families in both groups, fail to confirm this difference.

In summary, analysis of the data in Tables 7.3, 7.4 and 7.5 gives support to the evidence previously discussed for genetic heterogeneity within the group of families with ocular lesions, but leaves open the question of heterogenity as between these families and those without ocular lesions. This remains so irrespective of the pattern of inheritance.

A more general consideration of age of onset and at death among the non-ocular lesion families reveals that, although most conform to the typical pattern of early onset and death in males, there are a minority in which survival of males beyond 30 years is a consistent feature. This is seen especially among a minority of the families with clear autosomal inheritance (Mulrow *et al.* 1963; Tiliakos *et al.* 1964, family A; Maurer *et al.* 1968; Chazan *et al.* 1970, 1971, family A; Felts *et al.* 1970, family E), or X-linked inheritance (Chazan *et al.* 1971, family L; Pashayan *et al.* 1971). It has long been recognized that, apart from the fact that females are generally more mildly affected than males, there are some obligate female heterozygotes who show no clinical symptoms or abnormal urinary findings, even on repeat testing.

7.4.3. Renal pathology and pathogenesis

Early histopathological studies of the kidneys in Alport's disease revealed an essentially non-specific chronic pyelonephritis or glomerulo-nephritis. In the very earliest autopsy study Perkoff and colleagues (1951,

Table 7.5. *Comparison of various parameters in families with Alport's disease, with and without ocular lesions, and with various patterns of inheritance*

Group	Incidence		Sex ratio		Ratio		
	Ocular lesions	Perceptive deafness	A, B, and C	A and C only	All children of affected fathers to affected mothers	Affected to unaffected children of affected mothers	
						Sons	Daughters
With ocular lesions							
A (AD)	0.11	0.27	0.86		0.80	0.48	0.65
B (XD)[1]	0.17	1.00	1.00		1.00	—	—
C (AD or XD)	0.33	0.55	1.36		0.013	1.55	0.91
Mean	0.22	0.42	1.05	1.05			
Without ocular lesions			*I, II, and III*	*I and III only*			
I (AD)	—	0.31	0.86		0.62	1.10	1.22
II (XD)	—	0.20	0.61		0.33	0.91	1.02
III (AD or XD)	—	0.49	0.87		0.043	1.94	1.30
Mean		0.33	0.79	0.86			

[1] One family only.

1958) noted both chronic glomerulonephritis and chronic pyelonephritis but were more impressed by the latter. They also observed focal thickening of the basement membrane of Bowman's capsule, and commented on a feature subsequently highlighted by many authors: the presence of excess numbers of foam cells. Similar observations were made by Goldbloom (1957), but Whalen and associates (1961) were more struck by a glomerulonephritic (Fig. 7.1) rather than a pyelonephritic picture. Mulrow and others (1963) and Krickstein and coworkers (1966) both emphasized the mixed nature of the histopathological picture with combined features of chronic glomerulonephritis, pyelonephritis, and interstitial nephritis. The latter group of workers found lipid-laden foam cells in the great majority of cases, often forming macroscopically visible yellow streaks in the lower cortex (Fig. 7.2). They also noted that foam cells may be seen in renal biopsies relatively early in the disease, and demonstrated positive staining of these foam cells for lipid (oil red O stain), cholesterol (Schultz reaction), and phospholipid (Nile-blue sulphate stain). The foam cells are mainly tubular epithelial cells, although some are also found in glomeruli (Fig. 7.3).

Other workers have also examined renal biopsies relatively early in the

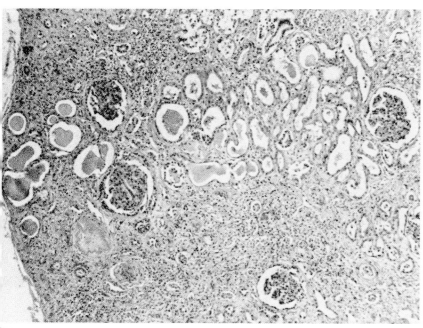

Fig. 7.1. Glomerulonephritic changes in Alport's disease (× 145). From Whalen *et al.* (1963) *Am. J. Med.* **31**, 171–86 (this figure p. 172) with the kind permission of Dr Whalen and the *American Journal of Medicine.*

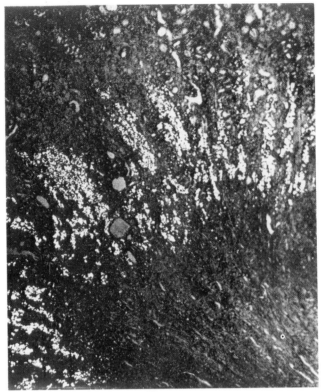

Fig. 7.2. Yellow streaks (the lighter areas in the photograph) in renal cortex due to lipid foam cells in Alport's disease (× 15). From Krickstein *et al.* (1966), *Arch. Pathol.*, **82**, 510–15, Fig. 10, Copyright 1966, American Medical Association, with the permission of Dr Krickstein and the American Medical Assocition.

disease and described a more focal picture of glomeruonlephritis than is seen in autopsy material (Rosenkranz 1963; White *et al.* 1964). Chaptal and colleagues (1965) performed serial renal biopsies in one case and demonstrated a slow progression of glomerular changes, with interstitial nephritis a relatively late development. Similar studies on patients early in the disease were reported by Antonovych and coworkers (1969) who described the persistence of 'fetal-like glomeruli', with reduced numbers of capillaries and crowding of visceral epithelium at the periphery, the presence of red cells and red-cell casts in distal tubular and collecting ducts, infrequent foam cells in the absence of interstitial fibrosis, and focal glomerular hypercellularity. They argued that interstitial fibrosis, especially periglomerular, is a later development. Kaufman and colleagues (1970) examined renal tissue by light microscopy from 23 patients, 15 of them serially, and found that glomerular basement

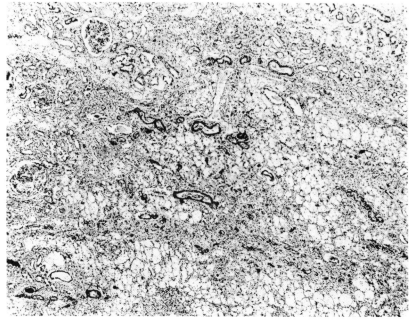

Fig. 7.3. Lipid foam cells (the large pale cells in the photograph) in a kidney in Alport's disease (×45). From Krickstein *et al.* (1966), *Arch. Pathol.*, **82**, 506–15, Fig. 11, Copyright 1966, American Medical Association, with the permission of Dr Krickstein and the American Medical Association.

membrane thickening was the earliest and most common lesion, being present in 18 out of 23 initial biopsies. In their serial studies a progressive interstitial fibrosis, with or without inflammatory changes, was the most prominent feature.

Numerous authors have sought evidence for involvement of immune mechanisms in the pathogenesis of Alport's disease. Wasserman and associates (1965) studied nine patients and found normal serum complement activity, both in acute episodes of haematuria and in quiescent stages of the disease. Since serum complement activity is nearly always reduced in acute postinfectious glomerulonephritis these authors suggest that its determination is a useful diagnositic procedure. Immunofluorescent studies of renal biopsies also fail to demonstrate evidence for glomerular deposition of specific immunoglobulins (Chiricosta *et al.* 1970; Kaufman *et al.* 1970; Spear *et al.* 1970; Hinglais *et al.* 1972). However, Spear's group did find anti-β-1^{C}/$\beta1^{A}$ globulin glomerular deposits, probably reacting with $C^{1}3$ complement component, whose fixation does not necessarily imply an immune mechanism. An exceptional report records the detection of IgA and IgG in mesangial fibrinoid deposits from a patient with Alport's disease (Sessa *et al.* 1973). The authors suggest that their patient has an acquired focal glomerulo-nephritis superimposed on hereditary nephritis. Conflicting results have been reported with regard to the detection of antithyroid antibodies in Alport's disease. Miyoshi and colleagues (1975) reported the finding of such antibodies in all patients and some relatives in two Alport's disease families. Zeromski and coworkers (1976), using different techniques, confirmed this observation in five Alport's cases but failed to demonstrate such antibodies in patients with other forms of glomerulo-nephritis. In contrast Schmidt and others (1976) also studied two Alport's families but could demonstrate no antithyroid antibodies and suggested that the antibodies detected by Miyoshi and colleagues were not due to their patients' Alport's disease.

Over the last two decades there has been a steadily increasing body of evidence pointing to glomerular basement membrane (GBM) lesions as the primary lesion in the kidney. As early as 1966 David and colleagues reported glomerular basement membrane thickening on electron microscopy in Alport's disease, and as mentioned above this was noted even on light microscopy as the earliest renal lesion by Kaufman and colleagues (1970). Similar thickening with splitting and distortion of the lamina densa, leaving intervening clear spaces which in some cases contain electron-dense particles, has been repeatedly observed on electron microscopy of both autopsy and biospy renal tissue from patients with Alport's disease, and also some with apparently pure hereditary nephritis (Kinoshita *et al.* 1969; Hinglais *et al.* 1972; Spear and Slusser 1972; Churg and Sherman 1973; Grunefeld *et al.* 1973; Gaboardi *et al.* 1974; Sherman *et al.* 1974; Kohaut *et al.* 1976; Farboody *et al.* 1979; O'Neill *et al.* 1980; Habib *et al.* 1982). The earliest report of both thickening of the GBM and splitting and splintering of the lamina densa on the ultrastructural study is that of Spear and Slusser (1972). These lesions were focal and sometimes separated by areas of extreme thinning of the lamina densa (Fig. 7.4). They did not observe electron-dense particles, such as were described by Hinglais and others (1972) as 50 nm diameter granules lying within electron-lucent areas within the split lamina densa of the GBM (Fig. 7.5). Churg and Sherman (1973) examined tissue from seven patients with Alport's disease from four families, and 10 patients from five families with pure hereditary or other non-Alport forms of familial nephritis. The characteristic GBM splitting was seen in all the Alport patients and one family with pure hereditary nephritis. Its presence or absence was in all cases consistent among affected members of any one family. Tubular membrane splitting, which was also seen, was less consistent. Kohaut and coworkers (1976) compared electron-microscopic changes of renal tissue in hereditary

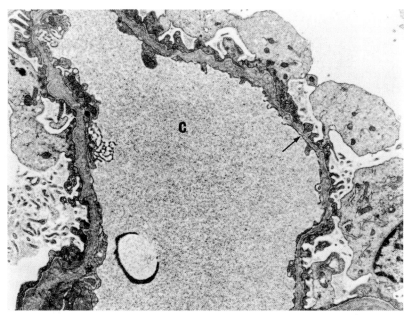

Fig. 7.4. Irregular width and (arrowed) splitting of the glomerular basement membrane in Alport's disease (×5600). C=capillary lumen. From Spear and Slusser (1972) *Am. J. Path.* **69**, 213–24 (this figure p. 223) with the permission of the *American Journal of Pathology.*

nephritis, with or without deafness, with those in nephrotic syndrome, glomerulonephritis, or benign familial haematuria blindly. Although focal splitting of GBMs was seen in benign familial haematuria, nephrotic syndrome, and glomerulonephritis it was never widespread as in hereditary nephritis, apparently confirming that widespread GBM splitting is specific for hereditary nephritis. However, Farboody and colleagues (1979) found GBM splitting with granular particles in kidneys from patients with IgA nephropathy and benign familial haematuria, and even in a kidney from a normal donor. O'Neill and colleagues (1980) undertook electron microscopy of renal tissue from affected members of two families with hereditary nephritis, one with associated deafness and the other without, but both showing a pattern of inheritance consistent with X-linked dominant inheritance. The findings in the two families were similar with focal GBM lamina densa thickening as the characteristic lesion. Lamination and dense granules were seen only in the two patients, one from each family, with impaired renal function. Their observations raised the possibility that these less severe GBM changes observed by them are characteristic of a form of hereditary nephritis with X-linked

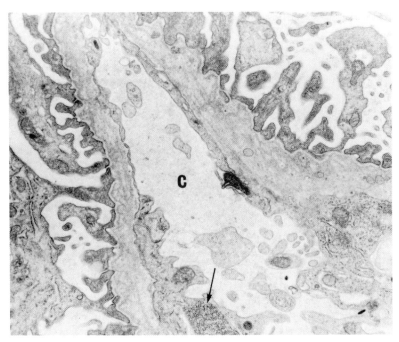

Fig. 7.5. 50 nm diameter granules (seen as fine dark dots) within lucent areas of the lamina densa of the glomerular basement membrane in Alport's disease (×11 250). C=capillary lumen, arrow=focal thickening of lamina densa. From Spear and Slusser (1972) *Am. J. Path.* **69**, 213–24 (this figure p. 224) with the permission of the *American Journal of Pathology.*

dominant inheritance. This suggestion requires confirmation or refutation in future studies. The most recent reports on the renal ultrastructural changes in Alport's disease come from Habib and Gubler's group. They confirm that the characteristic lesions among their families are diffuse, or more often focal, thickening of the GBM with splitting of the lamina densa, with in most cases interspersed areas of GBM thinning or normal basement membrane. In young children the predominant feature was often a thin, irregular GBM. They observed a few patients with either diffuse GBM thinning alone or with normal GBMs. In both of these groups the patients, male and female, had relatively mild clinical features and fell into an older age group, the males being $8\frac{1}{2}$ to 48 years and the females being 31 to 79 years. In summary these varied observations suggest that widespread but usually focal GBM thickening with lamination of the lamina densa is the characteristic ultrastructural renal lesion in most families with Alport's disease and in some families with pure hereditary nephritis. This is a progressive lesion, tends to be interspersed with areas of thickening alone, thinning, or normal basement membrane giving rise to an irregular outline. Because of its progressive nature younger patients may show only the less specific thickening or thinning without splitting. Patients with advanced disease may show electron-dense granules in clear spaces between parallel strands in the lamina densa. Although more characteristic of patients with hereditary nephritis, none of these lesions are wholly specific. Finally genetic heterogeneity is suggested by a minority of families with differing forms of atypical lesion.

Several research groups have looked for GBM antigens, either excreted in urine or in histological preparations or renal tissue, with anti-GBM antisera. Using such an antibody Lubec and colleagues (1978) undertook immunoelectrophoresis of urinary proteins in 12 children in whom the diagnosis of Alport's disease was suspected. The eight children who proved to have typical basement membrane changes on electron microscopy also showed an immunoprecipitation band not obtained from unaffected subjects, and with a more anodal migration (β-zone) than was seen from patients with nephrotic syndrome who gave a band in the α_1-zone. Six affected relatives of the Alport's disease children gave a similar precipitation band. Following the demonstration that the sera of patients with Goodpasture's syndrome contain anti-GBM antibodies which are not bound by glomeruli of patients with hereditary nephritis (McCoy *et al.* 1976), Lubec and Shabbir (1984) have developed a diagnostic test for Alport's disease involving affinity chromatography, using Goodpasture antiserum, of urinary proteins followed by polyacryl-amide gel electrophoresis. They found that, whereas controls and patients with glomerulonephritis revealed two major bands, one of 30 000 μ and its probable dimer, Alport's disease patients do not excrete this protein. Immunofluorescent studies of renal tissue from patients with hereditary nephritis using anti-GBM antisera from patients with Good-pasture's syndrome have shown either a complete failure to bind anti-GBM antibodies, in contrast to normal renal tissue (McCoy *et al.* 1976; Olson *et al.* 1980), or reduced binding (Jenis *et al.* 1981; Habib *et al.* 1982). Jenis and coworkers observed a failure to bind anti-GBM antibody in only four out of nine cases of hereditary nephritis, with absence of binding positively correlated with the severity of ultra-structural lesions. Similarly, Savage and colleagues (1986) obtained no binding with a monoclonal Goodpasture antibody in nine patients with hereditary nephritis, reduced binding in three and normal binding in one. Habib and others (1982), on the other hand, obtained positive binding using rabbit and guinea pig anti-GBM antisera in 11 patients with Alport's disease. However, the intestity of immunofluorescent staining was variable and did not correlate with the severity of the disease process. They obtained positive reactions with antisera to types IV and V collagen, laminin, fibronectin, and proteoglycan but negative reactions with anti-types I and III collagen antisera, a pattern similar to that obtained with normal kidney. It may of course be that Goodpasture antisera recognize an antigen not recognized by any of the antisera used by Habib and others. The GBM antigen recognized by Goodpasture antisera has been located within the noncollagenous globular domain of type IV collagen (Wieslander *et al.* 1984; Kashtan *et al.* 1986). Kashtan and colleagues used Goodpasture anti-sera, and an anti-serum from an Alport's disease patient, to demonstrate X-linked dominant inheritance of the antigenic anomaly in Alport's disease families; and also expression, with the latter anti-serum, in epidermal basement membrane. The studies using Goodpasture antisera certainly raise the possibility that a specific GBM antigen is lacking in the GBM of patients with hereditary nephritis, although the work of Jenis and associates suggests that, at least in pure hereditary nephritis if not Alport's disease, this may be a secondary rather than a primary abnormality.

Others have investigated the biochemical composition of GBMs in hereditary nephritis. DiBona and colleagues (1976) isolated GBMs from a patient with Alport's disease in renal failure who underwent nephrectomy. They found slight increases in proline and glycine content and slight decreases in half-cystine and hydroxyproline, and in the hydroxyproline:proline ratio. Carbohydrate composition was normal. They concluded that these observations suggest a decreased collagen content of GBM in Alport's disease. This idea received support from the observation of increased urinary excretion of hydoxylysine glycosides by seven patients with hereditary nephritis, including at least two with Alport's disease (Tina *et al.* 1979). This observation suggests an accelerated degradation of collagen in this disease. Yet further support for the concept of an abnormality of GBM biochemical composition comes from the findings of Habib and associates (1982). They found that GBM from Alport's disease, compared with normal controls, contained less sialic acid, glucosyl–galactosyl–hydroxylysine, hydroxylysine, hydroxyproline and half-cystine. Hydroxyproline is found only in collagen and its reduction can be viewed as an indicator of a reduced amount of collagen. Gubler and colleagues have suggested that there is persistence of a fetal GBM protein in Alport's disease but as yet there is no evidence to test their hypothesis. All that can be said at present is that the ultrastructural lesions of the GBM are paralleled by a replacement of a normal GBM antigen by one not normally detectable, associated with increased degradation of collagen. Further elucidation must await more detailed biochemical study of GBM collagen and other protein constituents in normal subjects, fetal kidneys, and patients.

7.4.4. Genetics

Alport's disease has been the subject of more genetic hypotheses and controversy than probably any other inherited disease. It is generally accepted as being a single gene defect, and several authors who have undertaken chromosomal analysis have not detected any abnormality (Mulrow *et al.* 1963; White *et al.* 1964; Onisawa *et al.* 1965; Lachhein *et al.* 1969). Cecil Alport (1972) himself merely referred to the disease in the family he reported as 'hereditary'. Subsequent authors who have attempted genetic analysis have found their task complicated by the tendency to much greater severity in males, with the consequential paucity of children of affected men. This probably accounts in part for some of the curious segregation ratios, and the unique hypotheses that have been proposed to account for them. Another reason is that almost certainly earlier authors have treated series of families that were genetically heterogeneous as homogeneous.

The earliest attempt at a genetic analysis was that of Perkoff and his colleagues (Perkoff *et al.* 1951; Stephens *et al.* 1951; Perkoff *et al.* 1958) on their large Utah family (referred to in many later papers as family P). Their analysis inevitably suffers from the weakness of being confined to a single family which can retrospectively be seen to be atypical in the late age at death of affected males. This single family has dominated genetic analysis of Alport's disease for many years since it has been the subject of attention by a succession of authors. On the basis of finding only 2 affected to 15 unaffected sons of affected fathers, and 18 affected to 4 unaffected daughters of affected fathers, Perkoff and colleagues postulated partial X-linkage with crossing over between the X and Y chromosomes. In their follow-up study published in 1958 the revised figures were 2 to 18 for sons, and 24 to 5 for daughters of affected fathers. Despite criticism by Morton (1957) of their hypothesis of partial sex linkage, hitherto unknown in humans, but postulated by Haldane (1936), they maintained that this was still the most likely explanation of their findings. Morton (1957) preferred the hypothesis of dominant complete sex linkage, with some other disease accounting for the two exceptional apparent father-to-son transmissions. Another alternative hypothesis for the inheritance in this family was proposed by Graham (1959) who like Morton found partial sex linkage difficult to accept. Graham suggested that inheritance was autosomal dominant with incomplete penetrance and sex influence, being more severe in males with intra-uterine death of half of the affected males. The argument was continued inconclusively in the correspondence columns of the *American Journal of Human Genetics* (Graham 1960; Perkoff *et al.* 1960). Shaw and Glover (1961) reanalysed the data from family P, along with data from a family of their own, the Virginia kindred. Like Graham they favoured autosomal dominant inheritance with intra-uterine loss of affected male zygotes for both family P and the Virginia family. However, in order to explain still unaccounted peculiarities of the segregation ratios in these two families they made the further suggestion of an abnormality at gametogenesis whereby non-random disjunction leads to preferential segregation of the chromosome bearing the mutant gene. They proposed that in oogenesis the mutant chromosome goes to the oocyte rather than the polar body, and that in spermatogenesis the mutant chromosome segregates preferentially with the X rather than the Y chromosome. They offered no suggestions as to the possible mechanisms for such an extraordinary phenomenon. Twelve years later Shaw included family P in a wider analysis of 35 published pedigrees (MacNeill and Shaw 1973). Their analysis excluded partial sex linkage but gave partial support to the hypothesis of Preus and Fraser, discussed below, of autosomal dominant inheritance with increased penetrance of the gene in sons of affected mothers due to an unfavourable intra-uterine milieu. They claimed that their pooled data also supported the preferential segregation hypothesis that Shaw had earlier put forward with Glover, with the modification that the proportion of affected to normal offspring of affected mothers was greater when the mother was symptomatic. Oliver Mayo (1973) showed that the pedigrees used by MacNeill and Shaw were heterogeneous. He suggested that they should not be pooled in the way MacNeill and Shaw had done, and that Alport's disease may well be genetically hetero-geneous. In response to Mayo's comments Shaw (1973) nailed his colours more firmly to the mast of his own hypothesis. Nevertheless Mayo's comment was the first firm suggestion of genetic heterogeneity in Alport's disease, a truly prophetic suggestion. This remarkable Utah family was reinvestigated, 20 years after Perkoff and colleagues' (1958) second study, by O'Neill and coworkers (1978). They used haematuria as their diagnostic criterion, rather than proteinuria or pyuria, and on this basis excluded the apparent instances of father-to-son transmission accepted by Perkoff and colleagues. This removed any need to involve partial sex linkage. O'Neill and coworkers also found a 2:1 ratio of affected female-to-male subjects making out a very good case for simple X-linked dominant inheritance as originally proposed by Morton (1957). Commenting on O'Neill and coworkers' paper, Tishler (1978) considered that a deficiency of sons of affected fathers was still unexplained. This prompted O'Neill and Atkin (1978) to suggest that the mutant gene may confer an advantage on the X-chromosome-bearing sperm compared with the Y-bearing sperm to account for this. A further recent segregation analysis, using O'Neill and coworkers' data and the method of likelihood analysis with correction for ascertainment bias, has confirmed X-linked dominant inheritance of the disease in family P (Hasstedt and Atkin 1983). They obtained a penetrance of 1.0 in males and 0.85 in females, and failed to confirm many of the abnormal segregation ratios found in earlier studies which formed the basis for the several unusual genetic hypotheses proposed for inheritance in family P.

The same group collaborating with workers in Boston have very recently reported, in abstract form, a linkage study of three large Utah families using 12 X-linked DNA probes. These presumably include, or embrace, family P although this is not stated. Their preliminary results suggest that the gene for X-linked dominant Alport's disease is located near the centromere of the X chromosome, the most significant LOD scores for linkage of the disease locus being 1.8 at a value of $\theta = 0.11$ for linkage to D X S7 (L1.28), 0.75 at $\theta = 0.21$ to D X S3 (ρ19–2), and 0.79 at $\theta = 0.0$ to D X S 67 (ρB24). In their pedigrees L1.28 and ρB24 are tightly linked and the data also give significant LODs in three point linkages for the disease locus and pairs of the same three markers (Menlove *et al.* 1984).

Feingold and Bois (1971) analysed 10 small families and also failed to obtain any abnormal segregation ratios. As a point of historical interest Cohen and Cassady described seven families with Alport's disease (Cassady *et al.* 1965; Cohen *et al.* 1961) with father-to-son transmission in five of these families. In a genetic analysis of the first five families (Cohen *et al.* 1961) they lent support to Shaw and Glover's (1961) non-random segregation hypothesis, as did Mulrow and associates (1963) in their analysis of another large family without father-to-son transmission, and also Purriel and coworkers (1970) for a very large South American family.

Apart from O'Neill and colleagues' reinterpretation of a family P as showing dominant X linkage, several other families have been reported as showing this type of inheritance, as listed in Tables 7.3 and 7.4. One of the earliest such families was that of Hobday and Jones (1969) in which two out of six affected males had children consisting of two normal sons and four affected daughters. Four affected mothers had six affected to three normal sons, and four affected to seven normal daughters. These findings, as the authors state, are strongly in favour of dominant X linkage. A very similar family, apart from six apparently unaffected daughters of affected fathers, was reported by Patton (1970). However, this family does contain four apparently normal females who have transmitted the disease to or through offspring, indicating a rather low penetrance in females. Gaboardi and others (1974) in a study of 19 families observed father-to-son transmission in only two or possibly three families. The authors suggested X-linked dominant inheritance for most of their other families and their pedigrees are certainly compatible with this. However, in many there are no children born to affected fathers and in only three can the evidence for X linkage be said to be strong. Evans and colleagues (1980) analysed 14 Michigan families and reported in detail on one large family (the Grand Rapids kindred) which shows probably X-linked dominance, and one small family with father-to-son transmission, confirming genetic heterogeneity.

A recent paper describes an animal model, with GBM splitting, for X-linked Alport's syndrome in Samoyed dogs (Jansen *et al.* 1986).

There are many other pedigrees in the literature showing clear evidence of father-to-son transmission, and therefore autosomal dominant inheritance, as listed in Tables 7.3 and 7.4. There were no affected males with children in Alport's pedigree in which the mode of inheritance therefore remains unknown. The earliest family with clearly autosomal inheritance was that of Poli (1953) in which there were five examples of male-to-male transmission, including one instance of transmission by grandfather to father to two out of three sons where the father was apparently unaffected. Crawfurd and colleagues (Arnott *et al.* 1966; Crawfurd and Toghill 1968) described three families in one of which there was transmission from an affected father to two, and possibly four, sons. In their earlier paper they analysed 37 published families, eight with lens defects and 29 without, and found that unaffected transmitting mothers had an excess of unaffected sons and daughters. They suggested on this basis that inheritance was autosomal dominant with modification of penetrance and expression by a common X-linked modifier gene. Unfortunately the Utah family P was included in their analysis and is now known to be X linked, and a further 27 families fell into the autosomal or X-linked category as listed in Tables 7.3 and 7.4. There has been no further evidence to support this hypothesis.

Clark Fraser and colleagues using a large French-Canadian family of their own, together with previous published reports, found no evidence to support partial sex linkage, preferential segregation, nor an X-linked modifier (Pashayan *et al.* 1971; Preus and Fraser 1971). They could not exclude genetic heterogeneity including the possibility that some families might show X-linked dominant inheritance. They proposed that their findings fitted autosomal dominant inheritance, with reduced penetrance in the sons of affected fathers, and that an unfavourable intra-uterine milieu of the symptomatic affected mother increases penetrance in affected sons to the full penetrance of affected daughters. Penetrance for sons only of affected fathers was reduced to about 60 per cent. This finding was not confirmed in a small study of six families (Dziuba *et al.* 1975).

Tishler has analysed ages at death of male patients in 37 families, including two new families and a series of published families, and has confirmed that these correlate within families (Tishler 1972; Tishler and Rosner 1974). Furthermore there are two groups with separate age ranges at death of 16 to 28 years and $33\frac{1}{2}$ to $52\frac{1}{2}$ years. Tishler accepts autosomal dominant inheritance for all of these families but proposes genetic heterogeneity on the basis of one major gene determining the disorder in each age at death group. His figures largely agree with those presented in Tables 7.3 and 7.4 which of course include the families analysed by Tishler, but the wider analysis in Tables 7.1 and 7.2 shows a few families in which the ages bridge Tishler's two groups and some overlap of the age ranges for the early and late death groups. This is true of the autosomal dominant, X-linked dominant, and unassignable families.

Habib and coworkers (1982) analysed data from 24 French and Belgian families, including results of electron microscopy of glomerular basement membranes. They found only one instance of father-to-son transmission and confirmed the excess of unaffected compared with affected sons of affected fathers noted by many previous workers. Among a further 11 families, without renal biopsies, there were three further instances of male-to-male transmission. They concluded that their data were compatible with either autosomal dominance with abnormal segregation, or genetic heterogeneity with both autosomal and X-linked dominant patterns of inheritance. Analysis of age at renal death in their 35 families provided further evidence of genetic heterogeneity.

Very few families have been reported that lend any support to the hypothesis of an autosomal recessive group of cases. Wood and Knight (1966) described a family in which four out of six sibs were affected but both parents were unaffected. However, the mother had a history of albuminuria in childhood. The parents were unrelated. Feingold and Bois (1971) included two families, in their series of 10, in which only sibs were affected although in one of these families the mother had an isolated proteinuria.

Grunefeld and coworkers have reported families with hereditary nephritis, with and without perceptive deafness (Hinglais *et al.* 1972; Grunefeld *et al.* 1973). Among their true Alport's disease families there were four in which only sibs were affected (the families of case 2, of cases 7 and 8, and cases 9 and 10 in the 1972 paper, and family 6 of the 1973 paper), including two families with parental consanguinity (cases 7 and 8, and family 6). However, in the family of cases 7 and 8 the father had perceptive deafness, and in family 6 anterior lenticonus was also present. Acecka and Dowbor (1972) have also reported a family with only sibs affected, four sons out of a family of five boys and three girls. Gaboardi and colleagues (1974) in reporting a series of 19 families with hereditary nephritis included two families each with Alport's disease in two out of three sibs (families 8 and 19), in one of which (family 8) the parents were first cousins. However, in these families either the mother cannot be excluded as being a carrier or pedigree data is incomplete. Habib and coworkers (1982) mentioned two families with typical Alport's disease in childhood but unaffected consanguineous parents. These dozen families do not provide sufficient evidence to establish a recessive form of the disease, especially in view of the known incomplete penetrance in females. However, there was parental consanguinity in five out of these 12 families and a very rare recessive type cannot be excluded.

Hasstedt and colleagues (1986), in a review of 23 Utah families, put the case for genetic heterogeneity of Alport's syndrome. They propose six dominant types based on mode of inheritance, age of expression, and presence of deafness or thrombocytopathia. Their type I is a provisional one for families in which juvenile Alport's syndrome is present but the inheritance is unclear. Their type IV is pure hereditary nephritis without deafness, as described in the last section. Their type V is Epstein syndrome to be described later (p. 379). Their remaining types are X-linked and autosomal juvenile Alport's syndrome, and X-linked adult Alport's syndrome (types II, VI, and IV respectively), all associated with deafness. As is evident from Table 19 there is also an autosomal adult type. Autosomal and X-linked families with lenticular defects may represent further types, as would an autosomal recessive type if it truly exists. A very tentative provisional classification of Alport's syndrome with deafness is presented in Table 7.6.

Surprisingly few instances of concordantly affected twins have been reported. Rosenkranz (1963) described a family in which dizygotic twin girls were the index patients, Raszeja-Wanic and colleagues (1969) reported monozygotic male twins with Alport's disease and hyper-prolinaemia, and Felts (1970) a monozygotic pair with uncomplicated Alport's disease. There have been no reports of discordant monozygotic twins.

Sporadic cases of Alport's disease are seldom reported, doubtless partially because of the difficulty in making such a diagnosis in the absence of a positive family history, but also because such cases are generally not felt to be worth publishing. Nevertheless male patients with the classical clinical picture of Alport's disease are not infrequently seen by clinicians with an interest in this disease (e.g. the present author), and have occasionally been reported as part of larger series of cases (e.g. Kaufman *et al.* 1970, one case out of 24). Presumably some of these sporadic cases represent fresh mutations. Shaw and Kallen (1976), making several assumptions including autosomal dominant inheritance, have calculated that at equilibrium frequencies of heterozygotes of between approximately 100 and 500 per million the mutation rate is

Table 7.6. *Syndromes of hereditary nephritis with deafness (Alport's syndrome)*

Type	Hasstedt type	Description with inheritance
I	VI ⎫	Autosomal dominant juvenile
II	II ⎬ Uncertain families: I	X-linked dominant juvenile
III	—	Autosomal dominant adult
IV	III	X-linked dominant adult
V	—	Autosomal dominant with lenticular lesions
VI	—	X-linked dominant with lenticular lesions (one family only)
VII	—	Autosomal recessive (not confirmed)
VIII	V	Autosomal dominant with thrombocytopathia

between 10 and 50 per million gametes, and the proportion of new mutants among affected individuals is 18.3 to 18.4 per cent. Since this is the proportion among all newborns with the Alport phenotype then clearly the proportion of new mutants among sporadic cases will be higher. They point out that the recent observation of glomerular basement membrane splitting as a characteristic feature of the disease should provide a basis for the confirmation of the diagnosis in suspected sporadic cases.

Theoretically there should be exceedingly rare homozygous affected individuals in whom the disease would be expected to be exceptionally severe. One such claim has been made for a boy and his sister, two of three affected children of consanguineous parents, one of whom had nephritis and the other of whom, the father, had hearing loss (Hanicki *et al.* 1970). However, since these two died at the ages of 17 and 11 years respectively, and the father did not have haematuria, the case must be considered unproved.

Alport's disease has been reported from many different populations throughout the world. Apart from Caucasian populations it has been reported in American Blacks (Grace *et al.* 1970), Amerindians (Westley 1970) and Japanese (Sato and Sawada 1962).

In final summary Alport's disease is a inherited nephritis associated in about a third of all affected individuals with perceptive deafness, and in a minority of families with macular and/or lens defects. There is a characteristic, but not specific, splitting of the glomerular basement membrane, and also some evidence for an abnormality of membrane collagen, or of a noncollagenous component of type IV collagen. It is more severe in males than females, with early renal death in the former at either late teenage to twenties, or less commonly in the late twenties to thirties or later. In a proportion of females there is a failure of penetrance. There is evidence for genetic heterogeneity, apart from the above clinical variations, in the pattern of inheritance. There are certainly families with autosomal dominant inheritance, and X-linked dominant families, and possibly a few autosomal recessive families. However, there is no indication of gene assignment for autosomal families. Probably about 18 per cent of all new cases have a fresh mutation. The disease has been reported from most of the major populations in the world. Future advances in our understanding of Alport's disease will come from further biochemical analysis of membrane components to establish the pathogenesis of the disease, or diseases, and molecular studies with DNA probes to resolve the genetic basis of this group of diseases. A start in this direction has already been made by Menlove and colleagues (1984) in the study mentioned earlier.

References

Acecka, H. and Dowbor, B. (1972). Nefropatia rodzinna. *Wiad. Lek.* **25**, 133–6.

Advisory Committee to the Renal Transplant Registry (1972). The Ninth Report of the Human Renal Transplant Registry. *JAMA* **220**, 253–60.

Alport, A. C. (1927). Hereditary familial congenital haemorrhagic nephritis. *Br. Med. J.* **1**, 504–6.

Antonovych, T. T., Deasy, P. F., Tina, L. U., D'Albora, J. B., Hollerman, C. E. and Calcagno, P. L. (1969). Hereditary nephritis: early clinical, functional, and morphological studies. *Paediatr. Res.* **3**, 545–56.

Arnott, E. J., Crawfurd, M.d'A. and Toghill, P. J. (1966). Anterior lenticonus and Alport's syndrome. *Br. J. Ophthalmol.* **50**, 390–403.

Asperti, G. (1964). Lentico anteriore bilaterale con lenticono posteriore mono-laterale in nefritico cronico iperazotemico. *Annali di Ottalmologia* **90**, 107–11.

Beathard, G. A. and Granholm, N. A. (1977). Development of the characteristic ultrastructural lesion of hereditary nephritis during the course of the disease. *Am. J. Med.* **62**, 751–6.

Beaudoing, A., Gachon, J., Gilbert, Y., Dieterlen, M. and Bertolo, J. (1970). Le syndrome d'Alport: étude clinique et génétique. *Ann. Pédiatr. (Paris)* **17**, 271–8.

Bodalski, J. and Margolis, A. (1966). Nefropatia rodzinna. *Ped. Pol.* **41**, 835–41.

Bouchet, M. and Paquelin. (1956). Syndrome familial de néphropathie avec surdité. Étude clinique et génétique. *Annales d'Oto-laryngologie* **73**, 895–905.

Brownell, R. D. and Wolter, J. R. (1964). Anterior lenticonus in familial hemorrhagic nephritis. *Arch. Ophthalmol.* **71**, 481–3.

van Buchem, F. S. P. and Beetstra, A. (1966). Hereditary renal disease associated with deafness—Alport's syndrome. *Acta Med. Scand.* **179**, 319–28.

Burguet, W., Lefebyre, P., Booz, G., Delwaide, P. J. and van Cauwenberge, H. (1966). Le syndrome d'Alport ou néphropathie héréditaire avec surdite. *J. Génét. Hum.* **15**, 7–20.

Cassady, G., Brown, K., Cohen, M. and De Maria, W. (1965). Hereditary renal dysfunction and deafness. *Pediatrics* **35**, 967–79.

Case Records of the Massachusset's General Hospital (Case 43511) (1957). *New Engl. J. Med.* **257**, 1231–7.

Chappel, J. A. and Kelsey, W. M. (1960). Hereditary nephritis. *Am. J. Dis. Child.* **99**, 401–7.

Chaptal, J., Jean, R., Pages, A. and Bonnet, H. (1965). Néphropathie hématurique familiale avec surdité (syndrome d'Alport): a propos de 2 séries d'observations. *Pédiatrie* **20**, 649–64.

Chavis, R. M. and Groshong, T. (1973). Corneal arcus in Alport's syndrome. *Am. J. Ophthal.* **75**, 793–4.

Chazan, J. A., Ambler, M., Kalderon, A., Cohen, J. J. and Zacks, J. (1970). Vascular deposits causing ischemic myopathy in uremia. Two brothers with hereditary nephritis. *Ann. Intern. Med.* **73**, 73–9.

——, Zacks, J., Cohen, J. J. and Garella, S. (1971). Hereditary nephritis. Clinical spectrum and mode of inheritance in five new kindreds. *Am. J. Med.* **50**, 764–71.

Chiricosta, A., Jindel, S. L., Metuzals, J. and Koch, B. (1970). Hereditary nephropathy with hematuria. (Alport's syndrome). *Can. Med. Assoc. J.* **102**, 396–401.

Chuang, V. P. and Reuter, S. R. (1974). Angiographic features of Alport's syndrome: hereditary nephritis. *Am. J. Roentgenol.* **121**, 539–43.

Churg, J. and Sherman, R. L. (1973). Pathologic characteristics of hereditary nephritis. *Arch. Pathol.* **95**, 374–9.

Cohen, M. M., Cassady, G. and Hanna, B. L. (1961). A genetic study of hereditary renal dysfunction with associated nerve deafness. *Am. J. Hum. Genet.* **13**, 379–89.

Cohen-Solal, J., Delepierre, M., Delepierre, F. and Herrault, A. (1970). A propos de deux familles atteintes de syndrome d'Alport. *Ann. Pediatr.* **17**, 734–49.

Crawfurd, M. d'A. and Toghill, P. J. (1968). Alport's syndrome of hereditary nephritis and deafness. *Quart. J. Med.* **37**, 563–76.

David, H., Grossman, P., Marx, I. and Natusch, R. F. (1966). Electronenmikroskopische Befunde an der Niere beim Alport-Syndrom. *Frankfurter Z. Pathol.* **76**, 12–20.

Delepierre, M. M. (1969). Syndrome d'Alport et néphropathie hématurique sans surdité. Revue de la littérature. Thése, Paris.

DiBona, G. F. (1983). Alport's syndrome: a genetic defect in biochemical composition of basement membrane of glomerulus, lens, and inner ear? (editorial). *J. Lab. Clin. Med.* **101**, 817–20.

——, Beisswenger, P. J. and Spear, G. S. (1976). Glomerular basement membrane composition in hereditary glomerulonephritis. *Clin. Res.* **24**, 398A.

Dziuba, P., Kobierska-Szczepanska, A. and Jonczyk, K. (1975). Genetical investigations of familial nephropathy. *Gen. Pol.* **16**, 229–33.

Eason, J., Smith, G. L. M. and Buchanan, G. (1924). Hereditary and familial nephritis. *Lancet* **2**, 639–46.

Ehrlich, L. H. (1946). Spontaneous rupture of the lens capsule in anterior lenticonus. *Am. J. Ophthalmol.* **29**, 1274.

Ellis, J. G. and Yaffe, S. J. (1964). Hereditary nephropathy (Alport's syndrome). A cause of haematuria in childhood. *Calif. Med.* **100**, 289–93.

Evans, S. H., Erickson, R. P., Kelsch, R. and Peirce, J. C. (1980). Apparently changing patterns of inheritance in Alport's hereditary nephritis: genetic heterogeneity versus altered diagnostic criteria. *Clin. Genet.* **17**, 285–92.

Farboody, G. H., Valenzuela, L. J., Kallen, R. and Osborne, D. G. (1979). Chronic hereditary nephritis: a clinico-pathologic study of 23 new kindreds and review of the literature. *Hum. Pathol.* **10**, 655–68.

Feingold, J. and Bois, E. (1971). Génétique du syndrome d'Alport. *Humangenetik* **12**, 29–34.

Felts, J. H. (1970). Hereditary nephritis with the nephrotic syndrome. *Arch. Intern. Med.* **125**, 459–61.

Ferguson, A. C. and Rance, C. P. (1972). Hereditary nephropathy with nerve deafness (Alport's syndrome). *Am. J. Dis. Child.* **124**, 84–8.

Flower, R. M. (1964). Familial coincident renal disease and hearing loss. *J. Speech and Hearing Disorders* **29**, 329–33.

Gaboardi, F., Edefonti, A., Imbasciati, E., Tarantino, A., Mihatsch, M. J. and Zollinger, H. U. (1974). Alport's syndrome (progressive hereditary nephritis). *Clin Nephrol.* **2**, 143–56.

Giacomelli, F. (1963). Considerazioni sulla sindrome nefrococleare ereditaria (Sindrome di Alport). *Minerva Otorinolaringologica* **13**, 336–45.

Gobin, C., Porge, J.-F., and Maréchar, A. (1958). Néphropathies familiales avec surdité. *J. de Méd. et Chir. Prat.* **129**, 1077–82.

Goetz, O., Karl, H. J. and Dattenberg, T. (1965). Familiäre Hämaturie und Innenohrsch-Werhörigkeit (Alport-Syndrom). *Z. Kinderheilk.* **94**, 63–79.

Goldman, R. and Haberfelde, G. C. (1959). Hereditary nephritis—report of a kindred. *New Engl. J. Med.* **261**, 734–8.

Goldbloom, R. B., Fraser, F. C., Waugh, D., Aronovitch, M. and Wiglesworth, F. W. (1957). Hereditary renal disease associated with nerve deafness and ocular changes. *Pediatrics* **20**, 241–52.

Grace, S. G., Suki, W. N., Spjut, H. J., Ecknoyan, G. and Martinez-Maldonado, M. (1970). Hereditary nephritis in the Nego. *Arch. Intern. Med.* **125**, 451–8.

Graham, J. B. (1959). Hereditary chronic kidney disease: an alternative to partial sex-linkage in the Utah kindred. *Am. J. Hum. Genet.* **11**, 333–8.

—— (1960). Chronic hereditary nephritis: not shown to be partially sex-linked. *Am. J. Hum. Genet.* **12**, 382–4.

Gregg, J. B. and Becker, S. F. (1963). Concomitant progressive deafness, chronic nephritis and ocular lens disease. *Arch. Ophthalmol.* **69**, 293–9.

Grunefeld, J.-P., Bois, E. P. and Hinglais, N. (1973). Progressive and non-progressive hereditary chronic nephritis. *Kidney Int.* **4**, 216–27.

Gubler, M., Levy, M., Brozer, M., Naizot, C., Gonzales, G., Perrin, D. and Habib, R. (1981). Alport's syndrome, a report of 58 cases and a review of the literature. *Am. J. Med.* **70**, 493–505.

Guthrie, L. G. (1902). 'Idiopathic', or congenital, hereditary and family haematuria. *Lancet* **1**, 1243–6.

Habib, R., Gubler, M.-C., Hinglais, N., Noel, L.-H., Droz, D., Levy, M., Mahieu, P., Fordart, J. M., Perrin, D., Bois, E. and Grunefeld. J.-P. (1982). Alport's syndrome: experience at Hôpital Necker. *Kidney Int.* **21**, Suppl. 11, S-20–S-28.

Haldane, J. B. S. (1936). A search for incomplete sex-linkage in man. *Ann. Eugen.* **7**, 28–57.

Hallberg, A. (1976). Alport's syndrome: a report of three Swedish families. *Acta Paediatr. Scand.* **65**, 49–56.

Hamburger, J., Crosnier, J., Lissac, J. and Naffah, J. (1956). Sur un syndrome familial de néphropathie avec surdite. *J. Urol. Med. (Paris)* **62**, 113–24.

Hanicki, Z., Hanicka, M. and Mieyzynski, W. (1970). Nefropatia rodzinna z gluchota neurogenna (zespol Alporta). *Pol. Arch. Med. Wewn.* **45**, 635–9.

Hasstedt, S. J. and Atkin, C. L. (1983). X-linked inheritance of Alport syndrome: family P revisited. *Am. J. Hum. Genet.* **35**, 1241–51.

——, —— and San Juan, A. C. (1986). Genetic heterogeneity among kindreds with Alport syndrome. *Am. J. Hum. Genet.* **38**, 940–53.

Hinglais, N., Grünefeld, J. P. and Bois, E. (1972). Characteristic ultrastructural lesion in the glomerular basement membrane in progressive hereditary nephritis (Alport's syndrome). *Lab. Invest.* **27**, 473–87.

Hobday, J. D. and Jones, G. D. T. (1969). Hereditary nephritis with deafness. *Med. J. Austr.* **2**, 1140–3.

Hobolth, N. (1963). Hereditary nephropathy with haematuria. *Acta. Paediatr.* **52**, 581–7.

Hooft, C., Acker, K. and van de Verbeeck, J. (1962). Familiale hematurie. *Maandschr. Kindergeneesk.* **30**, 357–68.

Howe, H. G. Jr., and Smythe, C. M. (1982). Hereditary nephropathy associated with nerve deafness and ocular lesions. *Clin. Res.* **10**, 43.

Hurst, A. F. (1923). Hereditary familial congenital haemorrhagic nephritis occurring in sixteen individuals in three generations. *Guy's Hosp. Rep.* **73**, 368–70.

Iversen, U. M. (1974). Hereditary nephropathy with hearing loss (Alport's syndrome). *Acta Paediatr. Scand.* (suppl 245), 1–23.

Jain, P. (1970). A family with Alport's syndrome. *Postgrad. Med. J.* **46**, 83–5.

Jansen, B., Tryphonas, L., Wong, J., Thorner, P., Maxie, M. G., Valli, V. E., Baumal, R. and Basrur, P. K. (1986). Mode of inheritance of Samoyed hereditary glomerulopathy: an animal model for hereditary nephritis in humans. *J. Lab. Clin. Med.* **107**, 551–5.

Jaworski, A. (1910). Ein fall von Lenticonus anterior und ueber dessen Entstehen. *Arch. f. Augenheilk.* **65**, 313.

Jenis, E. H., Valeski, J. E. and Calcagno, P. L. (1981). Variability of anti-GBM binding in hereditary nephritis. *Clin. Nephrol.* **15**, 111–14.

Johnson, W. J. and Hagan, P. J. (1965). Hereditary nephropathy and loss of hearing. *Arch. Otolanyng.* **82**, 166–72.

Junod, J. P. (1963). La néphropathie héréditaire avec surdité et atteinte oculaire. *Actualités Néphrologiques de l'hôpital Necher, Paris. Flammaron*, 29–45.

Kashtan, C., Fish, A. J., Kleppel, M., Yoshioka, K. and Michael, A. F. (1986). Nephritogenic antigen determinants in epidermal and renal basement membranes of kindreds with Alport-like familial nephritis. *J. Clin. Invest.* **78**, 1035–44.

Kaufman, D. B., McIntosh, R. M., Smith, F. G., Jr. and Vernier, R. L. (1970). Diffuse familial nephropathy: a clinicopathological study. *J. Pediatr.* **77**, 37–47.

Kendall, G. and Hertz, A. F. (1912). Hereditary familial congenital haemorrhagic nephritis. *Guy's Hosp. Rep.* **66**, 137–41.

Kenya, P. R., Asal, N. R., Pederson, J. A. and Lindemann, R. D. (1977). Hereditary (familial) renal disease: clinical and genetic studies. *S. Med. J.* **70**, 1049–51.

Kienecher, R. (1929). Ueber einem fall Doppelseitigen sog: Lentiglobus anterior. *Klin. Monatsbl. f. Augenheilk.* **82**, 55.

Kinoshita, Y., Morita, T., Wada, J., Watanabe, M., Osawa, G., Kobayashi, M.,

Ebe, T., Murohashi, K. and Murayama, M. (1969). Hereditary chronic nephritis (Alport) complicated by nephrotic syndrome. Light, fluorescent and electron microscopic studies of renal biopsy specimens. *Acta Med. Biol.* **17**, 101–17.

Klotz, R. E. (1959). Congenital hereditary kidney disease and hearing loss. *Arch. Otolaryng., Chicago.* **69**, 560–2.

Kohaut, E. C., Singer, D. B., Nevels, B. K. and Hill, L. L. (1976). The specificity of split renal membranes in hereditary nephritis. *Arch. Pathol.* **100**, 475–9.

Krickstein, H. I., Gloor, F. J. and Balogh, K. (1966). Renal pathology in hereditary nephritis with nerve deafness. *Arch. Pathol.* **82**, 506–17.

Kryzmanski, M., Czekalski, S., Zych, J. and Wojtczak, A. (1973). Ocena czynnosci nerek a 5 rodzin z zespolem rodzinnej nefropatii. *Pol. Tyg. Lek.* **26**, 1793–6.

Lachhein, L., Kemnitz, P., Buttner, H., Thial, W. and Witkowski, R. (1968). Erbliche Nephritis mit Inenohrschwerhörigkeit (Alport-Syndrom). *Dtsch. Med. Wschr.* **93**, 1891–6.

——, ——, ——, ——, and —— (1969). Hereditary nephritis with perceptive deafness (Alport's syndrome). *Germ. Med. Monthly* **14**, 218–22.

Lemoyne, J. and Fleury, P. (1962). Un nouveau cas de surdité familiale avec néphropathie. *Ann. Oto-laryngol.* **79**, 599–601.

Lubec, G. and Shabbir, C. (1984). Non-invasive diagnosis of Alport's syndrome. *Lancet* **1**, 1119.

——, Balzar, E., Weissenbacher, G. and Syré, G. (1978). Urinary excretion of glomerular basement membrane antigens in Alport's syndrome: a new diagnostic approach. *Arch. Dis. Child.* **53**, 401–6.

McCoy, R. C., Johnson, H. K., Stone, W. J. and Wilson, C. B. (1976). Variation in glomerular basement membrane antigens in hereditary nephritis (abs.). *Lab. Invest.* **34**, 325–6.

McKennan Hospital Clinical-Pathological conferences (1963). Concurrent progressive deafness, nephritis and outer lens disease. *S. Dak. J. Med. Pharm.* **16**, 23–8.

McKusick, V. A. (1960). Pedigree of a family with hereditary nephritis. *J. Chron. Dis.* **12**, 174–5.

MacNeill, E. and Shaw, R. E. (1973). Segregation ratios in Alport's syndrome. *J. Med. Genet.* **10**, 23–6.

Mamou, H. (1966). Maladie périodique familiale avec nephropathie et surdité. *Sem. Hôp. Paris* **42**, 3363–6.

Marie, J., Royer, P., Habib, R., Mathieu, H. and Reveillaud, R.-J. (1960). La néphropathie hématurique héréditaire avec surdité. *Ann. de Pédiatr.* **36**, 84–103.

Maurer, W., Fritz, R. D. and Madison, F. W. (1968). Hereditary hematuria. *Wis. Med. J.* **67**, 378–81.

Mayo, O. (1973). Alport's syndrome. *J. Med. Genet.* **10**, 396–7.

Menlove, L., Aldridge, J., Schwartz, C., Atkin, C., Hasstedt, S., Kunkel, L., Bruns, G., Latt, S. and Skolnick, M. (1984). Linkage between Alport syndrome-like hereditary nephritis and X-linked RFLPs (abs.). *Am. J. Hum. Genet.* **36**, 146S.

Mettier, S. R. (1961). Ocular defects associated with familial renal disease and deafness. *Arch. Ophthalmol.* **65**, 386–91.

Miller, G. W., Joseph, D. J., Cozad, R. L. and McCabe, B. F. (1970). Alport's syndrome. *Arch. Otolaryngol.* **92**, 419–32.

Milliner, D. S., Pierides, A. M. and Holley, K. E. (1982). Renal transplantation in Alport's syndrome: anti-glomerular basement membrane glomerulonephritis in the allograft. *Mayo Clin. Proc.* **57**, 35–43.

Minder, F. C., Dubach, U. C. and Antener, I. (1965). Hereditäre Nephropathie und Schwerhörigkeit. *Z. Klin. Med.* **158**, 601.

Miyoshi, K., Suzuki, M., Ohno, F., Yamano, T., Yagi, F. and Khono, H. (1975). Antithyroid antibodies in Alports syndrome. *Lancet* **2**, 480–2.

Morton, N. E. (1957). Further scoring types in sequential linkage tests with a critical review of autosomal and partial sex linkage in man. *Am. J. Hum. Genet.* **9**, 55–75.

Mulrow, P. J., Aron, A. M., Gathman, G. E., Yesner, R. and Lubb, H. A. (1963). Hereditary nephritis: report of a kindred. *Am. J. Med.* **35**, 737–48.

Myers, G. J. and Tyler, H. R. (1972). The etiology of deafness in Alport's syndrome. *Arch. Otoloryngol.* **96**, 333–40.

Naffah, J. (1956). Sur un syndrome familial de nephropathie avec surdité. Thése, Paris.

Nichol, K. P. and Miller, A. (1965). Hereditary nephritis and deafness. *Lancet* **85**, 236–40.

Nielsen, C. E. (1978). Lenticonus anterior and Alport's syndrome. *Acta Ophthalmol.* **56**, 518–30.

Nieth, H. (1959). Beitrag zum Syndrome der hereditären. Hämatarie, Nephropathie und Schwerhörigkeit. *Verh. Dtsch. Ges. Inn. Med.* **65**, 664–7.

Oberiter, V. (1966). Familijarna nefropatija s gluhocom (syndroma Alport). *Arch. Zastitu Majke Djetata* **10**, 285–9.

Ohlsson, L., (1963). Congenital renal disease, deafness and myopia in one family. *Acta Med. Scand.* **174**, 77–84.

Olson, D. L., Anand, S. K., Landing, B. H., Heuser, E., Gruskin, C. M. and Lieferman, E. (1980). Diagnosis of hereditary nephritis by failure of glomeruli to bind anti-glomerular basement membrane antibodies. *J. Pediatr.* **96**, 697–9.

O'Neill, W. M. Jr. and Atkin, C. L. (1978). Hereditary nephritis. *Ann. Intern. Med.* **89**, 286.

——, —— and Bloomes, H. A. (1978). Hereditary nephritis: a re-examination of its clinical and genetic features. *Ann. Intern. Med.* **88**, 176–82.

——, Mennemeyer, R. P., Bloomer, H. A. and Atkin, C. L. (1980). Early pathologic features of hereditary nephritis: a clinicopathologic correlation. *Pathol. Res. Pract.* **168**, 146–62.

Onisawa, J., Sato, H., Suzuki, Y. and Takatsu, T. (1965). Aminoaciduria in Alport's syndrome. *Paediatr. Univ. Tokyo* **11**, 9–17.

Pashayan, H., Fraser, F. C. and Goldbloom, R. B. (1971). A family showing hereditary nephropathy. *Am. J. Hum. Genet.* **23**, 555–67.

Patton, R. B. (1970). Chronic hereditary nephritis with nerve deafness; a Nebraska kindred. *Ann. Otol. Rhinol. Laryng.* **79**, 194–202.

Perkoff, G. T. (1964). Familial aspects of diffuse renal diseases. *Ann. Rev. Med.* **15**, 115–24.

——, Stephens, F. E., Dolowitz, D. A. and Tyler, F. H. (1951). A clinical study of hereditary interstitial pyelonephritis. *Arch. Intern. Med.* **88**, 191–200.

——, Nugent, C. A. Jr., Dolowitz, D. A., Stephens, F. E., Carnes, W. H., and Tyler, F. H. (1958). A follow up study of hereditary chronic nephritis. *Arch. Intern. Med.* **102**, 733–46.

——, Stephens, F. E. and Tyler, F. H. (1960). Chronic hereditary nephritis and Y-chromosome linkage: reply to Graham. *Am. J. Hum. Genet.* **12**, 381–2.

Perrin, D. (1964). Le syndrome d'Alport (Néphropathies héréditaires avec surdite et atteinte oculaire. *Ann. Oculist., Paris.* **197**, 329–46.

——, Jungers, P., Grünefeld, J. P., Delons, S., Noël, L. H. and Zenatti, C. (1980). Perimacular changes in Alport's syndrome. *Clin. Nephrol.* **13**, 163–7.

Peters, R. (1964). Syndroom van Alport a hereditaire chronische nefritis. *Maandershr. Kindergeneesk.* **32**, 18–28.

Polak, B. C. P. and Hogewind, B. L. (1977). Macular lesions in Alport's disease. *Am. J. Ophthalmol.* **84**, 532–5.

Poli, M. (1953). Nefropatie mediche bilaterale familiari. *51st Congr. Soc. Ital. Med. Intern., Montecatini, 1950.* Ed. Minerva Med., Torino. p. 358.

—— (1955). Néphropathie médicale bilatérale familiale a évolution chronique. *Helv. Med. Acta* **22**, 109–22.

Preus, M. and Fraser, F. C. (1971). Genetics of hereditary nephropathy with deafness (Alport's disease). *Clin. Genet.* **2**, 331–7.

Purriel, P., Drets, M., Pascale, E., Cestau, R. S., Borras, A., Ferreira, W. A., Delucca, A. and Fernandez, L. (1970). Familial hereditary nephropathy (Alport's syndrome). *Am. J. Med.* **49**, 753–73.

Raszeja-Wanic, B., Wachowiak, A. and Kosicka, M. (1969). Nefropatia rodzinna u blizniat. *Pol. Tyg. Lek.* **24**, 124–6.

Reyersbach, G. C. and Butler, A. M. (1954). Congenital hereditary haematuria. *New Engl. J. Med.* **251**, 377–80.

Robin, E. D., Gardner, F. H. and Levine, S. A. (1957). Hereditary factors in chronic Bright's disease. *Trans. Assoc. Am. Phys.* **70**, 140–7.

Rones, B. (1934). Anterior lenticonus. *JAMA* **103**, 327–30.

Rosenkranz, von A. (1963). Hereditäre Nephritis (Alport's Syndrom). *Ann. Paediatr.* **201**, 365–80.

Royer, P. (1968). Familial nephropathy with deafness. In *Nephrology*, eds. Hamburger, J. *et al.* pp. 803–10. Saunders, Philadelphia.

Sato, H. and Sawada, K. (1962). Shonika, *Shinryo* **25**, 699–707.

Savage, C. O. S., Reed, A., Kershaw, M., Pincott, J., Pusey, C. D., Dillon, M. J., Barratt, J. M. and Lockwood, C. M. (1986). Use of a monoclonal antibody in differential diagnosis of children with haematuria and hereditary nephritis. *Lancet* **1**, 1459–61.

Schmidt, P., Kopsa, H., Zazgornik, J. and Pils, P. (1976). Antithyroid antibodies in Alport's syndrome. *Lancet* **1**, 968.

Schneegans, E., Rohmer, A., Levy-Silagy, J., Elmejjati, A., Sengel, P., Stoebner, P. and Laforgue, D. (1971). Contribution a l'etude du syndrome d'Alport: a propos d'un cas. *Sem. Hôp. Paris. Ann. Pédiatr.* **18**, 757–69.

Schneider, R. G. (1963). Congenital hereditary nephritis with nerve deafness. *NY State J. Med.* **63**, 2644–8.

Sessa, A., Cioffi, A., Allaria, P., Conte, F. and D'Amico, G. (1973). Hereditary nephritis with immunofluorescent mesangial deposits. *Lancet* **2**, 853.

Shaw, R. F. (1973). Alport's syndrome. *J. Med. Genet.* **10**, 398.

—— and Glover, R. A. (1961). Abnormal segregation in hereditary renal disease with deafness. *Am. J. Hum. Genet.* **13**, 89–97.

—— and Kallen, R. J. (1976). Population genetics of Alport's syndrome. *Nephron* **16**, 427–32.

Sherman, R. L., Churg, J. and Yudis, M. (1974). Hereditary nephritis with a characteristic renal lesion. *Am. J. Med.* **56**, 44–51.

Sohar, E. (1954). Heredo-familial syndrome characterized by renal disease, inner ear deafness, and ocular changes. *Harefuah* **47**, 161.

—— (1956). Renal disease, inner ear deafness and ocular changes: a new heredo-familial syndrome. *Arch. Intern. Med.* **97**, 627–30.

Spear, G. S. (1973). Alport's syndrome: a consideration of pathogenesis. *Clin. Nephrol.* **1**, 336–7.

—— and Slusser, R. J. (1972). Alport's syndrome: emphasizing electron microscopic studies of the glomerulus. *Am. J. Pathol.* **69**, 213–24.

——, Whitworth, J. M. and Konigsmark, B. W. (1970). Hereditary nephritis with nerve deafness. Immunofluorescence studies on the kidney, with a consideration of discordant immunoglobulin-complement immunofluorescent reactions. *Am. J. Med.* **49**, 52–63.

Stephens, F. E., Perkoff, G. T., Dolowitz, D. A. and Tyler, F. H. (1951). Partially sex-linked dominant inheritance of interstitial pyelonephritis. *Am. J. Hum. Genet.* **3**, 303–13.

Sturtz, G. S. and Burke, E. C. (1956). Hereditary hematuria, nephropathy and deafness, a preliminary report. *New Engl. J. Med.* **254**, 1123–6.

—— and —— (1958). Syndrome of hereditary hematuria, nephropathy and deafness. *Mayo Clin. Proc.* **33**, 289–97.

Symboulidis, A., Voudiclaris, S., Mayopoulou-Symvoulidis, D., Oreopoulos, D. and Yatzidis, H. (1968). Alport's syndrome: a study of 7 families including 150 members. *Nosokomiaca Chronica* **30**, 491–506.

——, ——, —— and Katirtsoglou. A. (1972). Hereditary nephritis. *Br. Med. J.* **4**, 489.

Tiliakos, A., Voulgaridis, D. and Gialafos, T. (1964). Syndrome d'Alport ou néphrite héréditaire avec surdite. *Presse Méd.* **72**, 1567–70.

Tina, L. U., Lou, M. F., Dizio, D. and Calcagno, P. L. (1979). Alteration of collagen metabolism in hereditary nephritis. *Pediatr. Res.* **13**, 774–6.

Tishler, P. V. (1972). Hereditary nephritis. *Br. Med. J.* **4**, 269.

—— (1978). Genetics of hereditary nephritis. *Ann. Intern. Med.* **89**, 285–6.

—— (1979). Healthy female carriers of a gene for the Alport syndrome: importance for genetic counselling. *Clin. Genet.* **16**, 291–4.

Tishler, P. V. and Rosner, B. (1974). The genetics of the Alport syndrome. *Birth Defects* **10**, 93–9.

Tsukahara. (1930). Zwei Fälle von Lentiglobus anterior. Anhang: Resultate der Untersuchung der Tätigkeit des Vegitativen Nervensystems. *Acta Soc. Ophth. Jap.* **34**, 370. Abstracted in *Zentralbl. f. Ges Ophth.* (1931). **24**, 171.

Turner, J. S. Jr. (1970). Hereditary hearing loss with nephropathy (Alport's syndrome). *Acta Otolaryng.* **271**, (Suppl.), 7–26.

Unger, L. (1957). *Klin. Mbl. Augenheilk.* **130**, 696.

Wasserman, E., Schwarz, F., Wachstein, M. and Lange, K. (1963). Diagnostic value of complement determination in hereditary glomerulonephritis (abs.). *J. Pediatr.* **63**, 722.

——, ——, —— and —— (1965). Diagnostic value of serum complement determination in hereditary gomerulonephritis. *J. Lab. Clin. Med.* **65**, 589–99.

Westley, C. R. (1970). Familial nephritis and associated deafness in a southwestern Apache Indian family. *S. Med. J.* **63**, 1415–19.

Whalen, R. E., Huang, S.-S., Peschel, E. and McIntosh, H. D. (1961). Hereditary nephropathy, deafness and renal foam cells. *Am. J. Med.* **31**, 171–86.

White, R. H. R., Parsons, V. and Walt, F. P. (1964). The renal disorder in Alport's syndrome. *Guys Hosp. Rep.* **113**, 179–89.

Wieslander, J., Barr, J. F., Butkowski, R. J., Edwards, S. J., Byren, P., Heinegard, D. and Hudson, B. G. (1984). Goodpastures antigen of the glomerular basement membrane: localization to noncollagenous regions of type IV collagen. *Proc. Nat. Acad. Sci.* **81**, 3838–42.

Williamson, D. A. J. (1961). Alport's syndrome of hereditary nephritis with deafness. *Lancet* **2**, 1321–3.

Winter, L. E., Cram, B. M. and Banovetz, J. O. (1968). Hearing loss in hereditary renal disease. *Arch. Otolaryngol.* **88**, 238–41.

Wood, T. J. and Knight, L. W. (1966). A family with Alport's syndrome of hereditary nephritis and deafness. *Aust. Ann. Med.* **15**, 227–35.

Zavala, C., Villar-Puig, P., Garza, R., Lisker, R. and Dies, F. (1969). Nefropatia cronica hereditaria con hipoacusia y defectos oculares. Sobretiro de la Revista de Investigacion *Clin. Mex.* **21**, 369–82.

Zeromski, J. O., Górny, M. K. and Kryzmánski, M. (1976). Antithyroid antibodies in Alport's syndrome. *Lancet* **1**, 296.

7.5. FAMILIAL NEPHROTIC SYNDROME

7.5.1. Familial nephrosis

The earliest report of the familial occurrence of nephrotic syndrome is probably that of Benson (1893) who observed the disease in four out of six children of first-cousin parents. Onset varied between 1 and 4 years, and three out of the four affected children died, at about 1, 4 and 6 years respectively. Subsequent reports have been notable for the heterogeneity of the cases described (Lagrue and Bariéty 1963) although most fall into two groups: further instances of nephrosis of early childhood or later onset, and congenital or early infantile cases. Benson's, and several other early papers, do not distinguish the histological type of nephrosis but do include several examples of familial occurrence of the later onset type. There have been several reports of concordant monozygotic twin pairs (Forge 1950; Prader 1950; Kretchmer *et al.* 1960; Sereni and Careddu 1961; Jovanovic *et al.* 1962; Roy and Pitcock 1971; Bader *et al.* 1974a) and of families with at least two affected sibs (Blechmann and Taverner 1934; Fanconi *et al.* 1951; Barnett *et al.* 1952; Fanconi and Illig 1960; Marie *et al.* 1960; Sereni and Careddu 1961; Gentili and Tangheroni 1964; Mehls and Schärer 1970; Moncrieff *et al.* 1973; White 1973; Gekle *et al.* 1975; Gonzales *et al.* 1977). These and other examples of familial occurrence are reviewed by Norio (1969) who argues fairly convincingly that the family data point to a polygenic rather than a single gene inheritance. If this is indeed so then many sporadic cases too must be of polygenic aetiology. In 1974 Bader and associates (1974a) published a study of 70 patients with idiopathic nephrotic syndrome. Fifty-four of these were sporadic and 16 familial. Of 24 sporadic patients who had renal biopsy 16 had minimal change and eight had major glomerular changes, and of the 12 patients with familial disease who had biopsies nine had minimal change and three had focal global glomerulo-sclerosis, a late abnormality in minimal change disease to be distinguished from focal segmental glomerulosclerosis. The familial cases consisted of a pair of concordant monozygotic twins (one more severe than the other), five affected sib pairs, two single affected with cousin parents and two affected first cousins from a consanguineous family. They found no signficant differences between the familial and non-familial cases on either clinical or histopathological criteria. Segregation analysis excluded simple autosomal recessive inheritance and the authors support Norio (1969) in favouring a polygenic model with a threshold effect. Despite their rejection of a mixed aetiology with a small proportion of autosomal recessive cases among their families this would still seem to be likely for a few of the famlies in the literature, including Benson's (1893) original family, and one of the families of Fanconi and Illig (1960). In both of these families there were three or more affected sibs with cousin parents. Norio (1983) also accepts that at least some families are probably due to autosomal recessive inheritance. Whether or not this is true of the reported families of three (Schwarz *et al.* 1976) or two sibs (Naruse *et al.* 1980) with nephrotic syndrome with focal glomerular sclerosis is impossible to say. However, Naruse and colleagues' sibs did have first-cousin parents. Bader and colleagues (1974b) found an empirical risk at 0.06 for sibs of patients with nephrotic syndrome of minimal change type. Another form of idiopathic nephrosis, membranous nephropathy, shows a strong association with HLA-DRW3 (Klouda *et al.* 1979; Müller *et al.* 1981; Rashid *et al.* 1983) and is occasionally also associated with dermatitis herpetiformis (Davies and Davies 1979) or coeliac disease (Katz *et al.* 1979) both of which diseases are also associated with HLA-DRW3 and with one another.

References

Bader, P. I., Grove, J., Trygstad, C. W. and Nance, W. E. (1974a). Familial nephrotic syndrome. *Am. J. Med.* **56**, 34–43.
——, ——, Nance, W. E. (1974b). Inheritance of idiopathic nephrotic syndrome. In *Birth defects—urinary system and others*, ed. Bergsma, D. **10**, Pt. 16, pp. 73–9.
Barnett, H. L., Forman, C. W. and Lauson, H. D. (1952). The nephrotic syndrome in children. *Adv. Pediatr.* **5**, 53–128.

Benson, A. H. (1893). Nephritis of obscure origin in several children of one family. *Lancet* **1**, 588.

Blechmann, G. and Taverner, L. (1934). Néphrose lipoidique chez deux fréres. *Concours Méd.* **10** *bis*, 751.

Davies, M. G. and Davies, P. G. (1979). Dermatitis herpetiformis, glomerulonephritis, and HLA-DRW3. *Lancet* **2**, 911.

Devin, P. (1960). Syndromes nephrotiques familiaux et congénitaux. *Thése Médicale Nancy* No. 27.

Fanconi, G. and Illig, R. (1960). Das familiäre Vorkommen der Lipoidnephrose und der Nephronophthise. *Mod. Probl. Paediat. (Karger)* **6**, 298.

——, Kousmine, C. and Frischknecht, W. (1951). Die konstitutionelle Bereitschaft zum nephrosesyndrom. *Helv. Paediatr. Acta.* **6**, 199–218.

Forge, M. J.-F. (1950). A propos de 4 cas de néphrose lipoidique chez de jumeaux monozygotes. *Bull. Soc. Med. Hôp. (Paris)*, **48**, 87.

Gekle, D., Buchinger, G. and Könitzen, T. (1975). Untersuchungen zur Familiarität des nephrotischen Syndroms. *Monatsschr. f. Kinderheilk.* **123**, 106.

Gentili, A. and Tangheroni, W. (1964). Sindrome nefrosica congenita e sindrome nefrosica familiare del bambino. *Clin. Pediatr.* **46**, 385.

Gonzales, G., Kleinknecht, C., Gubler, M. C. and Lenoir, G. (1977). Syndromes néphrotiques familiaux. *La Revue de Pédiatrie* **13**, 427.

Jovanovic, V., Mirkovic, D. and Vukasinovic, N. (1962). Nephrotic syndrome in a pair of twins. *Sprski Arkh. Tselal. Lek.* **6**, 635.

Katz, A., Dyck, R. F. and Bear, R. A. (1979). Celiac disease associated with immune complex glomerulonephritis. *Clin. Nephrol.* **11**, 39–44.

Klouda, P. T., Manos, J., Acheson, E. J., Dyer, P. A., Goldby, F. S., Harris, R., Lawler, W., Mallick, N. P. and Williams, G. (1979). Strong association between idiopathic membranous nephropathy and HLA-DRW3. *Lancet* **2**, 770–1.

Kretchmer, N., Barnett, H. L. and Shibuya, M. (1960). Current problems associated with the nephrotic syndrome in children. *Mod. Probl. Paediatr. (Karger)* **6**, 273.

Lagrue, G. and Bariéty, J. (1963). Les syndromes néphrotiques de la premiere enfance et les syndromes néphrotiques familiaux. *Actualitiés Néphrologiques de l'Hôpital Necker, Paris, Flammarion* pp. 23–8.

Marie, J., Royer, P. and Leveque, B. (1960). Le syndrome néphrotique familiel de l'enfant. *Ann. Pédiatr., Paris.* **36**, 76.

Mehls, O. and Schärer, K. (1970). Familiäres nephrotisches syndrom. *Monatsschr. f. Kinderheilk.* **118**, 328.

Moncrieff, M. W., White, R. H. R., Glasgow, E. F., Winterborn, M. H., Cameron, J. S. and Ogg, C. S. (1973). The familial nephrotic syndrome: II. A clinicopatholgical study. *Clin. Nephrol.* **1**, 220.

Müller, G. A., Müller, C., Liebau, G., Kömpf, J., Ising, H. and Wernet, P. (1981). Strong association of ideopathic membraneous nephropathy (IMN) with HLA-DR3 and MT-2 without involvement of HLA-18 and no association to BfF1. *Tissue Antigens* **17**, 332–7.

Naruse, T., Hirokawa, N., Maekawa, T., Azato, H., Ito, K. and Kaya, H. (1980). Familial nephrotic syndrome with focal glomerular sclerosis. *Am. J. Med. Sci.* **280**, 109–13.

Norio, R. (1969). The nephrotic syndrome and heredity. *Hum. Hered.* **19**, 113–20.

—— (1983). The nephrotic syndromes, In *Principles and practice of medical genetics*, eds. Emery, A. E. H. and Rimoin, D. L. pp. 1011–18. Churchill Livingstone, Edinburgh.

Prader, A. (1950). Lipoidnephrose bei eineügen Zwellinger. *Helv. Paediatr. Acta* **5**, 392.

Rashid, H. U., Papiha, S. S., Agroyannis, B., Morley, A. R., Ward, M. K., Roberts, D. F. and Kerr, D. N. S. (1983). The association of HLA and other genetic markers with glomerulonephritis. *Hum. Genet.* **63**, 38–44.

Roy, S. and Pitcock, J. A. (1971). Idiopathic nephrosis in identical twins. *Am. J. Dis. Child.* **121**, 428–30.

Schwarz, R., Stoegmann, W. and Fischbach, H. (1976). Familiaeres nephritisches Syndrom mit fokaler Glomerulosklerose. *Wien Klin. Wschr.* **88**, 548–54.

Sereni, F. and Careddu, P. (1961). Attuali conoscenze sulla sindrome nefrosica infantile. *Minerva Pediatr.* **13**, 808.

White, R. H. R. (1973). The familial nephrotic syndrome: I. A European survey. *Clin. Nephrol.* **1**, 216.

7.5.2. Congenital (Finnish) or infantile nephrosis

Nephrosis with onset at birth or early infancy has been reported with high frequency from Finland and in infants of Finnish parentage elsewhere, although one of the earliest reports of congenital nephrosis was British (Giles *et al.* 1957), and congenital nephrosis, which is in all respects identical to the Finnish, has been reported at low frequency from all over the world, and in all races (Eiben *et al.* 1954; Kobayashi *et al.* 1961; Yamamoto *et al.* 1961; Kendall-Smith *et al.* 1968; Hallman *et al.* 1970; Habib and Bois 1973; Rajamma *et al.* 1974; George *et al.* 1976). The Finnish cases are sufficiently consistent in their clinical, pathological, and genetic features to be accepted as constituting a distinct entity. The non-Finnish cases present a less clear picture, some are probably due to the gene prevalent in Finland but others show appreciable differences from the Finish form and do not present any consistent picture.

Early reports of the Finnish congenital nephrosis (Hallman *et al.* 1956; Hallman and Hjelt 1959; Huttunen 1976; Hallman and Rapola 1978) established a characteristic clinical picture of onset at birth or within the first few weeks of life with peripheral oedema, abdominal distension, pronouced proteinuria (Huttunen *et al.* 1980), frequent premature birth, and a high incidence of early deaths of premature sibs, a large placenta (Inferrera *et al.* 1980), and death by 2 years, with a notable resistance to therapy. The family reported by Vernier and colleagues from Minesota appears to have the same or a very similar disorder (Vernier *et al.* 1957; Worthen *et al.* 1959).

Pathologically fatty degeneration of renal tubular cells and proliferative glomerular changes, with loss of epithelial foot processes and basement membrane splitting on electron microscopy, typical of nephrotic syndrome, were noted. Despite these glomerular changes many early pathological studies concentrated on the tubular changes. Oliver (1960) and Fetterman and Feldman (1960) who both undertook micro-dissection studies in American cases, and Ongre (1961) who did the same in two Finnish sibs, all describe proximal tubular dilation with formation of 'microcysts'. Another early suggestion, based on the rapid rejection of skin grafts from affected infants by their mothers, was that of maternal sensitization as an aetiological factor (Kouvalainen *et al.* 1962; Kouvalainen 1963). Lange and coworkers (1963) claimed to find immunoglobulin and complement deposits in glomeruli of an infant with congenital nephrosis from New York. However, none of Griswold and McIntosh (1972), Hoyer and associates (1967), or Rapola and Savilahti (1971) could in careful studies confirm any evidence for such immune mechanisms. The latter group studied three sibs, including a pair of monozygotic twins, from a family of Finnish extraction. They contrasted these cases with a fourth non-Finnish case with onset at 6 months, a lack of microcysts in the kidneys and responding to adrenocorticotrophic hormone (ACTH) therapy. A similar distinction has been made by McCrory and colleagues (1966).

More recent pathological research has placed the emphasis on glomerular changes and indicates that the tubular changes are secondary. Hallman and colleagues (1967, 1973) describe a proliferative glomerular lesion with thickening of glomerular walls and crescent formation, as well as the microcystic dilation of proximal tubules. They also note that these changes are initially slight but develop over the immediate postnatal period. Others have described the ultrastructural changes in the Finnish type in more detail: a narrow width to the lamina densa, a lack of immune complex deposits, epithelial foot process fusion, increased amounts of fibrillar material in epithelial cytoplasm adjacent to the basement membrane, vacuoles, and heteromorphic bodies in mesangial cell cyto-plasm (Rapola and Savilahti 1971; Mahieu *et al.* 1976; Autio-Harmainen 1981; Autio-Harmainen and Rapola 1983). Studies of the chemical composition of the glomerular basement membrane also point to this as the site of the basic defect, although there is not complete agreement on the precise changes. Tryggvason (1977) in a study of 3-hydroxy- to 4-hydroxy proline ratios concluded that there was less collagen than normal in basement membranes from glomeruli of patients with the Finnish type, in contrast to an increase in collagen-specific amino acids in the non-Finnish type (Mahieu *et al.* 1976). However, Risteli and associates (1982) found increased type IV (basement membrane) collagen in renal cortices of Finnish patients with an increased collagen:laminin ratio. Furthermore they found a slow accumulation of the collagenous component of the glomerular basement membrane with time, not seen in control kidneys. Vernier and colleagues (1983) have found a decreased concentration of heparan sulphate rich anionic sites which they have demonstrated in the lamina rara externa of normal human glomerular basement membrane. These anionic sites are formed by side chains of membrane proteoglycans. These observations, if confirmed, are of profound importance for the pathogenesis of congenital nephrosis but unfortunately leave open a wide range of options for the genetic defect.

Norio and his colleagues found an incidence of congenital nephrosis in Finland of 1 in 10 000 births and demonstrated its autosomal recessive inheritance (Norio *et al.* 1964; Norio 1966). Huttunen (1976) found a Finnish birth incidence of 12.2 per 100 000.

Among the non-Finnish cases a series of nine from Liverpool (Bouton and Coulter 1974) including two pairs of sibs contains five cases (their cases 1, 2, 4, 6, and 9) consistent with the diagnosis of the Finnish type. Of their remaining cases one (case 5) had a normal birth weight, late onset but rapidly fatal course; another (case 3) showed a distinctive pathological picture; a sib pair (case 7 and 8) showed survival to 5 years in one case. Hoyer and colleagues (1973) in a further study from Minneapolis report successful renal transplantation in four cases but in at least two of these survival was already too long for diagnosis of the Finnish type. Mahan and colleagues (1984) have reported their experience of 41 cases of nephrotic syndrome, with onset within the first 3 months of life, from Minneapolis. Nine of these were of Finnish ancestry and 18 had a positive family history. Seventeeen of their patients had undergone renal transplantation without recurrence of nephrotic syndrome, and with a 2-year survival rate of 82 per cent.

A possibly distinct but also autosomal recessive form of infantile nephrosis is that showing diffuse mesangial sclerosis. Onset is neonatal to just over 1 year and is fatal by 4 years (Habib and Bois 1973; Hallman *et al.* 1973; Kaplan *et al.* 1974; Richard *et al.* 1975; Seelig *et al.* 1975; Gonzales *et al.* 1977; Rumpelt and Bachmann 1980). In two of Habib and Bois' families, in Gonzales and colleagues' family and in one other probable family (Rossenbeck *et al.* 1966) there have been affected sibs.

Seppälä and Ruoslahti (1972) observed a grossly raised amniotic fluid α-fetoprotein (AFP) in a pregnancy which resulted in the birth of an infant with congenital nephrosis of Finnish type. This observation has stimulated an appreciable literature on the prenatal diagnosis of this disorder. Kjessler and coworkers (1975a and b) reported the first prospective prenatal diagnoses and terminations. They also reported pathological changes in the fetal kidneys on electron microscopy. Seppälä's group have undertaken prenatal diagnosis in 23 at-risk pregnancies and found normal amniotic fluid AFP in 16 followed by the birth of healthy infants, and a raised AFP in seven which were terminated (Rapola *et al.* 1975; Seppälä *et al.* 1976; Aula *et al.* 1978). They confirmed the electron microscopic changes observed by Kjessler and associates, and in five of their cases with raised AFP in the amniotic fluid found it to be also raised in maternal serum. Similar prenatal diagnoses have been reported from the United States (Milunsky *et al.* 1977) and Britain (Thom *et al.* 1977; Batstone *et al.* 1981). Thom and colleagues also demonstrated elevated albumin, AFP, α_2-macroglobulin, and IgG in the fetal urine in their case. In a case reported by Spritz and associates (1978), clearly not of Finnish type (Rapola and Hallman 1979) the amniotic fluid AFP measured at 23 weeks was not elevated but the subsequent infant developed nephrosis at 5 months of age. Thus AFP is only reliable for the prenatal diagnosis of the Finnish type. Seppälä's group have shown that in both neural tube defect and Finnish-type congenital nephrosis it is the non-concanavilin A subfraction of AFP that is relatively increased, at least up to 18 weeks of pregnancy. The same group have used maternal serum AFP to screen over 10 000 pregnancies; 2.5 per cent had a persistently raised serum AFP, and out of these 2.1 per cent had an amniocentesis. Sixteen mothers (0.15 per cent) had amniotic fluid AFP greater than 10 standard deviations above the normal mean, of which six had fetuses with nephrotic syndrome and none were missed (Ryynänen *et al.* 1983). Brock and Hayward (1980) observed that the raised amniotic fluid AFP, seen in pregnancies with a fetus affected by Finnish-type congenital nephrosis, is associated with absence of an acetylcholinesterase band on acrylamide gel electrophoresis. Morin and colleagues (1984) demonstrated raised amniotic fluid trehalase activity in two affected pregnancies. Trehalase is an enzyme located in renal brush border membranes and it is released into urine whenever there is damage to such membranes, as in nephrosis or infantile polycystic kidney (Morin *et al.* 1981).

References

Aula, P., Rapola, J., Karjalainen, O., Lindgren, J., Hartikainen, A. L. and Seppälä, M. (1978). Prenatal diagnosis of congenital nephrosis in 23 high-risk families. *Am. J. Dis. Child.* **132**, 984–7.

Autio-Harmainen, H. (1981). Renal pathology of fetuses with congenital nephrotic syndrome of the Finnish type. 2. A qualitative and quantitative electron microscopic study. *Acta Pathol. Microbiol. Scand.* **89A**, 215–22.

—— and Rapola, J. (1983). The thickness of the glomerular basement membrane in congenital nephrotic syndrome of the Finnish type. *Nephron* **34**, 48–50.

Batstone, G. F., Goldie, D. J., Letchworth, A. T. and McIver, A. (1981). Congenital (Finnish) nephrosis as a cause of abnormal amniotic fluid alpha-fetoprotein. *Lancet* **1**, 664

Bouton, J. M. and Coulter, J. B. S. (1974). The nephrotic syndrome of infancy. *Acta Paediatr. Scand.* **63**, 769–76.

Brock, D. J. H. and Hayward, C. (1980). Gel electrophoresis of amniotic fluid acetylcholinesterase as an aid to the prenatal diagnosis of fetal defects. *Clin. Chim. Acta* **108**, 135–41.

Eiben, R. M., Kleinerman, J. and Cline, J. C. (1954). Nephrotic syndrome in a neonatal premature infant. *J. Pediatr.* **44**, 195–202.

Fetterman, G. H. and Feldman, J. D. (1960). Congenital anomalies of renal tubules in a case of 'infantile nephrosis'. *Am. J. Dis. Child.* **100**, 319–32.

George, C. R. P., Hickman, R. O. and Stricker, G. E. (1976). Infantile nephrotic syndrome. *Clin. Nephrol.* **5**, 20.

Giles, H. McC., Pugh, R. C. B., Darmady, E. M., Stranack, F. and Woolf, L. I. (1957). The nephrotic syndrome in early infancy: a report of 3 cases. *Arch. Dis. Child.* **32**, 167–80.

Griswold, W. and McIntosh, R. M. (1972). Immunological studies in congenital nephrosis. *J. Med. Genet.* **9**, 245–7.

Habib, R. and Bois, E. (1973). Hétérogénéité des syndromes néphrotiques a debut précoce du nourisson (syndrome néphrotique 'infantile'). Etude anatomo-clinique et génetique de 37 observations. *Helv. Pediatr. Acta* **28**, 910–1007.

Hallman, N. and Hjelt, L. (1959). Congenital nephrotic syndrome. *J. Pediatr.* **55**, 152–62.

—— and Rapola, J. (1978). In *Pediatric kidney disease* ed. Edelmann, C. M. Jr. p. 711. Little Brown, Boston.

——, Hjelt, L. and Ahvenainen, E. K. (1956). Nephrotic syndrome in newborn and young infants. *Ann. Paediatr. Fenn.* **2**, 227–41.

——, Norio, R. and Kouvalainen, K. (1967). Main features of the congenital nephrotic syndrome. *Acta Paediatr. Scand. Suppl.* **172**, 75–8.

——, ——, ——, Vilska, J. and Kojo, N. (1970). Das kongenitale nephrotische Syndrom. *Ergerbnisse Inn. Med. Kinderheilk.* **30**, 3.

——, —— and Rapola, J. (1973). Congenital nephrotic syndrome. *Nephron* **11**, 101–10.

Hoyer, J. R., Michael, A. F., Good, R. A. and Vernier, R. L. (1967). The nephrotic syndrome of infancy: clinical, morphologic and immunologic studies of four infants. *Pediatrics.* **40**, 233–46.

——, Mauer, S. M., Kjellstrand, C. M., Buselmeier, T. J., Simmons, R. L., Michael, A. F., Najarian, J. S. and Vernier, R. L. (1973). Successful renal transplantation in 3 children with congenital nephrotic syndrome. *Lancet* **1**, 1410–12.

Huttunen, N.-P. (1976). Congenital nephrotic syndrome of Finnish type. Study of 75 patients. *Arch. Dis. Child.* **51**, 344–8.

——, Vehaskari, M., Vükari, M. and Laipio, M.-L. (1980). Proteinuria in congenital nephrotic syndrome of Finnish type. *Clin. Nephrol.* **13**, 12–19.

Inferrera, C., Barresi, G., Chimicata, S., DeLuca, F., Baviera, G., Gulli, V. and Gemelli, M. (1980). Morphologic considerations on the placenta in congenital nephrotic syndrome of Finnish type. *Virchow's Arch.* **A389**, 13–26.

Kaplan, B. S., Bureau, M. A. and Drummond, K. N. (1974). The nephrotic syndrome in the first year of life: is a pathologic classification possible? *J. Pediatr.* **85**, 615–21.

Kendall-Smith, I. M., Pullon, D. H. H. and Tomlinson, B. E. (1968). Congenital nephrotic syndrome in Maori siblings. *NZ Med. J.* **68**, 156–60.

Kjessler, B., Johansson, S. G. O., Sherman, M., Gustavson, K.-H. and Hultquist, G. (1975a). Alpha-fetoprotein in antenatal diagnosis of congenital nephrosis. *Lancet* 1, 432–3.

——, Johansson, S. G. O., Sherman, M., Gustavsson, K.-H. and Hultquist, G. (1975b). Antenatal diagnosis of congenital nephrosis. *Lancet* 2, 553.

Kobayashi, N., Imahori, K. and Wakao, H. (1961). The congenital nephrotic syndrome, a case report and a review. *Paediatria Universitatis Tokyo* 6, 27.

Kouvalainen, K. (1963). A clinical and experimental study. *Ann. Pediatr. Fenn.* Suppl. 22, 9–23.

——, Vainio, T., Hjelt, L. and Hallman, H. (1962). Behaviour of skin grafted from infants to mothers in congenital nephrosis families. *Ann. Pediatr. Fenn.* 8, 173–80.

Lange, K., Wachstein, H., Wasserman, E., Alptekin, F. and Slobody, L. B. (1963). The congenital nephrotic syndrome. An immune reaction? *Am. J. Dis. Child.* 105, 338–45.

McCrory, W. W., Shibuya, M. and Worthen, H. G. (1966). Hereditary renal glomerular disease in infancy and childhood. *Adv. Pediatr.* 14, 253–80.

Mahan, J. D., Maver, S. M., Sibley, R. K. and Vernier, R. L. (1984). Congenital nephrotic syndrome: evolution of medical management and results of renal transplantation. *J. Pediatr.* 105, 549–57.

Mahieu, P., Monnens, L. and van Haelst, U. (1976). Chemical properties of glomerular basement membrane in congenital nephrotic syndrome. *Clin. Nephrol.* 5, 134–9.

Milunsky, A., Alpert, E., Frigoletto, F. D., Driscoll, S. G., McCluskey, R. T. and Colvin, R. B. (1977). Prenatal diagnosis of the congenital nephrotic syndrome. *Pediatrics.* 59, 770–3.

Morin, P. R., Potier, M., Dallaire, L., Melancon, S. B. and Boisvert, J. (1981). Prenatal detection of the autosomal recessive type of polycystic kidney disease by trehalase assay in amniotic fluid. *Prenatal Diagnosis* 1, 75–9.

——, ——, —— and —— (1984). Prenatal detection of the congenital nephrotic syndrome (Finnish type) by trehalase assay in amniotic fluid. *Prenatal Diagnosis* 4, 257–60.

Norio, R. (1966). Heredity in the congenital nephrotic syndrome. A genetic study of 57 Finnish families with a review of reported cases. *Ann. Pediatr. Fenn.* 12 (Suppl. 27), 1–94.

——, Hjelt, L. and Hallman, N. (1964). Congenital nephrotic syndrome: an inherited disease. A preliminary report. *Ann. Paediatr. Fenn.* 10, 223–7.

Oliver, J. (1960). Microcystic renal disease and its relation to 'infantile' nephrosis. *Am. J. Dis. Child.* 100, 312–18.

Ongre, A. A. (1961). Nephrotic syndrome with cyst-like dilations of renal tubules: report of 2 cases in siblings in early infancy. *Acta. Pathol. Microbiol. Scand.* 51, 1–8.

Rajamma, K., Balasundaram, D. and Rao, B. N. (1974). Congenital nephrotic syndrome: a case report. *Ind. Pediatr.* 11, 149.

Rapola, J. and Hallman, N. (1979). A. F. P. and congenital nephrosis Finnish type. *Lancet* 1, 274–5.

—— and Savilahti, E. (1971). Immunofluorescent and morphological studies in congenital nephrotic syndrome. *Acta Paediatr. Scand.* 60, 253–63.

——, Aula, P., Huttunen, N.-P. and Seppälä, M. (1975). Antenatal diagnosis of congenital nephrosis. *Lancet* **1**, 981.

Richard, P., Déchellete, E., Gilly, J., Bouvier, R. and Larbre, F. (1975). Syndrome néphrotique infantile. A propos de 14 observations. *Pédiatrié* **30**, 581–9.

Risteli, L., Autio-Harmainen, H., Huttunen, N.-P. and Risteli, J. (1982). Slow accumulation of basement membrane collagen in kidney cortex in congenital nephrotic syndrome. *Lancet* **1**, 712–14.

Rossenbeck, H. G., Margraf, O. and Hofmann, D. (1966). Über das infantile nephrotische Syndrom bei kongenitaler Glomerulonephritis. *Dtsch. Med. Wchsr.* **91**, 348–55.

Rumpelt, H. J. and Bachmann, H. J. (1980). Infantile nephrotic syndrome with diffuse mesangial sclerosis: a disturbance of glomerular basement membrane development? *Clin. Nephrol.* **13**, 146–50.

Ruoslahti, E., Pekkala, A., Comings, D. E. and Seppälä, M. (1970). Determination of subfractions of amniotic fluid alpha-fetoprotein in diagnosing spina bifida and congenital nephrosis. *Br. Med. J.* **3**, 768–9.

Ryynänen, M., Seppäläa, M., Kuusela, P., Rapola, J., Aula, P., Seppä, A., Jokela, V. and Castren, O. (1983). Antenatal screening for congenital nephrosis in Finland by maternal serum α-fetoprotein. *Br. J. Obstet. Gynaecol.* **90**, 437–42.

Seelig, H. P., Seelig, R. and Schärer, K. (1975). Immunohistologische Untersuchungen bei der diffusen mesangialen Sklerose mit nephrotischen Syndrom im Sauglingsalter. *Z. f. Kinderheilk* **120**, 111–20.

Seppälä, M. and Ruoslahti, E. (1972). Alpha fetoprotein in amniotic fluid: an index of gestational age. *Am. J. Obstet. Gynecol.* **114**, 595–8.

——, Aula, P., Rapola, J., Karjalainen, O., Huttunen, N.-P. and Ruoslahti, E. (1976). Congenital nephrotic syndrome: prenatal diagnosis and genetic counselling by estimation of amniotic-fluid and maternal serum alpha-fetoprotein. *Lancet* **2**, 123–5.

Spritz, R. A., Soiffer, S. J., Siegel, N. J. and Mahoney, M. J. (1978). False-negative A. F. P. screen for congenital nephrosis Finnish type. *Lancet* **2**, 1251.

Thom, H., Johnstone, F. D., Gibson, J. I., Scott, G. B. and Noble, D. W. (1977). Fetal proteinuria in diagnosis of congenital nephrosis detected by raised alpha-fetoprotein in maternal serum. *Br. Med. J.* **1**, 16–18.

Tryggvason, K. (1977). Composition of the glomerular basement membrane in the congenital nephrotic syndrome of the Finnish type. *Eur. J. Clin. Invest.* **7**, 177–80.

Vernier, R. L., Brunson, J. and Good, R. A. (1957). Studies on familial nephrosis. I. Clinical and pathologic study of four cases in a single family. *Am. J. Dis. Child.* **93**, 469–85.

——, Klein, D. J., Sisson, S. P., Mahan, J. D., Oegema, T. R. and Brown, D. M. (1983). Heparan sulfate-rich anionic sites in the human glomerular basement membrane. Decreased concentration in congenital nephrotic syndrome. *New Engl. J. Med.* **309**, 1001–9.

Worthen, H. G., Vernier, R. L. and Good, R. A. (1959). Infantile nephrosis: clinical, biochemical, and morphologic studies of the syndrome. *Am. J. Dis. Child.* **98**, 731–48.

Yamamoto, Y., Kuroda, T., Kanamura, S. and Sawada, S. (1961). A case of 'congenital nephrotic syndrome'. *Ann. Paediatr. Japon.* **7**, 391.

7.5.3. Familial nephrosis associated with non-renal abnormalities

There have been several reports of the familial occurrence of syndromes with multiple abnormalities including nephrosis. Braun and Bayer (1962) described a family in which two brothers had nephrosis with onset at 18 months and $2\frac{1}{2}$ years. Three other brothers had bilateral conductive deafness and short, broad thumbs and great toes with bifurcation of the distal phalanx. Two of these deaf brothers also have congenital urinary tract anomaly—ureteric obstruction in one and a duplication of the renal pelvis and upper ureter in the other. It is impossible to say from this isolated report that there is any connection between the nephrosis in two brothers and the different abnormalities in the other three brothers; nor can we deduce the mode of inheritance of the disorder, or disorders, present. A similar difficulty arises over a single family in which four sisters had nephrosis and pulmonary stenosis (Fournier *et al.* 1963), which represent a single unique disorder or two disorders segregating together, and also another family in which three sibs had nephrosis, with onset ranging from 1 week to 14 months, and epicanthus.

One is on slightly surer ground with the association of nephrotic syndrome, congenital microcephaly, and hiatus hernia. This combination has been reported in two families. In the first nephrosis started in a brother and sister at 9 months and 2 years respectively, with death at 20 and 28 months (Galloway and Mowat 1968), and in the second there were again a brother and sister who had proteinuria from birth and died at 14 days and 3 years respectively. Autopsy revealed microcystic renal dysplasia and focal glomerulosclerosis (Shapiro *et al.* 1976). In neither family were the parents related to one another. Daentl and colleagues (1978) reported two brothers with a syndrome of fatal nephrosis, hydrocephalus, thin skin, blue sclerae, growth retardation, abnormal T-lymphocyte function, and unusual dysmorphic facies. This picture is sufficiently distinctive to assume *prima facie* that the association is not coincidental. In none of the families described above was there parental consanguinity.

Barakat and colleagues (1977) reported the association of steroid-resistant nephrosis, deafness, and hypoparathyroidism in four brothers. This Barakat syndrome is probably autosomal recessive but could be X-linked recessive.

Opitz and others (1985) have described two sisters, with consanguineous parents from a Hutterite community, who have a syndrome of dwarfism, severe mental retardation and neurological disturbance, and renal impairment with a terminal nephrotic syndrome. They term this disorder 'Hutterite cerebro-osteo-nephrodysplasia' and propose autosomal recessive inheritance. Detailed investigation of the renal lesion, and indeed other aspects, was not possible.

Another new syndrome has been reported in which two male sibs were affected, the first dying at under 3 years, and the second a termination of pregnancy at 22 weeks of gestation (Palm *et al.* 1986). The boy had a glomerular disease with proteinuria and nephrosis, associated with central nervous system abnormalities including paraventricular heteropias, central canal abnormalities, and hydrocephalus. The second affected pregnancy was diagnosed on the finding of a grossly raised amniotic fluid AFP level and an ultrasound observation of widening of the upper vertebral column. The fetal kidneys showed numerous small cysts at the corticomedullary junction and, on electron microscopy, fusion of podocytes and irregularity of the glomerular basement membrane. The parents were well and unrelated, and there were two normal sibs. Inheritance could be either autosomal or X-linked recessive.

References

Barakat, A. Y., D'Albora, J. B., Martin, M. M. and Jose, P. A. (1977). Familial nephrosis, nerve deafness, and hypoparathyroidism. *J. Pediatr.* **91**, 61–4.

Braun, F. C. Jr. and Bayer, J. F. (1962). Familial nephrosis associated with deafness and congenital urinary tract anomalies in siblings. *J. Pediatr.* **60**, 33–41.

Daentl, D. L., Townsend, J. J., Siegel, R. C., Goodman, J. R., Piel, C. F., Wara, D. W. and Bachmann, R. P. (1978). Familial nephrosis, hydrocephalus, thin skin, blue sclerae syndrome: clinical structural and biochemical studies. *Birth Defects Orig. Art. Series* **14**, (6B), 315–39.

Fournier, A., Paget, M., Pauli, A. and Devin, P. (1963). Syndromes nephrotiques familiaux. Syndrome nephrotique associe à une cardiopathie congenitale chez quatre soeurs. *Pédiatrie* **18**, 677–85.

Galloway, W. H. and Mowat, A. P. (1968). Congenital microcephaly with hiatus hernia and nephrotic syndrome in two sibs. *J. Med. Genet.* **5**, 319–21.

Opitz, J. M., Lowry, R. B., Holmes, T. M. and Morgan, K. (1985). Hutterite cerebro-osteo-nephrodysplasia: autosomal recessive trait in a Lehrerleut Hutterite family from Montana. *Am. J. Med. Genet.* **22**, 521–9.

Palm, L., Hägerstrand, I., Kristoffersson, U., Blennow, G., Brun, A. and Jörgensen, C. (1986). Nephrosis and disturbances of neuronal migration in male siblings—a new hereditary disorder? *Arch. Dis. Child.* **61**, 545–8.

Shapiro, L. R., Duncan, P. A., Farnsworth, P. B. and Lefkowitz, M. (1976). In *Cytogenetics, environment and malformation syndromes*, ed. Bergsma, D. Alan R. Liss for the Nat. Found.—March of Dimes, New York. *Birth Defects Orig. Art. Series* **12**, 275–8.

7.6. HYPERPROLINAEMIA WITH HEREDITARY NEPHRITIS, A NON-DISEASE

Hyperprolinaemia is an inborn error of metabolism with raised plasma proline concentrations and increased excretion of proline, hydroxy-proline, and glycine. These amino acids share a common pathway of renal tubular reabsorption and are excreted in excess whenever the plasma level of proline exceeds 11 mg per 100 ml (Scriver *et al.* 1961). Two types with different enzyme defects and associated abnormalities have been described. In type I proline dehydrogenase (or oxidase) activity is deficient (Efron 1965), whereas in type II the defect involves Δ'-pyrroline-5-carboxylic-acid dehydrogenase (Valle *et al.* 1974, 1976, 1979). Type II has been associated with mental retardation and epilepsy (Berlow and Efron 1964; Simila 1970) but not renal abnormality in the earlier reported cases, but has been symptomless in some more recent cases and is probably benign (Applegarth *et al.* 1974; Pavone *et al.* 1975); it is associated with higher plasma levels of proline than in type I. It need not concern us here any further.

Type I hyperprolinaemia has been described in association with a variety of clinical abnormalities including several forms of renal abnormality, epilepsy, and mental retardation. However, like type II it is probably a benign asymptomatic condition with the observed abnormalities being coincidental. There is a precisely homologous animal model in the Pro/Re mouse (Scriver *et al.* 1983).

In the first reported family with hyperprolinaemia and renal disease there was a remarkable cluster of abnormalities including Alport's syndrome, hyperprolinaemia, renal hypoplasia, mental retardation, and photogenic epilepsy (Schafer *et al.* 1962; Scriver *et al.* 1961, 1964). The authors were careful to point out that the Alport's disease and the hyperprolinaemia appeared to be segregating independently in this family with the former showing dominant and the latter recessive inheritance.

Other families with Alport's disease and hyperprolinaemia, presumed to be type I, have been reported (Fuhrmann 1963; Kopelman *et al.* 1964; Minder *et al.* 1965; Dubach *et al.* 1966; Goyer *et al.* 1968; Raszeja-Wanic *et al.* 1969; Zavala *et al.* 1969). Minder and Dubach's family was first reported before the hyperprolinaemia had been noted (Dubach and Gsell 1962). Raszeja-Wanic and colleagues reported monozygotic twins with Alport's disease and hyperprolinaemia. Zavala and coworkers described a family with Alport's disease and probable male-to-male transmission in which one of two sib probands with second-cousin parents had hyperprolinaemia. Despite this rather large number of families in which the association of Alport's disease and hyperprolinaemia has been reported a close examination of the reports does not provide evidence that the two conditions are related.

There is even less reason to suppose that other renal abnormalities reported in patients with hyperprolinaemia, that is congenital ureteral obstruction and uraemia (Efron 1965), Wilms' tumour (Perry *et al.* 1968) and pyelonephritis, are other than chance associations (Scriver *et al.* 1983).

Types I and II hyperprolinaemia both appear to be inherited in an autosomal recessive manner with affected sibs, and in some families parental consanguinity, although of course due to genes at different loci. Parental consanguinity has been reported in four families with type I hyperprolinaemia (Perry *et al.* 1968; Goyer *et al.* 1969; Woody *et al.* 1969; Zavala *et al.* 1969). However, in type I recessivity is incomplete with some obligate heterozygotes having hyperprolinaemia (Scriver *et al.* 1983). In none of the families in which there is an associated renal abnormality do the two defects consistently segregate together. Indeed in those with nephritis this is in most cases clearly dominant in contrast to the recessive hyperprolinaemia.

References

Applegarth, D. A., Ingram, P., Hingston, J. and Hardwick, D. F. (1974). Hyper-prolinemia type II. *Clin. Biochem.* **7**, 14–28.

Berlow, S. and Efron, M. L. (1964). A new cause of hyperprolinemia associated with the excretion of Δ'-pyrroline-5-carboxylic acid. *Proc. Soc. Pediat. Res.* 34th Ann. Meet. Seattle, p. 43.

Dubach, U. C. and Gsell, O. R. (1962). Alport's syndrome. *Lancet* **1**, 159–60.

——, Minder, F. C. and Antener, I. (1966). Familial nephropathy and deafness: first observation of family and close relatives in Switzerland. *Helv. Med. Acta.* **33**, 36–43.

Efron, M. L. (1965). Familial hyperprolinemia. Report of a second case, associated with congenital renal malformations, hereditary hematuria and mild mental retardation, with demonstration of any enzyme defect. *New Engl. J. Med.* **272**, 1243–54.

Fuhrmann, W. (1963). Das Syndrom der erblichen Nephropathie mit Innenohr-schwerhörigkeit (Alport-Syndrom). *Dtsch. Med. Wschr.* **88**, 525–32.

Goyer, R. A., Reynolds, J., Burke, J. and Burkholder, P. (1968). Hereditary renal disease with neurosensory hearing loss, prolinuria and ichthyosis. *Am. J. Med. Sci.* **256**, 166–79.

Kopelman, H., Asatoor, A. M. and Milne, M. D. (1964). Hyperprolinaemia and hereditary nephritis. *Lancet* **2**, 1075–9.

Minder, F. C., Dubach, U. C. and Antener, I. (1965). Familiäre nephropathie und Schwerhörigkeit: erste Beobachtung in der Schweiz. *Helv. Med. Acta.* **32**, 404–5.

Pavone, L., Mollica, F. and Levy, H. L. (1975). Asymptomatic type II hyper-prolinemia associated with hyperglycinaemia in three sibs. *Arch. Dis. Child.* **50**, 637–41.

Raszeja-Wanic, B., Wachowiak, A. and Kosicka, M. (1969). Nefropatia rodzinna u blizniat. *Pol. Tyg. Lek.* **24**, 124–6.

Perry, T. L., Hardwick, D. F., Lowry, R. B. and Hansen, S. (1968). Hyper-prolinaemia in two successive generations of a North American Indian family. *Ann. Hum. Genet.* **31**, 401–7.

Schafer, I. A., Scriver, C. R. and Efron, M. L. (1962). Familial hyperprolinaemia, cerebral dysfunction and renal anomalies occurring in a family with hereditary nephritis and deafness. *New Engl. J. Med.* **267**, 51–60.

Scriver, C. R., Schafer, I. A. and Efron, M. L. (1961). New renal tubular amino acid transport system and a new hereditary disorder of amino acid metabolism. *Nature* **192**, 672–3.

——, Efron, M. L. and Schafer, I. A. (1964). Renal tubular transport of proline, hydroxyproline and glycine in health and in familial hyperprolinaemia. *J. Clin. Invest.* **43**, 374–85.

——, Smith, R. J. and Phang, J. M. (1983). Disorders of proline and hydroxy-proline metabolism. Chapter 18 in *The metabolic basis of inherited disease*, 5th edn. eds. Stanbury, J. B., Wyngaarden, J. B., Fredrickson, D.S., Goldstein, J. L. and Brown, M. S. pp. 360–81. McGraw-Hill, New York.

Simila, S. (1970). Intravenous proline tolerance in a patient with hyperprolin-aemia type II and his relatives. *Helv. Paediatr. Acta* **3**, 287–92.

Valle, D., Goodman, S. I., Applegarth, D. A., Shih, V. E. and Phang, J. M. (1976). Type II hyperprolinemia. Δ′-pyrroline-5-carboxylic acid dehydrogenase defi-ciency in cultured skin fibroblasts and circulating lymphocytes. *J. Clin. Invest.* **58**, 598–603.

——, ——, Harris, S. C. and Phang, J. M. (1979). Genetic evidence for a common enzyme catalyzing the second step in the degradation of proline and hydroxy-proline. *J. Clin. Invest.* **64**, 1365–70.

——, Phang, J. M. and Goodman, S. I. (1974). Type II hyperprolinemia: absence of Δ′-pyrroline-5-carboxylic acid dehydrogenase activity. *Science* **185**, 1053–4.

Woody, N. C., Snyder, C. H. and Harris, J. A. (1969). Hyperprolinemia: clinical and biochemical family study. *Pediatrics* **44**, 554–63.

Zavala, C., Villar-Puig, P., Garza, R., Lisker, R. and Dies, F. (1969). Nefropatia cronica hereditaria con hipoacusia y defectos oculares. Sobretiro de la Revista de Investigacion. *Clin. Mex.* **21**, 369–82.

7.7. FAMILIAL HYPERURICAEMIC NEPHROPATHY

A disease comprising familial chronic interstitial nephritis, gout and hyperuricaemia not associated with partial deficiency of hypoxanthine-guanine phosphoribosyltransferase activity, nor with phosphoribosyl-pyrophosphate synthetase overactivity, has been described. Probably the first family to be reported with this distinct disorder was that of Duncan and Dixon (1960). Other reports have shown a familial pattern either consistent with autosomal dominant inheritance or without a clear mendelian pattern (Rosenbloom *et al.* 1967; Treadwell 1971; van Goor *et al.* 1971; Thompson *et al.* 1978; Massari *et al.* 1980; Simmonds *et al.* 1980; Richmond *et al.* 1981; Warren *et al.* 1981; Leumann and

Wegmann 1983). MacDermot and colleagues (1984) investigated five such families in which affected members all had hyperuricaemia, with or without renal failure. These families were all either strongly suggestive of, or compatible with, autosomal dominant inheritance. Since they were unable to demonstrate increased *de novo* purine synthesis *in vitro* they suggest that the pathogenesis may lie in a reduced renal tubular net excretion of urate. Such a mechanism would be the opposite of that proposed in hyperuricosuric nephrolithiasis described in Chapter 5.

A variant is a syndrome comprising renal insufficiency, hyperuricaemia, ataxia, and deafness reported in five members of a family (Rosenberg *et al.* 1970). Males and females were equally severely affected and serum urate levels were raised in relatives with normal renal function. The genetics of the condition is uncertain.

References

Duncan, H. and Dixon, A. St. J. (1960). Gout, familial hyperuricaemia and renal disease. *Quart. J. Med.* **29**, 127–35.

Leumann, E. P. and Wegmann, W. (1983). Familial nephropathy with hyperuricemia and gout. *Nephron* **34**, 51–7.

MacDermot, K. D., Allsop, J. and Watts, R. W. E. (1984). The rate of purine synthesis *de novo* in blood mononuclear cells *in vitro* from patients with familial hyperuricaemic nephropathy. *Clin. Sci.* **67**, 249–58.

Massari, P. U., Hsu, C. H., Barnes, R. V., Fox, I. H., Gikas, P. W. and Weller, J. M. (1980). Familial hyperuricemia and renal disease. *Arch. Intern. Med.* **140**, 680–4.

Richmond, J. M., Kincaid-Smith, P., Whitworth, J. A. and Becker, G. J. (1981). Familial urate nephropathy. *New Engl. J. Med.* **304**, 535–6.

Rosenberg, A. L., Bergstrom, L., Troost, B. T. and Bartholomew, B. A. (1970). Hyperuricemia and neurologic deficits: a family study. *New Engl. J. Med.* **282**, 992–7.

Rosenbloom, F. M., Kelley, W. N., Carr, A. A. and Seegmiller, J. E. (1967). Familial nephropathy and gout in a kindred (abs.). *Clin. Res.* **15**, 270.

Simmonds, H. A., Warren, D. J., Cameron, J. S., Potter, C. F. and Farebrother, D. A. (1980). Familial gout and renal failure in young women. *Clin. Nephrol.* **14**, 176–82.

Thompson, G. R., Weiss, J. J., Goldman, R. J. and Rigg, G. A. (1978). Familial occurrence of hyperuricemia, gout, and medullary cystic disease. *Arch. Intern. Med.* **138**, 1614–17.

Treadwell, B. L. (1971). Juvenile gout. *Ann. Rheum. Dis.* **30**, 279–84.

van Goor, W., Kooiker, C. J. and Dorhout Mees, E. J. (1971). An unusual form of renal disease associated with gout and hypertension. *J. Clin. Pathol.* **24**, 354–9.

Warren, D. J., Simmonds, H. A., Gibson, T. and Naik, R. B. (1981). Familial gout and renal failure. *Arch. Dis. Child.* **56**, 699–704.

7.8. LOWE'S OCULO-CEREBRO-RENAL SYNDROME

Lowe and colleagues (1952) were the first to describe this syndrome in a family with affected brothers. The principal features as described by them are gross mental retardation with *grand mal* epilepsy, hyporeflexia, hypotonia, and behavioural disturbance; cataracts with nystagmus leading on to glaucoma; rickets or osteomalacia, which may result in fractures; and a renal tubular abnormality with proteinuria, a Fanconi type of aminoaciduria with mild glycosuria and an inability of the kidney to produce ammonia with a consequent hyperchloraemic acidosis. Similar families, with only minor clinical variation, were reported by others over the following years (Fanconi 1954; Schoen and Young 1959; Dent and Smellie 1961 and many others). Abbassi and colleagues (1968) provided a valuable review of 70 cases up to that date including several new cases. The brothers reported by McCance and colleagues (1960) were probably suffering from a distinct disorder. Acker and coworkers (1967) described the renal histopathology, and Witzleben and associates (1968) reported progressive renal histological changes. Schoen and Young (1959) were the first to note the presence of structural changes in the mitochondria of the renal tubular epithelium. Ores and others have confirmed that there are mitochondrial abnormalities in an electron microscopical study (Ores 1970; Sagel *et al.* 1970); and recently Gobernado and others (1984) have demonstrated markedly diminished mitochondrial respiration with substrates reducing NAD and with a flavoprotein-linked substrate, suggesting a defect in electron transport prior to the cytochromes. In addition, a reduction in procollagen synthesis by cultured fibroblasts from patients has been demonstrated (Palmieri *et al.* 1985).

Most of the reported patients have been boys. Among the few exceptions are girls reported by Svorc and others (1967), Harris and colleagues (1970), and Sagel and associates (1970). Strieff and colleagues (1958) first suggested that the disorder was inherited in an X-linked recessive manner. This would appear to be the mode of inheritance in the great majority of families. It is not clear whether the few reported girls are from families with a rare autosomal genocopy of the X-linked disorder, or represent extreme manifestation in a female heterozygote of the X-linked disorder itself. Certainly there is evidence of expression in female heterozygotes, such as lens opacities on slit lamp examination (Richards *et al.* 1965; Martin and Carson 1967; Delleman *et al.* 1977), or aminoaciduria on ornithine loading (Chutorian and Rowland 1966). On the other hand genetic heterogeneity is suggested by families other than that of McCance and colleagues (1960). Matusda and colleagues (1969, 1970) reported a Japanese boy in whom there appeared to be a defect of bicarbonate reabsorption rather than of urinary acidification, and in which the father developed an aminoaciduria or ornithine loading, suggesting autosomal recessive inheritance. The family of Oetliker and Rossi (1969) may have been similar.

References

Abbassi, V., Lowe, C. U. and Calcalgno, P. L. (1968). Oculocerebro-renal syndrome: a review. *Am. J. Dis. Child.* **115**, 145–68.

Acker, K. J., Roels, H., Beelaerts, W., Pasterwack, A. and Valcke, R. (1967). The histological lesions of the kidney in the oculo-cerebro-renal syndrome of Lowe. *Nephron* **4**, 193–214.

Chutorian, A. and Rowland, L. P. (1966). Lowe's syndrome. *Neurology* **16**, 115–22.

Delleman, J. W., Bleeker-Wagemakers, E. M. and van Veelen, A. W. C. (1977). Opacities of the lens indicating carrier status in the oculo-cerebro-renal (Lowe) syndrome. *J. Pediatr. Ophthal.* **14**, 205–12.

Dent, C. E. and Smellie, J. M. (1961). Two children with the oculo-cerebro-renal syndrome of Lowe, Terrey and MacLachlan. *Proc. R. Soc. Med.* **54**, 335–6.

Fanconi, G. (1954). Tubular insufficiency and renal dwarfism. *Arch. Dis. Child.* **29**, 1–6.

Gobernado, J. J., Lousa, M., Gimeno, A. and Gonsalvez, M. (1984). Mitochondrial defects in Lowe's oculocerebrorenal syndrome. *Arch. Neurol.* **41**, 208–9.

Harris, L. S., Gitter, K. A., Galin, M. A. and Plechaty, G. P. (1970). Oculocerebro-renal syndrome: report of a case in a baby girl. *Br. J. Ophthalmol.* **54**, 278–80.

Lowe, C. U., Terrey, M. and MacLachlan, E. A. (1952). Organic-aciduria, decreased ammonia production, hydrophthalmos and mental retardation: a clinical entity. *Am. J. Dis. Child.* **83**, 164–84.

McCance, R. A., Matheson, W. J., Gresham, G. A. and Elkinton, J. R. (1960). The cerebro-ocular-renal dystrophies: a new variant. *Arch. Dis. Child.* **35**, 240–9.

Martin, V. A. F. and Carson, N. A. J. (1967). Inborn metabolic disorders with associated ocular lesions in Northern Ireland. *Trans. Ophthalmol. Soc. UK* **87**, 847–70.

Matsuda, I., Takeda, T., Sugai, M. and Matsuura, N. (1969). Oculocerebrorenal syndrome: in a child with normal urinary acidification and a defect in bicarbonate reabsorption. *Am. J. Dis. Child.* **117**, 205–12.

——, Sugai, M. and Kajii, T. (1970). Ornithine loading test in Lowe's syndrome. *J. Pediatr.* **77**, 127–9.

Oetliker, O. and Rossi, E. (1969). The influence of extracellular fluid volume on the renal bicarbonate threshold: a study of two children with Lowe's syndrome. *Pediatr. Res.* **3**, 140–8.

Ores, R. O. (1970). Renal changes in oculo-cerebro-renal syndrome of Lowe: electron microscopic study. *Arch. Pathol. Lab. Med.* **89**, 221–5.

Palmieri, M. J., O'Hara, J., States, B. and Segal, S. (1985). Decreased procollagen production in cultured fibroblasts from patients with Lowe's syndrome. *J. Inher. Metab. Dis.* **8**, 187–92.

Richards, W., Donnell, G. N., Wilson, W. A., Stowens, D. and Perry, T. (1965). The oculo-cerebro-renal syndrome of Lowe. *Am. J. Dis. Child.* **109**, 185–203.

Sagel, I., Ores, R. O. and Yuceoglu, A. M. (1970). Renal function and morphology in a girl with oculo-cerebrorenal syndrome. *J. Pediatr.* **77**, 124–7.

Schoen, E. J. and Young, G. (1959). 'Lowe's syndrome'. Abnormalities of renal tubular function in combination with other congenital defects. *Am. J. Med.* **27**, 781–92.

Strieff, E. B., Straub, W. and Golay, L. (1958). Les manifestations oculaires du syndrome de Lowe. *Ophthalmologica* **135**, 632–9.

Svorc, J., Masopust, J., Komarkova, A., Macek, M. and Hyanek, J. (1967). Oculo-cerebrorenal syndrome in a female child. *Am. J. Dis. Child.* **114**, 186–90.

Witzleben, C. L., Schoen, E. J., Tu, W. H. and McDonald, L. W. (1968). Progressive morphologic renal changes in the oculo-cerebro-renal syndrome of Lowe. *Am. J. Med.* **44**, 319–24.

7.9. ONYCHO-OSTEODYSPLASIA, THE NAIL–PATELLA SYNDROME

Nail–patella syndrome is chiefly of genetic interest because it is one of the earliest disorders for which linkage to a genetic marker, the ABO blood group system, was established (Renwick and Lawler 1955; Renwick and Schulze 1965). This linkage group has since been extended to include adenylate kinase-1 and assigned to the long arm of chromosome 9, at 9q 34 (Ferguson-Smith *et al.* 1976; Westerveld *et al.* 1976). Inheritance is autosomal dominant.

The principal clinical findings are dysplastic nails and absent or hypoplastic patellae, limited pronation supination, and on X-ray iliac horns (Hawkins and Smith 1950; Zimmerman 1961). Nephropathy is a variable feature which tends to show familial aggregation suggesting genetic heterogeneity. However, if the nephropathic and non-nephropathic forms are due to different genes these are likely to be allelic as the linkage studies do not reveal any heterogeneity. The earliest description of a renal abnormality resembling glomerulonephritis, was that of Hawkins and Smith (1950). Several other authors have described renal changes which are usually mild (Darlington and Hawkins 1967; Eisenberg *et al.* 1972; Bennett *et al.* 1973; Morita *et al.* 1973) but may lead to renal failure (Myers *et al.* 1980) or even early death (Leahy 1966). Cohen and Berant (1976) reported duplication of the renal collecting system in the nail–patella syndrome. Electron microscopy has demonstrated increased numbers of collagen fibrils in glomerular basement membranes (Morita *et al.* 1973; Sabnis *et al.* 1980). The patient reported by Similä and colleagues (1970) was unusual in presenting with congenital nephrosis.

References

Bennett, W. M., Musgrave, J. E., Campbell, R. A., Elliot, D., Cox, R., Brooks, R. E., Lovrien, E. W., Beals, R. K. and Porter, G. A. (1973). The nephropathy of the nail–patella syndrome: clinico-pathologic analysis of 11 kindreds. *Am. J. Med.* **54**, 304–19.

Cohen, N. and Berant, M. (1976). Duplications of the renal collecting system in the hereditary osteo-onycho-dysplasia syndrome. *J. Pediatr.* **89**, 261–3.

Darlington, D. and Hawkins, C. F. (1967). Nail patella syndrome with iliac horns and hereditary nephropathy: necropsy report and anatomical dissection. *J. Bone Jt. Surg.* **49B**, 164–74.

Eisenberg, K. S., Potter, D. E. and Bovill, E. G. Jr. (1972). Osteo-onycho-dystrophy with nephropathy and renal osteodystrophy: a case report. *J. Bone Jt. Surg.* **54**, 1301–5.

Ferguson-Smith, M. A., Aitken, D. A., Turleau, C. and De Grouchy, J. (1976). Localisation of the human ABO: Np-1: AK-1 linkage group by regional assignment of AK-1 to 9q34. *Hum. Genet.* **34**, 35–43.

Hawkins, C. F. and Smith, O. E. (1950). Renal dysplasia in a family with multiple hereditary abnormalities including iliac horns. *Lancet* **1**, 803–8.

Leahy, M. S. (1966). The hereditary nephropathy of osteo-onychodysplasia (nail–patella syndrome). *Am. J. Dis. Child.* **112**, 237–41.

Morita, T., Laughlin, O., Kawano, K., Suzuki, Y., Kimmelstiel, P. and Churg, J. (1973). Nail–patella syndrome: light and electron microscopic studies of the kidney. *Arch. Intern. Med.* **131**, 271–7.

Myers, H. S., Gregory, M. and Beighton, P. (1980). Clinical pathologic conference: renal failure in a 44-year old female. *Urol. Raidol.* **1**, 251–3.

Renwick, J. H. and Lawler, S. D. (1955). Genetical linkage between the ABO and nail patella loci. *Ann. Hum. Genet.* **19**, 312–31.

—— and Schulze, J. (1965). Male and female recombination fractions for the nail patella: ABO linkage in man. *Ann. Hum. Genet.* **28**, 379–92.

Sabnis, S. G., Antonovych, T. T., Argy, W. P., Rakowski, T. A., Gandy, D. R. and Salcedo, J. R. (1980). Nail–patella syndrome. *Clin. Nephrol.* **14**, 148–53.

Similä, S., Vesa, L. and Wasz-Höchert, O. (1970). Hereditary onycho osteo-dysplasia (the nail–patella syndrome) with nephrosis-like renal disease in a new-born boy. *Pediatrics* **46**, 61–5.

Westerveld, A., Jongsma, A. P. M., Meera Khan, P., van Someren, H. and Bootsma, D. (1976). Assignment of the AK(1):Np:ABO linkage group to human chromosome 9. *Proc. Nat. Acad. Sci.* **73**, 895–9.

Zimmerman, C. (1961). Iliac horns: a pathognomonic roentgen sign of familial onycho-osteodysphasia. *Am. J. Roentgenol.* **86**, 478–83.

7.10. HEREDITARY NEPHRITIS, DEAFNESS, AND MACROTHROMBOCYTOPATHIA

This rare disorder was described by Epstein and colleagues (1972) in two unrelated families. The renal disease and deafness are indistinguishable from Alport's disease except that it is more severe in females. Six further families have been reported (Eckstein *et al.* 1975; Bernheim *et al.*

1976; Parsa *et al.* 1976; Hansen *et al.* 1978; Clare *et al.* 1979; Peterson *et al.* 1985). Inheritance is probably autosomal dominant, although male-to-male transmission was not observed in three of the eight reported families. There is heterogeneity among even this small group of families. In most reports the platelets have been functionally abnormal as well as large. However, at least in the family reported by Eckstein and coworkers platelet function was normal. In Hansen and coworkers' family aortic cystic medionecrosis was also present. In Peterson and colleagues' large family cataracts and leucocyte inclusions constituted additional features. They introduced the term 'Fechtner syndrome', after the name of their propositus, for the particular constellation of findings in their family. Alving and associates (1986) have reported successful renal transplantation in a patient with this disease, which they term 'Epstein syndrome'.

References

Alving, B. M., Tarassoff, P. G., Moore, J. Jr., Leissenger, C. A. and Fernandez-Bueno, C. (1986). Successful renal transplantation for Epstein syndrome. *Am. J. Hematol.* **21**, 111–13.

Bernheim, J., Dechavanne, M., Byron, P. A., Labarde, M., Colon, S., Pozet, N. and Traeger, J. (1976). Thrombocytopenia, macrothrombocytopathia, nephritis and deafness. *Am. J. Med.* **61**, 145–50.

Clare, N. M., Montiel, M. M., Lifschitz, M. D. and Bannayan, G. A. (1979). Alport's syndrome associated with macrothrombopathic thrombocytopenia. *Am. J. Clin. Pathol.* **72**, 111–17.

Eckstein, J. D., Filip, D. J., and Watts, J. C. (1975). Hereditary thrombocytopenia, deafness and renal disease. *Ann. Intern. Med.* **82**, 639–45.

Epstein, C. J., Sahud, M. A., Piel, C. F., Goodman, J. R., Bernfield, M. R., Kushner, J. H. and Ablin, A. R. (1972). Hereditary macrothrombocytopathia, nephritis and deafness. *Am. J. Med.* **52**, 299–310.

Hansen, M. S., Behnke, O., Pedersen, N. T. and Videbaek, A. (1978). Mega-thrombocytopenia associated with glomerulonephritis, deafness and aortic cystic medionecrosis. *Scand. J. Haemat.* **21**, 197–205.

Parsa, K. P., Lee, D. N., Zamboni, L. and Glassock, R. J. (1976). Hereditary nephritis, deafness and abnormal thrombopoiesis: study of a new kindred. *Am. J. Med.* **60**, 665–72.

Peterson, L. C., Rao, K. Y., Crosson, J. T. and White, J. G. (1985). Fechtner syndrome—a variant of Alport's syndrome with leukocyte inclusions and macrothrombocytopenia. *Blood* **65**, 397–406.

7.11. OCULO-RENAL-CEREBELLAR (ORC) SYNDROME

A single family has been reported in which three boys and two girls, from a Mennonite family of 11 children with parents who were fifth and sixth cousins, had this syndrome (Hunter *et al.* 1982). The features were severe mental subnormality, choreoathetosis with progressive spastic diplegia, progressive tapetoretinal degeneration, and nephropathy leading to renal failure with death in the late first or early second decade. At autopsy one of the boys showed absence of the granular layer of the cerebellum. A renal biopsy on another of the affected boys revealed atretic glomeruli in the superficial layer of the cortex. On electron microscopy there was irregular thickening of the glomerular basement membrane with electron-dense deposits up to 2.2 μm in diameter, containing round closely packed fine particles or curved linear structures, a unique structural change. Inheritance must be presumed to be autosomal recessive.

Reference

Hunter, A. G. W., Jurenka, S., Thompson, D. and Evans, J. A. (1982). Absence of the cerebellar granular layer, mental retardation, tapetoretinal degeneration and progressive glomerulopathy: an autosomal recessive oculo-renal-cerebellar syndrome. *Am. J. Hum. Genet.* **11**, 385–95.

7.12. HEREDITARY INTERSTITIAL NEPHRITIS AND POLYNEUROPATHY

Marin and Tyler (1961) reported a single family with this combination.

Reference

Marin, O. S. M. and Tyler, H. R. (1961). Hereditary interstitial nephritis associated with polyneuropathy. *Neurology* **11**, 999–1005.

7.13. FAMILIAL NEPHRITIS AND ERYTHROMELALGIA

Cross (1962) reported a single family with hereditary nephritis present over four generations. The renal pathology was non-specific apart from the observation of foam cells. Affected individuals also had a generalized aminoaciduria, and affected males died at 31 to 40 years. There was no mention of deafness in any member of the family. Despite the title of the paper, and the fact that erythromelalgia was in many instances present in individuals with nephritis, the two phenomena segregated independently. No male-to-male transmission was observed so that the mode of inheritance of the nephritis remains uncertain.

Reference

Cross, E. G. (1962). The familial occurrence of erythromelalgia and nephritis. *Can. Med. Assoc. J.* **87**, 1–4.

7.14. NEPHROCALCINOSIS AND AZOTAEMIA

A remarkable family was described by Stanbury and Castleman in the *New England Journal of Medicine's* Case Records of the Massachusetts General Hospital (1968). The index case was a young man with a nephropathy with foam cells in the glomeruli, renal osteodystrophy, secondary parathyroid hyperplasia, and unilateral deafness. He had hypophosphataemia, hypercalcaemia, and nephrocalcinosis. At least seven members of the family over three generations were affected, although male-to-male transmission was not observed.

Reference

Stanbury, S. W. and Castleman, B. (1968). Nephrocalcinosis and azotaemia in a young man. *New Engl. J. Med.* **278**, 839–46.

7.15. CARPOTARSAL OSTEOLYSIS WITH NEPHROPATHY

Early reports of this disease established a clinical and radiological picture of progressive osteolysis of the carpal and tarsal bones, usually starting at around 2 to 3 years (Francois and Detrait 1950; Marie *et al.* 1951; Neyroud *et al.* 1955; Thieffrey and Sorrel-Dejerine 1958; Caffey 1961), or earlier (Fryns *et al.* 1980). This osteolysis may eventually lead to complete disappearance of the bones. It was subsequently realized that hypertension and renal failure, associated with arteriolar thickening, are a feature of the disorder (Neyroud *et al.* 1955; Derot *et al.* 1961; Mahoudeau *et al.* 1961; Marie *et al.* 1963; Shurtleff *et al.* 1964; Lagier and Rutishauser 1965; Torg and Steel 1968; Berthoux *et al.* 1971; McManus *et al.* 1972; MacPherson *et al.* 1973; Beals and Bird 1975; Counahan *et al.* 1976; Whyte *et al.* 1978; Fryns *et al.* 1980). However, families have been reported without nephropathy (Kohler *et al.* 1973), and it is unclear whether or not such families are due to the same mutant genes as those with nephropathy.

Caffey (1961) reported a father and son affected. Further reports of hereditary occurrence followed involving three generations (Shurtleff *et al.* 1964; Gluck and Miller 1972), or two generations (Kohler *et al.* 1973; Whyte *et al.* 1978). Sporadic cases (Lagier and Rutishauser 1965; Torg and Steel 1968) may represent new mutations of the gene responsible for autosomal dominant inheritance in the familial cases or may be due to a separate gene with autosomal recessive inheritance, as suggested by Torg and colleagues (1969) whose patient's parents were consanguineous.

References

Beals, R. K. and Bird, C. B. (1975). Carpal and tarsal osteolysis. *J. Bone Jt. Surg.* **25A**, 681–6.

Berthoux, F., Robert, J. M., Zech, P., Fries, D. and Traeger, J. (1971). Acro-ostéolyse essentialle a début carpien et tarsien avec néphropathie. *Arch Pediatr.* **28**, 615–29.

Caffey, J. P. (1961). Idiopathic familial multiple carpal necrosis. In *Pediatric X-ray diagnosis*, 4th edn. p. 984. Year Book Med. Publ., Chicago.

Counahan, R., Simmons, M. J. and Charlwood, G. J. (1976). Multifocal osteolysis with nephropathy. *Arch. Dis. Child.* **51**, 717–19.

Derot, M., Rathery, M., Rosseling, G. and Catellier, C. (1961). Acro-ostéolyse du carpe, pied creux, scoliose et strabisme chez une jeune fille atteinte d'une insuffisance renale. *Bull. Mém. Soc. Méd. Hôp. Paris* **77**, 223–8.

Francois, J. and Detrait, C. (1950). Dystrophie démochondrocornéenne familiale. *Ann. Paediatr.* **174**, 145–74.

Fryns, J. P., Pedersen, J. C., Hauglustaine, D., Michielsen, P. and van den Berghe, H. (1980). Carpal and tarsal osteolysis. *Ann. Génét.* **23**, 123–5.

Gluck, J. and Miller, J. J. (1972). Familial osteolysis of the carpal and tarsal bones. *J. Pediatr.* **81**, 506–10.

Kohler, E., Babbit, D., Huizenga, B. and Good, T. A. (1973). Hereditary osteolysis. A clinical, radiological and chemical study. *Radiology* **108**, 99–106.

Lagier, R. and Rutishauser, E. (1965). Osteoarticular changes in a case of essential osteolysis. An anatomical and radiological study. *J. Bone Jt. Surg.* **47B**, 339–53.

McManus, L. F., Ballard, A., Walton, S. and Omer, G. E. (1972). Carpal and tarsal agenesis with features of essential and hereditary osteolysis. *J. Bone Jt. Surg.* **54A**, 1099–104.

MacPherson, R. I., Walker, R. D. and Kowall, M. H. (1973). Essential osteolysis with nephropathy. *J. Can. Assoc. Radiol.* **24**, 98–103.

Mahoudeau, D., Dubrisay, D., Elissalde, B. and Sraer, C. (1961). A propos du procés-verbal: osteolyse essentielle et néphrite. *Bull. Mém. Soc. Méd. Hôp. Paris* **77**, 229–34.

Marie, J., Scalet, J. and Leveque, B. (1951). Polydystrophies squelettiques avec osteolyse progressive. *Arch. Fr. Pédiat.* **8**, 725–53.

——, Leveque, B., Lyon, G., Bebe, M. and Watchi, J. M. (1963). Acro-ostéolyse essentielle compliquée d'insuffisance rénale d'évolution fatale. *Presse Méd.* **71**, 249–55.

Neyroud, M., Baumgartner, J. and Lenoir, A. (1955). Un cas d'ostéolyse essentielle. *Helv. Paediatr. Acta* **11**, 1551–71.

Shurtleff, D. B., Sparkes, R. S., Clawson, D. K., Guntheroth, W. G. and Mottet, N. K. (1964). Hereditary osteolysis with hypertension and nephropathy. *JAMA* **188**, 363–8.

Thieffrey, S. and Sorrel-Dejerine, J. (1958). Forme spéciale d'ostéolyse essentielle hereditaire et familiale á stabilisation spontanée, survenant dans l'enfance. *Presse Méd.* **66**, 1858–61.

Torg, J. S. and Steel, H. N. (1968). Essential osteolysis with nephropathy. A review of the literature and case report of an unusual syndrome. *J. Bone Jt. Surg.* **50A**, 1629–38.

——, DiGeorge, A. M., Kirkpatrick, J. A. and Trujillo, M. M. (1969). Hereditary multicentric osteolysis with recessive transmission: a new syndrome. *J. Pediatr.* **75**, 243–52.

Whyte, M. P., Murphy, W. A., Kleerekoper, M., Teitelbaum, S. L. and Avioli, L. V. (1978). Idiopathic multicentric osteolysis: report of an affected father and son. *Arthritis Rheum.* **21**, 367–76.

7.16. AMELOGENESIS IMPERFECTA AND NEPHROCALCINOSIS

MacGibbon (1972) described a new syndrome, in a brother and sister, comprising dental enamel agenesis and nephrocalcinosis with normal calcium metabolism, but eventual death from renal failure. A second such family has recently been reported, also in a brother and sister, with a lack of enamel, renal medullary nephrocalcinosis, and impaired renal-concentrating ability (Lubinsky *et al.* 1985). In both families the parents were normal and non-consanguineous. It would seem likely that this is an autosomal recessive disorder.

References

Lubinsky, M., Angle, C., Marsh, P. W. and Witkop, C. J. Jr. (1985). Syndrome of amelogenesis imperfecta, nephrocalcinosis, impaired renal concentration and possible abnormality of calcium metabolism. *Am. J. Med. Genet.* **20**, 233–43.

MacGibbon, D. (1972). Generalized enamel hypoplasia and renal dysfunction. *Aust. Dent. J.* **17**, 61–3.

7.17. FACI-OCULO-ACOUSTICO-RENAL (FOAR) SYNDROME

A combination of facial anomalies, myopia, telecanthus and hyper-telorism, perceptive deafness, epiphyseal dysplasia of the femoral heads and proteinuria was reported in a brother and sister (Holmes and Schepens 1971; Murdoch and Mengel 1971). Further cases were discussed by Ozer (1974) and Fraser (1976). The latter's patient had a heavy proteinuria of 250 mg/100 ml of urine.

Inheritance is probably autosomal recessive.

References

Fraser, G. R. (1976). *The causes of profound deafness in childhood.* A study of 3535 individuals with severe auditory handicaps present at birth or of childhood onset. Johns Hopkins University Press, Baltimore.
Holmes, L. B. and Schepens, C. L. (1971). Syndrome of ocular and facial anomalies, telecanthus and deafness. *J. Pediatr.* **81**, 552–5.
Murdoch, J. L. and Mengel, M. C. (1971). An unusual eye–ear syndrome with renal abnormality. *Birth Defects Orig. Art. Series* 7(4), 136.
Ozer, F. L. (1974). A possibly 'new' syndrome with eye and renal abnormalities. *Birth Defects Orig. Art. Series.* **10**(4), 168.

7.18. HAEMOLYTIC URAEMIC SYNDROME

The great majority of patients with this syndrome of acute renal failure, thrombocytopenia, and 'burr cell' haemolytic anaemia are of sporadic occurrence. There is a high incidence in certain endemic areas such as Argentina, South Africa, the West Coast of the United States, and the Netherlands. There is some evidence for a viral aetiology (Gianantonio *et al.* 1968), and this may even lead to familial occurrence. Indeed Kaplan and colleagues (1975) found that familial cases with onset in sibs close together in time are more common in endemic areas and have a relatively good prognosis. They suggest that such cases are of environmental origin, but that where affected sibs are born more than a year apart that prognosis is worse, origin is usually from a non-endemic area, and aetiology is likely to be genetic. There have been numerous reports of affected sibs of both sexes (Hagge *et al.* 1967; Bergstein *et al.* 1974; Tune 1974; Blattler *et al.* 1975; Hellman *et al.* 1980; Hymes and Warshaw 1981), and one of concordant monozygotic twins (Campbell and Carre 1965). However, there have also been reports of more than one generation being involved (Farr *et al.* 1975; Perret *et al.* 1979) and even affected adopted, unrelated sibs (Chan *et al.* 1969). Hence the question as to whether a minority of cases may be genetically determined remains open. Merrill and colleagues (1985) have pointed out the clinicopathological similarity of haemolytic–uraemic syndrome and thrombotic thrombocytopenic purpura, in both of which a thrombotic microangiopathy is the characteristic lesion. They report a family in which two adult sisters developed haemolytic uraemic syndrome with thrombotic microangiopathy. One sister died but the other survived on dialysis. The twin sister of one of them and their father may have also been affected.

References

Bergstein, J., Michael, A., Kjellstrand, C., Simmons, R. and Najarian, J. (1974). Hemolytic–uremic syndrome in adult sisters. *Transplantation* **17**, 487–90.

Blattler, W., Wegmann, W., Herold, H. and Straub, P. W. (1975). Familiaeres haemolytisch-uraemisches Syndrom: Untersuchungen zur Pathogenesis bei den ueberlebenden. *Schweiz. Med. Wschr.* **105**, 1773–4.

Campbell, S. and Carre, I. J. (1965). Fatal haemolytic uraemic syndrome and idiopathic hyperlipaemia in monozygotic twins. *Arch. Dis. Child.* **40**, 654–8.

Chan, J. C. M., Eleff, M. G. and Campbell, R. A. (1969). The hemolytic–uremic syndrome in non-related adopted siblings. *J. Pediatr.* **75**, 1050–3.

Farr, M. J., Roberts, S., Morley, A. R., Dewar, P. J., Roberts, D. F. and Uldall, P. R. (1975). The haemolytic uraemic syndrome—a family study. *Quart. J. Med.* 161–88.

Gianantonio, C. A., Vitacco, M., Mendilaharzu, F. and Gallo, G. (1968). The hemolytic–uremic syndrome: renal status of 76 patients at long-term follow-up. *J. Pediatr.* **72**, 757–65.

Hagge, W. W., Holley, K. E., Burke, E. C. and Stickler, G. B. (1967). Hemolytic-uremic syndrome in two siblings. *New Engl. J. Med.* **277**, 138–9.

Hellman, R. M., Jackson, D. V. and Buss, D. H. (1980). Thrombotic thrombo-cytopenic purpura and hemolytic–uremic syndrome in HLA-identical siblings. *Ann. Intern. Med.* **93**, 283–4.

Hymes, L. C. and Warshaw, B. L. (1981). Hemolytic–uremic syndrome in two siblings from a non endemic area. *Am. J. Dis. Child.* **135**, 766–7.

Kaplan, B. S., Chesney, R. W. and Drummond, K. N. (1975). Hemolytic–uremic syndrome in families. *New Engl. J. Med.* **292**, 1090–3.

Merrill, R. H., Knupp, C. L. and Jennette, J. C. (1985). Familial thrombotic microangiopathy. *Quart. J. Med.* **57**, 749–59.

Perret, B., Gaze, H., Zimmerman, A. and Detliker, O. (1979). Syndrome hemo-lytique uremique familial non-endemique: nephrectomie et transplantation. *Helv. Paediatr. Acta.* **34**, 167–76.

Tune, B. M. (1974). Hemolytic–uremic syndrome in siblings—prospective survey. *J. Pediatr.* **85**, 682–3.

7.19. CONGENITAL ICHTHYOSIS, MENTAL RETARDATION, DWARFISM, AND RENAL IMPAIRMENT

This combination of features was found in two sisters and a brother in an Iranian family, and in a half-sister of both parents born to the paternal grandfather and maternal grandmother (Passwell *et al.* 1975).

Reference

Passwell, J. H., Goodman, R. M., Ziprkowski, M. and Cohen, B. E. (1975). Congenital ichthyosis, mental retardation, dwarfism and renal impairment: a new syndrome. *Clin. Genet.* **8**, 59–65.

7.20. IMERSLUND–GRASBECK SYNDROME OF JUVENILE PERNICIOUS ANAEMIA WITH SELECTIVE MALABSORPTION OF VITAMIN B_{12} AND PROTEINURIA

Several forms of juvenile pernicious anaemia including defective ileal transport of vitamin B_{12} have been described. Grasbeck (1960) described a family in which there was a megaloblastic anaemia of juvenile onset, which he attributed to a selective intestinal malabsorption of vitamin B_{12}. There was an associated proteinuria and urinary tract malformation. Subsequently further cases were reported, predominantly from Finland (Lamy *et al.* 1961; Imerslund and Bjornstad 1963; Spurling *et al.* 1964). Grasbeck (1972) commented that of 47 cases reported at that time 21 were Finnish, and more recently Nevanlinna (1980) has reviewed 27 Finnish cases in 17 sibships. Sib occurrence is indicative of autosomal recessive inheritance.

References

Grasbeck, R. (1960). Familjar selectiv B12-malabsorption with proteinuri ett perniciosaliknande syndrome. *Nord. Med.* **63**, 322–3.

—— (1972). Familial selective vitamin B12 malabsorption (letter). *New Engl. J. Med.* **287**, 358.

Imerslund, O. and Bjornstad, P. (1963). Familial vitamin B12 malabsorption. *Acta Haemat.* **30**, 1–7.

Lamy, M., Besancon, F., Loverdo, A. and Afifi, F. (1961). Specific malabsorption of vitamin B12 and proteinuria. Megaloblastic anemia of Imerslund–Grasbeck: study of 4 cases. *Arch. Fr. Pédiatr.* **18**, 1109–20.

Nevanlinna, H. R. (1980). Selective malabsorption of vitamin B12. In *Population structure and genetic disorders*, eds. Eriksson, A. W., Forsius, H. R., Nevanlinna, H. R., Workman, P. L. and Norio, R. K. pp. 680–2. Academic Press.

Spurling, C. L., Sachs, M. S. and Jiji, R. M. (1964). Juvenile perniceous anaemia. *New Engl. J. Med.* **271**, 995–1003.

7.21. MYOCLONUS–NEPHROPATHY SYNDROME

Andermann and colleagues (1981) have briefly reported a French-Canadian family in which two sibs, and another member of the family with consanguineous parents, all developed tremors of the fingers and hands, and proteinuria at the age of 17 to 18 years. The disorder was progressive, developing into a severe action clonus with ataxia, dysarthria, and occasional generalized seizures, accompanied by renal failure requiring dialysis or renal transplantation by 19 to 23 years. Intelligence remained unimpaired. Nephrosialidosis was excluded. The patients all had a common family name and the disorder is presumed to show autosomal recessive inheritance.

Reference

Andermann, F., Andermann, E., Carpenter, S., Wolfe, L., Nelson, R., Patry, G., Boileau, J., Warren, Y. and Barcelo, R. (1981). Action myoclonus–renal failure: a new autosomal recessive syndrome in three families (abs.). *Proc. 6th Int. Congr. Hum. Genet.* p. 199. Jerusalem.

7.22. DYSCHONDROSTEOSIS AND NEPHRITIS

A family has been reported showing inheritance of typical dyschondrosteosis and a nephritis over four generations (Funderburk *et al.* 1976). Both sexes were involved but no male-to-male transmission was observed.

Reference

Funderburk, S. J., Smith, L., Falk, R. E., Bergstein, J. M. and Winter, H. (1976). A family with concurrent mesomelic shortening and hereditary nephritis. *Birth Defects Orig. Art. Series.* **12**(6), 47–61.

7.23. THYROTOXICOSIS AND RENAL DISEASE

A single case report describes a syndrome of thyrotoxicosis, proteinuria, and absent frontal sinuses (Wochner *et al.* 1969). The authors observed this combination in a pair of young adult female identical twins. Renal biopsy in one of them showed subacute proliferative glomerulonephritis with glomerular immune deposits. Since their mother also had absent frontal sinuses that finding may be unrelated to the apparently auto-immune thyrotoxicosis and renal disease. At least one of the twins became euthyroid on treatment, making it unlikely that this is a single gene defect.

Reference

Wochner, R. D., Silverman, D., Germuth, F., Kaufman, R., Kechijian, P. and Perkoff, G. T. (1969). An apparently hereditary syndrome of thyrotoxicosis, renal disease and absent frontal sinuses. *Clin. Res.* **17**, 530.

7.24. ARTERIAL HEPATIC DYSPLASIA (ALAGILLE'S SYNDROME)

Alagille and colleagues (1978) described a syndrome of hepatic ductular hypoplasia with chronic cholestasis and a characteristic facies with prominent forehead, deep set mildly hyperteloric eyes, a straight nose and a small pointed chin giving a rather startled appearance. Additional features include a mid-systolic cardiac murmur associated with pulmonary stenosis or even co-arctation, vertebral arch defects giving a 'butterfly' appearance to the vertebrae radiologically, retardation of physical and mental development, hypogonadism in males with absence of spermatogenic cells on testicular biopsy. Chung Park and coworkers (1982) noted that in addition some patients had renal artery stenosis and glomerular foam cells. A more extensive study of the renal changes, in 6 autopsy cases and 20 living cases, revealed large glomeruli with mesangial foam cells in all of the autopsy cases and in 12 out of the 20 living cases. Glomerular filtration rate was reduced in half of the total cases and a few showed proteinuria or hyperchloraemic acidosis (Habib, 1987). Inheritance appears to be autosomal dominant.

References

Alagille, D., Odievre, M., Gautier, M. and Dommergues, J. P. (1975). Hepatic ductular hypoplasia associated with characteristic facies, vertebral malformations, retarded physical, mental and sexual development, and cardiac murmur. *J. Pediatr.* **86**, 63–71.

Chung-Park, M., Petrelli, M., Tavill, A. S., Hall, P. W., III, Henoch, M. S. and Dahms, B. B. (1982). Renal lipidosis associated with arteriohepatic dysplasia (Alagille's syndrome). *Clin. Nephrol.* **18**, 314–20.

Habib, R. (1987). Renal lesions in Alagille's syndrome. *Pediatr. Nephrol.* (in press).

8. Nephropathy secondary to systemic disorders

8.1. ESSENTIAL HYPERTENSION

There is a long history of genetic hypotheses for the aetiology of essential hypertension. As early as 1923 Weitz postulated dominant inheritance, a view supported by many others subsequently (Allan 1933; Hines 1940; Platt 1947; Sobye 1948; Thomas and Cohen 1955; Wear 1956). In the 1950s to 1960s there was a major controversy between Platt (1959, 1960, 1961, 1963) who maintained his view that there is a single major gene involved in the determination of hypertension, or at least arterial disease, and Miall and Oldham (1955, 1958, 1963) and Pickering and colleagues (Hamilton *et al.* 1954a, b, and c, 1963; Pickering 1955a and b) who argued that blood pressure is a continuous variable. Platt observed that the distribution of blood pressure values among sibs of hypertensive subjects showed an irregular bimodality or even trimodality, with an excess number of individuals to the right of the curve, rather than a Gaussian distribution. From this, and the finding of concordance in three monozygotic twin pairs, he concluded that a single gene with incomplete dominance and a frequency of about 0.24 determined severe essential hypertension in homozygotes and moderate hypertension in heterozygotes. Morrison and Morris (1959) working with London busmen also interpreted their data in single dominant gene terms. Pickering's group, Miall and Oldham and others (Ostfeld and Paul 1963; Parnell 1963, 1965) have pointed out that irregularities of distribution of a multifactorially determined variable may be due to chance variation in small samples or even correlated with varying distribution of blood pressure among parents and grandparents of propositi (Parnell 1965), rather than to the action of a single major determinant; in their own studies they obtained data wholly consistent with polygenic inheritance. Miall and Oldham (1963) estimated a value for heritability of essential hypertension, at best, of 63 per cent for systolic and only 36 per cent for diastolic pressure, and Pickering also concluded that environmental factors were of greater importance than genetic predisposition. This view receives strong support from the observation that hypertension is virtually non-existent among the inbred inhabitants of Easter Island but readily develops among those islanders who migrate to mainland Chile (Cruz-Coke *et al.* 1964).

However, Acheson and Fowler (1967) in a critique of Pickering's conclusions point out weaknesses in his comparison of blood pressure distribution with that for height, and express their own belief that inheritance is a more important determinant of blood pressure than environment. Feinleib (1975) in a twin study found a correlation coefficient for male monozygotic twins of 0.55 but for dizygotic pairs of only 0.25. He suggests that systolic heritability is 82 per cent and diastolic 64 per cent. A recent statistical reassessment of the single-gene:multifactorial controversy (McManus 1982) questions the generally accepted view that Pickering and the multifactorial school won the debate. The best fit for the distribution of blood pressure in the general population is the logarithm of a bimodal distribution. Moreover, when blood pressures are remeasured in a given population, although there is a tendency for the high and low extremes to regress towards the population mean there is evidence that a subgroup with initially high pressures regress towards a higher mean. These observations suggest that there may after all be a subpopulation of patients with essential hypertension in whom single gene factors are important. A recent analysis of blood pressure in a national cohort at the age of 36 years has confirmed that familial factors are involved (Wadsworth *et al.* 1985). One possible single gene factor may be that proposed by Chesley and Cooper (1986) as the major determinant of pre-eclampsia. They present the results of a family study carried out over a fifty-year period which demonstrates a high heritability for pre-eclampsia consistent with the recessive action of a single autosomal gene.

Nephropathy is a common complication of essential hypertension, which must be clearly distinguished from primary renal or renal arterial disease as a cause of secondary hypertension. The renal complications of essential hypertension differ markedly between the benign and malignant phases of the disease. The renal changes in the benign phase are characterized by arteriolar changes whose severity is correlated with the degree of elevation of the blood pressure. They may induce minor degrees of renal impairment but never sufficiently severe as to result in uraemia. In contrast the renal changes in the malignant phase are characterized by proteinuria, microscopic haematuria, and declining renal function associated with medial and internal fibrinoid lesions of small arteries and arterioles with narrowing of the vascular lumen. This fibrinoid necrosis progressively reduces the renal blood flow leading to renal failure and eventual uraemic death and appears in both humans and experimental animals to be a direct, and in its early stages reversible, consequence of very high arterial pressures. Experimental studies, in which the kidneys of genetically hypertensive rats transplanted into normotensive rats induce hypertension and those of normotensive rats reduce it when transplanted into hypertensive rats, suggest that the hereditary factor in hypertension operates through the kidney (Bianchi *et al.* 1974). Their hypertensive and normotensive animals differed in their sensitivity to dietary salt, suggesting that it may be this sensitivity which is genetically determined. These observations on rats have been confirmed in more recent studies, and parallel observations were made in humans by Skrabal and associates (1981). They found in a study of 20 medical students that a low-sodium–high-potassium diet reduced blood pressure more effectively in those with a hypertensive parent. A group from the London Hospital (Holly *et al.* 1981; Parfrey *et al.* 1981a and b) obtained similar results. Similar studies by other groups have yielded negative results (Watt *et al.* 1985) and even in those studies with positive results the magnitude of the effect is small (Grobbee and Hofman 1986). There is a suggestion that susceptibility to the hypertensive effects of dietary salt may show racial variation, being greater in West Africans in whom it may be associated with an uncoupling of the correlation between urinary sodium and dopamine excretion seen in normotensive Caucasians (Critchley and Lee 1986).

These observations on the possible role of cations in hypertension form part of a wider interest in several aspects of this topic that has given rise to an extensive literature in recent years, only a part of which relates to familial factors. Garay and Meyer's group from Paris have demonstrated a defect in erythrocyte sodium–potassium cotransport in hypertensive patients and in a high proportion of normotensive subjects with hypertensive parents (54 per cent of those with one hypertensive parent and 74 per cent of those with two) (Garay *et al.* 1980a; Canessa *et al.* 1981; Meyer *et al.* 1981). They postulated that this defect is determined by a single gene with autosomal dominant inheritance. Other groups, without postulating a single gene effect, have obtained similar, but not always as clear-cut, results as the Paris group in both red and white blood cells (Canessa *et al.* 1980; Woods *et al.* 1981; Heagerty *et al.* 1982; Zidek *et al.* 1982). More recently the Paris group have produced evidence for heterogeneity in cation transport defects in hypertension (Garay 1983; Garay *et al.* 1983), and propose that individual blood pressure levels are the product of such functional disturbances when present, hormonal and other homeostatic mechanisms, and environmental factors such as salt intake. One such factor is the comparatively recently discovered atrial natriuretic peptide (Sagnella and MacGregor 1984) whose plasma concentration is raised in patients with essential hypertension (Sagnella *et al.* 1986). MacDonald and colleagues (1986) have suggested that this elevation of atrial natriuretic peptide in hypertensives may be due to sodium overload associated with a defect in renal sodium handing due to impaired mobilization of dopamine in the proximal tubule. This they suggest might result in ineffective renal vasodilatation and ineffective natriuresis. They quote unpublished evidence that such a fault is more common in the first-degree relatives of hypertensive patients.

Further evidence for heterogeneity comes from the work of Hollenberg and colleagues (1986). They found that about half of a group of 61 patients with essential hypertension failed to modulate their renal and adrenal responses to infusion of angiotensin II, as measured by para-aminohippurate clearance and plasma aldosterone level respectively. The other half showed similar modulatory responses to normotensives. The 'non-modulators' had a delay in the achievement of external sodium balance following a shift from low to high sodium intake compared to the other two groups. 84.6 per cent of the non-modulators had a history of hypertension in a first degree relative compared to 27.3 per cent of the modulating hypertensives.

Apart from the ouabain-sensitive sodium pump (Edmondson *et al.* 1975), the furosemide-sensitive sodium–potassium cotransport system may be impaired (Garay *et al.* 1980b; Davidson *et al.* 1982), as may also the sodium-dependent lithium efflux, or lithium–sodium counter-transport system (Canessa *et al.* 1980; Clegg *et al.* 1982). It has to be said that several groups have not been able to confirm these various claims of defects in sodium flux. For example Watt and colleagues (1983) in a comparison of children of parents with high or low blood pressure confirmed a positive parent–child correlation, but found no differences in 24-hour urinary electrolyte excretion, and Gudmundsson and associates (1984a, b) have found no difference between normotensive subjects with and without familial predisposition to hypertension in changes in sodium elimination rate on a high sodium intake.

Experimental and clinical studies have suggested that essential hypertension, in both laboratory animals and humans, may be due to inhibition of the Na^+–K^+–ATPase pump by a circulating ouabain-like substance (de Wardener *et al.* 1961; Dahl *et al.* 1969; Haddy and Oberbeck 1976; Blaustein 1977a and b; de Wardener and MacGregor 1980; de Wardener *et al.* 1981; de Wardener and MacGregor 1982; MacGregor *et al.* 1981; Poston *et al.* 1981). De Wardener and his colleagues at Charing Cross Hospital have postulated that the underlying defect is a genetically determined renal difficulty in excreting sodium the expression of which is related to sodium intake and which leads to a transient hypervolaemia and increased hypothalamic secretion of Na^+–K^+–ATPase inhibitor, which in turn tends to restore the balance of sodium excretion but also increases vascular smooth muscle tone, resulting in increased arterial pressure (de Wardener and MacGregor 1982). They have not put forward any suggestions as to the nature of the renal genetic defect other than by reference to twin studies on renal excretion of a sodium load indicating that variation in this capacity is genetically determined and that normotensive relatives of hypertensives excrete sodium less efficiently than controls (Grim *et al.* 1979a and b). How these hypotheses correlate with those of MacDonald and colleagues (1986), discussed above, is as yet unclear.

Several workers, as for example Blaustein (1977a), have suggested that intracellular calcium plays a central role in the mechanism of increased smooth muscle tone in essential hypertension. Blaustein suggests that reduced activity of the sodium pump, with its consequent rise in intra-cellular sodium, interferes with the normal exchange of sodium for calcium across the cell membrane and results in a rise in intracellular calcium. Corroborative evidence for a role for calcium comes from epidemiological evidence for a positive correlation between serum calcium and both systolic and diastolic blood pressure (Kesteloot and Geboers 1982), and from evidence that effective treatment of hypertension with calcium antagonists does not alter cellular sodium content or efflux rate (Heagerty *et al.* 1983).

There is also epidemiological evidence for a protective role for potassium in the prevention of hypertension (Meneely and Battarbee 1976; Khaw and Rose 1982). Khaw and Thom (1982) demonstrated a lowering of both systolic and diastolic pressures in healthy males during potassium oral supplementation.

In summary, there is now a considerable body of evidence implicating alterations in cellular electrolyte flux and a natriruetic hormone in the aetiology of essential hypertension, at both genetic and environmental levels, with a postulated primary defect in renal excretion of sodium and a secondary affect of dietary high sodium or low potassium intake. The evidence regarding the importance of these factors is conflicting and the genetic mechanisms proposed are obscure. Clearly there is still much research to be done before the picture becomes clear.

It must also be remembered that there are many inherited disorders involving the kidney in which secondary hypertension may occur. These are mostly discussed elsewhere in this book and include inborn errors of metabolism such as Fabry's disease, renal tubular disorders such as familial pseudohyperaldosteronism, Alport's disease and other heredi-tary nephritides, diabetic nephropathy, lupus nephritis, severe juvenile arterial sclerosis, haemolytic uraemic syndrome, and neurofibromatosis. It is also seen in renal failure associated with familial obstructive renal disease, familial phaeochromocytoma and some forms of congenital adrenal hyperplasia.

References

Acheson, R. M. and Fowler, G. B. (1967). On the inheritance of stature and blood pressure. *J. Chron. Dis.* **20**, 731–45.

Allan, W. (1933). Heredity in hypertension: a statistical study. *Arch. Intern. Med.* **52**, 954–8.

Bianchi, G., Fox, U., DiFrancesco, G. F., Giovanetti, A. M. and Pagetti, D. (1974). Blood pressure changes produced by kidney cross transplantation between spontaneously hypertensive rats and normotensive rats. *Clin. Sci. Mol. Med.* **47**, 435–48.

Blaustein, M. P. (1977a). Sodium ions, calcium ions, blood pressure regulation, and hypertension: a reassessment and a hypothesis. *Am. J. Physiol.* **232**, C165–73.

—— (1977b). The role of Na–Ca exchange in the regulation of tone in vascular smooth muscle. In *Excitation contraction coupling in smooth muscle*, eds. Castees, R. *et al.* pp. 101–7. Elsevier/North Holland, Amsterdam.

Canessa, M., Adragna, N., Solomon, H. S., Connolly, T. M. and Tosteson, D. C. (1980). Increased sodium–lithium countertransport in red cells of patients with essential hypertension. *New Engl. J. Med.* **302**, 772–6.

——, Bize, I., Solomon, H., Adragna, N., Tosteson, D. C., Dagher, G., Garay, R. and Meyer, P. (1981). Na countertransport and cotransport in human red cells: dysfunction and genes in essential hypertension. *Clin. Exp. Hypertension* **3**, 783–95.

Chesley, L. C. and Cooper, D. W. (1986). Genetics of hypertension in pregnancy: possible single gene control of pre-eclampsia in the descendants of eclamptic women. *Br. J. Obstet. Gynaecol.* **93**, 898–908.

Clegg, G., Morgan, B. D. and Davidson, C. (1982). The heterogeneity of essential hypertension. *Lancet* **2**, 891–4.

Critchley, J. J. H. and Lee, M. R. (1986). Salt-sensitive hypertension in West Africans: an uncoupling of the renal sodium-dopamine relation. *Lancet* **2**, 460.

Cruz-Coke, R., Etcheverry, R. and Nagel, R. (1964). The influence of migration on blood pressure of Easter Islanders. *Lancet* **1**, 697–9.

Dahl, L. K., Knudsen, K. D. and Iwai, J. (1969). Humoral transmission of hypertension: evidence from parabiosis. *Circ. Res.* **24** and **25**, Suppl. I, I.23–I.33.

Davidson, J. S., Opie, L. H. and Keding, B. (1982). Sodium–potassium co-transport activity as genetic marker in essential hypertension. *Br. Med. J.* **284**, 539–41.

Edmondson, R. P. S., Thomas, R. D., Jilton, P. J., Patrick, J. and Jones, N. F. (1975). Abnormal leucocyte composition and sodium transport in essential hypertension. *Lancet* **1**, 1003–5.

Feinleib, M. (1975). In *Epidemiology and control of hypertension*, ed. Paul, O. Stratton, New York.

Garay, R. P. (1983). Neither Platt, nor Pickering (letter). *Lancet* **1**, 932.

——, Dagher, G., Pernollet, M. G., Devynck, M. A. and Meyer, P. (1980a). Inherited defect in Na^+-K^+ co-transport system in erythrocytes from essential hypertensive patients. *Nature* **284**, 281–3.

——, Elghozi, J. L., Dagher, G. and Meyer, P. (1980b). Laboratory distinction between essential and secondary hypertension by measurement of erythrocyte cation fluxes. *New Engl. J. Med.* **302**, 769–71.

——, Nazaret, C., Hannaert, P. and Price, M. (1983). Abnormal Na$^+$, K$^+$ co-transport function in a group of essential hypertensive patients. *Eur. J. Clin. Invest.* **13**, 311–20.

Grim, C. E., Luft, F. C., Fineberg, N. S. and Weinberger, M. H. (1979a). Responses to volume expansion and contraction in categorised hypertensive and normotensive man. *Hypertension* **1**, 476–85.

——, Miller, J. Z., Luft, F. C., Christian, J. C. and Weinberger, M. H. (1979b). Genetic influences of renin, aldosterone, and the renal excretion of sodium and potassium following volume expansion and contraction in man. *Hypertension* **1**, 583–90.

Grobbee, D. E. and Hofman, A. (1986). Does sodium restriction lower blood pressure? *Br. Med. J.* **293**, 27–9.

Gudmundsson, O. (1984a). Sodium and blood pressure: studies in young and middle-aged men with a positive family history of hypertension. *Acta Med. Scand.* Suppl. **688**, 1–65.

——, Cederblad, A., Wikstrand, J. and Berglund, G. (1984b). Sodium elimination rate and blood pressure during normal and high salt intake in subjects with and without familial predisposition to hypertension. *Acta Med. Scand.* **216**, 345–52.

Haddy, F. J. and Overbeck, H. W. (1976). The role of humoral agents in volume expanded hypertension. *Life Sci.* **19**, 935–48.

Hamilton, M., Pickering, G. W., Fraser Roberts, J. A. and Sowry, G. S. C. (1954a). The aetiologyy of essential hypertension. 1. The arterial pressure in the general population. *Clin. Sci.* **13**, 11–35.

——, ——, —— and —— (1954b). The aetiology of essential hypertension. 2. Scores for arterial blood pressures adjusted for differences in age and sex. *Clin. Sci.* **13**, 37–49.

——, ——, —— and —— (1954c). The aetiology of essential hypertension. 4. The role of inheritance. *Clin. Sci.* **13**, 273–304.

——, ——, —— and —— (1963). Arterial pressure of relatives of patients with secondary and malignant hypertension. *Clin. Sci.* **24**, 91–108.

Heagerty, A. M., Bing, F. R., Milner, M., Thurston, H. and Swales, J. D. (1982). Leucocyte membrane sodium transport in normotensive populations: dissociation of abnormalities of sodium efflux from raised blood pressure. *Lancet* **2**, 894–6.

——, ——, Thurston, H. and Swales, J. D. (1983). Calcium antagonists in hypertension: relation to abnormal sodium transport. *Br. Med. J.* **287**, 1405–7.

Hines, E. A. (1940). Hereditary factor and subsequent development of hypertension. *Mayo Clin. Proc.* **15**, 145–6.

Hollenberg, N. K., Moore, T., Shoback, D., Redgrave, J., Rabinowe, S. and Williams, G. H. (1986). Abnormal renal sodium handling in essential hypertension: relation to failure of renal and adrenal modulation of responses to angiotensin II. *Am. J. Med.* **81**, 412–18.

Holly, J. M. P., Goodwin, F. J., Evans, S. J. W., Vandenburg, M. J. and Ledingham, J. M. (1981). Re-analysis of data in two Lancet papers on the effect of dietary sodium and potassium on blood pressure. *Lancet* **2**, 1384–7.

Kesteloot, H. and Geboers, J. (1982). Calcium and blood pressure. *Lancet* **1**, 813–15.

Khaw, K. T. and Rose, G. (1982). Population study of blood pressure and associated factors in St Lucia, West Indies. *Int. J. Epidemiol.* **11**, 372-7.

—— and Thom, S. (1982). Random double-blind cross-over trial of potassium on blood-pressure in normal subjects. *Lancet* **2**, 1127-9.

MacDonald, T. M., Jeffrey, R. F. and Lee, M. R. (1986). Atrial natriuretic peptides in essential hypertension. *Lancet* **1**, 562.

MacGregor, G. A., Fenton, S., Alaghband-Zadeh, J., Markandu, R., Roulston, J. E. and de Wardener, H. E. (1981). Evidence for a raised concentration of a circulating sodium transport inhibitor in essential hypertension. *Br. Med. J.* **283**, 1355-7.

McManus, I. C. (1982). The distribution of blood pressure. *Clin. Sci.* **62**, 30p-31p.

Meneely, G. R. and Battarbee, H. D. (1976). High sodium–low potassium environment and hypertension. *Am. J. Cardiol.* **38**, 768-84.

Meyer, P., Garay, R. P., Nazaret, C., Dagher, G., Bellet, M., Broyer, M. and Feingold, J. (1981). Inheritance of abnormal erythrocyte cation transport in essential hypertension. *Br. Med. J.* **282**, 1114-17.

Miall, W. E. and Oldham, P. D. (1955). A study of arterial blood pressure and its inheritance in a sample of the general population. *Clin. Sci.* **14**, 459-88.

—— and —— (1958). Factors influencing arterial blood pressure in the general population. *Clin. Sci.* **17**, 409-44.

—— and —— (1963). The hereditary factor in arterial blood-pressure. *Br. Med. J.* **1**, 75-80.

Morrison, S. L. and Morris, J. N. (1959). Epidemiological observations on high blood-pressure without evident cause. *Lancet* **2**, 864-70.

—— and —— (1960). Nature of essential hypertension. *Lancet* **2**, 829-32.

Oldham, P. D., Pickering, G., Roberts, J. A. F. and Sowry, G. S. C. (1960). The nature of essential hypertension. *Lancet* **1**, 1085-93.

Ostfeld, A. M. and Paul, O. (1963). The inheritance of hypertension. *Lancet* **1**, 575-9.

Parfrey, P. S., Condon, K., Wright, P., Vandenburg, M. J., Holly, J. M. P., Goodwin, F. J., Evans, S. J. W. and Ledingham, J. M. (1981a). Blood pressure and hormonal changes following alterations in dietary sodium and potassium in young men with and without a familial predisposition to hypertension. *Lancet* **1**, 113-17.

——, Vandenburg, M. J., Wright, P., Holly, J. M. P., Goodwin, F. J., Evans, S. J. W. and Ledingham, J. M. (1981b). Blood pressure and hormonal changes following alteration in dietary sodium and potassium in mild essential hypertension. *Lancet* **1**, 59-63.

Parnell, R. W. (1963). Heredity in hypertension (letter). *Lancet* **1**, 1213.

—— (1965). Hyperpiesis. *Br. Med. J.* **2**, 1180-1.

Pickering, G. W. (1955a). The genetic factor in essential hypertension. *Ann. Intern. Med.* **43**, 457-64.

—— (1955b). *High blood pressure.* Churchill Livingstone, London.

—— (1963). Heredity in hypertension (letter). *Lancet* **1**, 1213-14.

—— (1965). Hyperpiesis: high blood pressure without evident cause: essential hypertension. *Br. Med. J.* **2**, 959-68, 1021-6.

Platt, R. (1947). Heredity in hypertension. *Quart. J. Med.* **16**, 111-33.

—— (1959). The nature of essential hypertension. *Lancet* **2**, 55–7.

—— (1961). Essential hypertension: incidence, course, and heredity. *Ann. Intern. Med.* **55**, 1–11.

—— (1963). Heredity in hypertension. *Lancet* **1**, 899–904, 1269.

Poston, L., Sewell, R. B., Wilkinson, S. P., Clarkson, E. M., MacGregor, G. A. and de Wardener, H. E. (1981). Evidence for a circulating sodium transport inhibitor in essential hypertension. *Br. Med. J.* **282**, 847–9.

Sagnella, G. A. and MacGregor, G. A. (1984). Cardiac peptides and the control of sodium excretion. *Nature* **309**, 666–7.

——, Markandu, N. D., Shore, A. C. and MacGregor, G. A. (1986). Raised circulating levels of atrial natriuretic peptides in essential hypertension. *Lancet* **1**, 179–81.

Skrabal, F., Aubock, J. and Hortnagel, H. (1981). Low sodium/high potassium diet for prevention of hypertension. Probable mechanisms of action. *Lancet* **2**, 895–900.

Sobye, P. (1948). *Heredity in hypertertension and nephrosclerosis.* Nyt Nordisk Forlag, Arnold Burck, Copenhagen.

Thomas, C. B. and Cohen, B. H. (1955). The familial occurrence of hypertension and coronary artery disease, with observations concerning obesity and diabetes. *Ann. Intern. Med.* **42**, 90–127.

Wadsworth, M. E. J., Cripps, H. A., Midwinter, R. E. and Colley, J. R. T. (1985). Blood pressure in a national birth cohort at the age of 36 related to social and familial factors, smoking, and body mass. *Br. Med. J.* **291**, 1534–8.

de Wardener, H. E. and MacGregor, G. A. (1980). Dahl's hypothesis that a saluretic substance may be responsible for a sustained rise in arterial pressure: its possible role in hypertension. *Kidney Int.* **18**, 1–9.

—— and —— (1982). The natriuretic hormone and essential hypertension. *Lancet* **1**, 1450–4.

——, Mills, I. H., Clapham, W. F. and Hayter, C. J. (1961). Studies on the efferent mechanism of the sodium diuresis which follows the administration of intravenous saline in the dog. *Clin. Sci.* **21**, 249–58.

——, MacGregor, G. A., Clarkson, E. M., Alaghband-Zadeh, J., Bitensky, L. and Chayen, J. (1981). Effect of sodium intake on ability of human plasma to inhibit renal Na$^+$–K$^+$-adenosine triphosphate *in vitro*. *Br. Med. J.* **282**, 847–9.

Watt, G. C. M., Foy, C. J. W. and Tudor Hart, J. (1983). Comparison of blood pressure, sodium intake, and other variables in offspring with and without a family history of high blood pressure. *Lancet* **1**, 1245–8.

——, ——, ——, Bingham, G., Edwards, C., Hart, M., Thomas, E. and Walton, P. (1985). Dietary sodium and arterial blood pressure: evidence against genetic susceptibility. *Br. Med. J.* **291**, 1525–8.

Wear, L. E. (1956). A hypertensive family. *Lancet* **1**, 83.

Weitz, W. (1923). Zur Aetiologie der genuinen oder vascularen Hypertension. *Z. Klin. Med.* **96**, 151–81.

Woods, K. L., Beevers, D. G. and West, M. (1981). Familial abnormality of erythrocyte cation transport in essential hypertension. *Br. Med. J.* **282**, 1186–8.

Zidek, W., Vetter, H., Dorst, K. G., Zumkley, H. and Losse, H. (1982). Intracellular Na$^+$ and Ca^{2+} activities in essential hypertension. *Clin. Sci.* **63**, 41S–43S.

8.2. DIABETES MELLITUS IN ITS RENAL COMPLICATIONS

8.2.1. Insulin-dependent diabetes

Genetic factors play an important role in the aetiology of diabetes mellitus of all types.

An early family study of insulin-dependent, juvenile onset or type 1, diabetes mellitus (IDDM) provided evidence for polygenic inheritance or at least susceptibility (Simpson 1962). HLA identical sibs of IDDM patients have poorer glucose tolerance than HLA non-identical sibs (Orchard *et al.* 1986); and affected sibs of index patients also tend to share HLA haplotypes (Bhata *et al.* 1986). Numerous studies over the last decade have shown statistically significant associations of IDDM with specific HLA, properdin (Bf) or complement component four (C4) phenotypes. Early work indicated an association with HLA-B8 and BW15 (Singal and Blajchman 1973; Cudworth and Woodrow 1974, 1976; Nerup *et al.* 1974; Cathelinau *et al.* 1975; Jansen *et al.* 1975). This association is stronger for patients with a family history of IDDM (Cudworth and Woodrow 1974; Cudworth and Woodrow 1975; Löw *et al.* 1975), or of impaired glucose tolerance (Landgraf *et al.* 1976). Genetic heterogeneity in this predisposition is indicated by the observation that, whereas the frequency of BW15 is increased in both concordant and discordant identical twin pairs for IDDM, that of HLA-B8 is increased only for concordant pairs (Nelson *et al.* 1975). An even stronger association with HLA-DR3 and DR4 has been demonstrated (Nerup *et al.* 1976; Schernthaner *et al.* 1977), and the latter is transmitted by diabetic parents to their diabetic children with a greater than expected frequency (MacDonald *et al.* 1986a). Other genetic markers linked to the HLA gene cluster on the short arm of chromosome 6, such as the BfFl phenotype of the properdin factor B (Raum *et al.* 1979) especially in a haplotype association with HLA-B18 (Bertrams *et al.* 1979; Deschamps *et al.* 1979; Weitkamp *et al.* 1979), and several nul alleles of C4 resulting in a low serum C4 level (de Mouzon *et al.* 1979; Bertrams *et al.* 1982; Dawkins *et al.* 1983; Uko *et al.* 1983; Vergani *et al.* 1983; Mijovic *et al.* 1985). Mijovic and colleagues (1985) also demonstrated an association in IDDM of another variant of C4, C4B3, with the presence of microangiopathic complications. However, a low serum C4 level is not itself associated with such complications (Jacob *et al.* 1986). Several studies indicate that certain haplotype combinations of these inherited factors, segregating in particular families, especially predispose to IDDM (Cudworth *et al.* 1977; Walker and Cudworth 1980). It has also been confirmed that these markers must be linked to at least two genes, possibly immune response genes, determining susceptibility. One new line of evidence is the observation that the BfFl association is with early, rather than late, onset IDDM (Barbosa *et al.* 1979; Bernal *et al.* 1979; Kirk *et al.* 1979). Another is the finding that among patients with IDDM who are HLA-DR3 or 4 the heterozygous phenotype DR3/DR4 is more common than would be expected from the allele frequencies (Anderson *et al.* 1983; Johnston *et al.* 1983; Morton *et al.* 1983; Rotter *et al.* 1983; Thomson 1983; Louis and Thomson 1986), and that DR3 is associated with a more slowly progressive disease (Ludrigsson *et al.* 1986). These studies lead to the rejection of a simple single gene hypothesis of susceptibility and indicate that the DR3 and DR4 alleles must be independently in linkage disequilibrium with susceptibility genes. Further evidence for the independent association of DR3 and DR4 comes from the observation that the association of DR3 is as strong with IDDM in Yorubas in Nigeria as in Caucasians, whereas that for DR4 is weaker (MacDonald *et al.* 1986b). Another study looking at HLA-B determinants came to similar conclusions (Walsh *et al.* 1983).

A further complication is introduced by the demonstration that IDDM is also associated with DNA polymorphisms within the HLA-D region (Owerbach *et al.* 1984), and HLA-DR2 associated Dw subtypes correlate with such DNA polymorphisms (Cohen *et al.* 1986).

Identical twin studies have shown that the immune changes observed in IDDM may remit without causing the disease (Millward *et al.* 1986), although this has not been the experience of other workers (Dib *et al.* 1986). Furthermore lymphocytoxic antibodies are detectable in non-consanguineous, as well as consanguineous, relatives (Charlesworth *et al.* 1986). These observations point to the role of an environmental agent, presumably viral, in the immediate causation of the disease.

References

Anderson, C. E., Hodge, S. A., Rubin, R., Rotter, J. I., Terasaki, P. I., Irvine, W. J. and Rimoin, D. L. (1983). A search for heterogeneity in insulin dependent diabetes mellitus (IDDM): HLA and antoimmune studies in simplex, multiplex and multigenerational families. *Metabolism* **32**, 471–7.

Barbosa, J., Weitkamp, L., Guttermsen, S., Johnson, S. and Szalapski, E. Jr. (1979). Bf in early-onset insulin-dependent diabetes. *Lancet* **2**, 1239–40.

Bernal, J. E., Ellis, D. A. and Haigh, J. (1979). Bf in insulin-dependent diabetes mellitus. *Lancet* **2**, 961.

Bertrams, J., Baur, M. P., Gruneklee, D. and Gries, F. A. (1979). Association of BfFl, HLA-B18 and insulin-dependent diabetes mellitus. *Lancet* **2**, 98.

——, Hintzen, U., Schlicht, V. and Schoeps, S. (1982). C4: another marker for type 1 diabetes. *Lancet* **1**, 41.

Bhata, E., Mehra, N. K., Maloviya, A. N. and Ahiya, M. M. S. (1986). HLA and autoimmunity in North Indian type I (insulin-dependent) diabetic multiplex families. *Horm. Metab. Res.* **18**, 331–4.

Cathelinau, G., Cathelinau, L., Hors, J., Schmid, M. and Dausset, J. (1975). HL-A and juvenile diabetes. *Diabetologia* **11**, 335.

Charlesworth, J. A., Peake, P., Campbell, L. V., Rumma, J., Pussell, B. A., Howard, N. and Elder, G. J. (1986). Detectioni of lymphocytotoxic antibodies in relatives of patients with type 1 diabetes. *Br. Med. J.* **292**, 292–4.

Cohen, N., Brautbar, C., Font, M.-P., Dausset, J. and Cohen, D. (1986). HLA-DR2-associated Dw subtypes correllate with RFLP clusters: most DR2 IDDM patients belong to one of these clusters. *Immunogenetics* **23**, 84–9.

Cudworth, A. G. and Woodrow, J. C. (1974). HL-A antigens and diabetes mellitus. *Lancet* **2**, 1153.

—— and —— (1975). Evidence for HL-A-linked genes in 'juvenile' diabetes mellitus. *Br. Med. J.* **3**, 133–5.

—— and —— (1976). Genetic susceptibility in diabetes mellitus: analysis of the HLA association. *Br. Med. J.* **4**, 846–8.

——, Gamble, D. R., White, G. B. B., Lendrum, R., Woodrow, J. C. and Bloom, A. (1977). Aetiology of juvenile onset diabetes: a prospective study. *Lancet* **1**, 385–8.

Dawkins, R. L., Uko, G., Christiansen, F. T. and Kay, P. H. (1983). Low C4 concentrations in insulin dependent diabetes mellitus. *Br. Med. J.* **287**, 839.

Deschamps, I., Lestradet, H., Marcelli-Barge, A., Benajam, A., Busson, M., Hors, J. and Dausset, J. (1979). Properdin factor B alleles as markers for insulin-dependent diabetes. *Lancet* **2**, 793.

Dib, S., Vardi, P., Connelly, J., Eisenborth, G. S. and Soeldner, J. S. (1986). Immune changes associated with insulin dependent diabetes may remit without causing disease: a study in identical twins. *Br. Med. J.* **292**, 1670.

Jacob, B. G., Richter, W. O., Schwandt, P., Fateh-Moghadam, A. and Witt, Th.N. (1986). Low serum C4 concentrations and peripheral neuropathy in type I and type II diabetes. *Br. Med. J.* **292**, 1671.

Jansen, F. K., Bertrams, J., Grüneklee, D., Drost, H., Reis, H. E., Bever, J., Kuwert, E., Gries, F. A. and Altrock, E. (1975). Genetic association of the insulin-antibody production with histocompatibility (HL-A) antigens in diabetics. *Diabetologia* **11**, 352–3.

Johnston, C., Pyke, D. A., Cudworth, A. G. and Wolf, E. (1983). HLA-DR typing in identical twins with insulin-dependent diabetes: difference between concordant and discordant pairs. *Br. Med. J.* **1**, 253–5.

Kirk, R. L., Serjeantson, S. W., Theophilus, J., Zimmet, P., Whitehouse, S. and Court, J. M. (1979). Age relationship between insulin-dependent diabetes and rare alleles of properdin factor B. *Lancet* **2**, 537.

Landgraf, R., Landgraf-Leurs, M. M. C., Lander, T., Scholz, S., Kuntz, B. and Albert, E. D. (1976). HLA haplotypes and glucose tolerance in families of patients with juvenile-onset diabetes mellitus. *Lancet* **2**, 1084–5.

Louis, E. J. and Thomson, G. (1986). Three-allele synergistic mixed model for insulin-dependent diabetes mellitus. *Diabetes* **35**, 958–63.

Löw, B., Schersten, B., Sartor, G., Thulin, T. and Mitelman, F. (1975). HL-A8 and W15 in diabetes mellitus and essential hypertension. *Lancet* **1**, 695.

Ludvigsson, J., Samuelsson, U., Beauforts, C., Deschamps, I., Dorchy, H., Drash,

A., Francois, R., Herz, G., New, M. and Schober, E. (1986). HLA-DR3 is associated with a more slowly progressive form of type 1 (insulin-dependent) diabetes. *Diabetologia* **29**, 207–10.

MacDonald, M. J., Gottschall, J., Hunter, J. B. and Winter, K. L. (1986a). HLA-DR4 in insulin-dependent diabetic parents and their diabetic children: a clue to dominant inheritance. *Proc. Nat. Acad. Sci.* **83**, 7049–53.

——, Famuyiwa, O. O., Nwabuebo, I. A., Bella, A. F., Junaid, T. A., Marrari, M. and Duquesnoy, R. J. (1986b). HLA-DR associations in Black type I diabetic in Nigeria: further support for models of inheritance. *Diabetes* **35**, 583–9.

Mijovic, C., Fletcher, J., Bradwell, A. R., Harvey, T. and Barnett, A. H. (1985). Relation of gene expression (allotypes) of the fourth component of complement to insulin dependent diabetes and its microangiopathic complications. *Br. Med. J.* **291**, 9–10.

Millward, B. A., Aviggi, L., Hoskins, P. J., Johnston, C., Heaton, D., Bottazzo, G. F., Vergani, D., Leslie, R. D. G. and Pyke, D. A. (1986). Immune changes associated with insulin dependent diabetes may remit without causing the disease: a study in identical twins. *Br. Med. J.* **292**, 793–6.

Morton, N. E., Green, A., Dunsworth, T., Svejgaard, A., Barbosa, J., Rich, S. S., Iselius, L., Platz, P. and Ryder, L. P. (1983). Heterozygous expression of insulin-dependent diabetes mellitus (IDDM) determinants in the HLA system. *Am. J. Hum. Genet.* **35**, 201–13.

de Mouzon, A., Ohayon, E., Ducos, J. and Hauptmann, G. (1979). Bf and C4 markers for insulin-dependent diabetes in Basques. *Lancet* **2**, 1364.

Nelson, P. G., Pyke, D. A., Cudworth, A. G., Woodrow, J. C. and Batchelor, J. R. (1975). Histocompatibility antigens in diabetic identical twins. *Lancet* **2**, 193–4.

Nerup, J., Platz, P., Andersen, O. O., Christy, M., Lyngsoe, J., Poulsen, J. E., Ryder, L. P., Nielsen, L. S., Thomsen, M. and Svejgaard, A. (1974). HLA-A antigens and diabetes mellitus. *Lancet* **2**, 864–6.

——, ——, Ortved Andersen, O., Christy, M., Egeberg, J., Poulsen, J. E., Ryder, L. P., Thomsen, A. and Svejgaard, A. (1976). In *Genetics of diabetes mellitus*, eds. Creutzfeldt, W., Kobberling, J. and Neel, J. V. p. 106. Springer-Verlag, Berlin.

Orchard, T. J., Wagner, D. K., Rabin, B. S., La Porte, R. E. Cavender, D., Kuller, L. H., Drash, A. L. and Becker, D. J. (1986). Glucose tolerance in siblings of type 1 diabetic patients: relationship to HLA status. *Diabetologia* **29**, 39–45.

Owerbach, D., Hagglof, B., Lernmark, A. and Holmgren, G. (1984). Susceptibility to insulin-dependent diabetes defined by restriction enzyme polymorphism of HLA—D region genomic DNA. *Diabetes* **33**, 958–65.

Raum, D., Alper, C. A., Stein, R. and Gabbay, K. H. (1979). Genetic marker for insulin-dependent diabetes mellitus. *Lancet* **1**, 1208–10.

Rotter, J. I., Anderson, C. E., Rubin, R., Congleton, J. E., Terasaki, P. I. and Rimoin, D. L. (1983). HLA genotypic study of insulin-dependent diabetes: the excess of DR3/DR4 heterozygotes allows rejection of the recessive hypothesis. *Diabetes* **32**, 169–74.

Schernthaner, G., Ludwig, H. and Mayr, W. R. (1977). B-lymphocyte alloantigens and insulin-dependent diabetes mellitus. *Lancet* **2**, 1128.

Simpson, N. E. (1962). The genetics of diabetes: a study of 233 families of juvenile diabetics. *Ann. Hum. Genet.* **26**, 1–21.

Singal, D. P. and Blajchman, M. A. (1973). Histocompatibility HL-A antigens, lymphocytotoxic antibodies and tissue antibodies in patients with diabetes mellitus. *Diabetes* **22**, 429–32.

Thomson, G., (1986). Investigation of the mode of inheritance of the HLA-associated diseases by the method of antigen genotype frequencies among diseased individuals. *Tissue Antigens* **21**, 81–104.

Uko, G., Christiansen, F. T., Dawkins, R. L. and Kay, P. H. (1983). Low serum C4 concentrations in insulin dependent diabetes mellitus. *Br. Med. J.* **286**, 1748–9.

Vergani, D., Johnston, C., B-Abdullah, N. and Barnett, A. H. (1983). Low serum C4 concentrations: an inherited predisposition to insulin dependent diabetes? *Br. Med. J.* **1**, 926–8.

Walker, A. and Cudworth, A. G. (1980). Type 1 (insulin dependent) diabetic multiplex families: mode of genetic transmission. *Diabetes* **29**, 1036–9.

Walsh, L. J., Ehrlich, R. M., Falk, J. A. and Simpson, N. E. (1983). HLA haplotype segregation in families of type 1 diabetes. *Hum. Hered.* **33**, 253–60.

Weitkamp, L. R., Barbosa, J., Guttormsen, S. A. and Johnson, S. (1979). Insulin-dependent diabetes mellitus and properdin factor B. *Lancet* **2**, 369–70.

8.2.2. Non-insulin-dependent diabetes

In contrast to IDDM no HLA associations have been observed in non-insulin-dependent diabetes mellitus (type II or maturity onset diabetes). Nevertheless, non-insulin-dependent diabetes mellitus (NIDDM), although not inherited in a simple mendelian manner, is almost wholly genetically determined. The evidence for this statement comes from a series of monozygotic twin studies in diabetes by David Pyke and his colleagues at King's College Hospital (Pyke and Taylor 1967; Pyke *et al.* 1970; Tattersall and Pyke 1972; Pyke and Tattersall 1973; Lendrum *et al.* 1976; Barnett *et al.* 1981a and b). These studies show that for NIDDM identical twin pair concordance, including impaired metabolic response to glucose, is near 100 per cent, indicating a polygenic determination since it is difficult to imagine an environmental determinant which would produce such a high concordance. In contrast only about half of monozygotic cotwins are concordant in IDDM. An association has been reported between NIDDM and Rh blood group and haptoglobin phenotypes (Stern *et al.* 1986). There was also evidence for linkage disequilibrium between the Hp-1 allele and a major susceptibility gene for NIDDM, in that heterozygosity for Hp-1 was associated with a 50 per cent increase and homozygosity with a 100 per cent increase in prevalence of NIDDM.

There has for many years been controversy as to whether type II diabetes is due to insulin insensitivity or to a defect in insulin secretion by the pancreatic β-cells. Recently a study of 154 first degree relatives of 55 type II patients, using continuous glucose infusion with assay of both plasma glucose and insulin, found impaired glucose tolerance in 20 per cent of the relatives (O'Rahilly *et al.* 1986a). Insulin secretion was impaired in all the glucose intolerant relatives, but insulin resistance was found only in the more severely hyperglycaemic relatives. The authors interpret their results as demonstrating a primary β-cell dysfunction in type II diabetes. They defended this view (O'Rahilly *et al.* 1986b) in the face of suggestions that the effect was secondary (Ferner 1986; Jarrett 1986; Leslie 1986).

References

Barnett, A. H., Eff, C., Leslie, R. D. G. and Pyke, D. A. (1981a). Diabetes in identical twins. A study of 200 pairs. *Diabetologia* **20**, 87–93.
——, Spiliopoulos, A. J., Pyke, D. A., Stubbs, W. A., Burrin, J. and Alberti, K. G. M. M. (1981b). Metabolic studies in unaffected co-twins of non-insulin-dependent diabetics. *Br. Med. J.* **282**, 1656–8.
Ferner, R. E. (1986). Beta-cell function in type II diabetes. *Lancet* **2**, 628.
Jarrett, R. J. (1986). Beta-cell function in type II diabetes. *Lancet* **2**, 628.
Lendrum, R., Nelson, P. G., Pyke, D. A., Walker, G. and Gamble, D. R. (1976). Islet-cell, thyroid, and gastric autoantibodies in diabetic identical twins. *Br. Med. J.* **1**, 553–5.
Leslie, R. D. G. (1986). Beta-cell function in type II diabetes. *Lancet* **2**, 628.
O'Rahilly, S. P., Nugent, Z., Rudenski, A. S., Hasker, J. P., Burnett, M. A., Darling, P. and Turner, R. C. (1986a). Beta-cell dysfunction, rather than insulin insensitivity, is the primary defect in familial type 2 diabetes. *Lancet* **2**, 360–364.
O'Rahilly, S. P., Nugent, Z., Rudenski, A. S., Hasker, J. P. and Turner, R. G. (1986b). Beta-cell function in type II diabetes. *Lancet* **2**, 629.
Pyke, D. A. and Tattersall, R. B. (1973). Diabetic retinopathy in identical twins. *Diabetes* **22**, 613–18.
—— and Taylor, K. W. (1967). Glucose tolerance and serum insulin in unaffected identical twins of diabetics. *Br. Med. J.* **2**, 21–4.
——, Cassar, J., Todd, J. and Taylor, K. W. (1970). Glucose tolerance and serum insulin in identical twins of diabetics. *Br. Med. J.* **2**, 649–52.
Stern, M. P., Ferrell, R. E., Rosenthal, M., Haffner, S. M. and Hazuda, H. P. (1986). Association between NIDDM, RH blood group and haptoglobin phenotype: results from the San Antonio heart study. *Diabetes* **35**, 387–91.
Tattersall, R. B. and Pyke, D. A. (1972). Diabetes in identical twins. *Lancet* **2**, 1120–5.

MODY

There is one comparatively uncommon form of non-insulin-dependent diabetes, maturity onset diabetes of the young (MODY), which shows a classical autosomal dominant pattern of inheritance (Tattersall 1974; Johansen and Gregersen 1977; Fajans *et al.* 1979). However, there is evidence of genetic heterogeneity in this form of diabetes, with a minority of sporadic cases (Panzram and Adolph 1981); but the possibility that such sporadic cases represent fresh mutations of the usual MODY allele cannot be excluded. As in typical NIDDM there is no association with HLA phenotypes in MODY (Nelson and Pyke 1976; Faber *et al.* 1978; Panzram and Adolph 1981), despite evidence suggesting that the gene might be within the HLA cluster on chromosome 6 (Falk *et al.* 1978). This type of diabetes is mild, with complications, including nephropathy, being rare.

References

Faber, O. K., Thomsen, M., Binder, C., Platz, P. and Svejgaard, A. (1978). HLA antigens in a family with maturity-onset type diabetes mellitus. *Acta Endocrinol.* **88**, 329–38.

Fajans, S. S., Cloutier, M. C. and Crowther, R. L. (1979). Clinical and etiological heterogeneity of idiopathic diabetes mellitus. *Schweiz. Med. Wschr.* **109**, 1774–85.

Falk, C. T., Suciu-Foca, N. and Rubinstein, P. (1978). Possible localization of the gene(s) for juvenile diabetes mellitus (JDM) to the HLA region of chromosome 6. *Cytogenet. Cell Genet.* **22**, 298–300.

Johansen, K. and Gregersen, G. (1977). A family dominantly inherited mild juvenile diabetes. *Acta Med. Scand.* **201**, 567–70.

Nelson, P. G. and Pyke, D. A. (1976). Genetic diabetes is not linked to the HLA locus. *Br. Med. J.* **1**, 196–7.

Panzram, G. and Adolph, W. (1981). Heterogeneity of maturity onset diabetes at young age (MODY). *Lancet* **2**, 986.

Tattersall, R. B. (1974). Mild familial diabetes with dominant inheritance. *Quart. J. Med.* **43**, 339–57.

8.2.3. DIDMOAD syndrome

Another rare inherited form of diabetes is that described by Wolfram and Wagener in 1938, and known as the Wolfram or DIDMOAD syndrome. The syndrome consists of non-renal diabetes insipidus, diabetes mellitus, optic atrophy, and nerve deafness. Inheritance is autosomal recessive (Cremers *et al.* 1977; Page *et al.* 1976). The diabetes mellitus is of the insulin dependent type, although onset is often less abrupt than in IDDM (Peden *et al.* 1986), and not all patients need insulin therapy (Gunn *et al.* 1976). Families with parental consanguinity have been reported by several authors (Tyrer 1943; Rose *et al.* 1966; Ikkos *et al.* 1970; Page *et al.* 1976), and many more families with affected sibs of both sexes but no parental consanguinity (Shaw and Duncan 1958; Raiti *et al.* 1963; Rorsman and Soderstrom 1967; Bretz *et al.* 1970; Gunn *et al.* 1976; Pilley and Thompson 1976). This disease is not linked to HLA (Stanley *et al.* 1979; Blasi *et al.* 1982). However HLA association has been reported, to HLA-DR2, but not to the DR3 and 4 phenotypes involved in the association with IDDM (Blasi *et al.* 1982; Deschamps *et al.* 1983; Monson and Boucher 1983); but Bertrams and colleagues (1983) did find this association in two sibs studied by them. Apart from diabetic nephropathy patients with DIDMOAD syndrome have been reported with atonia of the urinary tract and bladder (Cremers *et al.* 1977; Najjar *et al.* 1985), probably due to degeneration of the nerves to the ureters and bladder (Peden *et al.* 1986). Renal failure associated with recurrent urinary tract infection (Carson *et al.* 1977; Khardori *et al.* 1983) may be preventable by active management (Peden *et al.* 1986).

References

Bertrams, J., Wendel, U. and Koletzko, S. (1983). HLA and Wolfram (DIDMOAD) syndrome. *Lancet* **2**, 573.

Blasi, C., Andreani, D., Lulli, P., Scherbaum, W. and Bottazzo, G. F. (1982). DIDMOAD syndrome: an hereditary form of juvenile diabetes not HLA-linked. *Excerpta Med. Int. Congr. Ser.* No. 577, 160.

Bretz, G. W., Baghdassarian, A., Graber, J. D., Zacherle, B. J., Norum, R. A. and Blizzard, R. M. (1970). Co-existence of diabetes mellitus and insipidus and optic atrophy in two male siblings: studies and review of literature. *Am J. Med.* **48**, 398–403.

Carson, M. J., Slager, U. T. and Steinberg, R. M. (1977). Simultaneous occurrence of diabetes mellitus, diabetes insipidus and optic atrophy in a brother and sister. *Am. J. Dis. Child.* **131**, 1385–8.

Cremers, C. W. R. J., Wijdeveld, P. G. A. B. and Pinckers, A. J. L. G. (1977). Juvenile diabetes mellitus, optic atrophy, hearing loss, diabetes insipidus, atonia of the urinary tract and bladder, and other abnormalities (Wolfram syndrome): a review of 88 cases from the literature with personal observations on 3 new patients. *Acta. Paediatr. Scand. Suppl.* **264**, 1–16.

Deschamps, I., Lestradet, H., Schmid, M. and Hors, J. (1983). HLA-DR2 and DIDMOAD syndrome. *Lancet* **2**, 109.

Gunn, T., Bortolussi, R., Little, J. M., Andermann, F., Fraser, F. C. and Belmonte, M. M. (1976). Juvenile diabetes mellitus, optic atrophy, sensory nerve deafness, and diabetes insipidus—a syndrome. *J. Pediatr.* **89**, 565–70.

Ikkos, D. G., Fraser, G. R., Matsouki-Gavra, E. and Petrochilos, M. (1970). Association of juvenile diabetes mellitus, primary optic atrophy and perceptive hearing loss in three sibs, with additional idiopathic diabetes insipidus in one case. *Acta Endocr. (Kbh.)* **65**, 95–102.

Khadori, R., Stephens, J. W., Page, O. C. and Dow, R. S. (1983). Diabetes mellitus and optic atrophy in two siblings: a report on a new association and a review of the literature. *Diabetes Care* **6**, 67–70.

Monson, J. P. and Boucher, B. J. (1983). HLA type and islet cell antibody status in family with (diabetes insipidus and mellitus, optic atrophy, and deafness) DIDMOAD syndrome. *Lancet* **1**, 1286–7.

Najjar, S. S., Saikaly, M. G., Zaytoun, G.-M. and Abdelnoor, A. (1985). Association of diabetes insipidus, diabetes mellitus, optic atrophy, and deafness: the Wolfram or DIDMOAD syndrome. *Arch. Dis. Child.* **60**, 823–8.

Page, M. McB., Asmal, A. C. and Edwards, C. R. W. (1976). Recessive inheritance of diabetes: the syndrome of diabetes insipidus, diabetes mellitus, optic atrophy and deafness. *Quart. J. Med.* **45**, 505–20.

Peden, W. R., Gay, J. D. L., Jung, R. T. and Kuwayti, K. (1986). Wolfram (DID-MOAD) syndrome: a complex long-term problem in management. *Quart. J. Med.* **58**, 167–80.

Pilley, S. F. J. and Thompson, H. S. (1976). Familial syndrome of diabetes insipidus, diabetes mellitus, optic atrophy, and deafness (DIDMOAD) in child-hood. *Br. J. Ophthalmol.* **60**, 294–8.

Raiti, S., Plotkin, S. and Newns, G. H. (1963). Diabetes mellitus and insipidus in two sisters. *Br. Med. J.* **2**, 1625–9.

Rorsman, G. and Soderstrom, N. (1967). Optic atrophy and juvenile diabetes mellitus with familial occurrence. *Acta Med. Scand.* **182**, 419–25.

Rose, F. C., Fraser, G. R., Friedmann, A. I. and Kohner, K. M. (1966). The association of juvenile diabetes mellitus and optic atrophy: clinical and genetical aspects. *Quart. J. Med.* **35**, 385–405.

Shaw, D. A. and Duncan, L. J. P. (1958). Optic atrophy and nerve deafness in diabetes mellitus. *J. Neurol. Neurosurg. Psychiat.* **21**, 47–9.

Stanley, C. A., Spielman, R. S., Zmijewski, C. M. and Baker, L. (1979). Wolfram syndrome not HLA linked (letter). *New Engl. J. Med.* **301**, 1398–9.

Tyrer, J. H. (1943). A case of infantilism with goitre, diabetes mellitus, mental defect and bilateral primary optic atrophy. *Med. J. Aust.* **2**, 398–401.

Wolfram, D. J. and Wagener, H. P. (1938). Diabetes mellitus and simple optic atrophy among siblings: report of four cases. *Mayo Clin. Proc.* **13**, 715–18.

8.2.4. Studies on the insulin gene and its 5′ flanking region

Recent studies have investigated the relationship between various types of diabetes mellitus and the insulin gene on the short arm of chromosome 11, or a DNA polymorphism in its 5′ flanking region. Rotwein and colleagues (1981, 1983) observed DNA insertions of 0.6 to 5.5 kb within the 5′ flanking region of the insulin gene. These were present in a significantly higher proportion of non-insulin-dependent diabetics than in insulin-dependent diabetics or non-diabetics. Because of their proximity to the 5′ end of the insulin gene it was suggested that they may influence the expression of that gene. Owerbach and associates (1982b) studied the segregation of such DNA insertions in a large family and found that the different-sized insertions in this family behaved as alleles. They also observed that the two large insertions, of 4.6 and 4.8 kb, were associated with high haemoglobin A_{1C} levels in non-diabetic family members, suggesting that they may affect glucose regulation. The same group (Owerbach *et al.* 1982a) found that the larger insertions, termed U alleles and defined as being larger than 1600 bp, were also strongly associated with macroangiopathy as evidenced by a history of myocardial infarction, angina pectoris, intermittent claudication, or cerebrovascular disease. They interpreted this finding as indicating a possible association of these U alleles with atherosclerosis and subsequently demonstrated a higher frequency of these alleles among non-diabetic atherosclerotic patients (Mandrup-Poulson *et al.* 1984). However, as yet other groups have not confirmed the association with either diabetes (Yokoyama 1983; Dobs *et al.* 1986) or atherosclerosis (Jowett *et al.* 1984a). Furthermore, these insertional polymorphisms have a low incidence in Japanese NIDDM patients (Aoyama *et al.* 1986). Nor is there any linkage of these polymorphisms with insulin-dependent diabetes (Ferns *et al.* 1986). In contrast to the findings of Owerbach's group, who put the association with atherosclerosis as primary and that with diabetes as secondary, Jowett and associates found a strong association of the allele(s) determining the larger insertion with NIDDM and with diabetic hypertriglyceridaemia (Hitman *et al.* 1984; Jowett *et al.* 1984b). Owerbach's group, in association with Pyke's group at Kings College Hospital, have shown that there is no association of either the larger or small insertions with Mason-type NIDDM (Johnston *et al.* 1984), nor with MODY (Owerbach *et al.* 1983). Furthermore, Bell and colleagues (1983) have shown that MODY shows no linkage to DNA polymorphisms recognized by a probe to the insulin gene itself.

References

Aoyama, N., Nakamura, T., Doi, K., Baba, S., Takahashi, R. and Sugiyama, T. (1986). Low frequency of 5′-flanking insertion of human insulin gene in Japanese non-insulin dependent diabetic subjects. *Diabetes Care* **9**, 365–9.

Bell, J. I., Wainscot, J. S., Old, J. M., Chlouverakis, C., Keen, H., Turner, R. C. and Weatherall, D. J. (1983). Maturity onset diabetes of the young is not linked to the insulin gene. *Br. Med. J.* **1**, 590–2.

Dobs, A. S., Phillips, J. A. III, Mallonnee, R. L., Saudek, C. D. and Ney, R. L. (1986). Pedigree analysis of the 5′ flanking region of the insulin gene in familial diabetes mellitus. *Metabolism* **35**, 13–17.

Ferns, G. A. A., Hitman, G. A., Trembath, R., Williams, L., Tarn, A., Gale, E. A. and Galton, D. J. (1986). DNA polymorphic haplotypes on the short arm of chromosome 11 and the inheritance of type I diabetes mellitus. *J. Med. Genet.* **23**, 210–16.

Hitman, G. A., Jowett, N. I., Williams, L. G., Humphries, S., Winter, R. M. and Galton, D. J. (1984). Polymorphisms in the 5′-flanking region of the insulin gene and non-insulin-dependent diabetes. *Clin. Sci.* **66**, 383–8.

Johnston, C., Owerbach, D., Leslie, R. D. G., Pyke, D. A. and Nerup, J. (1984). Mason-type diabetes and DNA insertion polymorphism. *Lancet* **1**, 280.

Jowett, N. I., Rees, A., Caplin, J., Williams, L. G. and Galton, D. J. (1984a). DNA polymorphisms flanking insulin gene and atherosclerosis. *Lancet* **2**, 348.

——, Williams, L. G., Hitman, G. A. and Galton, D. J. (1984b). Diabetic hypertriglyceridaemia and related 5′ flanking polymorphism of the human insulin gene. *Br. Med. J.* **1**, 96–9.

Mandrup-Poulsen, T., Owerbach, D., Mortensen, S. A., Johansen, K., Meinertz, H., Sorensen, H. and Nerup, J. (1984). DNA sequences flanking the insulin gene on chromosome 11 confer risk of atherosclerosis. *Lancet* **1**, 250–2.

Owerbach, D., Johansen, K., Billesbolle, P., Poulsen, S., Schroll, M. and Nerup, J. (1982a). Possible association between DNA sequences flanking the insulin gene and atherosclerosis. *Lancet* **2**, 1291–3.

——, Poulsen, S., Billesbolle, P. and Nerup, J. (1982b). DNA insertion sequences near the insulin gene affect glucose regulation. *Lancet* **1**, 880–2.

——, Thomsen, B., Johansen, K., Lamm, L. U. and Nerup, J. (1983). DNA insertion sequences near the insulin gene are not associated with maturity-onset diabetes of young people. *Diabetologia* **25**, 18–20.

Rotwein, P., Chyn, R., Chirgwin, J., Cordell, B., Goodman, H. M. and Permutt, M. A. (1981). Polymorphism in the 5'-flanking region of the human insulin gene and its possible relation to type 2 diabetes. *Science* **213**, 1117–20.

——, Chirgwin, J., Province, M., Knowler, W. C., Pettitt, D. J., Cordell, B., Goodman, H. M. and Permutt, M. A. (1983). Polymorphism in the 5' flanking region of the human insulin gene: a genetic marker for non-insulin-dependent diabetes. *New Engl. J. Med.* **308**, 65–71.

Yokoyama, S. (1983). Polymorphism in the 5'-flanking region of the human insulin gene and the incidence of diabetes. *Am. J. Hum. Genet.* **35**, 193–200.

8.2.5. Diabetic nephropathy

Theories regarding the involvement of the kidney in diabetes mellitus have a centuries long history, as outlined by Parsons and Watkins (1979) in their excellent review of the subject to which the reader is referred, and also to that of Beyer (1984) for a fuller account. Proteinuria has been recognized as a complication of diabetes for over 200 years, and in 1936 the first description of a specific pathological lesion was published by Kimmelstiel and Wilson in the form of the spherical hyaline glomerular masses of nodular glomerulosclerosis. Allen (1941) demonstrated a specific laminated fibrillar lesion in the glomerular lobules in diabetic nodular glomerulosclerosis that stains positively with silver. Diffuse glomerulosclerosis was described by Fahr in 1942, and in the same year Bell reported arteriolar lesions. A decade later it was recognized that the glomerulosclerosis of diabetes was a feature of a more generalized microangiopathy (Lundbaek 1953).

The earliest clinical sign of renal involvement is proteinuria, at first intermittent and of mild degree. This gradually becomes more marked and continuous and eventually signs of impaired renal function develop. Proteinuria is an important indicator of eventual renal failure in diabetes and recent studies have concentrated on the quantitative assessment of excretion of specific proteins. Before proteinuria becomes detectable by the usual methods such as 'Albustix', at a level of about 0.5 g/24 h, lesser increases can be detected by more sensitive methods. At the earliest stage radioimmunoassays may show microproteinuria with increased excretion of albumin and of IgG, related to the level of glycosylated haemoglobin and found by some to be reversible by strict glycaemic control (Viberti *et al.* 1979, 1982c), but not by others (Feldt-Rasmussen *et al.* 1986b). The presumption is that this microalbuminuria and gammaglobulinuria are due to glycosylation of glomerular proteins or merely to an increased glomerular pressure gradient associated with the increased glomerular filtration rate, which is the earliest functional change. Feldt-Rasmussen (1986a) has demonstrated increased trans-capillary escape of albumin in patients with microalbuminuria. Subsequently the microalbuminuria progressively exceeds the gamma-globulinuria, indicating selective filtration of the polyanionic albumin molecule, which suggests a depletion of the normal polyanionic barrier of the glomerular basement membrane (Viberti *et al.* 1983). This excess albuminuria persists into the stage of routinely detectable proteinuria until the glomerular filtration rate begins to fall when IgG excretion rises further to match that of albumin, and an increased excretion of β_2-microglobulin also develops (Viberti *et al.* 1983), which is associated with the development of large pores in the glomerular basement membrane (Carrie and Myers 1980; Myers *et al.* 1982). Viberti and colleagues (1982b) and also Mogensen and Christensen (1984), have shown that microalbuminuria is a reliable indicator of the eventual development of clinical nephropathy in insulin-dependent diabetes, and the same groups of workers have also shown that it is an indicator of early death in both non-insulin-dependent (Jarrett *et al.* 1981; Mogensen 1984) and insulin-dependent diabetes (Borch-Johnsen *et al.* 1985), and of proliferative diabetic retinopathy (Mogensen *et al.* 1985). However, once nephropathy has developed strict glycaemic control is more difficult to maintain and cannot reverse the declining renal function (Bending *et al.* 1984, 1986). A pathological increase in albuminuria in response to exercise is seen in non-insulin-dependent diabetes, even at the time of initial diagnosis (Mohamed *et al.* 1984). The finding of Mohamed and coworkers that, if detected sufficiently early, this abnormality was correctable by dietary therapy alone supports the view that screening for subclinical NIDDM and its early treatment may be beneficial.

One of the earliest signs of impaired renal function is the development of peripheral oedema, although true nephrotic syndrome as described by Kimmelstiel and Wilson (1936) is a rare late complication which when present does not remit. During the phase of chronic renal impairment hyperkalaemic renal acidosis (type IV renal acidosis) may develop. Only a minority of diabetic patients actually die of uraemia, mainly younger patients with long-standing diabetes. The commonest cause of death among older patients with nephropathy is in fact coronary artery disease.

Myocardial ischaemia occurs as part of a generalized atheroma that may also affect the renal arteries and contribute to impaired renal function. It is possible that this atherosclerosis is related to the reduced level of serum apolipoprotein B that has been reported in patients with IDDM (Winocour *et al.* 1986). Atheroma of interlobular renal arteries is a frequent striking autopsy appearance in patients with diabetic renal disease (Hall 1952). Medial calcification is also a common complication of diabetes but is probably not specifically related to diabetic nephropathy. However, symptomatic neurogenic bladder due to sacral nerve autonomic neuropathy is a rare complication in diabetics with advanced neuropathy.

At a functional level the earliest change in diabetic nephropathy is an increased microvascular vasodilatation and blood flow resulting in increased glomerular filtration rate (GFR) and T_{m_G}. This is not associated with raised plasma glucagon or growth hormone levels (Wiseman *et al.* 1985). The factors that are involved in these early microvascular changes are not fully understood, but potential factors have been recently reviewed (Tooke 1986; Zatz and Brenner 1986).

Next follows a phase of stable GFR during which proteinuria first appears and is associated histologically with the development of glomerulosclerosis. The proteinuria is correlated with duration of disease and with glycosylated haemoglobin level (Davies *et al.* 1985). During this phase the normal autoregulation of GFR in response to hypotension is impaired (Parving *et al.* 1984, 1985). Finally GFR and T_{m_G} both fall, and eventually renal plasma flow and $T_{m_{PAH}}$ also fall, there is fluid retention, and end-stage renal failure. Another indicator of nephropathy, especially in hypertensive diabetics, is a decreased urinary excretion of kallikrein (Baba *et al.* 1986).

Histologically the earliest change is a microangiopathy manifested as glomerular basement membrane thickening, which is seen in all cases of IDDM. It is associated with an increased hydroxylsine content of the GBM along with increased glucosyl–galactosyl disaccharide moieties, which may be related to increased membrane permeability (Spiro 1973). This is followed by mesangial proliferation at the stage of irreversible proteinuria (Silverstein *et al.* 1985), and then by diffuse and nodular glomerulosclerosis, and by ischaemic lesions. A recent autopsy study comparing renal changes in insulin-dependent diabetes with and without clinical nephropathy found severe glomerulosclerosis even in the group without clinical nephropathy, and a similar frequency of arterial lesions and Kimmelstiel–Wilson lesions in both diabetic groups. The distinguishing feature of kidneys from the patients with clinical nephropathy was a greater increase in mesangium and in interstitial tissue of the glomerulus (Thomsen *et al.* 1984). Biopsy ultrastructural studies have shown that breaks in the paramesangial basement membrane may be associated with the formation of saccular glomerular microaneurysms in adolescents with IDDM (Vogler *et al.* 1986).

A Danish follow-up study of IDDM found that 45 per cent of patients developed clinical nephropathy by 40 years duration of diabetes, with increasing prevalence with duration of the disease (Andersen *et al.* 1983). The development of proteinuria is influenced by metabolic control but subsequent progression to renal failure is more related to blood pressure (Hasslacher *et al.* 1985; Krolewski *et al.* 1985). No such clear relationship of incidence of nephropathy with duration of disease has emerged in NIDDM.

There is only limited evidence for inheritance of liability to nephropathy in diabetes other than that for the inheritance of diabetes itself (Barbosa and Saner 1984). Most of the evidence, including reversibility of the nephropathy in kidneys transplanted from a diabetic donor into non-diabetic recipients (Abouna *et al.* 1983, 1986; Abouna and Al-Adnani 1984), seems to point to environmental factors, such as the strictness of diabetic control, as the primary determinants for the initiation of nephropathy and other microangiopathic complications. There is, however, some circumstantial evidence, particularly from twin studies, for a genetic contribution to susceptibility to small blood vessel disease (Barbosa and Saner 1984). In particular, despite some conflicting earlier reports, there do not seem to be any HLA antigen associations with nephropathy in IDDM (Walton *et al.* 1984), although as mentioned earlier there is an association of diabetic microangiopathy with the C4 variant C4B3 (Mijovic *et al.* 1986). A report that C4 concentrations are lower in insulin-dependent diabetics with nephropathy compared with those without (Barnett *et al.* 1984) was not confirmed, for either IDDM or NIDDM, in a more recent study (Cooper *et al.* 1986). However, the latter group did observe lower values in IDDM patients, with or without nephropathy, compared with NIDDM patients. Another potential association with nephropathy in diabetes is with the Gm phenotype of the immunoglobulin heavy chain. Mijovic and colleagues (1986) found a significantly higher incidence of the Gm (zafnbg) phenotype in insulin-dependent diabetics with nephropathy (33 per cent) than in those without (9 per cent), and also found a greater risk of complications in patients with both C4B3 and Gm(zafnbg) than in those with only one of these phenotypes, or neither.

Several groups have reported a higher incidence of proteinuria in Asian patients with NIDDM compared to Caucasian patients (Samata *et al.* 1986; Jayarajah *et al.* 1986; Jialal 1986). However, the observation does not necessarily reflect any genetic difference, indeed several possible environmental explanations have been proposed by these groups.

Insulin-dependent diabetes is relatively common in older patients with cystic fibrosis. Most such patients do not live long enough to develop vascular complications of diabetes. However, two reports of diabetic nephropathy and retinopathy in adult patients with cystic fibrosis have recently appeared (Dolan 1986; Allen 1986).

References

Abouna, G. M. and Al-Adnani, M. S. (1984). Reversibility of diabetic nephropathy after transplantation of affected kidney. *Lancet* 1, 162–3.

——, Al-Adnani, M. S., Kremer, G. D., Kumar, S. A., Daddah, S. K. and Kusma, G. (1983). Reversal of diabetic nephropathy in human cadaveric kidneys after transplantation into non-diabetic recipients. *Lancet* 2, 1274–6.

——, Adnani, M. S., Kumar, M. S. A. and Samhan, S. A. (1986). Fate of transplanted kidneys with diabetic nephropathy. *Lancet* 1, 622–3.

Allen, A. C. (1941). So-called intercapillary glomerulosclerosis-lesion associated with diabetes mellitus: morphogenesis and significance. *Arch. Pathol.* 32, 35–51.

Allen, J. L. (1986). Progressive nephropathy in a patient with cystic fibrosis and diabetes. *New Engl. J. Med.* 315, 764.

Andersen, A. R., Christiansen, J. S., Andersen, J. K., Kreiner, S. and Deckert, T. (1983). Diabetic nephropathy in type 1 (insulin-dependent) diabetes: an epidemiological study. *Diabetologia* 25, 496–501.

Baba, T., Murabayashi, S., Ishizaki, T., Ido, Y., Aoyagi, K. and Takebe, K. (1986). Renal kallikrein in diabetic patients with hypertension and nephropathy. *Diabetologia* 29, 162–7.

Barbosa, J. and Saner, B. (1984). Do genetic factors play a role in the pathogenesis of diabetic microangiopathy? *Diabetologia* 27, 487–92.

Barnett, A. H., Mijovic, C., Fletcher, J., Chesner, I., Kulkuska-Langlands, B. M., Holder, R. and Bradwell, A. R. (1984). Low plasma C4 concentrations: association with microangiopathy in insulin dependent diabetes. *Br. Med. J.* 289, 943–5.

Bell, E. T. (1942). Renal lesions in diabetes mellitus. *Am. J. Pathol.* 18, 744.

Bending, J. J., Pickup, J. C., Viberti, G. C. and Keen, H. (1984). Glycaemic control in diabetic nephropathy. *Br. Med. J.* 288, 1187–91.

——, Viberti, G. C., Watkins, P. J. and Keen, H. (1986). Intermittent clinical proteinuria and renal function in diabetes: evolution and the effect of glycaemic control. *Br. Med. J.* 292, 83–6.

Beyer, M. M. (1984). Diabetic nephropathy. *Pediatr. Clin. N. Am.* 31, 635–51.

Borch-Johnsen, K., Andersen, P. K. and Deckert, T. (1985). The effect of proteinuria on relative mortality in type 1 (insulin-dependent) diabetes mellitus. *Diabetologia* 28, 590–6.

Carrie, B. J. and Myers, B. D. (1980). Proteinuria and functional characteristics of the glomerular barrier in diabetic nephropathy. *Kidney Int.* 17, 669–76.

Cooper, M. E., Duff, R., Buchanan, R., McPherson, J. and Jerums, G. (1986). Low serum C4 concentrations and microangiopathy in type I and type II diabetes. *Br. Med. J.* 292, 801.

Davies, A. G., Price, D. A., Postlethwaite, R. J., Addison, G. M., Burn, J. L. and Fielding, B. A. (1985). Renal function in diabetes mellitus. *Arch. Dis. Child.* **60**, 299–304.

Dolan, T. F. (1986). Microangiopathy in a young adult with cystic fibrosis and diabetes mellitus. *New Engl. J. Med.* **314**, 991–2.

Fahr, T. (1942). Ueber Glomerulosklerose. *Virchow's Arch. Path. Anat. Physiol. Klin. Med.* **309**, 16–33.

Feldt-Rasmussen, B. (1986a). Increased transcapillary escape rate of albumin in type I (insulin-dependent) diabetic patients with microalbuminuria. *Diabetologia* **29**, 282–6.

——, Mathiesen, E. R., Hegedus, L. and Deckert, T. (1986b). Kidney function during 12 months of strict metabolic control in insulin-dependent diabetic patients with incipient nephropathy. *New Engl. J. Med.* **314**, 665–70.

Hall, G. F. M. (1952). The significance of atheroma of the renal arteries in Kimmelsteil–Wilson's syndrome. *J. Pathol. Bact.* **64**, 103–20.

Hasslacher, Ch., Stech, W., Wahl, P. and Ritz, E. (1985). Blood pressure and metabolic control as risk factors for nephropathy in type 1 (insulin-dependent) diabetes. *Diabetologia* **28**, 6–11.

Jarrett, R. J., Viberti, G. C., Argyropoulos, A. (1981). Microalbuminuria predicts mortality in non-insulin-dependent diabetes. *Diab. Med.* **1**, 17–19.

Jeyarajah, R., Jayatissa, S. K., Gunawardena, J. N., Bandara C. D. J., Gamage, K. M. K., and Perera, P. L. A. P. (1986). Diabetic renal disease: differences between Asian and white patients. *Br. Med. J.* **293**, 629–30.

Jialal, I. (1986). Diabetic renal disease: differences between Asian and white patients. *Br. Med. J.* **293**, 696.

Kimmelstiel, P. and Wilson, C. (1936). Intercapillary lesions of glomeruli of kidney. *Am. J. Pathol.* **12**, 83–98.

Krolewski, A. S., Warram, J. H., Christlieb, A. R., Busick, E. J. and Kahn, C. R. (1985). The changing natural history of nephropathy in type 1 diabetes. *Am. J. Med.* **78**, 785–94.

Lundbaek, K. (1953). *Long-term diabetes.* Munkgaard, Kbh.

Mijovic, C., Fletcher, J. A., Bradwell, A. R. and Barnett, A. H. (1986). Phenotypes of the heavy chains of immunoglobulins in patients with diabetic microangiopathy: evidence for an immunogenetic predisposition. *Br. Med. J.* **292**, 433–5.

Mogensen, C. E. (1984). Microalbuminuria predicts clinical proteinuria and early mortality in maturity onset diabetes. *New Engl. J. Med.* **310**, 356–60.

—— and Christensen, C. K. (1984). Predicting diabetic nephropathy in insulin-dependent patients. *New Engl. J. Med.* **311**, 89–93.

——, Vigstrup, J. and Ehlers, N. (1985). Microalbuminuria predicts proliferative diabetic retinopathy. *Lancet* **1**, 1512–13.

Mohamed, A., Wilkin, T., Leatherdale, B. A. and Rowe, D. (1984). Response of urinary albumin to submaximal exercise in newly diagnosed non-insulin dependent diabetes. *Br. Med. J.* **288**, 1342–3.

Myers, B. D., Winetz, J. A., Chui, F. and Michaels, A. S. (1982). Mechanisms of proteinuria in diabetic nephropathy: a study of glomerular barrier function. *Kidney Int.* **21**, 633–41.

Parsons, V. and Watkins, P. J. (1979). Diabetes and the kidney. Chapter 23 in *Renal disease*, 4th edn. eds. Black, Sir Douglas and Jones, N. F. pp. 687–712.

Blackwell Scientific, Oxford.

Parving, H.-H., Kastrup, H., Smidt, U. M., Anderson, A. R., Feldt-Rasmussen, B. and Christiansen, J. S. (1984). Impaired auto-regulation of glomerular filtration rate in type 1 (insulin-dependent) diabetic patients with nephropathy. *Diabetologia* **27**, 547–52.

——, Kastrup, J. and Smidt, U. M. (1985). Reduced transcapillary escape of albumin during acute blood pressure lowering in type 1 (insulin-dependent) diabetic patients with nephropathy. *Diabetologia* **28**, 797–801.

Silverstein, J. H., Fenell, R., Donnelly, W., Banks, R., Stratton, R., Spillar, R. and Rosenbloom, A. L. (1985). Correlates of biopsy-studied nephropathy in young patients with insulin-dependent diabetes mellitus. *J. Pediatr.* **106**, 196–201.

Samanta, A., Barden, A. C., Feehally, J. and Walls, J. (1986). Diabetic renal disease: differences between Asian and white patients. *Br. Med. J.* **293**, 366–7.

Spiro, R. G. (1973). Biochemistry of the renal glomerular basement membrane in diabetes mellitus. *New Engl. J. Med.* **288**, 1377–42.

Thomsen, O. F., Andersen, A. R., Christiansen, J. S. and Deckert, T. (1984). Renal changes in long-term type 1 (insulin-dependent) diabetic patients with and without clinical nephropathy: a light microscopic, morphometric study of autopsy material. *Diabetologia* **26**, 361–5.

Tooke, J. E. (1986). Editorial review: microvascular haemodynamics in diabetes mellitus. *Clin. Sci.* **70**, 119–25.

Viberti, G. C., Pickup, J. C., Jarrett, R. J. and Keen, H. (1979). Effect of control of blood glucose on urinary excretion of albumin and β_2-microglobulin in insulin-dependent diabetes. *New Engl. J. Med.* **300**, 638–41.

——, Bilous, R. W., Keen, H. and MacKintosh, D. (1982a). Failure of long-term correction of hyperglycemia to effect the progression of clinical nephropathy. *Diabetes* **31** (Suppl. 2), 11A.

——, Hill, R. D., Jarrett, R. J., Argyropoulos, A., Mahmud, U. and Keen, H. (1982b). Microalbuminuria as a predictor of clinical nephropathy in insulin-dependent diabetes mellitus. *Lancet* **1**, 1431–2.

——, Mackintosh, D., Bilous, R. W., Pickup, J. C. and Keen, H. (1982c). Proteinuria in diabetes mellitus: role of spontaneous and experimental variation in glycaemia. *Kidney Int.* **11**, 714–20.

——, —— and Keen, H. (1983). Determinants of the penetration of proteins through the glomerular barrier in insulin-dependent diabetes mellitus. *Diabetes* **32** (Suppl. 2), 92–5.

Vogler, C., McAdams, A. J. and McEnery, P. (1986). Glomerular membranopathy in adolescents with insulin-dependent diabetes. *Hum. Pathol.* **17**, 308–13.

Walton, C., Dyer, P. A., Davidson, J. A., Harris, R., Mallick, N. P. and Oleesky, S. (1984). HLA antigens and risk factors for nephropathy in type 1 (insulin-dependent) diabetes mellitus. *Diabetolotia* **27**, 3–7.

Winocour, P. H., Durrington, P. N., Ishola, M. and Anderson, D. C. (1986). Lipoprotein abnormalities in insulin-dependent diabetes mellitus. *Lancet* **1**, 1176–8.

Wiseman, M. J., Redmond, S., House, F., Keen, H. and Viberti, G. C. (1985). The glomerular hyperfiltration of diabetes is not associated with elevated plasma levels of glucagon and growth hormone. *Diabetologia* **28**, 718–21.

Zatz, R. and Brenner, B. M. (1986). Pathogenesis of diabetic microangiopathy: the hemodynamic view. *Am. J. Med.* **80**, 443–53.

8.3. GOUT

Gout is a heterogeneous disorder in which hyperuricaemia is associated with acute arthritis, and in which renal disease is a common, and sometimes serious, complication. The acute arthritic attack is precipitated by the formation of crystals of monosodium urate, which produce an acute inflammatory reaction within the joint. It may occur as a secondary phenomenon in any disorder with a greatly increased turnover of purines, such as in leukaemia or polycythaemia; or it may be secondary to specific enzyme defects associated with overproduction of uric acid such as complete (Lesch–Nyhan disease) or partial hypoxanthine–guanine phosphoribosyltransferase deficiency, glucose 6-phosphatase deficiency (Von Gierke's disease), and PP-ribose-P synthetase overactivity. These specific enzyme defects are discussed elsewhere in this book.

Primary gout may be associated with overproduction of uric acid (Seegmiller *et al.* 1961) with normal or increased excretion, although the mechanism of such overproduction remains uncertain, or with reduced renal clearance of uric acid, or with both of these factors (Wyngaarden and Kelley 1983). Simkin (1979) in an analysis of six published studies noted impaired excretion of uric acid in patients with idiopathic gout, whether they were uric acid overproducers or not. Uric acid is filtered by the glomerulus, partially reabsorbed in the proximal tubule, followed by tubular secretion and finally post-secretory reabsorption (Rieselbach and Steele 1974). Impaired excretion of uric acid could be due to reduced filtration, increased reabsorption, or impaired secretion. Evidence as to which of these possible factors are involved is conflicting.

Overt renal disease although common in gout is only rarely due to hyperuricaemia itself (Berger and Yü 1975; Yü *et la.* 1979). Rather it is associated with secondary renal disease such as renal calculi, pyelonephritis, renal vascular disease, or hypertension. It is also correlated with age. This variable aetiology of renal disease is reflected in the observation that the GFR is maintained in many gouty patients but is progressively impaired in others (Gutman and Yü 1957), and in a great diversity of histopathological changes which may include deposition of urate cyrstals (Talbott and Terplan 1960). Urate crystals may be present in the interstitial tissue, the medulla, or pyramids, and may give rise to a giant-cell reaction. There may also be uric acid stones in the renal pelves. Crystals are seen in about half of patients examined postmortem, with evidence of consequent renal damage in about a quarter of these (Talbott and Terplan 1960). Renal biopsy studies indicate that the earliest renal lesions in gout are an interstitial reaction in the cortex and a fibrillar thickening of glomerular basement membranes, followed by atrophy of Henle's loops (Greenbaum *et al.* 1961; Gonick *et al.* 1965). Widely varying figures have been reported for the incidence of uric acid stones in gout. In a large American study Yü and Gutman (1967) found an incidence of 22 per cent in primary gout and an increasing incidence with rise in serum urate. Mortality in gout does not greatly exceed that of the general population, with a small percentage, about 7 per cent, of total mortality being attributable to gouty nephropathy (Gutman 1972; Yü and Talbott 1980).

Although the familial occurrence of idiopathic gout has been recognized for centuries, there is still controversy as to whether the genetic component in the aetiology is multifactorial or single gene. Most modern studies have analysed the genetic determination of hyperuricaemia, as determined by the assay of uric acid with uricase, rather than symptomatic gout. British and American studies have given widely varying figures for the proportion of cases with familial occurrence up to a maximum of 75 to 80 per cent (Talbott 1955). Among the relatives of patients with gout, reported in five separate studies, Smyth (1957) found that about 25 per cent were hyperuricaemic and a fifth of these actually had gout. In the earliest of the studies reviewed by Smyth, 34 out of 136 relatives of 27 gouty subjects were hyperuricaemic (Talbott 1940), and similar frequencies were found in Smyth's own study (Smyth *et al.* 1948) and that of Hauge and Harvald (1955).

Early workers postulated that hypercuricaemia was due to a single autosomal gene with dominant expression with low penetrance, especially in females (Smyth *et al.* 1948; Stecher *et al.* 1949; Emmerson 1960). Smyth and colleagues observed a bimodal distribution of serum uric acid values among relatives of patients with gout. Emmerson observed early onset and unusual severity of gout in the children of parents who were both affected themselves. He suggested that such children were homozygotes for an autosomal dominantly inherited gout. Others have questioned the single gene hypothesis and favoured multifactorial inheritance (Hauge and Harvald 1955; Mikkelsen *et al.* 1965; Neel *et al.* 1965; Burch *et al.* 1966; O'Brien *et al.* 1966; French *et al.* 1967; Hall *et al.* 1967; Healy *et al.* 1967; Morton 1979). The studies on uric acid production and excretion in gout confirm that idiopathic gout is heterogeneous so that although uric acid levels in normal subjects are polygenically determined the situation in gout is more complex. In all probability both the uric acid overproducing and non-overproducing groups are multifactorial, but there may well be single genes playing a major role in individual families or even isolated populations. As discussed elsewhere gout associated with specific enzyme defects is clearly monogenic.

References

Berger, L. and Yü, T. F. (1975). Renal function in gout. IV. An analysis of 524 gouty subjects including long term follow up studies. *Am. J. Med.* **59**, 605–13.

Burch, T. A., O'Brien, W. M., Need, R. and Kurland, L. T. (1966). Hyperuricemia and gout in Mariana Islands. *Ann. Rheum. Dis.* **25**, 114–16.

Emmerson, B. T. (1960). Heredity in primary gout. *Aust. Ann. Med.* **9**, 168–75.

French, J. G., Dodge, H. J., Kjelsberg, M. O., Mikkelsen, W. M. and Schull, W. J. (1967). A study of familial aggregation of serum uric acid levels in the population of Tecumseh, Michigan, 1959–1960. *Am. J. Epidemiol.* **86**, 214–24.

Gonick, H. C., Rubini, M. E., Gleason, I. O. and Sommers, S. C. (1965). The renal lesion in gout. *Ann. Intern. Med.* **62**, 667–74.

Greenbaum, D., Ross, J. H. and Steinberg, V. L. (1961). Renal biopsy in gout. *Br. Med. J.* **1**, 1502–4.

Gutman, A. B. (1972). Views on the pathogenesis and management of primary gout—1971. *J. Bone Jt. Surg.* **54A**, 357–72.

—— and Yü, T. F. (1957). Renal function in gout: with a commentary on the renal regulation of urate excretion and the role of the kidney in the pathogenesis of gout. *Am. J. Med.* **23**, 600–22.

Hall, A. P., Barry, P. E., Dawber, T. R. and McNamara, P. M. (1967). Epidemiology of gout and hyperuricemia: a long-term population study. *Am. J. Med.* **42**, 27–37.

Hauge, M. and Harvald, B. (1955). Heredity in gout and hyperuricemia. *Acta Med. Scand.* **152**, 247–57.

Healy, L. A., Skeith, M. D., Decker, J. L. and Bayani-Sioson, P. S. (1967). Hyperuricemia in Filipinos: interaction of heredity and environment. *Am. J. Hum. Genet.* **19**, 81–5.

Mikkelsen, W. M., Dodge, H. J. and Valkenburg, H. (1965). The distribution of serum uric values in a population unselected as to gout or hyperuricemia. Tecumseh, Michigan, 1959–1960. *Am. J. Med.* **39**, 242–51.

Morton, N. E. (1979). Genetics of hyperuricemia in families with gout. *Am. J. Med. Genet.* **4**, 103–6.

Neel, J. V., Rakik, M. T., Davidson, R. T., Valkenburg, H. L. and Mikkelson, W. M. (1965). Studies on hyperuricemia. II. A reconsideration of the distribution of serum uric acid values in the families of Smyth, Cotterman and Freyburg. *Am. J. Hum. Genet.* **17**, 14–22.

O'Brien, W. M., Burch, T. A. and Bunim, J. J. (1966). Genetics of hyperuricaemia in Blackfeet and Pima Indians. *Ann. Rheum. Dis.* **25**, 117–19.

Rieselbach, R. E. and Steele, T. H. (1974). The influence of the kidney upon urate homeostasis in health and disease. *Am. J. Med.* **56**, 665–75.

Seegmiller, J. E., Grayzel, A. I., Laster, L. and Liddle, L. (1961). Uric acid overproduction in gout. *J. Clin. Invest.* **40**, 1304–14.

Simkin, P. A. (1979). Uric acid excretion in patients with gout. *Arthritis Rheum.* **22**, 98–9.

Smyth, C. J. (1957). Hereditary factors in gout: a review of recent literature. *Metabolism* **6**, 218–29.

——, Cotterman, C. W. and Freyburg, R. H. (1948). The genetics of gout and hyperuricemia: analysis of nineteen families. *J. Clin. Invest.* **27**, 749–59.

Stecher, R. M., Hersh, A. H. and Solomon, W. M. (1949). The heredity of gout and its relationship to familial hyperuricemia. *Ann. Intern. Med.* **31**, 595–614.

Talbott, J. H. (1940). Serum urate in relatives of gouty patients. *J. Clin. Invest.* **19**, 645–8.

—— (1955). Gout. *J. Chron. Dis.* **1**, 338–45.

—— and Terplan, K. L. (1960). The kidney in gout. *Medicine* **39**, 405–68.

Wyngaarden, J. B. and Kelley, W. N. (1983). Gout. Chapter 50 in *The metabolic basis of inherited disease*, 5th edn. eds. Stanbury, J. B., Wyngaarden, J. B., Fredrickson, D. S., Goldstein, J. L. and Brown, M. S. pp. 1043–114. McGraw-Hill, New York.

Yü, T.-F. and Gutman, A. B. (1967). Uric acid nephrolithiasis in gout: predisposing factors. *Ann. Intern. Med.* **67**, 1133–48.

—— and Talbott, J. H. (1980). Changing trends in mortality in gout. *Sem. Arthritis Rheum.* **10**, 1–9.

——, Berger, L., Dorph, D. J. and Smith, H. (1979). Renal function in gout. V. Factors influencing the renal hemodynamics. *Am. J. Med.* **67**, 766–71.

8.4. HAEMOGLOBINOPATHIES

Renal complications of haemoglobinopathy relate mainly to sickle cell disease and its variants, that is, possession of the HbSS, HbSC, and HbSThal genotypes. In conditions of low oxygen tension, as may occur in the renal medulla, haemoglobin S polymerizes to form a viscous gel, which in turn induces the relatively rigid abnormal 'sickle' shape of the red blood cells, which impedes their free circulation. Although the only data for the incidence of renal complications in sickle cell disease are from Jamaica there is general agreement that these are common, and may be serious in older patients. As might be expected it is medullary and papillary functions that are most affected, but recent studies have demonstrated glomerular functional impairment as a late manifestation. Several excellent reviews of renal disturbance in sickle cell disease have been published (Buckalew and Someren 1974; Serjeant 1974; Alleyne *et al.* 1975; Vaamonde *et al.* 1981) so only a brief summary of the observations will be given here.

The earliest description of renal involvement in sickle cell disease was that of Herrick (1910) in his paper describing sickle cells. His patient had white blood cells and casts in the urine, and a low urinary specific gravity. Renal abnormalities may be either acute episodes occurring in a sickle cell crisis, or a progressive age-related deterioration in renal function.

Total body water and extracellular fluid volume are increased during sickling crises as is the GFR. Urine flow and sodium excretion rates are diminished (Wilson and Alleyne 1975, 1976). There may also be haematuria. Some patients in a sickling crises have metabolic acidosis

(Barreras and Diggs 1964), which itself exacerbates sickling; however, metabolic acidosis probably does not play a major role in initiating crises (Ringelhan and Konetey-Ahulu 1971).

The principal abnormalities of renal function in sickle cell disease are impaired urine concentration and acidification, and hyperuricaemia. Haematuria, papillary necrosis, proteinuria, impaired erythropoietin synthesis, and a late impairment of glomerular function are also seen, as is exceptionally even renal infarction (Granfortuna *et al.* 1986).

Reduced concentrating ability, probably due to altered medullary blood flow, is well documented (Keitel *et al.* 1956; Hatch *et al.* 1967; Statius van Eps *et al.* 1970). In both sickle cell anaemia and sickle cell–HbC disease maximal urine osmolality is usually less than 600 mosmol/kg H_2O, and falls with age, but is reduced from infancy. It is also present even in patients with a high level of HbF (Statius van Eps *et al.* 1970). The defect is correctable only in children by exchange transfusion, indicating that it is indeed due to the presence of red blood cells that sickle. A lesser impairment of concentrating ability has also been observed in sickle cell trait (Statius van Eps *et al.* 1967). Urine dilution is not impaired.

The other major renal tubular function to be impaired, acidification, is affected in varying proportions of patients in different studies, ranging from 29 to 100 per cent (Ho Ping Kong and Alleyne 1971; Goosens *et al.* 1972; Oster *et al.* 1976). In general the defect is only partial, resulting in a renal tubular acidosis only on acid loading, a finding termed 'incomplete renal tubular acidosis' by Buckalew and colleagues (1968).

Patients with sickle cell disease, like any patient with a chronic haemolytic anaemia with increased red-cell turnover, have an increased rate of uric acid production (Diamond *et al.* 1979). Indeed Diamond and colleagues (1974) have demonstrated that mean uric acid excretion is above normal in over half of adult sickle cell disease patients, and that there is an increased urinary uric acid to creatine ratio. However, serum uric acid levels are usually not raised in children and are mildly raised in only about a third of adult patients with homozygous sickle cell disease (Gold *et al.* 1968; Jarvis 1968; Walker and Alexander 1971; Diamond *et al.* 1975). Moreover secondary gout is rare (Gold *et al.* 1968; Ball and Sorensen 1970). Glomerular failure in older patients also tends to increase serum uric acid levels, and may lead to decreased uric acid excretion (Jarvis 1968; Walker and Alexander 1971). Morgan and associates (1984) have shown that serum urate concentration is dependent on both renal urate clearance and creatinine clearance. In a series of patients they found that fractional excretion and absolute urate excretion per millilitre of urine increased while creatinine clearance was falling, indicating a preservation of tubular urate secretion despite other evidence of impaired tubular function (Diamond *et al.* 1975).

Haematuria may be gross, especially when associated with a sickle cell crisis, or persistent and it may produce significant symptoms (Abel and Brown 1948; Goodwin *et al.* 1950; Lucas and Bullock 1960; Allen 1964). Haematuria may also occur as a symptomless microscopic finding (Schlitt and Keitel 1960). One cause of persistent haematuria in sickle cell disease is renal papillary necrosis (Mostofi *et al.* 1957; Akinkugbe 1967), usually of the medullary type (Schmidt and Flocks 1971).

The increase in erythropoietin concentrations in sickle cell disease is less than might be expected for the degree of anaemia. Morgan and colleagues (1982) in a study of 31 patients found that none had erythropoietin levels above the normal range. They observed that haemoglobin concentration was negatively correlated with creatinine clearance and positively correlated with erythropoietin level. They concluded that erythropoietin concentration was the limiting factor in red-cell production in sickle cell disease with renal insufficiency. They argued against inhibition of erythropoietin by uraemic toxins, implying that impaired glomerular function reduced renal capacity for synthesis of erythropoietin.

Impaired renal function associated with proteinuria, and sometimes referred to as 'sickle cell nephropathy', has comparatively recently been recognized as frequent complication of sickle cell disease in older patients. The nephropathy usually presents with proteinuria and occasionally even with nephrotic syndrome (Miller *et al.* 1964; Walker *et al.* 1971). Proteinuria may lead on to eventual renal insufficiency and even death from renal failure. Morgan and Sergeant (1981) investigated 25 Jamaican patients aged 40–64 years and observed higher blood urea concentrations than in a similar 18–39 years age group. Intravenous pyelography showed caliceal cupping, irregular renal outline, or cystic extension of the calix in 15 patients. Creatinine clearance was low in six patients and was inversely related to age. Proteinuria was common in patients with renal insufficiency. They suggested that this falling renal function was associated with cortical scarring. The same group (Thomas *et al.* 1982) in a review of the causes of death of 276 Jamaican patients found that, although the greatest mortality is in the first 5 years of life, about a quarter were aged over 30 years at the time of death. Among these older patients the commonest causes of death were cerebrovascular accidents and renal failure. Twenty-one out of 241 patients with homozygous sickle cell disease died from renal failure, all but four aged 20 years or over and eight aged 30 or over.

Histologically the kidneys from patients with sickle cell nephropathy show distended glomerular capillaries, especially involving the juxtamedullary glomeruli (Bernstein and Whitten 1960; Pitcock *et al.* 1970). Glomerular fibrosis (Bernstein and Whitten 1960), periglomerular fibrosis, and cortical infarction may be seen (Kimmelstiel 1948).

Glomeruli may show the changes of membrano-proliferative glomerulo-nephritis (Miller *et al.* 1964) with immune deposits (Pardo *et al.* 1975). McCoy (1969) has demonstrated focal fusion of epithelial foot processes on electron microscopy, along with basement membrane thickening. Others have confirmed and extended these observations on ultra-structural changes (Pitcock *et al.* 1970; Antonovych 1972; Pardo *et al.* 1975; Strauss *et al.* 1975).

The genetics of the haemoglobinopathies is of course better under-stood than that for virtually any other group of diseases, and will not be elaborated here. Homozygous sickle cell disease with HbSS is inherited in an autosomal recessive manner, being due to a structural gene mutation within the β-haemoglobin gene on chromosome 11. HbSC and HbSThal are double heterozygous situations. Carrier detection for the HbAS, as well as for HbSC and HbSThal can be readily detected post-natally by haemoglobin electrophoresis and estimation of the percentage of HbF in the red blood cells. Prenatal diagnosis of the affected, or of the heterozygous, fetus is best performed using recombinant DNA methods on trophoblast obtained by first-trimester chorionic villus sampling. The older biochemical methods performed on fetal blood had the disadvan-tage of relatively late and hazardous fetoscopy with blood sampling. Fortunately the DNA probes now available for the detection of sickle cell disease recognize the HbS mutation directly and do not depend on a linked polymorphism which might or might not be informative.

A study of 45 patients with β-thalassaemia major revealed haematuria in 67 per cent (Khalifa *et al.* 1985). Blood urea and serum creatinine were normal but serum β_2-microglobin levels were raised, especially in patients with haematuria. Both ultrasonography and renal biopsy revealed abnormalities in some patients. The ultrasonographic abnor-mities, found in 15.5 per cent, all with haematuria, included poor demarcation of the renal parenchyma and pelvi-calyceal system, and multiple cyst formation. Renal biopsy, performed on five patients, revealed moderate diffuse thickening of capillary walls with segmental and focal cellular proliferation in glomeruli, interstitial round cell infiltration, and tubular atrophy. The authors attributed these renal changes to the siderosis which treated patients develop. They recommend serum β_2-microglobulin assay as a screening test for renal damage in β-thalassaemia.

References

Abel, M. S. and Brown, C. R. (1948). Sickle cell disease with severe hematuria simulating renal neoplasm. *JAMA* **136**, 624–5.
Akinkugbe, O. O. (1967). Renal papillary necrosis in sickle-cell haemo-globinopathy. *Br. Med. J.* **3**, 283–4.

Allen, T. D. (1964). Sickle cell disease and hematuria: a report of 29 cases. *J. Urol.* **91**, 177–83.

Alleyne, G. A. O., Statius van Eps, L. W., Addae, S. K. (1975). The kidney in sickle cell anaemia. *Kidney Int.* **7**, 371–9.

Antonovych, T. T. (1972). Ultrastructural changes in glomeruli of patients with sickle cell disease and the nephrotic syndrome. *Abs. Am. Soc. Nephrol.* **5**, 3.

Ball, G. V. and Sorensen, L. B. (1970). The pathogenesis of hyperuricemia and gout in sickle cell anemia. *Arthritis Rheum.* **13**, 846–8.

Barreras, L. and Diggs, L. W. (1964). Bicarbonates, pH and percentage of sickled cells in venous blood of patients in sickle cell crisis. *Am. J. Med. Sci.* **247**, 710–18.

Bernstein, J. and Whitten, C. F. (1960). A histologic appraisal of the kidney in sickle cell anemia. *Arch. Pathol.* **20**, 407–18.

Buckalew, V. M. Jr. and Someren, A. (1974). Renal manifestations of sickle cell disease. *Arch. Intern. Med.* **133**, 660–9.

——, McCurdy, D. K., Ludwig, G. D., Chaykin, L. B. and Elkinton, J. R. (1968). Incomplete renal tubular acidosis: physiologic studies in three patients with a defect in lowering urine pH. *Am. J. Med.* **45**, 32–42.

Diamond, H., Sharon, E., Holden, D. and Cacatian, A. (1974). Renal handling of uric acid in sickle cell anemia. *Adv. Exp. Med. Biol.* **41**, 759–62.

——, Miesel, A., Sharon, E., Holden, D. and Cacatian, A. (1975). Hyperuricosuria and increased tubular secretion of urate in sickle cell anemia. *Am. J. Med.* **59**, 796–802.

——, —— and Holden, D. (1979). The natural history of urate overproduction in sickle cell anaemia. *Ann. Intern. Med.* **90**, 752–7.

Gold, M. S., Williams, J. C., Spivak, M. and Grann, V. (1968). Sickle cell anemia and hyperuricemia. *JAMA* **206**, 1572–3

Goodwin, W. E., Alston, E. F. and Semans, J. H. (1950). Hematuria and sickle cell disease: unexplained gross unilateral renal hematuria in Negroes, coincident with the blood sickling trait. *J. Urol.* **63**, 79–96.

Goosens, J. P., Statius van Eps, L. W., Schouten, H. and Giterson, A. L. (1972). Incomplete renal tubular acidosis in sickle cell disease. *Clin. Chim. Acta.* **41**, 149–56.

Granfortuna, J., Zamhoff, K. and Urrutia, E. (1986). Acute renal infarction in sickle cell disease. *Am. J. Hematol.* **23**, 59–64.

Hatch, F. E., Culbertson, J. W. and Diggs, L. W. (1967). Nature of the renal concentrating defect in sickle cell disease. *J. Clin. Invest.* **46**, 336–45.

Herrick, J. B. (1910). Peculiar elongated and sickle-shaped red blood corpuscles in a case of severe anemia. *Arch. Intern. Med.* **6**, 517–21.

Ho Ping Kong, H. and Alleyne, G. A. O. (1971). Studies on acid excretion in adults with sickle-cell anaemia. *Clin. Sci.* **41**, 505–18.

Jarvis, M. A. B. (1968). Hyperuricemia and gout in sickle cell disease. *Harper Hosp. Bull.* **26**, 140.

Keitel, H. G., Thompson, D. and Itano, H. A. (1956). Hyposthenuria in sickle cell anemia: a reversible renal defect. *J. Clin. Invest.* **35**, 998–1007.

Khalifa, A. S., Sheir, S., El Magd, L. A., El Tayeb, H., El Lamie, O., Khalifa, A. and Mokhtar, G. (1985). The kidney in beta-thalassaemia major. *Acta Haemat.* **74**, 60.

Kimmelstiel, P. (1948). Vascular occlusion and ischemic infarction in sickle cell disease. *Am. J. Med. Sci.* **216**, 11–19.

Lucas, W. M. and Bullock, W. H. (1960). Hematuria in sickle cell disease. *J. Urol.* **83**, 733–41.

McCoy, R. C. (1969). Ultrastructural alterations in the kidney of patients with sickle cell disease and the nephrotic syndrome. *Lab Invest.* **21**, 85–95.

Miller, R. E., Hartley, M. W., Clark, E. C. and Lupton, C. H. (1964). Sickle cell nephropathy. *Ala. J. Med. Sci.* **1**, 233–8.

Morgan, A. G. and Serjeant, G. R. (1981). Renal function in patients over 40 with homozygous sickle cell disease. *Br. Med. J.* **282**, 1181–3.

——, Gruber, C. A. and Serjeant, G. R. (1982). Erythropoietin and renal function in sickle-cell disease. *Br. Med. J.* **285**, 1686–8.

——, De Ceulaer, K. and Serjeant, G. R. (1984). Glomerular function and hyperuricaemia in sickle cell disease. *J. Clin. Pathol.* **37**, 1046–9.

Mostofi, K. F., Vorderbruegge, C. F. and Diggs, L. W. (1957). Lesions of the kidneys, removed for unilateral hematuria in sickle cell disease. *Arch. Pathol. Lab. Med.* **63**, 336–51.

Oster, J. R., Lespier, L. E., Lee, S. M., Pellegrini, E. L. and Vaamonde, C. A. (1976). Renal acidification in sickle-cell disease. *J. Lab. Clin. Med.* **88**, 389–401.

Pardo, V., Strauss, J., Kramer, H., Ozawa, T. and McIntosh, R. M. (1975). Nephropathy associated with sickle cell anemia: an autologous immune complex nephritis. II. Clinicopathologic study of seven patients. *Am. J. Med.* **59**, 650–9.

Pitcock, J. A., Muirhead, E. E., Hatch, F. E., Johnson, J. C. and Kelly, B. J. (1970). Early renal changes in sickle cell anemia. *Arch Pathol.* **90**, 403–10.

Ringelhann, B. and Konotey-Ahulu, F. I. D. (1971). Sickle cell crisis and acid-base balance. *Clin. Chim. Acta.* **34**, 63–6.

Schlitt, L. E. and Keitel, H. G. (1960). Renal manifestations of sickle cell disease: a review. *Am. J. Med. Sci.* **239**, 773–8.

Schmidt, J. D. and Flocks, R. H. (1971). Urologic aspects of sickle cell hemoglobin. *J. Urol.* **106**, 740–4.

Serjeant, G. R. (1974). *The clinical features of sickle cell disease.* North-Holland/Elsevier, New York.

Statius van Eps, L. W., Schouten, H., La Porte-Wijsman, L. W. and Struyker Boudier, A. M. (1967). The influence of red blood cell transfusions on the hyposthenuria and renal hemodynamics of sickle cell anemia. *Clin. Chim. Acta.* **17**, 449–61.

——, ——, Ter Harr Romeny-Wachter, C. Ch. and La Porte-Wijsman, L. W. (1970). The relation between age and renal concentrating capacity in sickle cell disease and hemoglobin C disease. *Clin. Chim. Acta* **27**, 501–11.

Strauss, J., Pardo, V., Koss, M. N., Griswold, W. and McIntosh, R. M. (1975). Nephropathy associated with sickle cell anemia: an autologous immune complex nephritis. I. Studies on nature of the glomerular-bound antibody and antigen identification in a patient with sickle cell disease and immune deposit glomerulonephritis. *Am. J. Med.* **58**, 382–7.

Thomas, A. N., Pattison, C. and Serjeant, G. R. (1982). Causes of death in sickle-cell disease in Jamaica. *Br. Med. J.* **285**, 633–5.

Vaamonde, C. A., Oster, J. R. and Strauss, J. (1981). The kidney in sickle cell disease. In *The kidney in systemic disease*, 2nd edn. eds. Suki, W. N. and Eknoyan, G. pp. 159–95. John Wiley, Chichester.

Walker, B. R. and Alexander, F. (1971). Uric acid excretion in sickle cell anemia. *JAMA* **215**, 255–8.

——, ——. Birdsall, T. R. and Warren, R. L. (1971). Glomerular lesions in sickle cell nephropathy. *JAMA* **215**, 437–40.

Wilson, W. A. and Alleyne, G. A. O. (1975). Renal function during painful sickle cell crisis. *West Indian Med. J.* **24**, 84–9.

—— and —— (1976). Total body water, extracellular and plasma volume compartments in sickle cell anaemia. *West Indian Med. J.* **25**, 241–50.

8.5. LUPUS ERYTHEMATOSUS

Renal disease is a common complication of lupus erythematosus and can cause serious morbidity or death. The pathology, clinical course, and response to treatment of lupus nephritis have been extensively documented and several classifications of the changes observed have been proposed, including a relatively recent WHO classification that defines five classes (Pollack *et al.* 1964; Comerford and Cohen 1967; Baldwin *et al.* 1977; Appel *et al.* 1978; Cameron *et al.* 1979; Karsh *et al.* 1979; Glassock and Goldstein 1981; Wallace *et al.* 1981, 1982; Magil *et al.* 1982; Austin *et al.* 1983; Coplon *et al.* 1983; Jarrett *et al.* 1983; Rubin *et al.* 1985). Berlyne (1979) in a review of lupus nephritis found that the incidence of renal involvement in systemic lupus erythematosus varies from 56 per cent to 75 per cent in different series, depending partially on the criteria, and averaging around two-thirds of patients. A higher incidence is recorded when histological rather than biochemical evidence is used. It is also higher in autopsy series. When present renal involvement is usually, but not invariably, detectable from the onset of the disease, and may be the only clinical manifestation of systemic lupus.

Apart from transient proteinuria during pyrexial episodes persistent proteinuria is the most common clinical presentation of lupus nephritis, with progressive deterioration of renal function in lupus glomeruloneph-ritis, or without deterioration in membranous lupus glomerulonephritis or lupus glomerulitis. Lupus glomerulonephritis may also present as an acute glomerulonephritis, and when renal function does deteriorate during the course of the disease the deterioration tends to be acute (Yeung *et al.* 1985). In about one-fifth of cases of lupus nephritis there is a nephrotic syndrome but in many of these the serum cholesterol remains normal. Death in renal failure tends to be associated with rapid decline in renal function within the first 2 years following the onset of the disease, and is usually associated with active lupus. However, most deaths of patients with lupus nephritis, especially now that these patients receive dialysis or transplantation for their renal failure, are due to vascular disease, infection or lupus itself, especially central nervous system lupus

(Cameron *et al.* 1979; Karsh *et al.* 1979; Correia *et al.* 1985; Yeung *et al.* 1985).

The renal histopathology on light microscopy was described by Pollak and his colleagues (Muehrcke *et al.* 1957; Pollak *et al.* 1964), and more recently Donadio and associates (1977) have described the picture in membranous nephropathy. The characteristic 'wire loop' lesions, which were first described by Baehr and colleagues (1935), consist of localized areas of glomerular basement membrane with intense eosinophilic staining due to fibrinoid change. Fibrinoid change may also be seen in capillary basement membranes and in arterioles. Another common glomerular lesion is basement membrane thickening, which is usually focal, but may be diffuse. It may be associated with fibrinoid change or even necrosis. Other glomerular lesions observed include tuft hyper-cellularity, fibro-epithelial crescents, capsular adhesions, and hyaline thrombi of the glomerular capillaries. Tubular degeneration and eventual atrophy are also common. Oedema of the interstitial tissue and, in chronic cases, focal fibrosis with or without cellular infiltration are also seen.

Electron microscopy may reveal electron-dense deposits of immune complexes (Comerford and Cohen 1967), which when present are either subepithelial or subendothelial, the latter being associated with a poor prognosis. The wire loop lesion is formed by deposits on the endothelial side of the basement membrane or within a split membrane. In membranous lupus glomerulonephritis, deposits are seen on the epithelial side of the basement membrane.

Pollak and colleagues (1964) classified lupus nephritis into four categories: focal glomerulitis with mild focal basement membrane thickening and hypercellularity; diffuse proliferative glomerulonephritis with more severe lesions including fibrinoid change and necrosis, crescent formation, wire loops, tubular, and interstitial changes; membranous lupus glomerulonephritis with diffuse basement membrane thickening; and mesangioproliferative glomerulonephritis. The WHO classification differs slightly comprising: I—with no glomerular changes, II—mesangial lupus nephritis, III—focal proliferative glomerulonephritis, IV—diffuse proliferative glomerulonephritis, and V—membranous nephritis with normocellular glomeruli but capillary wall thickening. Groups III and IV carry the worst prognosis. Pathogenesis is thought to be similar to that for other immune complex nephritides.

Transition from one type or renal lesion to another, either spontane-ously or in response to treatment, is frequent. Serial renal biopsy has revealed such transformations, usually from a more to a less severe lesion, in over half the cases of lupus nephropathy studied (Appel *et al.* 1978; Lee *et al.* 1985).

Familial occurrence of systemic lupus erythematosus, as of many auto-immune collagen disorders, is a frequent observation. However, it is not inherited in a simple Mendelian manner, despite early reports of both parent–child and sib–sib occurrence reviewed by Leonhardt (1964) in his extensive family study. His study was inspired by his own earlier report of one such family in which three sisters were affected (Leonhardt 1957). These three along with five further sibs, out of a family of 14 sibs, had hypergammaglobulinaemia. In his 1964 paper Leonhardt studied 225 first-degree relatives of 57 patients with definite lupus and observed an increased incidence of clinical features of lupus such as arthralgia and drug, cold, and sun sensitivity, and of immunological abnormalities such as positive tests for antinuclear factor. Pollak, also in 1964, made a similar observation of an increased incidence of antinuclear antibodies in relatives of patients. Other workers have since confirmed an increased incidence of autoantibodies among relatives of index patients, not only of lupus-related but also of other types of autoantibody such as those against thyroid (Siegel *et al.* 1965; Larsen 1972; Larsen and Godal 1972; De Horatius *et al.* 1975; Weinburg *et al.* 1980). There have also been further reports of familial occurrence of the disease itself (First 1973; Arnett and Shulman 1976; Brustein *et al.* 1977; Exner *et al.* 1980).

Essentially all that these reports demonstrate is a familial predisposition to autoimmune disease. There is some evidence for a viral aetiology of the disease, which if confirmed could account for both vertical and horizontal transmission within families. Lewis and colleagues (1974) produced evidence for involvement of C-type RNA viruses. Beaucher and coworkers (1977) demonstrated DNA antibodies in dogs in the households of patients with lupus. De Horatius and associates (1975) found anti-RNA antibodies only in relatives who were close household contacts of their patients, again supporting the theory of an infective agent. The viral, or other infective agent, induces autoantibody synthesis, and these antibodies render the cell surface DNA receptor defective (Bennett *et al.* 1986). Nevertheless twin studies (Kohler *et al.* 1974; Block *et al.* 1975; Yocum *et al.* 1975) have revealed a higher concordance for both clinical disease and immune defects in monozygotic than in dizygotic twin pairs. These observations indicate that genetic factors must play a significant, but in the light of some monozygotic discordance not exclusive, role in aetiology. Talal (1979) reviewed the evidence that the preponderance of female patients is associated with the higher oestrogen levels in women.

Most claims for single gene effects in lupus have related to specific variants of the disease, or to lupus-like diseases. Lappat and Cawein (1968) studied the family of a patient with procainamide-induced systemic lupus and found antinuclear antibodies, a coagulant defect, or other evidence of immune disturbance among the relatives. They suggested that their findings were due to a pharmacogenetic polymorphism. Schaller (1972) described a lupus-like illness in heterozygotes for X-linked chronic granulomatous disease. Tuffanelli and associates described an hereditary inflammatory vasculitis with lupus-like features (Tuffanelli 1971; Reed *et al.* 1972). Horn and colleagues (1978) reported a mixed connective tissue disease, with some features of lupus, in HLA-identical sibs.

The evidence for polygenic, or at least oligogenic, determination of systemic lupus comes from an animal model in mice in which Knight and Adams (1978) identified three genes involved in the development of lupus nephritis in the progeny of NZW × NZB crosses. Similar oligogenic models have been postulated in humans by Burch and Rowell for both discoid and systemic lupus, based on the former's approach of stochastic analysis of age and sex distribution. They postulate that manifestation of the disease is due to the accumulation of three random events, probably somatic mutations of X-linked genes in lymphoid cells, in individuals predisposed through being carriers of one of three X-linked dominant alleles and autosomal factors at one or more loci (Burch and Rowell 1965; Beck and Rowell 1966). More recently Miller and Schwartz (1979) have proposed that the development of systemic lupus requires the action of at least two functionally distinct classes of genes involved in suppressor cell function: class I genes determining defective T-cell function, and class II genes determining immunopathological lesions. There is little further evidence as to the nature of the genes involved apart from the observation of an association of hydralazine-induced lupus with HLA-DR4 (Batchelor *et al.* 1980), of the acetylator slow phenotype with idiopathic lupus (Batchelor *et al.* 1980; Reidenberg *et al.* 1980), and of HLA-B8 and DR3 in Hungarian patients (Stenszky *et al.* 1986). The Hungarian workers also noted that subjects homozygous for HLA-B8 and a Gm genotype were at greater risk for systemic lupus compared to heterozygotes. They also observed an increased frequency of a specific Gm type: 3,5,13, acting additively with HLA-B8, in lupus patients with renal disease.

References

Appel, G. B., Silva, F. G., Pirani, C. L., Meltzer, J. I. and Estes, D. (1978). Renal involvement in systemic erythematosus (SLE): a study of 56 patients emphasing histological classification. *Medicine* **57**, 371–410.

Arnett, F. C. and Shulman, L. E. (1976). Studies in familial systemic lupus erythematosus. *Medicine* **55**, 313–22.

Austin, H. A., Muenz, L. R., Joyce, K. M., Antonovych, T. A., Kullick, M. E.,

Klippel, J. H., Decker, J. L. and Balow, J. E. (1983). Prognostic factors in lupus nephritis: contribution of renal histological data. *Am. J. Med.* **75**, 382–91.

Baehr, G., Kleimperer, P. and Schifrin, A. (1935). A diffuse disease of the peripheral circulation (usually associated with lupus erythematosus and endocarditis). *Trans. Assoc. Am. Phys.* **50**, 139.

Baldwin, D. S., Gluck, M. C., Lowenstein, J. and Gallo, G. R. (1977). Lupus nephritis—clinical course related to morphologic forms and their transitions. *Am. J. Med.* **62**, 12–30.

Batchelor, J. R., Welsh, K. I., Tinoco, R. M., Dollery, C. T., Hughes, G. R. V., Bernstein, R., Ryan, P., Waish, P. F., Aber, G. M., Bing, R. F. and Russell, G. I. (1980). Hydralazine-induced systemic lupus erythematosus: influence of HLA-DR and sex on susceptibility. *Lancet* **1**, 1107–9.

Beaucher, W. N., Garman, R. H. and Condemi, J. J. (1977). Familial lupus erythematosus: antibodies to DNA in household dogs. *New Engl. J. Med.* **296**, 982–4.

Beck, J. S. and Rowell, N. R. (1966). Discoid lupus erythematosus. A study of the clinical features and biochemical and serological abnormalities in 120 patients with observations on the relationship of this disease to systemic lupus erythematosus. *Quart. J. Med.* **35**, 119–36.

Bennett, R. M., Peller, J. S. and Merritt, M. M. (1986). Defective DNA-receptor function in systemic lupus erythematosus and related diseases: evidence for an autoantibody influencing cell physiology. *Lancet* **1**, 186–8.

Berlyne, G. M. (1979). Renal involvement in collagen diseases. Chapter 22 in *Renal diseases*, 4th edn. eds. Black, D. and Jones, N. F. pp. 661–2. Blackwell Scientific, Oxford.

Block, S. R., Winfield, J. B., Lockshin, M. D., D'Angelo, W. A. and Christian, C. L. (1975). Studies of twins with systemic lupus erythematosus: a review of the literature and presentation of 12 additional sets. *Am. J. Med.* **59**, 533–52.

Brustein, D., Rodriguez, J. M., Minkin, W. and Rabhan, N. B. (1977). Familial lupus erythematosus. *JAMA* **238**, 2294–6.

Burch, P. R. J. and Rowell, N. R. (1965). Systemic lupus erythematosus: etiological aspects. *Am. J. Med.* **38**, 793–801.

Cameron, J. S., Turner, D. R., Ogg, C. S., Williams, D. G., Lessof, M. H., Chantler, C. and Liebowitz, S. (1979). Systemic lupus with nephritis: a long-term study. *Quart. J. Med.* **48**, 1–24.

Comerford, F. R. and Cohen, A. S. (1967). The nephropathy of systemic lupus erythematosus. *Medicine* **46**, 425–73.

Coplon, N. S., Diskin, C. J., Petersen, J. and Swenson, R. S. (1983). The long-term clinical course of systemic lupus erythematosus in end-stage renal disease. *New Engl. J. Med.* **308**, 186–90.

Correia, P., Cameron, J. S., Lian, J. D., Hicks, J., Ogg, C. S., Williams, D. G., Chantler, C. and Haycock, D. G. (1985). Why do patients with lupus nephritis die? *Br. Med. J.* **290**, 126–31.

De Horatius, R. J., Pillarisetty, R., Messner, R. P. and Talal, N. (1975). Antinucleic acid antibodies in systemic lupus erythematosus patients and their families: incidence and correlation with lymphocytoxic antibodies. *J. Clin. Invest.* **56**, 1149–54.

Donadio, J. V. Jr., Burgess, J. H. and Holley, K. E. (1977). Membranous lupus nephropathy: a clinicopathologic study. *Medicine* **56**, 527–36.

Exner, T., Barber, S., Kronenberg, H. and Rickard, K. A. (1980). Familial association of the lupus anticoagulant. *Br. J. Haemat.* **45**, 89–96.

First, M. R. (1973). Familial systemic lupus erythematosus. *S. Afr. Med. J.* **47**, 742–4.

Glassock, R. J. and Goldstein, D. A. (1981). Glomerulonephritis in systemic lupus erythematosus. *Am. J. Nephrol.* **1**, 53–67.

Horn, J. R., Kapur, J. J. and Walker, S. E. (1978). Mixed connective tissue disease in siblings. *Arthritis Rheum.* **21**, 209–714.

Jarrett, M. P., Santhanam, S. and Del Greco, F. (1983). The clinical course of end-stage renal disease in systemic lupus erythematosus. *Arch. Intern. Med.* **143**, 1353–6.

Karsh, J., Klippel, J. H., Balow, J. E. and Decker, J. L. (1979). Mortality in lupus nephritis. *Arthritis Rheum.* **22**, 764–9.

Knight, J. G. and Adams, D. D. (1978). Three genes for lupus nephritis in NZB×NZW mice. *J. Exp. Med.* **147**, 1653–60.

Kohler, P. F., Perry, J., Campion, W. M. and Smyth, C. J. (1974). Hereditary angioedema and 'familial' lupus erythematosus in identical twin boys. *Am. J. Med.* **56**, 406–11.

Lappat, E. J. and Cawein, M. J. (1968). A familial study of procainamide-induced systemic lupus erythematosus. A question of pharmacogenetic polymorphism. *Am. J. Med.* **45**, 846–52.

Larsen, R. A. (1972). Family studies in systemic lupus erythematosus (SLE). I. A proband material from central eastern Norway. *Acta Med. Scand.* **543** (Suppl.), 11–19.

—— and Godal, T. (1972). Family studies in systemic lupus erythematosus (SLE). IX. Thyroid diseases and antibodies. *J. Chronic Dis.* **25**, 225–33.

Lee, H. S., Mujais, S. K., Kasinath, B. S., Spargo, B. H. and Katz, A. I. (1985). Course of renal pathology in patients with systemic lupus erythematosus. *Am. J. Med.* **77**, 612–20.

Leonhardt, T. (1957). Familial hypergammaglobulinaemia and systemic lupus erythematosus. *Lancet* **2**, 1200–3.

—— (1964). Family studies in systemic lupus erythematosus. *Acta Med. Scand.* **176** (Suppl. 416), 1–156.

Lewis, R., Tannenberg, W., Smith, C. and Schwartz, R. (1974). Human systemic lupus erythematosus and C-type RNA viruses (abs.) *Clin. Res.* **22**, 422A.

Magil, A. B., Ballon, H. S. and Rae, A. (1982). Focal proliferative lupus nephritis: a clinicopathologic study using the WHO classification. *Am. J. Med.* **72**, 620–30.

Miller, K. B. and Schwartz, R. S. (1979). Familial abnormalities of suppressor-cell function in systemic lupus erythematosus. *New Engl. J. Med.* **301**, 803–9.

Muehrcke, R. C., Kark, R. M., Pirani, C. L. and Pollak, V. E. (1957). Lupus nephritis. A clinical pathological study based on renal biopsies. *Medicine* **36**, 1–145.

Pollak, V. E. (1964). Antinuclear antibodies in families of patients with systemic lupus erythematosus. *New Engl. J. Med.* **271**, 165–71.

——, Pirani, C. L. and Schwartz, F. D. (1964). The natural history of the renal manifestations of systemic lupus erythematosus. *J. Lab. Clin. Med.* **63**, 537–50.

Reed, W. B., Bergeron, R. F., Tuffanelli, D. and Jones, E. W. (1972). Hereditary inflammatory vasculitis with persistent nodules. A genetically-determined new entity probably related to lupus erythematosus. *Br. J. Dermatol.* **87**, 299–307.

Reidenberg, M. M., Levy, M., Drayer, D. E., Zylber-Katz, E. and Robbins, W. C. (1980). Acetylator phenotype in idiopathic systemic lupus erythematosus. *Arthritis Rheum.* **23**, 569–73.

Rubin, L. A., Urowitz, M. B. and Gladman, D. D. (1985). Mortality in systemic lupus erythematosus: the bimodal pattern revisited. *Quart. J. Med.* **55**, 87–98.

Schaller, J. (1972). Illness resembling lupus erythematosus in mothers of boys with chronic granulomatous disease. *Ann. Intern. Med.* **76**, 747–50.

Siegel, M., Lee, S. L., Widelock, D., Gwon, N. V. and Kravitz, H. (1965). A comparative family study of rheumatoid arthritis and systemic lupus erythematosus. *New Engl. J. Med.* **273**, 893–7.

Stenszky, V., Kozma, L., Svegedi, G. and Farid, N. R. (1986). Interplay of immunoglobulin G heavy chain markers (Gm) and HLA in predisposing to systemic lupus nephritis. *J. Immunogenet.* **13**, 11–17.

Talal, N. (1979). Systemic lupus erythematosus, autoimmunity, sex and inheritance. *New Engl. J. Med.* **301**, 838–9.

Tuffanelli, D. L. (1971). Lupus erythematosus panniculitis (profundus). Clinical and immunologic studies. *Arch. Dermatol.* **103**, 231–42.

Wallace, D. J., Podell, T., Weiner, J., Klinenberg, J. R., Forouzesh, S. and Dubois, E. L. (1981). Systemic lupus erythematosus: survival patterns. Experience with 609 patients. *JAMA* **245**, 934–8.

——, ——, ——, Cox, M. B., Klinenberg, J. R., Forouzesh, S. and Dubois, E. L. (1982). Lupus nephritis—experience with 230 patients in a private practice from 1950–1980. *Am. J. Med.* **72**, 209–20.

Weinberg, J. B., Hasstedt, S. J., Skolnick, M. H., Kimberling, W. J. and Baty, B. (1980). Analysis of a large pedigree with elliptocytosis, multiple lipomatosis, and biological false-positive serological test for syphilis. *Am. J. Med. Genet.* **5**, 57–67.

Yeung, C. K., Ng, W. L., Wong, W. S., Wong, K. L. and Chan, M. K. (1985). Acute deterioration in renal function in systemic lupus erythematosus. *Quart. J. Med.* **56**, 393–402.

Yocum, M. W., Grossman, J., Waterhouse, C., Abraham, G. N., May, A. G. and Condemi, J. J. (1975). Monozygotic twins discordant for systemic lupus erythematosus: comparison of immune response, autoantibodies, viral antibody titres, gamma globulin, and light chain metabolism. *Arthritis Rheum.* **18**, 193–9.

8.6. HAEMOPHILIA

Haematuria is an obvious common complication of haemophilia. It has been estimated that 20 per cent of asymptomatic haemophiliacs have microscopic haematuria (Prentice *et al.* 1971). Frank urinary tract bleeding is the second most common symptom of haemophilia after haemarthrosis (Rizza and Matthews 1972). In addition several studies have revealed a high incidence of renal abnormalities in haemophilia

(Prentice *et al.* 1971; Wright *et al.* 1971; Beck and Evans 1972; Dalinka *et al.* 1975; Forbes and Prentice 1977; Dholakia and Howarth 1979). Apart from haematuria the abnormalities noted include analgesic nephropathy, hypertension, urographic abnormalities including hydronephrosis and ureteric blood clot, impaired renal function, and renal enlargement. Small and colleagues (1982) have reported an assessment of 57 patients at the Glasgow and Birmingham haemophilia centres, 27 of whom had been assessed 11 years previously. They studied renal function in these patients biochemically and radiologically. Fewer new patients had haematuria or took analgesics, presumably because of improved treatment. Only one patient, a new one, had analgesic nephropathy and among the old patients haematuria was a less prominent complaint than it has been 11 years previously. In general haematuria was not associated with progressive loss of renal function. Only three patients had renal abnormalities, attributable to renal bleeding, persisting from the earlier assessment, hydronephrosis or pelvicalyceal dilation, which in one instance had gone on to retroperitoneal fibrosis.

Haemophilia A is an X-linked recessive disorder. The traditional method of heterozygote detection in females—measurement of factor VIII activity and factor VIII-like antigen—gives some false negatives and is not wholly reliable. Recent studies on DNA polymorphisms linked to the haemophilia locus (Harper *et al.* 1984; Oberle *et al.* 1985), and the molecular cloning and characterization of the haemophilia gene (Gitschier *et al.* 1984; Toole *et al.* 1984; Truett *et al.* 1985), open up possibilities for using recombinant DNA methods for both heterozygote detection and prenatal diagnosis, at least in those families that prove to be informative. Rall and colleagues (1985) have shown that factor VIII is synthesized in the kidney as well as in the liver.

References

Beck, P. and Evans, K. T. (1972). Renal abnormalities in patients with haemophilia and Christmas disease. *Clin. Radiol.* **23**, 349–54.

Dalinka, M. K., Lally, J. F., Rancier, L. F. and Mata, J. (1975). Nephromegaly in hemophilia. *Radiology* **115**, 337–40.

Dholakia, A. M. and Howarth, F. H. (1979). The urinary tract in haemophilia. *Clin. Radiol.* **30**, 533–8.

Forbes, C. D. and Prentice, C. R. M. (1977). Renal disorders in haemophilia A and B. *Scand. J. Haematol.* Suppl. **30**, 43–50.

Gitschier, J., Wood, W. I., Goralka, T. M., Wion, K. L., Chen, E. Y., Eaton, D. H., Vehar, G. A., Capon, D. J. and Lawn, R. M. (1984). Characterization of the human factor VIII gene. *Nature* **312**, 326–30.

Harper, K., Winter, R. M., Pembrey, M. E., Hartley, D., Davies, K. E. and Tuddenham, E. G. D. (1984). A clinically useful DNA probe closely linked to haemophilia A. *Lancet* **2**, 6–8.

Oberle, I., Camerino, G., Heilig, R., Grunebaum, L., Cazenave, J. P., Crapanzano, C., Mannucci, P. M. and Mandel, J.-L. (1985). Genetic screening for hemophilia A (classic hemophilia) with a polymorphic DNA probe. *New Engl. J. Med.* **312**, 682–6.

Prentice, C. R. M., Lindsay, R. M., Barr, R. D., Forbes, C. D., Kennedy, A. C., McNicol, G. P. and Douglas, A. S. (1971). Renal complications in haemophilia and Christmas disease. *Quart. J. Med.* **40**, 47–61.

Rall, L. B., Bell, G. I., Caput, D., Truett, M. A., Masiarz, F. R., Najarian, R. C., Valenzuela, P., Anderson, H. D., Din, N. and Hansen, B. (1985). Factor VIII: C synthesis in the kidney. *Lancet* **1**, 44.

Rizza, C. R. and Matthews, J. M. (1972). Management of the haemophiliac child. *Arch. Dis. Child.* **47**, 451–62.

Small, M., Rose, P. E., McMillan, N., Belch, J. J. F., Rolfe, E. B., Forbes, C. D. and Stuart, J. (1982). Haemophilia and the kidney: assessment after 11-year follow-up. *Br. Med. J.* **285**, 1609–11.

Toole, J. J., Knopf, J. L., Wozney, J. M., Sultzman, L. A., Buecker, J. L., Pittman, D. D., Kaufman, R. J., Brown, E., Shoemaker, C., Orr, E. C., Amphlett, G. W., Foster, W. B., Coe, M. L., Knutson, G. L., Fass, D. N. and Hewick, R. M. (1984). Molecular cloning of a cDNA encoding human antihaemophilic factor. *Nature* **312**, 342–7.

Truett, M. A., Blacher, R., Burke, R. L., Caput, D., Chu, C., Dina, D., Hartog, K., Kuo, C. H., Masiarz, F. R., Merryweather, J. P., Najavian, R., Pachl, C., Potter, S. J., Puma, J., Quiroga, M., Rall, L. B., Randolph, A., Urdea, M. S., Valenzuela, P., Dahl, H. H., Favalaro, J., Hansen, J., Nordfang, D. and Ezban, M. (1985). Characterization of the polypeptide composition of human factor VIIIK and the nucleotide sequence and expression of the human kidney cDNA. *DNA* **4**, 333–49.

Wright, F. W., Matthews, J. M. and Brock, L. G. (1971). Complications of haemophiliac disorders affecting the renal tract. *Radiology* **98**, 571–6.

8.7. CYSTIC FIBROSIS OF THE PANCREAS

The clinico-pathological picture in cystic fibrosis is dominated by the steatorrhoea secondary to loss of pancreatic enzyme secretion, recurrent respiratory infection, and in later childhood or adolescence hepatic cirrhosis. Mild proteinuria is a common finding on routine urine analysis of patients with cystic fibrosis, usually unexplained and not of any clinical significance. However, renal plasma flow and GFR in patients in a stable condition do not differ from the rates found in normal controls (Spiro *et al.* 1985). Nevertheless, fractional excretion of sodium has been reported as being higher in cystic fibrosis patients than in controls during saline diuresis, associated with a reduced ability to increase the GFR following saline loading (Aladjem *et al.* 1983). The authors conclude that this indicates a defect in sodium reabsorption in the proximal tubule. These observations directly contradict earlier claims that sodium reabsorption in cystic fibrosis is increased. (Robson *et al.* 1971; Berg *et al.* 1982; Strandvik 1982). Autopsy may reveal renal enlargement and congestion in about a half of all cases (Castile *et al.* 1985). Histologically there may be glomerular sclerosis, tubular degeneration, interstitial nephritis, or nephrocalcinosis (Abramowsky and Swinehart 1982; Castile *et al.* 1985). Thus in most cases the renal changes are non-specific.

A rare complication of cystic fibrosis, presumably related to the chronic pulmonary infection, is amyloidosis of the kidney, and other organs, with proteinuria. When present there is frequently progression to nephrotic syndrome and renal failure. Castile and colleagues (1985) have recently reviewed nine cases including three new cases of their own, and have shown that the amyloid present is of the secondary AA type (Travis *et al.* 1986). McGlennen and coworkers (1986) have also reviewed the literature and presented autopsy findings on 33 patients who died at 15 years or older. A third of these patients were found to have amyloidosis in multiple organs, including the kidneys. Only one of these patients had had symptoms relating to the amyloidosis.

A succession of recent reports from Canada, the USA, Britain and Denmark have established linkage of the gene for cystic fibrosis to several loci on the long arm of chromosome 7. These include para-oxonase (PON) (Eiberg *et al.* 1985; Schmiegelow *et al.* 1986), an oncogene *met* (White *et al.* 1985), a polymorphic DNA marker, DOCRI-917, which is also linked to PON (Knowlton *et al.* 1985; Tsui *et al.* 1985a), the COL1A2 gene, another polymorphic DNA marker pJ3.11, and the gene for the β-chain of the T-cell receptor, TCRβ (Scambler *et al.* 1985; Wainwright *et al.* 1985; Buchwald *et al.* 1986; Scambler *et al.* 1986a and b; Tsui *et al.* 1985; Wainwright *et al.* 1986). Lod scores of 2 to as high as 8.65 were obtained for values of θ ranging from 0.14 to 0. Cystic fibrosis is of course inherited in an autosomal recessive manner and is one of the commonest such disorders, at least in Caucasian populations, among which the disease has a birth incidence of about 1 in 2000. These new discoveries have already been used for carrier detection (Farrall *et al.* 1986a), and first trimester prenatal diagnosis (Farrall *et al.* 1986b). Others have discussed the problems associated with their use in these ways (Liechti-Gallati *et al.* 1986; Brock *et al.* 1986; Super *et al.* 1986; Colter 1986). Klinger and colleagues (1986), in a study of two large inbred families using chromosome 7 DNA markers, have confirmed linkage in a pattern similar to that established for outbred families, thereby supporting homogeneity of the gene for cystic fibrosis. Scambler and others (1986c) have transformed mouse NIH-3T3 cells, by chromosome mediated gene transfer, with chromosomes from a human cell line containing an activated *met* oncogene. Analysis of the transformed cells demonstrated the presence of known chromosome 7 cystic fibrosis linked markers, and others not previously known to be linked to *met* or cystic fibrosis.

It is hoped that these developments will lead to methods of carrier detection applicable on a population basis, eventually to the elucidation of the pathogenesis of the disease, and possibly even to effective treatment.

References

Aladjem, M., Lotan, D., Boichis, H., Orda, S. and Katznelson, D. (1983). Renal function in patients with cystic fibrosis. *Nephron* **34**, 84–6.

Ambramowsky, C. R. and Swinehart, G. L. (1982). The nephropathy of cystic fibrosis. *Hum. Pathol.* **13**, 934–9.

Berg, U., Kusoffsky, E. and Strandvik, B. (1982). Renal function in cystic fibrosis with special reference to the renal sodium handling. *Acta Paediatr. Scand.* **71**, 833–8.

Brock, D., Curtis, A., Holloway, S., Burn, J. and Nelson, D. (1986). DNA typing to avoid need for prenatal diagnosis of cystic fibrosis. *Lancet* **2**, 393.

Buchwald, M., Zsiga, M., Mariewicz, D., Plasvic, N., Kennedy, D., Zengerling, S., Willard, H. F., Tsipouras, P., Schmiegelow, K., Schwartz, M., Eiberg, H., Mohr, J., Barker, D., Donis-Keller, H. and Tsui, L.-C. (1986). Linkage of cystic fibrosis to the pro α2(I) collagen gene, COLIA2, on chromosome 7. *Cytogenet. Cell Genet.* **41**, 234–9.

Castile, R., Shwachman, H., Travis, W., Hadley, C. A., Warwick, W. and Missmahl, H. P. (1985). Amyloidosis as a complication of cystic fibrosis. *Am. J. Dis. Child.* **139**, 728–32.

Colten, H. R. (1986). Genetics of cystic fibrosis. *J. Pediatr.* **109**, 154–5.

Eiberg, H., Mohr, J., Schmiegelow, K., Neilsen, L. S. and Williamson, R. (1985). Linkage relationships of paraoxonase (PON) with other markers: indication of PON–cystic fibrosis synteny. *Clin. Genet.* **28**, 265–71.

Farrall, M., Scambler, P., Klinger, K. W., Davies, K., Worrall, C., Williamson, R. and Wainwright, B. (1986a). Cystic fibrosis carrier detection using a linked gene probe. *J. Med. Genet.* **23**, 295–9.

——, Law, H.-Y., Rodeck, C. H., Warren, R., Stainer, P., Super, M., Lissens, W., Scambler, P., Watson, E., Wainwright, B. and Williamson, R. (1986b). First-trimester prenatal diagnosis of cystic fibrosis with linked DNA probes. *Lancet* **1**, 1402–5.

Klinger, K., Stanislovitis, P., Hoffman, N., Watkins, P. C., Schwartz, R., Doherty, R., Scambler, P., Farrall, M., Williamson, R. and Wainwright, B. (1986). Genetic homogeneity of cystic fibrosis. *Nucl. Acids Res.* **14**, 8681–6.

Knowlton, R. G., Cohen-Haguenauer, O., Von Cong, N., Frezal, J., Brown, V. A., Barker, D., Braman, J. C., Schuman, J. W., Tsui, L.-P., Buchwald, M. and Donis-

Keller, H. (1985). A polymorphic DNA marker linked to cystic fibrosis is located on chromosome 7. *Nature* **318**, 380–2.

Liechti-Gallatis, S., Braga, S., Moser, H. and Hirsiger, H. (1986). How many families will be informative for prenatal prediction of cystic fibrosis with multiple linked DNA probes? *Lancet* **2**, 392–3.

McGlennen, R. C., Burke, B. A. and Dehner, L. P. (1986). Systemic amyloidosis complicating cystic fibrosis. *Arch. Pathol. Lab. Med.* **110**, 879–84.

Robson, A. M., Tateishi, S., Ingelfinger, J. R., Strominger, D. B. and Klahr, S. (1971). Renal function in patients with cystic fibrosis. *J. Pediatr.* **79**, 42–50.

Scambler, P. J., Wainwright, B. J., Farrall, M., Bell, J., Stanier, P., Lench, N. J., Bell, G., Kruyer, H., Ramirez, F. and Williamson, R. (1985). Linkage of COL1A2 collagen gene to cystic fibrosis and its clinical applications. *Lancet* **2**, 1241–2.

——, Bell, G., Watson, E., Farrall, M., Bates, G., Davies, K., Lench, N., Ashworth, A., Williamson, R., Tippett, P. and Wainwright, B. (1986a). Cystic fibrosis linkage exclusion data. *Cytogenet. Cell Genet.* **41**, 62–3.

——, Wainwright, B. J., Watson, E., Bates, G., Bell, G., Williamson, R. and Farrall, M. (1986b). Isolation of a further anonymous informative DNA sequence from chromosome seven closely linked to cystic fibrosis. *Nucl. Acids Res.* **14**, 1951–6.

——, Law, H.-Y., Williamson, R. and Cooper, C. S. (1986c). Chromosome mediated gene transfer of six DNA markers linked to the cystic fibrosis locus on human chromosome seven. *Nucl. Acids Res.* **14**, 7159–74.

Schmiegelow, K., Eiberg, H., Tsui, L.-C., Buchwald, M., Phelan, P. D., Williamson, R., Warwick, W., Niebuhr, E., Mohr, J., Schwartz, M. and Koch, C. (1986). Linkage between the loci for cystic fibrosis and paraoxonase. *Clin. Genet.* **29**, 374–7.

Spiro, M., Chai, R. P., Isles, A. F., Balfe, J. W., Brown, R. G., Thiessen, J. J. and MacLeod, S. M. (1985). Assessment of glomerular filtration rate and effective renal plasma flow in cystic fibrosis. *J. Pediatr.* **107**, 64–70.

Standvik, B. (1982). Renal disturbance in cystic fibrosis. *Lancet* **1**, 800.

Super, M., Hambleton, G., Elles, R., Schwartz, M. and Harris, R. (1986). Pre-conception counselling for parents who have a child with cystic fibrosis. *Lancet* **2**, 393–4.

Travis, W. D., Castile, R., Vawter, G., Schwachman, H., Warwick, W., Burke, B. A. and Skinner, M. (1986). Secondary (AA) amyloidosis in cystic fibrosis. *Am. J. Clin. Pathol.* **85**, 419–24.

Tsui, L.-P., Buchwald, M., Barker, D., Braman, J. C., Knowlton, R., Schumm, J. W., Eiberg, H., Mohr, J., Kennedy, D., Plavsic, N., Zsiga, M., Markiewicz, D., Akots, G., Brown, N., Helms, C., Gravius, T., Parker, C., Rediker, K. and Donis-Keller, H. (1985a). Cystic fibrosis locus defined by a genetically linked polymorphic DNA locus. *Science* **230**, 1054–7.

——, Zsiga, M., Kennedy, D., Plavsic, N., Markiewicz, D. and Buchwald, M. (1985b). Cystic fibrosis: progress in mapping the disease locus using polymorphic DNA markers. I. *Cytogenet. Cell Genet.* **39**, 299–301.

Wainwright, B. J., Scambler, P. J., Schmidtke, J., Watson, E. A., Law, H.-Y., Farrall, M., Cooke, H. J., Eisberg, H. and Williamson, R. (1985). Localisation of cystic fibrosis to human chromosome 7cen-q22. *Nature* **318**, 385–6.

——, ——, Farrall, M., Schwartz, M. and Williamson, R. (1986). Linkage between the cystic fibrosis locus and markers on chromosome 7q. *Cytogenet. Cell Genet.* **41**, 191–2.

White, R., Woodward, S., Leppert, M., O'Connell, P., Hoff, M., Herbst, J., Lalouel, J.-M., Dean, M. and Van de Woude, G. (1985). A closely linked genetic marker for cystic fibrosis. *Nature* **318**, 382–4.

8.8. ACUTE INTERMITTENT PORPHYRIA

Transient renal impairment is common during the acute attacks of acute intermittent porphyria (Stein and Tschudy 1970; Schley *et al.* 1970). Whitelaw (1974) reported the case of an 11-year-old girl who developed renal failure during an acute porphyric attack that could not be attributed to any other cause. Renal impairment persisted after the attack. Yeung and colleagues (1983) conducted a retrospective survey of patients with proved acute intermittent porphyria on the files of the Porphyria Research Unit at Glasgow Royal Infirmary, and diagnosed over a 20-year period. They identified six patients who also had early onset chronic renal failure. No other cause of the renal failure in these six patients could be detected, nor could it be attributed to porphyria-associated analgesic nephropathy or any nephrotoxic effects of porphyrins or their precursors. They concluded that porphyria-induced hypertension was the most important aetiological factor in this association. Acute intermittent porphyria is inherited in an autosomal dominant manner.

References

Schley, G., Bock, K. D., Hacevar, V. *et al.* (1970). Hypertension and tachycardia in acute intermittent porphyria [in German]. *Klin. Wschr.* **48**, 36–42.

Stein, J. A. and Tschudy, D. P. (1970). Acute intermittent porphyria—a clinical and biochemical study of 46 patients. *Medicine* **49**, 1–16.

Yeung Laiwah, A. A. C., Mactier, R., McColl, K. E. L., Moore, M. R. and Goldberg, A. (1983). Early-onset chronic renal failure as a complication of acute intermittent porphyria. *Quart. J. Med.* **52**, 92–8.

Whitelaw, A. G. L. (1974). Acute intermittent porphyria, hypercholesterolaemia, and renal impairment. *Arch. Dis. Child.* **49**, 406–7.

8.9. GOODPASTURE'S SYNDROME

Goodpasture's syndrome combines glomerulonephritis and pulmonary haemorrhage. It is generally regarded as an autoimmune disorder. Indeed anti-GBM antibodies obtained from patients with the disorder have been widely used in clinical research into GBM disorders. However,

Holdsworth and colleagues (1985), in a recent study of the variation in the clinico-pathological picture in 40 patients, have shown that only seven had anti-GBM antibodies. Twenty-two out of their 40 patients had a systemic vasculitis and five were idiopathic. All seven patients with anti-GBM antibodies had diffuse proliferative glomerulonephritis, with crescents in all of the glomeruli examined. All seven also had deposits of IgG immunoglobulin and C3 component of complement, 3 patients also had IgM deposits.

The syndrome is usually of sporadic occurrence. The observations of Holdsworth and colleagues suggest that it is heterogeneous in aetiology. However, there is little evidence for genetic factors in the great majority of cases, apart from the strong association with HLA-DRW2 mentioned earlier (p. 300) (Rees *et al.* 1978, 1984). There is a single report of the syndrome in identical twins (D'Apice *et al.* 1978), and only two other reports record familial occurrence (Maddock *et al.* 1967; Gossain *et al.* 1972).

References

D'Apice, A. J. F., Kincaid-Smith, P., Becker, G. J., Longhhead, M. G., Freeman, J. W. and Sands, J. M. (1978). Goodpasture's syndrome in identical twins. *Ann. Intern. Med.* **88**, 61–2.

Gossain, V. V., Gerstein, A. R. and Jones, A. W. (1972). Goodpasture's syndrome: a familial occurrence. *Am. Rev. Resp. Dis.* **105**, 621–4.

Holdsworth, S., Boyce, N., Thompson, N. M. and Atkins, R. C. (1985). The clinical spectrum of acute glomerulonephritis and lung haemorhage (Goodpasture's syndrome). *Quart. J. Med.* **55**, 75–86.

Maddock, R. K. Jr., Stevens, L. E., Reemtsma, K. and Bloomer, H. A. (1967). Goodpasture's syndrome: cessation of pulmonary hemorrhage after bilateral nephrectomy. *Ann. Intern. Med.* **67**, 1259–64.

Rees, A. J., Peters, D. K., Compston, D. A. S. and Batchelor, J. R. (1978). Strong association between HLA-DRW2 and antibody-mediated Goodpasture's syndrome. *Lancet* **1**, 966–8.

——, ——, Amos, N., Welsh, K. I. and Batchelor, J. R. (1984). The influence of HLA-linked genes on the severity of anti-GBM-antibody-mediated nephritis. *Kidney Int.* **26**, 445–50.

8.10. LAURENCE–MOON AND BARDET–BIEDL SYNDROMES

Laurence and Moon (1866) described four sibs with mental subnormality, retinitis pigmentosa, spastic paraplegia, and hypogenitalism. Further reports of this syndrome came from subsequent authors (Hutchinson 1882, 1900; Kapuscinski 1934; Bowen *et al.* 1965). A similar disorder of mental subnormality, retinitis pigmentosa, poly-dactyly, obesity, non-insulin-dependent diabetes, and hypogenitalism was reported by Bardet (1920) and by Biedl (1922). Many authors have regarded these two syndromes as varying manifestations of the same disorder (Solis-Cohen and Weiss 1925), usually termed Laurence–Moon–Biedl syndrome: others have considered them to be distinct disorders (Amman 1970; Schachat and Maumenee 1982). Both disorders appear to be inherited in an autosomal recessive manner. Renal abnormalities are common in at least the Bardet–Biedl syndrome, with more than one-third of patients dying from renal failure. Hydronephrosis and renal hypoplasia were reported by Nadjini and colleagues (1969), but calyceal dilation and clubbing, and medullary cysts, are the most frequently reported defects (Alton and McDonald 1973).

Many early reports, quoted by Kissane (1973), described shrunken kidneys with severe chronic glomerulonephritis. These were mostly autopsy reports of the terminal stage of the disease. An earlier stage of chronic nephritis has also been described in renal biopsies, with small, irregular kidneys with calyceal distortion, impaired urine concentration, and a variable histological picture (Hurley *et al.* 1975). In the early cases a mild to more marked increase in mesangial tissue was seen, and in later cases glomerular sclerosis. In the most advanced cases there was cystic dilation of tubules in both the cortex and medulla, and interstitial fibrosis and round-cell infiltration. It is not clear as to whether the medullary cysts seen on urography in earlier reports is the end-stage of the cystic change described by Hurley and colleagues.

Recent studies of the renal lesion have in general confirmed the above picture. Roussel and colleagues (1985) described a 6-year-old girl whose two elder brothers had been affected, and had died of renal failure. She presented with the features of the Bardet–Biedl variant of the syndrome. Her renal impairment necessitated dialysis. A renal biopsy showed a diffuse mixed tubular and interstitial nephritis with glomerulosclerosis. Linné and coworkers (1986) studied six patients, two of whom were sibs, all with the Bardet–Biedl syndrome. All six were found to have renal abnormalities; five had small kidneys with reduced GFR and concentrating ability. Two of them had developed end-stage renal failure, one of whom was successfully transplanted.

Alströms disease is a distinct disease with some similarities to Laurence–Moon–Bardet–Biedl syndrome. The main features are retinitis pigmentosa, type II diabetes mellitus, obesity, perceptive deafness, acanthosis nigricans, male hypogonadism, baldness, hypertriglyceri-daemia, and renal insufficiency (Alström *et al.* 1959; Weinstein *et al.* 1969; Goldstein and Fialkow 1973; Millay *et al.* 1986). Intelligence is normal. The renal disease is age related and is the commonest cause of death. Weinstein and colleagues (1969) reported two affected brothers, Goldstein and Fialkow (1973) three affected sisters, and Millay and coworkers (1986) a patient with consanguineous parents. These observations, and others, leave little doubt that inheritance is autosomal recessive.

References

Alström, C. H., Hallgren, B. and Nilsson, L. B. (1959). Retinal degeneration combined with obesity, diabetes mellitus and neurogenous deafness: a specific syndrome (not hitherto described) distinct from the Laurence–Moon–Biedl–Bardet syndrome. *Acta Psychiat. Neurol. Scand.* **34** (Suppl. 129), 1–35.

Alton, D. J. and McDonald, P. (1973). Urographic findings in Laurence–Moon–Biedl syndrome. *Radiology* **109**, 659–63.

Amman, F. (1970). Investigations cliniques et genetiques sur le syndrome de Bardet–Biedl en Suisse. *J. Genet. Hum.* **18** (Suppl.), 1–310.

Bardet, G. (1920). Sur un syndrome d'obesite infantile avec polydactylie et retinite pigmentaire (contribution à l'étude des formes cliniques de l'obesite hypophysaire). Thesis, Paris, No. 479.

Biedl, A. (1922). Ein Geschwisterpaar mit adiposo-genitaler Dystrophie. *Dtsch. Med. Wschr.* **48**, 1630.

Bowen, P., Ferguson-Smith, M. A., Moster, D., Lee, C. S. N. and Butler, H. G. (1965). The Laurence–Moon Syndrome: association with hypogonadotrophic hypogonadism and sex-chromosome aneuploidy. *Arch. Intern. Med.* **116**, 598–604.

Goldstein, J. L. and Fialkow, P. J. (1973). The Alström syndrome. Report of three cases with further delineation of the clinical, pathophysiological and genetic aspects of the disorder. *Medicine* **52**, 53–71.

Hurley, R. M., Dery, P., Nogrady, M. B. and Drummond, K. N. (1975). The renal lesion in the Laurence–Moon–Biedl syndrome. *J. Pediatr.* **87**, 206–9.

Hutchinson, J. (1882). On retinitis pigmentosa and allied affections, as illustrating the laws of heredity. *Ophthalmol. Rev.* **1**, 2–7, 26–30.

—— (1900). Slowly progressive paraplegia and disease of the choroids with defective intellect and arrested sexual development. *Arch. Surg.* **11**, 118–22.

Kapuscinski, W. (1934). Ueber familiaere Aderhautentartung mit ataktischen Stoerungen. *Ber. Dtsch. Ophthalmol. Ges.* **50**, 13–19.

Kissane, J. M. (1973). Hereditary disorders of the kidney. Part II: Hereditary nephropathies. *Perspect. Paediatr. Pathol.* **1**, 147–87.

Laurence, J. Z. and Moon, R. C. (1866). Four cases of retinitis pigmentosa occurring in the same family and accompanied by general imperfection of development. *Ophthalmol. Rev.* **2**, 32–41.

Linné, T., Wikstad, I. and Zetterstrom, R. (1986). Renal involvement in the Laurence–Moon–Biedl syndrome. *Acta Paediatr. Scand.* **75**, 240–4.

Millay, R. H., Weleber, R. G. and Heckenlively, J. R. (1986). Ophthalmologic and systemic manifestations of Alström's disease. *Am. J. Ophthalmol.* **102**, 482–90.

Nadjini, B., Flanagan, M. J. and Christian, J. R. (1969). Laurence–Moon–Biedl syndrome. *Am. J. Dis. Child.* **117**, 352–6.

Roussel, B., Leroux, B., Gaillard, D. and Fandre, M. (1985). Syndrome de Laurence–Moon–Bardet–Biedl, néphrite tubulo-interstitielle chronique diffuse et atteinte hépatique. *Helv. Paediatr. Acta* **40**, 405–13.

Schachat, A. P. and Maumenee, I. H. (1982). The Bardet–Biedl syndrome and related disorders. *Arch. Ophthalmol.* **100**, 285–8.

Solis-Cohen, S. and Weiss, E. (1925). Dystrophia adiposo-genitalis with atypical retinitis pigmentosa and mental deficiency: the Laurence–Biedl syndrome. *Am. J. Med. Sci.* **169**, 489–505.

Weinstein, R. L., Kliman, B. and Scully, R. E. (1969). Familial syndrome of primary testicular insufficiency with normal virilization, blindness, deafness and metabolic abnormalities. *New Engl. J. Med.* **281**, 967–77.

8.11. WISKOTT–ALDRICH SYNDROME AND FAMILIAL THROMBOCYTOPENIA WITH ELEVATED SERUM IgA AND GLOMERULONEPHRITIS

This immune deficiency syndrome is characterized by eczema, thrombo-cytopenic purpura, liability to infection, especially ear infections, and bloody diarrhoea in boys (Wiskott 1937; Aldrich *et al.* 1954; Van den Bosch and Drukker 1964). Death usually ensures under 4 years of age from infection or bleeding, and survivors tend to develop lymphomas or leukaemia. Perry and colleagues (1980) reported an incidence of 4 per million live male births in the United States of America. A variety of immune disorders have been described in Wiskott–Aldrich syndrome: low or absent ABO blood group haemagglutinins (Krivit and Good 1959), normal IgG, raised IgA and low IgM immunoglobulins (Cooper *et al.* 1968), delayed hypersensitivity, and impaired graft rejection but normal T-lymphocyte transformation by phytohaemagglutinin. These latter observations have led to the suggestion that antigen recognition and processing are impaired (Blaese *et al.* 1968; Cooper *et al.* 1968). This view received support from the evidence of Parkman and coworkers (1981) for the absence of a lymphocyte surface protein, and of a platelet surface glycoprotein, which may also account for the dual defect in this disorder.

Family studies have shown that the disorder is clearly X linked recessive. This is confirmed by Gealy and associates (1980) who demon-strated that in a female heterozygote, who was also heterozygous for the A and B variants of glucose 6-phosphate dehydrogenase, that only the B form of the enzyme was expressed in T lymphocytes and platelets, although both A and B forms were expressed in other tissues. This indicated that the X chromosome carrying the Wiskott–Aldrich gene was selected against in the T-lymphocyte and platelet cell compartments. Van den Bosch and Drukker (1964) observed low platelet counts in three out of five female obligate heterozygotes, and Shapiro and others (1978) demonstrated a defect in platelet oxidative phosphorylation that was expressed in heterozygotes.

Spitler and colleagues (1980) described a nephropathy in six out of 33 patients with Wiskott–Aldrich syndrome. The changes included haematuria, urine casts and proteinuria, raised blood urea and creatine, and reduced creatinine clearance. One patient became nephrotic and another died in hypertensive congestive heart failure. The latter patient showed an interstitial nephritis on renal biopsy and another a chronic proliferative glomerulonephritis at autopsy.

An earlier report described a family in which 12 members had thrombocytopenia, elevated serum IgA, and at least three of them had renal disease (Gutenberger *et al.* 1970). Inheritance appeared to be X linked. Standen and associates (1986) have recently described a very similar family in which 13 males have been affected over three generations. Five of the affected patients had suffered eczema since infancy. Minor abnormalities of immune function led the authors to conclude that both their family, and that of Gutenberger and coworkers, have a variant of Wiskott–Aldrich syndrome with partial expression. As they point out, confirmation will depend on the isolation of a DNA polymorphism linked to the Wiskott–Aldrich gene.

References

Aldrich, R. A., Steinberg, A. G. and Campbell, D. C. (1954). Pedigree demonstrating a sex-linked recessive condition characterized by draining ears, eczematoid dermatitis and bloody diarrhoea. *Pediatrics* **13**, 133–9.

Blaese, R. M., Strober, W., Brown, R. S. and Waldmann, T. A. (1968). The Wiskott–Aldrich syndrome: a disorder with a possible defect in antigen processing or recognition. *Lancet* **1**, 1056–61.

Cooper, M. D., Chae, H. P., Lowman, J. T., Krivit, W. and Good, R. A. (1968). Wiskott–Aldrich syndrome. An immunologic deficiency disease involving the afferent limb of immunity. *Am. J. Med.* **44**, 499–513.

Gealy, W. J., Dwyer, J. M. and Harley, J. B. (1980). Allelic exclusion of glucose-6-phosphate dehydrogenase in platelets and T lymphocytes from a Wiskott–Aldrich syndrome carrier. *Lancet* **1**, 63–5.

Gutenberger, J., Trygstad, C. W., Stiehm, E. R., Opitz, J. M., Thatcher, L. G., Bloodworth, J. M. B. Jr. and Setzkorn, J. (1970). Familial thrombocytopenia, elevated serum IgA levels and renal disease: a report of a kindred. *Am. J. Med.* **49**, 729–41.

Krivit, W. and Good, R. A. (1959). Aldrich's syndrome (thrombocytopenia, eczema and infection in infants). Studies of the defense mechanisms. *Am. J. Dis. Child.* **97**, 137–53.

Parkman, R., Remold-O'Donnell, E., Kenney, D. M., Perrine, S. and Rosen, F. S. (1981). Surface protein abnormalities in lymphocytes and platelets from patients with Wiskott–Aldrich syndrome. *Lancet* **2**, 1387–9.

Perry, G. S., Spector, B. D., Schuman, L. M., Mandel, J. S., Anderson, V. E., McHugh, R. B., Hanson, M. R., Fahlstrom, S. M., Krivit, W. and Kersey, J. H. (1980). The Wiskott–Aldrich syndrome in the United States and Canada (1892–1979). *J. Pediatr.* **97**, 72–8.

Shapiro, R. S., Gerrard, J. M., Perry, G. S., White, J. G., Krivit, W. and Kersey, J. H. (1978). Wiskott–Aldrich syndrome: detection of carrier state by metabolic stress of platelets. *Lancet* **1**, 121–3.

Spitler, L. E., Wray, B. B., Mogerman, S., Miller, J. J., O'Reilly, R. J. and Lagios, M. (1980). Nephropathy in the Wiskott–Aldrich syndrome. *Pediatrics* **66**, 391–8.

Standen, G. R., Lillicrap, D. P., Matthews, N. and Bloom, A. L. (1986). Inherited thrombocytopenia, elevated serum IgA and renal disease: identification as a variant of the Wiskott–Aldrich syndrome. *Quart. J. Med.* **59**, 401–8.

Van den Bosch, J. and Drukker, J. (1964). Het syndroom van Aldrich: een klinisch en genetisch Onderzoek van enige Nederlandse Families. *Maandschr. Kindergeneesk.* **32**, 359–73.

Wiskott, A. (1937). Familiärer, engelborener Morbus Werlhofii? *Monatschr. Kinderheilk.* **68**, 212–16.

8.12. MARFAN SYNDROME

This autosomal dominant syndrome is characterized by tall height, relative increase in length of the long bones of limbs and digits, joint laxity, myopia and ectopia lentis, mitral valve prolapse, and dilatation of the aortic root (Pyeritz and McKusick 1979). It is thought to be a connective tissue disorder (Pyeritz and McKusick 1981), although there is almost certainly genetic heterogeneity at the molecular level. For example Byers and colleagues (1981) detected an abnormality of one of the α_2-chains of type I collagen in one out of 11 cases studied.

The kidneys are not usually in any way abnormal in Marfan syndrome although renal duplication and ectopia have been reported in four patients, and chronic pyelonephritis in a further four patients (Loughridge 1959).

Expressivity of the syndrome is variable. About a quarter of cases are fresh mutations and such new mutant cases show a paternal age effect. The only one of several linkage studies to obtain a positive lod score, a low one of 1.17 at $\theta = 0.30$ for linkage to rhesus, was that of Mace (1979).

References

Byers, P. H., Siegel, R. C., Peterson, K. E., Rowe, D. W., Holbrook, K. A., Smith, L. T., Chang, Y.-H. and Fu, J. C. C. (1981). Marfan syndrome: abnormal α-2 chain in type I collagen. *Proc. Nat. Acad. Sci.* **78**, 7745–9.

Loughridge, L. W. (1959). Renal abnormalities in the Marfan syndrome. *Quart. J. Med.* **28**, 531–44.

Mace, M. (1979). A suggestion of linkage between the Marfan syndrome and the rhesus blood group. *Clin. Genet.* **16**, 96–102.

Pyeritz, R. E. and McKusick, V. A. (1979). The Marfan syndrome. *New Engl. J. Med.* **300**, 772–7.

—— and McKusick, V. A. (1981). Basic defects in the Marfan syndrome (editorial). *New Engl. J. Med.* **305**, 1011–12.

8.13. COCKAYNE SYNDROME

Patients with this syndrome show a prematurely senile appearance. They are dwarfed, and develop pigmentary tapeto-retinal degeneration, optic atrophy and deafness, light sensitivity, mental retardation, and marbled digital epiphyses (MacDonald *et al.* 1960; Paddison *et al.* 1963; Proops *et al.* 1981). Ultraviolet light sensitivity of cultured cells from patients has been observed by several groups (Schmickel *et al.* 1977; Andrews *et al.* 1978; Deschavanne *et al.* 1981).

Hypertension and renal disease are relatively common findings (MacDonald *et al.* 1960; Ohno and Hirooka 1966; Fujimoto *et al.* 1969; Higginbottom *et al.* 1979). Ohno and Hirooka studied three cases, all of whom had impaired renal function, and two of whom on renal biopsy showed glomerular basement membrane thickening, hyalinization of glomeruli, tubular atrophy, and interstitial fibrosis. Fujimoto and colleagues (1969) in a study of a single case demonstrated renal insufficiency and reduced creatinine clearance, azotaemia, and hyperchloraemic acidosis. Higginbottom and associates also studied three children, including two brothers, and observed similar changes to those described by Ohno and Hirooka in renal biopsies from two of them. They also demonstrated glomerular deposits of complement and immunoglobulins. Hernandez and coworkers (1975) reported a more advanced renal lesion with nephrosclerosis.

Inheritance is autosomal recessive (MacDonald *et al.* 1960; Paddison *et al.* 1963; Pearce 1972; Higginbottom *et al.* 1979; Proops *et al.* 1981).

References

Andrews, A. D., Barrett, S. F., Yoder, F. W. and Robbins, J. H. (1978). Cockayne's syndrome fibroblasts have increased sensitivity to ultraviolet light but normal rates of unscheduled DNA synthesis. *J. Invest. Dermatol.* **70**, 237–9.

Deschavanne, P. J., Diatloff-Zito, C., Macieira-Coelho, A. and Malaise, E.-P. (1981). Unusual sensitivity of two Cockayne's syndrome cell strains to both UV and gamma irradiation. *Mutat. Res.* **91**, 403–6.

Fujimoto, W. Y., Greene, M. L. and Seegmiller, J. E. (1969). Cockayne's syndrome: report of a case with hyperlipoproteinemia, hyperinsulinemia, renal disease, and normal growth hormone. *J. Pediatr.* **75**, 881–4.

Hernandez, A. L., DeLeon, B. and De La Puente, S. G. (1975). Lesiones renales ultraestructurales del sindrome de Cockayne. *Rev. Invest. Clin.* **27**, 153–8.

Higginbottom, M. C., Griswold, W. R., Jones, K. L., Vasquez, M. D., Mendoza, S. A. and Wilson, C. B. (1979). The Cockayne syndrome: an evaluation of hypertension and studies of renal pathology. *Pediatrics* **64**, 929–34.

MacDonald, W. B., Fitch, K. D. and Lewis, I. C. (1960). Cockayne's syndrome: a heredo-familial disorder of growth and development. *Pediatrics* **25**, 997–1007.

Ohno, T. and Hirooka, M. (1966). Renal lesions in Cockayne's syndrome. *Tohoku J. Exp. Med.* **89**, 151–66.

Paddison, R. M., Moosey, J., Derbes, V. J. and Kloepfer, H. W. (1963). Cockayne's syndrome: a report of five new cases with biochemical, chromosomal, dermatologic, genetic and neuropathologic observations. *Dermatol. Trop.* **2**, 195–203.

Pearce, W. G. (1972). Ocular and genetic features of Cockayne's syndrome. *Can. J. Ophthalmol.* **7**, 435–44.

Proops, R., Taylor, A. M. R. and Insley, J. (1981). A clinical study of a family with Cockayne's syndrome. *J. Med. Genet.* **18**, 288–93.

Schmickel, R. D., Chu, E. H. Y., Trosko, J. E. and Change, C. C. (1977). Cockayne syndrome: a cellular sensitivity to ultraviolet light. *Pediatrics* **60**, 135–9.

8.14. α_1-ANTITRYPSIN DEFICIENCY

Necrotizing angiitis and glomerulonephritis have been reported as complicating the autosomal recessive disorder α_1-antitrypsin deficiency with emphysema in a 53-year-old man (Miller and Kuschner 1969). At autopsy there was proliferative glomerulonephritis with crescent formation and capillary thrombi in the kidneys and arteritis in the lungs, skeletal muscle, and other tissues, with fibrinoid necrosis and destruction of the elastic lamina. A similar case involving a 44-year-old man with diffuse vasculitis of skin, kidneys, and colon has subsequently been reported (Lewis *et al.* 1985). The renal vasculitis resulted in a rapidly progressive glomerulonephritis with epithelial crescents in 97 per cent of glomeruli at autopsy. Alpha₁-antitrypsin has been demonstrated in blood vessel walls of skin in cutaneous vasculitis (Brandup and Ostergaard 1978), and glomeruli in membranoproliferative glomerulonephritis of childhood (Moroz *et al.* 1976), in association with cirrhosis and α_1-antitrypsin deficiency. Although glomerulonephritis is a rare complication of α_1-antitrypsin deficiency these observations suggest that it is more than just a chance association.

References

Brandup, F. and Ostergaard, P. A. (1978). Alpha₁-antitrypsin deficiency associated with persistent cutaneous vasculitis. *Arch. Dermatol.* **114**, 921–4.

Lewis, M., Kallenbach, J., Zaltzman, M., Levy, H., Lurie, D., Baynes, R., King, P. and Meyers, A. (1985). Severe deficiency of alpha$_1$-antitrypsin associated with cutaneous vasculitis, rapidly progressive glomerulonephritis, and colitis. *Am. J. Med.* **79**, 489–94.

Miller, F. and Kuschner, M. (1969). Alpha$_1$-antitrypsin deficiency, emphysema, necrotizing angiitis and glomerulonephritis. *Am. J. Med.* **46**, 615–23.

Moroz, S. P., Cutz, E., Williamson Balfe, J. and Sass-Kortsak, A. (1976). Membranoproliferative glomerulonephritis in childhood cirrhosis associated with alpha$_1$-antitrypsin deficiency. *Pediatrics* **57**, 232–8.

8.15. CHARCOT–MARIE–TOOTH DISEASE

Two brothers, and a further unrelated patient, have been described with Charcot–Marie–Tooth disease and renal abnormalities (Lemieux and Neemeh 1967). The elder brother, aged 34 years, had proteinuria, cylinduria, and microscopic haematuria, with foci of tubular atrophy and lymphocytic infiltration on renal biopsy. Some glomeruli showed thickened basement membranes, and there were foam cells in the interstitium. The younger brother, aged 25 years, had microscopic haematuria and on renal biopsy some lymphocytic infiltration and foci of tubular atrophy. The third patient was a 21-year-old woman with hypertension and persistent proteinuria. The brothers had nerve deafness and also had a further brother with gross haematuria but without Charcot–Marie–Tooth disease, and a sister with Charcot–Marie–Tooth disease alone. This raises the question as to whether Alport's disease may have been segregating independently of the Charcot–Marie–Tooth disease in this family. The affected woman's mother, brother, and sister also had Charcot–Marie–Tooth disease but no nephropathy, which again casts doubt on the significance of the association of the two disorders.

References

Lemieux, G. and Neemeh, J. A. (1967). Charcot–Marie–Tooth disease and nephritis. *Can. Med. Assoc. J.* **97**, 1193–8.

8.16. GENERALIZED NEUROFIBROMATOSIS

Renal tract involvement in generalized neurofibromatosis, or von Recklinghausen's disease, is rare. When it does occur the bladder is most commonly affected, causing urinary incontinence and in many cases hydroureteralnephrosis, frequently with simultaneous involvement of the genitalia (McDonnell 1936; Hess 1938; Labardini *et al.* 1967; Daneman and Gratten-Smith 1976; Jenson and Nissen 1976; Clark *et al.* 1977;

Forbes 1979; Borden and Shrader 1980; Elliott *et al.* 1981; Kramer *et al.* 1981; Rink and Mitchell 1983). In most of these cases the bladder is affected by a plexiform neuroma with a reduction of bladder capacity and urethral obstruction. The genitalia may be affected without bladder involvement (Dehner and Smith 1970; Fethiere *et al.* 1974; Greer and Pederson 1981; Dwosh *et al.* 1984). Genital involvement usually takes the form of penile and/or scrotal enlargement in the male or pseudo-masculinization of the clitoris in the female. The neurofibromata giving rise to these various lesions are thought to arise in the pelvic autonomic plexus (Pessin and Bodian 1964). Recently a typical patient has been reported with penile and scrotal hypertrophy, bladder wall hypertrophy, ureteral obstruction, and bilateral hydronephrosis due to a pelvic plexiform neurofibroma (Ogawa and Watanabe 1986).

Neurofibromata can develop in the kidney as elsewhere but are surprisingly uncommon. A rare association with neurofibromatosis is Wilm's tumour, which has been reported on three occasions (Miller 1969; Kung and Nyman 1973; Walden *et al.* 1977). A unique association described in a single family is with eosinophilic renal carcinoma (Valleteau de Moulliac *et al.* 1974), discussed in Chapter 12 (p. 632).

Hypertension may develop as a result of an associated phaeochromocytoma or from a plexiform neuroma causing renal artery stenosis.

References

Borden, T. A. and Shrader, D. A. (1980). Neurofibromatosis of the bladder in a child: unusual cause of enuresis. *Urology* **15**, 155–8.

Clark, S. S., Marlett, M. M., Prudencio, R. F. and DasGupta, T. K. (1977). Neurofibromatosis of the bladder in children: case report and literature review. *J. Urol.* **118**, 654–6.

Daneman, A. and Gratten-Smith, P. (1976). Neurofibromatosis involving the lower urinary tract in children. A report of three cases and a review of the literature. *Pediatr. Radiol.* **4**, 161–6.

Dehner, L. P. and Smith, B. H. (1970). Soft tissue tumors of the penis. A clinico-pathologic study of 46 cases. *Cancer* **25**, 1431–7.

Dwosh, J., Mininberg, D. T., Schlossberg, S. and Peterson, P. (1984). Neuro-fibroma involving the penis in a child. *J. Urol.* **132**, 988–9.

Elliott, F. G., Eid, T. C. and Lakey, W. H. (1981). Genitourinary neurofibromas: clinical significance. *J. Urol.* **125**, 725–7.

Fethiere, W., Carter, H. W. and Sturim, H. S. (1974). Elephantiasis neuromatosa of the penis. Light and electron microscopical studies. *Arch. Pathol.* **97**, 326–30.

Forbes, K. A. (1979). Neurofibromatous ureteral obstruction relieved by sigmoid conduit cytoplasty. *J. Urol.* **121**, 100–2.

Greer, D. M. Jr. and Pederson, W. C. (1981). Pseudomasculinisation of the phallus. *Plast. Reconstr. Surg.* **68**, 787–8.

Hess, E. (1938). Sarcoma of prostate and adjacent retrovesical structures. *J. Urol.* **40**, 629–40.

Jensen, A. and Nissen, H. M. (1976). Neurofibromatosis of the bladder. *Scand. J. Urol. Nephrol.* **10**, 157–9.

Kramer, S. A., Barrett, D. M. and Utz, D. C. (1981). Neurofibromatosis of the bladder in children. *J. Urol.* **126**, 693–4.

Kung, F. H. and Nyman, W. L. (1973). In *Cancer medicine*, eds. Holland, J. and Frei, E. III, pp. 188. Lee & Febiger, Philadelphia.

Labardini, M. M., Kallet, H. A. and Cerny, J. C. (1967). Urogenital neurofibromatosis simulating an intersex problem. *J. Urol.* **98**, 627–32.

McDonnell, C. H. (1936). Neurofibromatosis of bladder and prostate. *Am. J. Surg.* **34**, 90–3.

Miller, R. W. (1969). Childhood cancer and congenital defects. A study of US death certificates during the period 1960–1966. *Pediatr. Res.* **3**, 389–97.

Ogawa, A. and Watanabe, K. (1986). Genitourinary neurofibromatosis in a child presenting with an enlarged penis and scrotum. *J. Urol.* **135**, 755–7.

Pessin, J. I. and Bodian, M. (1964). Neurofibromatosis of the pelvic autonomic plexus. *Br. J. Urol.* **36**, 510–18.

Rink, R. C. and Mitchell, M. E. (1983). Genitourinary neurofibromatosis in childhood. *J. Urol.* **130**, 1176–9.

Valleteau de Moulliac, M., Ganansia, R., Hors, J., Letexier, A. and Morin, M. (1974). Cancer du rein familial et systeme HLA. Quatre cancers du rein gauche dans une fratrie. *La Nouv. Presse Méd.* **3**, 1539–42.

Walden, P. A. M., Johnson, A. G. and Bagshawe, K. D. (1977). Wilms' tumour and neurofibromatosis. *Br. Med. J.* **1**, 813.

8.17. SEVERE JUVENILE ARTERIAL SCLEROSIS

Severe juvenile arterial sclerosis, or familial calcific arterial sclerosis, is listed in McKusick's *Mendelian inheritance in man*, 6th edn (1983) as having been reported to McKusick by Kaitila (1981) in a personal communication. Kaitila observed eight patients, all but one male, in five families. The features were an early onset of medial arteriosclerosis with calcification, hypertension, short stature, delayed puberty, and anaemia. There may be vertebral and hip dysplasia. Radiologically there is extensive calcification of the aorta and peripheral arteries. The renal arteries may be involved with shrinkage of glomerular tufts and relative dilatation of Bowman's space, giving a cystic appearance, and a nephrocalcinotic radiological appearance. Kaitila's families all came from the same remote part of Finland and in one family the parents were first cousins, reinforcing the view that this must be an autosomal recessive disorder.

References

Kaitila, I. (1981). Personal communication to McKusick, V. A. cited in his *Mendelian inheritance in man*, 6th edn. (1983). pp. 609–10. Johns Hopkins University Press, Baltimore.

8.18. FAMILIAL DYSAUTONOMIA

This disorder, also known as the Riley–Day syndrome, is characterized clinically by paroxysmal hypertension, excessive sweating, lack of tear formation, progressive pain insensitivity and congenital corneal anaesthesia, skin blotching, a liability to aspiration pneumonia and its complications, and emotional lability (Riley *et al.* 1949; Riley 1952; Axelrod *et al.* 1981). Axelrod (1983) has written an excellent brief review of the disorder.

Pearson and colleagues (1980) have described progressive impairment of renal function leading to glomerulosclerosis and moderate azotemia, in association with a deficiency of sympathetic nerve endings on the kidney.

Pathologically there is demyelination in the medulla and dorsal spinal tracts, and degeneration, pigmentation, and loss of cells of autonomic ganglia (Brown *et al.* 1964). The basic defect would appear to consist in a failure in the development of the autonomic and sensory nervous systems. Sympathetic ganglia are only a third of normal size (Pearson and Pytel 1978). Abnormalities of the β-subunit of nerve growth factor in both serum (Siggers *et al.* 1976) and cultured fibroblasts (Schwartz and Breakefield 1980), and axonal depletion of substance P in the spinal cord and medulla (Pearson *et al.* 1982) have been reported.

The disorder shows autosomal recessive inheritance and occurs predominantly in Ashkenazi Jews, especially Polish Ashkenazim, with a birth incidence in that population of 1 in 10 000 to 20 000 (Goldstein-Nieviazhski and Wallis 1966; McKusick *et al.* 1967; Moses *et al.* 1967; Brunt and McKusick 1970). Hence the heterozygote frequency among Ashkenazi Jews can be estimated at 1 in 50. Neither heterozygote detection nor prenatal diagnosis is as yet available.

References

Axelrod, F. B. (1983). Autonomic and sensory disorders. Chapter 23 in *Principles and practice of medical genetics*, eds. Emery, A. E. H. and Rimoin, D. L. pp. 284–95. Churchill Livingstone, Edinburgh.
——, Iyer, K., Fish, I., Pearson, J., Sein, M. E. and Spielholz, N. (1981). Progressive sensory loss in familial dysautonomia. *Pediatrics* **67**, 517–22.
Brown, W. J., Beauchemin, J. A. and Linde, L. M. (1964). A neuropathological study of familial dysautonomia (Riley–Day syndrome) in siblings. *J. Neurol. Neurosurg. Psychiatry* **27**, 131–9.
Brunt, P. W. and McKusick, V. A. (1970). Familial dysautonomia: a report of genetic and clinical studies, with a review of the literature. *Medicine* **49**, 343–74.

Goldstein-Nieviazhski, C. and Wallis, K. (1966). Riley–Day syndrome (familial dysautonomia). Survey of 27 cases. *Ann. Paediatr.* **206**, 188–94.

McKusick, V. A., Norum, R. A., Farkas, H. J., Brunt, P. W. and Mahloudji, M. (1967). The Riley–Day syndrome: observations on genetics and survivorship. *Israel J. Med. Sci.* **3**, 372–9.

Moses, S. W., Rotem, Y., Jogoda, N., Talmor, N., Eichhorn, F. and Levin, S. (1967). A clinical genetic and biochemical study of familial dysautonomia in Israel. *Israel J. Med. Sci.* **3**, 358–71.

Pearson, J. and Pytel, B. (1978). Quantitative studies of sympathetic ganglia and spinal cord intermedio-lateral gray columns in familial dysautonomia. *J. Neurol. Sci.* **39**, 47–59.

——, Gallo, G., Gluck, M. and Axelrod, F. (1980). Renal disease in familial dysautonomia. *Kidney Int.* **17**, 102–12.

——, Brandeis, L. and Cuello, A. C. (1982). Depletion of substance P-containing axons in substantia gelatinosa of patients with diminished pain sensitivity. *Nature* **295**, 61–3.

Riley, C. M. (1952). Familial autonomic dysfunction. *JAMA* **149**, 1532–5.

——, Day, R. L., Greely, D. McL. and Langford, W. S. (1949). Central autonomic dysfunction with defective lacrimation. *Pediatrics* **3**, 468–77.

Schwartz, J. P. and Breakefield, X. O. (1980). Altered nerve growth factor in fibroblasts from patients with familial dysautonomia. *Proc. Nat. Acad. Sci.* **77**, 1154–8.

Siggers, D. C., Rogers, J. G., Boyer, S. H., Margolet, L., Dorkin, H., Benerjee, S. P. and Shooter, E. M. (1976). Increased nerve growth factor β-chain cross reacting material in familial dysautonomia. *New Engl. J. Med.* **270**, 704–7.

8.19. CHRONIC GRANULOMATOUS DISEASE

Urinary tract involvement has been reported in X-linked chronic granulomatous disease with either glomerulosclerosis or an interstitial cystitis (Kontras *et al.* 1971) in the typical childhood form of the disease. In an adult variant affecting three brothers the development of glomerulonephritis was described as one of several late sequelae (Dilworth and Mandell 1977).

References

Dilworth, J. A. and Mandell, G. L. (1977). Adults with chronic granulomatous disease of 'childhood'. *Am. J. Med.* **63**, 233–43.

Kontras, S. B., Bodenbender, J. G., McClare, C. R. and Smith, J. P. (1971). Interstitial cystitis in chronic granulomatous disease. *J. Urol.* **105**, 575–8.

9. Cystic kidneys: definition and classification

The term cystic kidneys, or renal cystic disease, has been widely used as a simple morphological description for a wide variety of disorders ranging from solitary renal cysts to the several forms of multicystic and polycystic kidneys. In some types such as 'adult type polycystic kidney' the kidneys are enlarged, in others such as cystic dysplastic kidneys they may be small and shrunken. Renal cysts in chromsomal disorders have already been discussed in Chapter 3, Zellweger's syndrome in Chapter 4, and microcysts as a histopathological feature of congenital nephrosis in Chapter 7, and cysts in renal tumours will be discussed in Chapter 12, and will not be considered further here.

From the discussion of normal renal embryology (in Chapter 2) it follows that renal cysts must develop either through dilatation of Bowman's capsule or the convoluted tubules when they are of meta-nephric origin, or through dilatation of collecting ducts when of ureteric bud origin. Unfortunately even when the origin can be defined this does not help greatly in understanding the pathogenesis of renal cysts, which largely remains obscure despite numerous hypotheses proposed from the mid 19th century on. In lower urinary tract obstruction blockage of urine outflow is the self-evident pathogenesis and it is reasonable to consider whether various mechanisms of intrarenal obstruction may play a role in some other forms of cystic disease. This concept does not preclude the blockage resulting from some malformation of the nephron or the ureteric bud during development. Alternatively dilatation could result from some inate or acquired weakness of the wall or overgrowth of the endothelial cells of the tubules. Another possibility, proposed in the past, that cysts in the nephron might be due to a failure of nephron and ureteric bud to meet up has not been supported by the evidence from microdissection studies.

A number of classifications have been proposed, none of which are wholly satisfactory. None the less several clear entities can be defined on the basis of pathological features and inheritance. One of the earliest classifications was that of Bell (1935, 1946) whose anatomical categories of cystic kidney were: cystic disease including adult and infantile varieties of a bilateral form and a unilateral form; large solitary cysts; and multiple small cysts associated with contracted kidneys. He recognized the existence of a strong hereditary tendency, which had of course been emphasized a decade earlier by Cairns (1925) in his study of a single family. Marquardt (1935, 1936a and b) writing at the same period was probably the first to recognize clearly the dominant inheritance of adult and recessive inheritance of infantile lethal polycystic kidney disease. Fergusson (1949), acknowledging the help of Prof. Lionel Penrose, made similar observations to those of Marquardt, and carried out a linkage study using blood groups and other markers in five families with the adult form, with negative results.

Dalgaard (1957, 1963) in an extensive Danish study including 242 proposita for adult and 24 for congenital polycystic kidneys, confirmed this distinction in the mode of inheritance for the two ages of onset. Furthermore he found virtually complete penetrance of the adult form for subjects who live long enough. He undertook a larger, but still negative, linkage study of the adult form. Dalgaard agrees with Potter (1952) in recognizing that congenital polycystic kidney takes at least two forms, one form with large 'spongy' kidneys and recessive inheritance, and the other with small cystic kidneys which is probably not genetically determined.

Lundin and Olow (1961) extended this subdivision of infantile cystic kidneys further in a study of 28 cases in newborns, infants, and children. They recognized at least three groups as well as individual cases not fitting any of their three main groups. Their group I comprised nine cases with large kidneys with radially arranged cysts giving a spongy appearance. Group II kidneys, with 10 cases, were also enlarged and contained areas of cysts surrounded by connective tissue interspersed with more or less normal renal tissue. Group III kidneys, of which they had only four cases, were hypoplastic with cysts of greatly varying size again surrounded by connective tissue but with little or no normal renal tissue.

Edith Potter has published a series of studies on cystic kidneys in succeeding editions of her book *Pathology of the fetus and infant* (Potter 1952, 1961; Potter and Craig 1975), with Osathanondh (Osathanondh and Potter 1964), and in another book, *Normal and abnormal development of the kidney* (Potter 1972). Her approach has been a pathological one combining conventional histology with microdissection. The findings from microdissection of 30 kidneys are described in detail in the series of papers with Osathanondh. They recognize four main types of polycystic kidney.

Their type 1 corresponds to the group I of Lundin and Olow, they recognize its recessive inheritance and comment on invariable early fatality. They make the important point that infants with this type represent only a small proportion of all infants with polycystic kidneys. Like Lundin and Olow they note an associated bile duct proliferation and dilatation in the hepatic portal tracts. They conclude that the cysts in this type result from a diffuse enlargement of developmentally normal collecting tubules associated with a cellular hyperplasia of the tubule wall of unknown cause.

Osathanondh and Potter's type 2 presents a more variable picture with large or small kidneys and bilateral, unilateral, or segmental involvement. Cysts also vary widely in size and number. When bilateral this type also is always fatal soon after birth. They regard this type as differing from type 1 in having an abnormal pattern of development. Unlike type 1 the liver is not involved in the cystic disease and the condition is not familial. There may be associated malformations of other organs. When only part of one kidney is involved the disorder is known as multilocular cystic disease but the pathology is similar to that seen when the whole kidney is abnormal. Histologically they found no normal renal parenchyma, only cysts of differing size, shape, and lining embedded in connective tissue containing primitive ducts surrounded by whorls of fibrous tissue, blood vessels, nerves, and occasionally aberrant tissue such as cartilage. Microdissection of nine cases revealed reduced branching of collecting tubules which nearly all terminated in cysts. This type probably corresponds to the two non-familial cases in group III of Lundin and Olow and perhaps at least some of the latter's group II (other cases in group II may represent examples of infantile presentation of 'adult type'). More recently Potter has subdivided type 2 into 2A with enlarged kidneys and 2B with small kidneys and small or even absent cysts, corresponding roughly to Lundin and Olow's groups II and III respectively (Potter and Craig 1975). Pathogenesis of this 'multicystic, dysplastic' disease is obscure and confused. Osathanondh and Potter (1964) suggested that the normal induction of nephron development by the ampullae of the collecting tubules is inhibited. Associated with this they suggest that there is a corresponding inhibition of the normal branching of the ureteric bud and conversion of the terminal ampullary portions into cysts. An alternative hypothesis of developmental error proposes, on the basis of experimental studies in chick embryos, that it is a lack of condensed metanephrogenic mesenchyme apposed to the ureteric ampullae that results in the primitive ducts of renal dysplasia (Maizels and Simpson 1983)— the reverse of Potter's theory. In two of Osathanondh and Potter's cases one kidney was clearly of type 2, but the other was of type 3. In the most recent edition of *Pathology of the fetus and newborn* (Potter and Craig 1975) such mixed cases are not mentioned, but 17 cases of mixed type 2A and 2B are described so perhaps some kidneys that Potter earlier termed type 3 she would now classify under type 2A. Potter implies that type 2 is a developmental anomaly, but in those cases which involve the whole kidney she describes irregular dilatation and constriction of the ureter (Osathanondh and Potter 1964) and recognizes that urethral obstruction when complete typically also results in type 2, but when incomplete in her type 4 (Potter and Craig 1975). Others have also favoured urinary tract obstruction as the primary cause of renal dysplasia (Bernstein 1968). It is clearly difficult, in our present state of knowledge about renal dysplasia in humans, to distinguish between developmental dysplasia secondary to urinary tract obstruction as a pathogenetic hypothesis and primary developmental error, whether of the ureteric bud or the metanephrogenic mesenchyme.

Potter's type 3 mainly comprises the misleadingly named adult polycystic kidneys. This is a long-recognized well-defined entity with autosomal dominant inheritance, again of unknown pathogenesis. Although typically of adult clinical onset, affected patients may present in childhood or even at birth. Unlike the earlier types there tends to be admixture of normal and abnormal renal parenchyma in the same portion of the kidney. It usually presents with bilateral progressively enlarging kidneys, owing to enlargement of cysts with age. There may also be dilated bile ducts and increased fibrous tissue in the portal tracts of the liver. Cysts are usually distributed throughout both kidneys, vary greatly in size, and show no ordered arrangement in contrast to the cysts in type 1. They may arise from the structure of the nephron or the collecting tubules and in the latter case may be surrounded by dense connective tissue. Microdissection confirms the variable proportion of normal and abnormal nephrons and collecting tubules, and variable site of origin of cysts. It also confirms that all cysts connect to the renal pelvis. Osathanondh and Potter attribute these abnormalities to impaired function of the ampullae of ureteral bud branches, leading to irregular ureteric bud division and failure of development of calyces and papillae. This impaired ampullary function is at least in part due to the ampulla becoming cystic and ceasing to divide. Despite defective branching ampullae may still induce normal numbers of nephrons, but some of these may develop local hyperplasia and cystic change. Others have rejected this interpretation of the cystic change being due to a branching defect or impaired ampullary function (Baert 1978). In addition to typical adult type polycystic kidney Osathanondh and Potter include under type 3 kidneys from some patients with renal dysplasia, as discussed above, and single cases of microcystic kidney associated with trisomy 13, and of cystic dilatation of the loops of Henle or the terminal portions of the collecting ducts in an infant with tuberous sclerosis. Further examples of these rare causes of type 3 cystic disease are described by Potter in her more recent studies (Potter and Craig 1975), along with infants with cerebrohepatorenal syndrome. Curiously the only instances of familial occurrence of type 3 reported by Potter were two pairs of affected sibs.

Potter's type 4 is renal cystic disease associated with urethral obstruction without gross renal pelvic dilatation, but with small sub-capsular cysts formed only within the last one or two generations of nephrons or terminal ends of collecting tubules. Although Potter placed her kidneys from an infant with trisomy 13 under type 3 the appearance more closely resembles her type 4. A more severe change, indistinguishable from type 2 or occasionally type 3 cystic disease, is also seen, which is probably due, according to Potter, to earlier or more severe obstruction of the urethra. An excellent updated review of the Potter classification is provided by Zerres and colleagues (1984), who also list a large number of syndromes in which renal cysts may be present. A brief review is given by Shaw and Pincott (1986).

Several subsequent authors have proposed more detailed classifications of renal cystic disease. Arey (1959) failed to recognize that different modes of inheritance do imply different disease entities. Bernstein and colleagues (Bernstein and Meyer 1967; Bernstein 1968; Elkin and Bernstein 1969) have produced evidence for the production of cystic dysplasia by ureteric obstruction at a critical stage of fetal development in experimental animals, confirming Potter's views from her clinico-pathological experience from human infants. They have also evolved a classification attempting to take into account clinical, genetic, pathological, and radiological features. Their major categories are: I—renal dysplasia including lower urinary tract obstruction; II—polycystic disease, infantile and adult; III—cortical cysts including trisomy 13 syndrome and tuberous sclerosis; IV—medullary cysts in medullary sponge kidney, medullary cystic disease, and others; V—miscellaneous intrarenal acquired cysts; and VI—extraparenchymal renal cysts.

Others have also recognized that environmental factors may play a role in inducing renal cyst formation (Resnick *et al.* 1976; Bommer *et al.* 1980; Werder *et al.* 1984). In contrast, although renal dysplasia is generally non-familial, affected sibs have been observed (Williams and Risdon 1982). Several rare disorders other than those already mentioned may show renal cystic change (Potter and Craig 1975; Williams and Risdon 1982). The increasing recognition of renal cystic disease has been greatly assisted by the ease and sensitivity of detection by diagnostic ultrasonography. It has been estimated that ultrasound will detect renal cysts in 97 per cent of affected patients (Sherwood 1975). Renal cystic disease has been reviewed in a monograph by Gardner (1976).

This chapter will describe those forms of renal cystic disease, and their inheritance, not discussed in other chapters.

The principal types of genetic or idiopathic renal cysts described in this chapter, or elsewhere in the book, are listed in Table 9.1. Single, or occasionally multiple, cysts are a common incidental finding. The division into primary and secondary cystic disease is a natural one, and placing renal dysplasia and lower urinary tract obstruction together in a category intermediate between the other two is a logical extension of such a classification.

Table 9.1 *Types of renal cystic disease*

Category	Disorder	Inheritance
Primary		
Simple cysts	Single	Non-mendelian
	multiple	Non-mendelian
Polycystic disease	Infantile (Potter type 1)	AR
	Congenital hepatic fibrosis	AR
	'Adult type' (Potter type 3)	AD
Medullary cysts	Medullary sponge kidney	AD (one form)
	Medullary cystic disease (nephronophthisis)	AR
	Other rare medullary cystic disorders	Most AR
Multisystem disease	Familial dysplasia of kidneys, liver and pancreas (Ivemark)	AR
	Cystic dysplasia of kidneys and liver and agenesis of vermis cerebelli	AR
	Renal dysplasia and asplenia	Probably AR
	Meckel–Gruber syndrome	AR
Dysplasia and lower urinary tract obstruction	Enlarged or small dysplastic cystic (or multicystic) kidneys (Potter types 2A and 2B)	Non-mendelian
	Renal cystic disease in early developmental obstruction	Non-mendelian
	Prune-belly syndrome	Non-mendelian
	Vesico-urethral reflux	Non-mendelian
Secondary		
Chromosomal anomaly (Ch. 3)	Trisomy 13 commonly	
	Trisomy 18, partial trisomy 10, triploidy, Turners syndrome, duplication/deletion defect of chromosome 3 occasionally	
Inherited metabolic disease (Ch. 4)	Cerebro-hepato-renal (Zellweger) disease	AR
Hereditary nephropathy (Ch. 7)	Congenital nephrosis (microcysts)	AR

Table 9.1.—*Continued*

Category	Disorder	Inheritance
Renal tumours (Ch. 12)	Wilms' tumour (embryonal carcinoma) Renal cell carcinoma (hypernephroma)	Non-mendelian
Systemic disorders	Tuberose sclerosis	AD
	Myotonic dystrophy	AD
	Von Hippel Lindau's disease	AD
	Dandy–Walker syndrome	AD
	Ehlers–Danlos syndrome	AD
	Wiedemann–Beckwith syndrome	AD

Abbreviations: AD = Autosomal dominant, AR = Autosomal recessive.

References

Arey, J. B. (1959). Cystic lesions of the kidney in infants and children. *J. Pediatr.* **54**, 429–45.

Baert, L. (1978). Hereditary polycystic kidney disease (adult form): a microdissection study of two cases at an early stage of the disease. *Kidney Int.* **13**, 519–25.

Bell, E. T. (1935). Cystic disease of the kidneys. *Am. J. Pathol.* **11**, 373–418.

—— (1946). *Renal disease.* W. B. Saunders, Philadelphia.

Bernstein, J. (1968). Developmental abnormalities of the renal parenchyma: renal hypoplasia and dysplasia. In *Pathology annual,* ed. Sommers, S. C. Appleton-Century-Crofts, New York.

———— and Meyer, R. (1967). Chapter 26. Parenchymal maldevelopment of the kidneys. In *Brennemann–Kelly practice of pediatrics,* Vol. III. Harper & Row, Maryland.

Bommer, J., Waldherr, R., van Kaick, G., Strauss, L. and Ritz., E. (1980). Acquired renal cysts in uremic patients—*in vitro* demonstration by computed tomography. *Clin. Nephrol.* **14**, 299–303.

Cairns, H. W. B. (1925). Heredity in polycystic disease of the kidneys. *Quart. J. Med.* **18**, 359–92.

Dalgaard, O. Z. (1957). Bilateral polycystic disease of the kidneys. A follow-up of two hundred and eighty four patients and their families. *Acta Med. Scand.* **158**, (Suppl. 328), 1–251.

—— (1963). Bilateral polycystic disease of the kidneys. In *Diseases of the Kidney,* eds. Strauss, M. and Welt, L. G. pp. 907–10. Little Brown, Boston.

Elkin, M. and Bernstein, J. (1969). Cystic disease of the kidney—radiological and pathological considerations. *Clin. Radiol.* **20**, 65–82.

Fergusson, J. D. (1949). Observations on familial polycystic disease of the kidney. *Proc. R. Soc. Med.* **42**, 806–14.

Gardner, K. D. (1976). *Cystic diseases of the kidney.* p. 173. John Wiley, New York.

Lundin, P. M. and Olow, I. (1961). Polycystic kidneys in newborns, infants and children. A clinical and pathological study. *Acta Paediatr.* **50**, 185–200.

Maizels, M. and Simpson, S. B. Jr. (1983). Primitive ducts of renal dysplasia induced by culturing urethral buds denuded by condensed renal mesenchyme. *Science* **219**, 509–10.

Marquardt, W. (1935). Cystenniere, Cystenleber und Cystenpankreas bei zwei Geschwistern. Dissertation, Tubingen.

—— (1936a). Die Verebung der congitalen doppelseitigen Cystennieren. *Der Erbarzt*, **3**, 69–70.

—— (1936b). Zur Kasuistik des familiären Auftretens der Cystennieren. *Der Erbarzt* **3**, 102–3.

Osathanondh, V. and Potter, E. L. (1964). Pathogenesis of polycystic kidneys. *Arch. Pathol.* **77**, 459–512.

Potter, E. L. (1952). *Pathology of the fetus and the newborn.* Year Book Medical Publishers, Chicago.

—— (1961). *Pathology of the Fetus and Infant*, 2nd edn. Year Book Medical Publishers, Chicago.

—— (1972). *Normal and abnormal development of the kidney.* Year Book Medical Publishers, Chicago.

—— and Craig, J. M. (1975). *Pathology of the fetus and the infant*, 3rd edn. Year Book Medical Publishers, Chicago.

Resnick, J. S., Brown, D. M. and Vernier, L. (1976). Normal development and experimental models of cystic renal disease. In *Cystic diseases of the kidney*, ed. Gardner, K. D. p. 221. John Wiley, New York.

Shaw, D. G. and Pincott, J. R. (1986). Renal cystic disease—problems in identification, inheritance and prognosis: a review. *J. R. Soc. Med.* **79**, 476–7.

Sherwood, T. (1975). Renal masses and ultrasound. *Br. Med. J.* **4**, 682–3.

Werder, A. A., Amos, M. A., Nielson, A. H. and Wolfe, G. H. (1984). Comparative effects of germfree and ambient environments on the development of cystic kidney disease in CFWwd mice. *J. Lab. Clin. Med.* **103**, 399–407.

Williams, D. I. and Risdon, R. A. (1982). Hypoplastic, dysplastic and cystic kidneys. Chapter 14 in *Paediatric urology*, 2nd edn. eds. Williams, D. I. and Johnston, J. H. pp. 137–50. Butterworths, London.

Zerres, K., Volpel, M.-C. and Weiss, H. (1984). Cystic kidneys: genetics, pathologic anatomy, clinical picture and prenatal diagnosis. *Hum. Genet.* **68**, 104–35.

9.1. PRIMARY RENAL CYSTIC DISEASE

9.1.1. Infantile (Potter type 1) polycystic kidneys

Probably the earliest recorded description of this type of polycystic kidney is that of Bunting (1906) who reported two sibs who died at 11 days and at 19 days. A further family was reported by Lightwood and Loots (1932) with sibs dying at 1 year 10 months, 4 years, and 1 year 11 months, clearly a less severe form than that present in Bunting's family.

Reference has been made above to the early studies of Bell, Cairns, Marquardt, Fergusson, Dalgaard, Potter, Lundin and Olow, and Bernstein. These and other authors have established the main clinico-pathological features and autosomal recessive mode of inheritance of this type (Parker 1956, case 1; Hooper 1958, who reported monozygotic female twins dying at 3 months; Lathrop 1959; Reilly and Neuhauser 1960, a radiological study of 11 cases from six families; Kerr *et al.* 1962, who recognized that congenital hepatic fibrosis is a separate entity from infantile polycystic kidney, as also did Reilly and Neuhauser). The characteristic radial pattern of the cysts is shown in Fig. 9.1.

In addition to Osathanondh and Potter's microdissection studies, mentioned above, others have carried out similar studies in infantile polycystic renal disease. Heggö and Natvig studied kidneys from five newborns, including two pairs of sibs, who died within 2 to 9 hours of birth, and dissected kidneys from three of these (Heggö and Natvig 1963, 1965; Heggö 1966). Like Potter they associated the tubular dilatation with a proliferation of the tubular epithelium. Baxter (1965) came to similar conclusions. More recent clinical reports include those of Aurich (1967) with five out of eight children in one family affected, Fasske (1967) who reported three stillborn sibs, Becker and colleagues (1969) who observed three out of four sibs affected with a maximal survival of 5 months, and Lee and Change (1970) who described a fetal death with uterine dystocia in labour due to infantile polycystic kidney. Whether or not the murine model described by Fry and coworkers (1985) is relevant to the human disease is unclear.

The various reports mentioned so far differ widely in the clinico-pathological severity of the renal disease and in the extent of hepatic

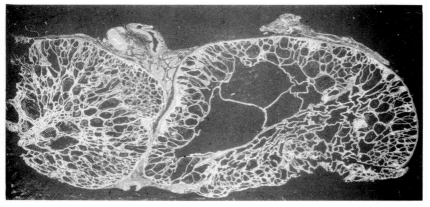

Fig. 9.1. Radial arrangement of renal cysts in infantile (Potter type I) polycystic kidneys.

involvement. This variability raises the possibility of heterogeneity within this type, and was the basis of a study by Blyth and Ockenden (1969, 1971) and Carter (1974). They separated the infantile type into four subgroups on the basis of age of onset and severity of renal involvement. They recognized the invariable hepatic involvement and preferred the term 'childhood type of polycystic disease of kidneys and liver'. They noted that the less severe the renal involvement the greater was the hepatic involvement. Their four subgroups, perinatal, neonatal, infantile, and juvenile, showed good sib correlation and all four appeared to be autosomal recessive from family data. The milder forms without Potter facies and with survival beyond the neonatal period seem to be very rare (Potter 1972; Adams *et al.* 1974), and have a relatively good prognosis with survival at least beyond childhood. Whether Blyth and Ockenden's four subgroups are, as they suggest, genetically distinct or at least allelic, or whether they are merely arbitrary divisions within a gradation as suggested by some later writers (Lieberman *et al.* 1971), remains to be determined.

More recent radiological studies include those of Thaler and coworkers (1973) who investigated a juvenile case, and Vuthibhagdee and Singleton (1973) who studied three juvenile and four infantile cases. Melson and colleagues (1985) have described the postnatal ultrasono-graphic findings in nine infants, and emphasize the variability.

Adams and coworkers (1974) characterized polycystic disease of the liver and kidney in an elegant study using three-dimensional reconstruction of hepatic portal tracts from serial sections to define the precise hepatic pathology. They concluded, from study of the liver of an infant who died with the neonatal form of infantile polycystic kidney, that the longitudinal ductules at the periphery of the portal tracts were irregularly dilated and anastomosed so extensively as almost to form an annular channel, whilst the main interlobular ducts appeared to be absent. Four other cases of infantile polycystic kidney, although not reconstructed, showed similar lesions in the liver and kidney, indicating that the findings in the first case are probably fairly typical. These findings contrast with those in congenital hepatic fibrosis in which reconstruction reveals a complex system of discrete longitudinal ductules and a normal main interlobular duct at the periphery of the portal tract, confirming that despite the apparent overlap with late onset infantile polycystic kidney this is a distinct disorder. The three-dimensional appearance in Meckel's syndrome and in Ivemark's syndrome of cystic disease of liver, kidney, and pancreas were also distinct.

Schmidt and colleagues (1982) have reported on ultrasonographic prenatal diagnosis of Potter syndrome in 23 cases with a variety of renal abnormalities including two cases of infantile polycystic kidney. Luthy and Hirsch (1985) described attempted ultrasound prenatal diagnosis of infantile polycystic kidney in three successive pregnancies of the same mother, with one correct positive, one false positive, and one false negative result. Romero and associates (1984) had better success with ultrasound prenatal diagnosis of 19 at-risk pregnancies. The fetus was affected in 10 of these pregnancies and was correctly diagnosed in nine with no false positives.

Prenatal diagnosis has also been claimed on the basis of a high amniotic fluid trehalase activity (Morin *et al.* 1981), in what the authors describe as 'autosomal recessive type of polycystic kidney disease (type II)', but would appear to be the infantile type of polycystic kidney disease (Potter type I). The trehalase activity at 21 weeks pregnancy was greater than two standard deviations above the mean for 18–21-week controls, although just within the range obtained for those controls. However, the trehalase to lactase ratio was well outside the control range, being 6.6. times the control mean. An ultrasound diagnosis had already been made at 19 weeks, and the fetus aborted spontaneously at 30 weeks when polycystic renal disease was confirmed histologically. The mother's one previous child had had a similar type of renal cystic disease.

Spurlock and Taylor (1984) reported an isolated case of a neonate who died at 20 minutes with infantile polycystic kidneys, and who also had male hermaphroditism with immature testes, ovary-like structures devoid of follicles and oocytes, masculinized external genitalia, and Müllerian internal structures. This may or may not be a purely chance association.

References

Adams, C. M., Danks, D. M. and Campbell, P. E. (1974). Comments upon the classification of infantile polycystic diseases of the liver and kidney, based upon three-dimensional reconstruction of the liver. *J. Med. Genet.* **11**, 234–43.

Aurich, G. (1967). Uber kongnitale zystische Dysplasien. *Pädiatrie und Grenzgebiate* **6**, 19–34.

Baxter, T. J. (1965). Cysts arising in the renal tubules. A microdissection study. *Arch. Dis. Child.* **260**, 464–73.

Becker, S. M., Finkel, J., Amboy, P. and Hyun, B. H. (1969). Polycystic kidney disease type I. *Arch. Pathol.* **88**, 265–8.

Blyth, H. M. and Ockenden, B. G. (1969). A clinico-pathological and family study of polycystic disease of the kidneys and liver in children (abs.). *J. Clin. Pathol.* **22**, 508.

—— and —— (1971). Polycystic disease of the kidney and liver presenting in childhood. *J. Med. Genet.* **8**, 257–84.

Bunting, C. H. (1906). Congenital cystic kidney and liver with family tendency. *J. Exp. Med.* **8**, 271–88.

Carter, C. O. (1974). Polycystic disease presenting in childhood. In *Clinical delineation of birth defects*. XVI. *Urinary system and others*, ed. Bergsma, D. *Birth Defects Orig. Art. Series*. X(**4**), 16–21.

Fasske, E. van, (1967). Hereditat angeborener Zystennieren? *Mediz. Klinik.* **62**, 1828–34.

Fry, J. L. Jr., Kock, W. E., Jennette, J. C., McFarland, E., Fried, F. A. and Mandell, J. (1985). A genetically determined murine model of infantile polycystic kidney disease. *J. Urol.* **134**, 828–33.

Heggö, O. (1966). A microdissection study of cystic disease of the kidneys in adults. *J. Pathol. Bact.* **91**, 311–15.

—— and Natvig, J. B. (1963). Microdissection studies of structural changes in cystic disease of the kidneys. *Lancet* **2**, 616–17.

—— and —— (1965). Cystic disease of the kidneys. A microdissection study. *Acta Pathol. Microbiol. Scand.* **63**, 500–12.

Hooper, J. W. Jr. (1958). Cystic disease of the kidney in infants. *J. Urol.* **79**, 917–24.

Kerr, D. N. S., Warrick, C. K. and Hartmercer, J. (1962). A lesion resembling medullary sponge kidney in patients with congenital hepatic fibrosis. *Clin. Radiol.* **13**, 85–91.

Lathrop, D. B. (1959). Cystic disease of the liver and kidney. *Pediatrics* **24**, 215–24.

Lee, K. H. and Chang, E. (1970). Dystocia due to congenital polycystic kidneys. *J. Obstet. Gynecol.* **71**, 1115–16.

Lieberman, E., Salinas-Madrigal, L., Gwinn, J. L., Brennan, L. P., Fine, R. N. and Landing, B. H. (1971). Infantile polycystic disease of the kidneys and liver. *Medicine* **50**, 277–318.

Lightwood, R. and Loots, G. H. (1932). Three cases of familial congenital cystic disease of the kidney and liver. *Proc. R. Soc. Med.* **25**, 1230–2.

Luthy, D. A. and Hirsch, J. H. (1985). Infantile polycystic kidney disease: observations from attempts at prenatal diagnosis. *Am. J. Med. Genet.* **20**, 505–17.

Melson, G. L., Shackleford, G. D., Cole, B. R. and McClennan, B. L. (1985). The spectrum of sonographic findings in infantile polycystic kidney disease with urographic and clinical correlations. *J. Clin. Ultrasound* **13**, 113–19.

Morin, P. R., Potier, M., Dallaire, L., Melançon, S. B. and Boisvert, J. (1981). Prenatal detection of the autosomal recessive type of polycystic kidney disease by trehalase assay in amniotic fluid. *Prenatal Diagnosis* **1**, 75–9.

Parker, R. G. F. (1956). Fibrosis of the liver as a congenital anomaly. *J. Pathol. Bact.* **71**, 359–68.

Potter, E. L. (1952). *Pathology of the fetus and the newborn*. Year Book Medical Publishers, Chicago.

Reilly, B. J. and Neuhauser, E. B. D. (1960). Renal tubular ectasia in cystic disease of the kidneys and liver. *Am. J. Roentgenol.* **84**, 546–54.

Romero, R., Cullen, M., Jeanty, P., Grannum, P., Reece, E. A., Venus, I. and Hobbins, J. C. (1984). The diagnosis of congenital renal anomalies with ultrasound. II. Infantile polycystic kidney disease. *Am. J. Obstet. Gynecol.* **150**, 259–62.

Schmidt, W., Schroeder, T. M., Buchinger, G. and Kubli, F. (1982). Genetics, pathoanatomy and prenatal diagnosis of Potter I syndrome and other urogenital tract disorders. *Clin. Genet.* **22**, 105–27.

Spurlock, R. G. and Taylor, F. M. (1985). Polycystic kidneys and male hermaphroditism in an infant: a case report and review of the literature. *Hum. Pathol.* **15**, 895–7.

Thaler, M. M., Ogata, E. S., Goodman, J. R., Piel, C. F. and Korobkin, M. T. (1973). Congenital fibrosis and polycystic disease of liver and kidneys. *Am. J. Dis. Child.* **126**, 374–80.

Vuthibhagdee, A. and Singleton, E. B. (1973). Infantile polycystic disease of the kidney. *Am. J. Dis. Child.* **125**, 167–70.

9.1.2. Congenital hepatic fibrosis

This disorder overlaps in its clinical and pathological features with the late onset, juvenile form of infantile polycystic kidney. In both disorders there is hepatic bile duct proliferation and fibrosis of periportal distribution, and mild renal cystic disease. These similarities have led several authors to regard the two disorders as minor variants of a single disease (Kerr *et al.* 1962; Blyth and Ockenden 1971). However, a renal cystic lesion is seen in only about half the cases of congenital hepatic fibrosis (Lieberman *et al.* 1971) and, as discussed below, is not necessarily that of infantile polycystic kidney. Three-dimensional reconstruction of the liver, as discussed above, confirms a pattern that is quite distinct from that of infantile polycystic kidney disease (Adams *et al.* 1974).

There have been a number of papers describing congenital hepatic fibrosis in sibs. An affected brother and two sisters have been the subject of several reports (Sweetnam 1955; Kerr *et al.* 1961; Sweetnam and Sykes 1961). The younger two sibs at least had polycystic kidneys. The eldest sib in this family was seen by the present author in 1972 for genetic counselling. Since the 1961 reports her brother had died, at the age of 14 years, in 1963 as well as her younger sister as already reported. Campbell and colleagues (1958) also described three sibs, all of whom had congenital hepatic fibrosis and cystic kidneys. Kerr and colleagues (1961) record a further family with two sibs with both hepatic and renal disease. Further families have been reported (Nathan and Batsakis 1969, two families; Boichis *et al.* 1973; Naveh *et al.* 1980). In the last two reports quoted there was parental consanguinity.

There is considerable confusion in the literature regarding the nature of the renal lesion in those patients with congenital hepatic fibrosis in whom the kidneys are involved. Early papers simply report cystic kidneys. Kerr and coworkers (1962) claim that the commonest renal lesion in congenital hepatic fibrosis is medullary sponge kidney, but that adult type polycystic kidney may also be seen. Clermont and his associates (1967) studied eight cases of whom five had renal lesions. Three of these had medullary sponge kidney radiographically, confirmed on histology in one; one had cortical microcysts histologically, but normal intravenous pyelogram; one had cysts of adult type histologically. The clearly inherited adult polycystic kidney disease and the congenital hepatic fibrosis present in two sibs in the family of Lee and Paes (1985) are probably segregating independently. Nathan and Batsakis (1969) observed polycystic kidney disease, without defining the type, in 11 out of 13 patients with congenital hepatic fibrosis. They argue for a unitary concept of polycystic liver disease and congenital hepatic fibrosis but do not discuss the relationship to cystic renal disease. Blyth and Ockenden (1971) regard congenital hepatic fibrosis as merely an accompaniment of any of their four types of childhood polycystic disease of liver and kidney. Boichis and colleagues (1973) describe the renal lesion in their family as nephronophthisis, otherwise known as medullary cystic kidney. Similar families with nephronophthisis and congenital hepatic fibrosis have been reported by others (Proesmans *et al.* 1975; Robins *et al.* 1976; Delaney *et al.* 1978). The families of Proesmans and colleagues (1975) and of Delaney and colleagues (1978) showed tapeto-retinal degeneration in addition to nephronophthisis and hepatic fibrosis, whereas that of Robins and colleagues (1976) showed skeletal abnormalities (see section 9.1.6). Doubtless some cases reported with a primary diagnosis of congenital hepatic fibrosis correspond to the juvenile or infantile forms of childhood polycystic disease of liver and kidneys of Blyth and Ockenden. Almost certainly other cases, with or without renal disease, are distinct. How many different genetic disorders are included within this group remains to be determined, and in particular it is not clear whether or not the distinction between medullary sponge kidney and nephronophthisis in association with hepatic fibrosis is valid.

Hunter and colleagues (1974) described a family with what is almost certainly a distinct, probably autosomal recessive, syndrome. They reported a French-Candian family with unrelated parents and two children, a brother and sister. Both children had congenital hepatic fibrosis, radiological renal tubular ectasia with histological findings in the elder child of small subcapsular and tubular cysts, developmental delay and dysmorphic features including frontal bossing, a high palate, anteverted nares, hypertelorism, carp mouth, and colobomata. A similar syndrome has recently been described in two sisters, one of whom also had an encephalocoele suggesting Meckel syndrome, and the other features of Smith–Lemli–Opitz syndome. However, both had congenital hepatic fibrosis, cystic kidneys, and moderate or severe mental retardation, and one had coloboma (Thompson and Baraitser 1986).

References

Adams, C. M., Danks, D. M. and Campbell, P. E. (1974). Comments upon the classification of infantile polycystic disease of the liver and kidney, based upon three dimensional reconstruction of the liver. *J. Med. Genet.* **11**, 234–43.

Blyth, H. and Ockenden, B. G. (1971). Polycystic disease of the kidneys and liver presenting in childhood. *J. Med. Genet.* **8**, 257–84.

Boichis, H., Passwell, J., David, R. and Miller, H. (1973). Congenital hepatic fibrosis and nephronophthisis: a family study. *Quart. J. Med.* **42**, 221–33.

Campbell, G. S., Bick, H. D., Paulsen, E., Lober, P.-H., Watson, C. J. and Varco, R. L. (1958). Bleeding esophageal varices with polycystic liver. Report of three cases. *New Engl. J. Med.* **259**, 904–10.

Clermont, R. J., Maillard, J. N., Benhamon, J. P. and Fauvert, R. (1967). Fibrose hepatique congenitale. *Can. Med. Assoc. J.* **97**, 1272–8.

Delaney, V., Mullaney, J. and Bourke, E. (1978). Juvenile nephronophthisis, congenital hepatic fibrosis and retinal hypoplasia in twins. *Quart. J. Med.* **47**, 281–90.

Hunter, A. G. W., Rothman, S. J., Hwang, W. S. and Deckelbaum, R. J. (1974). Hepatic fibrosis, polycystic kidney, colobomata and encephalopathy in siblings. *Clin. Genet.* **6**, 82–9.

Kerr, D. N. S., Harrison, C. V., Sherlock, S. and Milnes Walker, R. (1961). Congenital hepatic fibrosis. *Quart. J. Med.* **30**, 91–117.

——, Warrick, C. K. and Hart-Mercer, J. (1962). A lesion resembling medullary sponge kidney in patients with congenital hepatic fibrosis. *Clin. Radiol.* **13**, 85–91.

Lee, F. I. and Paes, A. R. (1985). Congenital hepatic fibrosis and adult-type autosomal dominant polycystic kidney disease in a child. *Postgrad. Med. J.* **61**, 641–2.

Lieberman, E., Salinas-Madrigala, L., Gwinn, J. L., Brennan, L. P., Fine, R. N. and Landing, B. H. (1971). Infantile polycystic disease of the kidneys and liver. *Medicine* **50**, 277–318.

Nathan, M. and Batsakis, J. G. (1969). Congenital hepatic fibrosis. *Surg. Gynecol. Obstet.* **128**, 1033–41.

Naveh, Y., Roquin, N., Ludatscher, R., Auslaender, L., Schramek, A. and Aharon, M. (1980). Congenital hepatic fibrosis with congenital heart disease: a family study with ultrastructural features of the liver. *Gut* **21**, 799–807.

Proesmans, W., van Damme, B. and Macken, J. (1975). Nephronophthisis and tapetoretinal degeneration associated with liver fibrosis. *Clin. Nephrol.* **3**, 160–4.

Robins, D. G., French, T. A. and Chakera, T. M. H. (1976). Juvenile nephronophthisis associated with skeletal abnormalities and hepatic fibrosis. *Arch. Dis. Child.* **51**, 799–801.

Sweetnam, W. P. (1955). Banti's syndrome in siblings treated by porta-caval anastamosis (two cases). *Proc. Roy. Soc. Med.* **48**, 1108.

—— and Sykes, C. G. W. (1961). Congenital fibrosis of the liver as a familial defect. *Lancet* **1**, 374–6.

Thompson, E. and Baraitser, M. (1986). An autosomal recessive mental retardation syndrome with hepatic fibrosis and renal cysts. *Am. J. Med. Genet.* **24**, 151–8.

9.1.3. 'Adult type' (Potter type 3) polycystic kidneys

Possibly the earliest description of this type of renal cystic disease was that of Virchow (1869) who postulated renal infection leading to tubular obstruction as the cause. Others have suggested a developmental non-union of the ureteric buds with the nephrogenic blastema as the origin of the cyst formation (Hildebrand 1894; Ribbert 1896). Probably the earliest accurate description was that of Steiner (1899) who reported two families. A number of early writers recognized that there are two age groups for the clinical onset of renal cystic disease: under 1 year and in the third to fourth decades (Bell 1935). Marquardt (1936) and Fergusson (1949) recognized that the infantile lethal type was recessive and the adult form dominant. The latter also undertook a linkage study of the dominant form with negative results.

Clinically onset is typically in the third or fourth decade, well into the reproductive period of life (Rall and Odel 1949; Funck-Brentano *et al.* 1964). The course of the disease is not affected by pregnancy (Milutinovic *et al.* 1983). Both later and much earlier onset have frequently been recorded, even in the early literature (Halbertsma 1932; Oppenheimer 1934). It has also been detected coincidentally at an early age (Savera 1946). More recently there have been numerous reports of presentation of 'adult type' polycystic kidney disease in childhood (Rall and Odel 1949; Kaplan *et al.* 1977), in infancy (Mehrizi *et al.* 1964; Blyth and Ockenden 1971; Ross and Travers 1975; Stickler and Kelalis 1975; Loh *et al.* 1977; McLean *et al.* 1980), or at birth (Kaye and Lewy 1974; Bengtsson *et al.* 1975; Fellows *et al.* 1976; Shokeir 1978; Fryns and van den Berghe 1979; Proesmans *et al.* 1982). It has even been diagnosed in premature stillborn infants (Eulderink and Hogewind 1978) and in fetuses from terminations (Carter 1974).

The clinical picture is typically one of a patient with pain in the loin or abdomen, urinary tract infection, hypertension or haematuria, who is found to have enlarged kidneys. Alternatively, enlarged kidneys may be found coincidentally, or because of examination for a family history of the disease. The disease is earlier in onset among female patients mainly because urinary tract infection and hypertension are more common early clinical manifestations in female patients. Sixty-six per cent of male patients under 30 years of age, but only 11 per cent of such female patients, are asymptomatic (Milutinovic *et al.* 1984). When account is taken of patients who must remain unrecognized even higher percentages must remain asymptomatic for many years (Churchill *et al.* 1984). A minority of patients present with nocturia, renal calculi, renal failure or non-specific symptoms of weight loss, vomiting or nausea, headache, and such like (Oppenheimer 1934; Rall and Odel 1949; Higgins 1952; Simon and Thompson 1955; Dalgaard 1957; Ward *et al.* 1967; Milutinovic *et al.* 1984). A recent study identified increased extracellular fluid volume in the early stages of the disease (Danielsen *et al.* 1986).

Many patients show associated abnormalities, some of which may be coincidental, as for example in all likelihood the myopia in Cairns's (1925) family. Others are clearly significant associations of which the most constant is cystic dilation of bile ducts in the liver (McMahon 1929). This has been noted in around 30 per cent of autopsies and was associated with palpable hepatic enlargement in a quarter of cases (Oppenhemier 1934; Rall and Odel 1949; Case Records Mass. Gen. Hosp. 1968). Conversely polycystic kidneys are found in about half of all cases of cystic disease of the liver (Poinso *et al.* 1954). Nevertheless, some workers still regard adult polycystic liver and kidney diseases as distinct disorders (Karhunen and Tenhu 1986).

Another frequent association is intracranial aneurysm, which may rupture causing a cerebral haemorrhage. Aneurysms may be observed clinically, as in cerebral haemorrhage, or as a coincidentally diagnosed cerebral artery aneurysm or malformation (Brown 1951; Poutasse *et al.* 1954; Dalgaard 1957; Ditlefsen and Tonjum 1960; Funck-Brentano and Vantelon 1963; Proesmans *et al.* 1982) or an autopsy association (Bigelow 1953). Abdominal aortic aneurysms are another significant association which positively contraindicate treatment by peritoneal dialysis (Chapman and Hilson 1980; Montoliu *et al.* 1980). The prevalence of cerebral aneurysm among patients with adult type polycystic kidney disease seen at autopsy has been estimated at 10–30 per cent (Levey *et al.* 1983), and Chapman and Hilson found aortic aneurysm in three out of 31 patients under their care. The propensity to such anomalies may well be greater in some families than others, as Ditlefsen and Tonjum observed cerebral haemorrhage in six out of 15 to 17 affected members of their family.

Other isolated reported associations include myocardial infarction and endocardial fibroelastosis (Mehrizi *et al.* 1964), hypertrophic pyloric stenosis (Loh *et al.* 1977), and liver disease with portal hypertension and oesophageal varices (Ratcliffe *et al.* 1984).

In the absence of dialysis or renal transplantation survival is typically to age 40 to 50 or 60 years (Oppenheimer 1934; Rall and Olsen 1969). The institution of these forms of therapy have improved prognosis, with about half of the renal transplants functioning after 1 year in the study of De Bono and Evans (1977). Nevertheless these authors had had 13 deaths out of 31 transplanted patients.

Microdissection studies have clarified the pathological changes in the kidneys. Osathanondh and Potter (1964) described their type 3 polycystic kidneys as having a mixed ampullary and interstitial abnormality of the collecting tubules, resulting in the formation of cysts of irregular size, involving Henle's loop, the proximal tubule, or even Bowman's capsule intermingled with areas of apparently normal nephrons (see Fig. 9.2). They attribute these abnormalities to impaired ampullary function. Heggö (1966) studied six typical adult cases, in contrast to the cases of mixed origin of Osanthanondh and Potter. Nevertheless he confirmed the origin of cysts from Bowman's capsule, Henle's loop, and collecting tubules and like them associated this with an abnormality of collecting-duct branching. Baert (1978) in a study of two cases at an early stage of the disease also confirmed the site of the cysts and the continuity with the collecting system, but could not confirm any abnormality of branching or of ampullary function. Milutinovic and colleagues (1980a) found that, in renal biopsies from asymptomatic relatives, early disease was expressed in dilatation of distal and collecting tubules and splitting of glomerular and tubular basement membranes.

The pathogenesis of these changes remains obscure, although Darmady and his associates (1970), on the basis of a comparison of microdissection and histological changes in patients with those in rats with experimentally induced cystic disease, proposed that a genetically determined toxic metabolite was responsible. Bernstein and his colleagues (Gardner *et al.* 1978; Evan *et al.* 1979) have drawn attention to a polypoid and papillary epithelial hyperplasia in outer medullary

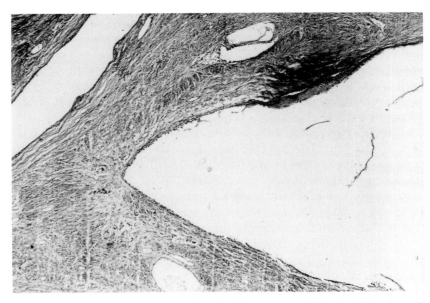

Fig. 9.2. Renal cysts (the light regions in the photograph) in 'adult' polycystic kidney disease ($\times 44$).

collecting tubules as a consistent finding, similar to those seen in experimental models. They suggest that this hyperplasia may cause a partial
obstruction with resultant cyst formation. Support for the idea that such
changes may be the result of a circulating metabolite comes from the
confirmation by computerized tomography that total renal volume
decreases on dialysis or after kidney transplantation (Thaysen and
Thomsen 1982). On the other hand the finding of ultrastructural
changes, especially splitting of the lamina densa of the glomerular
basement membrane (Milutinovic *et al.* 1980a), suggests a defect in
collagen or some other membrane protein.

An autosomal dominant animal model, in CFWwd mice, which fails to
develop in germ-free mice has been described (Werder *et al.* 1984),
raising the question as to whether the ambient environment may play a
role in the pathogenesis of human disease. An autosomal recessive
model, in cy/cy mice, is similar in clinicopathological features to the
human adult type disease, apart from a lack of cystic changes in the liver
(Takahashi *et al.* 1986). In neither of these mouse models is there any
description of epithelial hyperplasia.

An outstanding problem is that of presymptomatic diagnosis for
genetic counselling, or of prental diagnosis. Over the years a variety of
techniques have been used for this purpose. Initially radiological
techniques were employed, especially intravenous and to a less extent
retrograde pyelography. Evans and coworkers (1954), using tomography,
demonstrated renal lesions in patients who had had normal intravenous
pyelograms, and in other cases confirmed bilateral involvement where
previously only one kidney had been shown to be abnormal.
Tomography also facilitated the differentiation between a tumour and a
cyst better than pyelography, an advantage confirmed by Ward and
colleagues (1967). Hatfield and Pfister (1972) also found nephrotomography the method of choice. Fellows and colleagues (1976), using a
variety of radiological techniques in two newborns with abdominal
masses, obtained results in both suggestive of infantile polycystic kidney
but both proved histologically of adult type and both had relatives with
the typical adult type. Abrams and McNeil (1978) in a review of
computed tomography point out that cysts as small as 1 cm diameter
have been detected and that the method has localized cysts where
ordinary pyelography and angiography have failed to do so.

Sherwood (1975) showed that diagnostic ultrasound could be used for
the detection of renal cysts. He and others have shown that some 98 per
cent of known cysts can be detected with a high degree of accuracy by
ultrasound. Ultrasonic investigation of the clinically normal parents of an
infant who had had severe adult type polycystic renal disease revealed
the father to be affected (Begleiter *et al.* 1977). Davis and colleagues

(1977) described the use of β-mode ultrasound scanning for the detection of polycystic kidneys in subjects with a family history of the disease. Wolf and associates (1978) found six out of 17 at-risk children to have renal cysts, including two in whom nephrotomography had failed to do so. Others have reported similar experiences. Hogewind and associates (1980) found that 17 out of 52 at-risk subjects (14 out of 30 over the age of 20 years) had renal cysts detectable by ultrasound. Similarly, Milutinovic (1980b) also found the expected 50 per cent affected among at-risk children over the age of 19 years, but only 30 per cent among those aged 15–19 years. Rosenfield and others (1977), Kelsey and Bowie (1977), and Sahney and colleagues (1983) have all reported their experience of ultrasound and pointed out its advantages in patients with poor renal function, or in children or pregnant women. Bear and associates (1984), in contrast to several of the groups quoted above, found a progressive increase in positive ultrasound diagnosis with age rather than any specific age cut-off. The greater sensitivity of ultrasound, compared with pyelography, in the diagnosis of adult polycystic kidney disease has recently been confirmed (Gabow *et al.* 1984). Ultrasound presymptomatic diagnosis in genetic counselling is clearly of value in two situations. The first is the apparently normal couple who have had an infant with renal cystic disease that is, or could be, of the adult type, as in Begleiter and colleagues' (1977) case. The second is the adult with a parent known, or thought likely, to carry the gene, who has a compelling reason, such as contemplating starting a family, to know his or her own status. That such people at present mostly do not get adequate advice, or are not even aware of their risk, has been demonstrated in a survey of at-risk subjects by Sahney and colleagues (1982).

Zerres and associates (1982) reported the first ultrasound prenatal diagnosis of the disease at 33 weeks of pregnancy in a woman with a positive family history, and this was confirmed postpartum. Main and others (1983) have made prenatal diagnoses at 36 weeks, and in one of a pair of twins at 30 weeks. Scans at 21 weeks in the first of their cases and at 16 and 22 weeks in their second case had been normal. It would thus appear that ultrasound fails to detect the disease in the second trimester. Zerres and colleagues (1985) reported a further prenatal diagnosis of 32 weeks; and subsequently reported prenatal diagnosis at nine weeks from a chorionic villus biopsy using the hypervariable chromosome 16 DNA probe of Reeders described below (Reeders *et al.* 1986b).

Ultrasound along with scintillation has been used to detect hepatic cysts in a patient with polycystic renal disease (Igawa and Muyagishi 1972).

Adult type polycystic kidney is probably the most common inherited renal disease, although its true incidence is difficult to gauge as many cases only become apparent at autopsy. Early estimates that did not differentiate type, based on frequency among hospital admissions, are of the order of 1 in every 3500 admissions (Braasch and Schacht 1933; Oppenheimer 1934), whereas the frequency among autopsies is about 10 fold higher, ranging between 1 in 1000 (Braasch and Schacht 1933) and about 1 in 300 to 400 (Davis 1925; Oppenheimer 1934). Dalgaard (1957) estimated the risk of developing the disease, up to the age of 80, as about 1 in 1200 (80–90 cases per 100 000 population). The disease accounts for 7 to 8 per cent of patients with end-stage renal failure (Parsons *et al.* 1972; Jacobs *et al.* 1977), and 9 per cent of patients on chronic dialysis (Lowrie and Hampers 1981).

The presumption of autosomal dominant inheritance is based on numerous individual reports of families, small series, and the one large series of Dalgaard. Many observations have confirmed roughly equal proportions of affected males and females (Braasch and Schacht 1933; Hausman 1940; Rall and Odel 1949; Dalgaard 1957; Ward *et al.* 1967). One of the difficulties of the early reports of familial cases is that several of those involve affected sibs but lack sufficiently detailed histology to be sure that they represent true adult type polycystic kidney disease, as for example the family of Dunger (1904) in which there were five affected children in the same family. Nevertheless in many such families it is likely that there was an undetected affected parent. Other early family reports include those of Borelius (1901), Osler (1902), Bull (1910), Paus (1914), and Wobus (1918). Crawford (1923) reported a large family in which there were 17 cases among 40 members over five generations including seven out of nine sibs in the fifth generation. One of the largest reported single families was that of Cairns (1925) who studied an East London family with 10 out of 42 members affected over three generations, including male-to-male transmission. Three out of eight sibs were affected in the second generation, five out of 25 at-risk children in the third generation, but none in the fourth, and youngest, generation. Doubtless if Cairns had had modern investigative facilities he would have recognized a higher proportion of affected members. Although Cairns has often been credited with the first recognition of the heritable aetiology of adult polycystic renal disease it is clear that several of the earlier authors quoted above strongly suspected this. One remarkable family consisted of an affected father and six out of his 15 children. One of the affected children and one other child developed hypernephromas (Clemmesen 1942). Fuller (1929) and Cannon (1947) have also published large multigeneration families showing typical autosomal dominant inheritance.

Several authors have published small series, from general medical or surgical practice, in which a varying proportion of cases have had a definite or probable family history of the disease, ranging from 14 per cent of cases (Davis 1928; Oppenheimer 1934) to around 50 per cent definite and probable (Rall and Odel 1949; Higgins 1952). Other similar series include those of Cumming (1928), Arrigoni and colleagues (1954), Simon and Thompson (1955) who observed concordant monozygotic male twins, and Ward and others (1967). The relatively low proportion of patients with a family history in these series could be due to a number of factors. A small proportion of sporadic cases are probably due to new mutation. Non-genetic phenocopies, or misdiagnosis, cannot be excluded although there is no evidence for such heterogeneity. Probably most are due either to a failure to obtain a family history or to the presence in the family of asymptomatic gene carriers. Such gene carriers cannot be reliably detected under the age of 20 years, even with ultrasound and radiological investigation. It is perhaps of interest in this context that out of 14 families referred for genetic counselling to the present author there was more than one affected member diagnosed in all but three families. An early statistical study (Arrigoni *et al.* 1954) of 15 families concluded that the disease was inherited in a dominant manner with variable expression.

Dalgaard (1957) reviewed all cases of polycystic kidney seen in Copenhagen between 1920–1950. These included 242 index cases with the adult type, with a further 108 affected relatives. There were 193 females to 157 males. Mean age of onset was 40.7 years and mean age at diagnosis was 47.2 years. Mean age at death in 254 cases was 51.5 years, being due to renal failure (59 per cent), cerebral haemorrhage (13 per cent), or heart disease (6 per cent) in the great majority. The predominant clinical features were abdominal pain or discomfort, proteinuria, haematuria, pyuria, and palpable mass. Many patients developed an insidious anaemia, presumably due to renal insufficiency. Survival varied from 1 to 13 years. At autopsy hepatic cysts were seen in 75 out of 173 cases (43 per cent). Dalgaard was able to carry out a family study of 232 of his 242 propositi. The clinical case reports on the original 242 propositi mentioned relatives with polycystic kidney in only 15 cases, and with non-specified kidney disease in a further 26 cases. Dalgaard's study revealed the disease in the families of 162 propositi (70 per cent). He found no parental consanguinity. Analysis of his data on the basis of incomplete multiple selection by Weinberg's 'general propositus method' led him to the conclusion that at least the great majority of cases are due to an autosomal gene with dominant inheritance and high penetrance but variable expressivity. He also found a positive correlation within families in age at diagnosis, or death. Dalgaard estimated indirectly a mutation rate of between 6.5×10^{-5} and 12×10^{-5} per gene per generation but admitted the difficulty of making a direct estimate. Of his 80 sporadic cases, in only one did he feel reasonably certain that neither parent carried the gene.

A linkage study to various blood group systems gave negative results, as had Fergusson's earlier linkage study. Two French studies have found an association of adult type polycystic kidney disease and HLA-B5 (Dausset and Hors 1975; Noel *et al.* 1976). However, more recently Dyer and colleagues (1982) have shown that there is no linkage to HLA. This is confirmed by Reeders and his colleagues (1985, 1986a) in Oxford who have very recently reported recombinant DNA studies on nine families with adult polycystic kidney disease. They found linkage to the gene for paraoxonase, an enzyme polymorphism on starch gel electrophoresis, and to a highly variable region on the 3' side of the α-globin gene cluster on the short arm of chromosome 16. This region generates a large number of alleles from DNA rearrangements giving variable copy numbers of a tandem-repeat sequence. The maximum lod score for linkage of the disease locus, in males and females taken together, to this 3' hypervariable region gave $\tilde{z} = 25.85$ at $\theta = 0.05$.

There have been no other major genetic studies of adult polycystic kidney disease since Dalgaard's excellent Danish survey. A number of important questions remain unanswered. To what other gene loci or DNA probes on 16p is the locus linked, and could they be used for presymptomatic or prenatal diagnosis? What are the true mutation rate and gene frequencies? Are there indeed non-genetic phenocopies or is there genetic heterogeneity? And above all what is the gene product and what is its role in pathogenesis? The answers to these questions depend on the discovery of further linked DNA probes and on the eventual isolation and cloning of the disease gene itself. It also remains to be seen whether or not the elucidation of the gene product will eventually lead to specific therapy to arrest the disease process.

References

Abrams, H. L. and McNeil, B. J. (1978). Medical implications of computed tomography ('cat scanning'). *New Engl. J. Med.* **298**, 310–18.

Arey, J. B. (1954). Cystic lesions of the kidney in infants and children. *J. Pediatr.* **54**, 429–45.

Arrigoni, G., Cresseri, A. and Lovati, G. (1954). Genetic research in polycystic kidney. In *Genetica Medica. 1ᵘᵐ Symposium Internationale Geneticae Medicae, 6–7 September, 1953*, ed. Gedda. L. pp. 242–80. Gregor Mendel Institute, Rome.

Baert, L. (1978). Hereditary polycystic kidney disease (adult form): a micro-dissection study of two cases at an early stage of the disease. *Kidney Int.* **13**, 519–25.

Bear, J. C., McManamon, P., Morgan, J., Payne, R. H., Lewis, H., Gault, M. H. and Churchill, D. N. (1984). Age at onset and at ultrasonographic detection of adult polycystic kidney disease: data for genetic counselling. *Am. J. Med. Genet.* **18**, 45–53.

Begleiter, M. L., Smith, T. H., Harris, D. J. (1977). Ultrasound for genetic counselling in polycystic kidney disease (letter). *Lancet* **2**, 1073–4.

Bell, E. T. (1935). Cystic disease of the kidneys. *Am. J. Pathol.* **11**, 373–418.

Bengtsson, U., Hedman, L. and Svalander, C. (1975). Adult type of polycystic kidney disease in a new-born child. *Acta Med. Scand.* **197**, 447–50.

Bigelow, N. H. (1953). Association of polycystic kidneys with intracranial aneurysms and other related disorders. *Am. J. Med. Sci.* **225**, 485–94.

Blyth, H. and Ockenden, B. G. (1971). Polycystic disease of the kidneys and liver presenting in childhood. *J. Med. Genet.* **8**, 257–84.

Borelius, J. (1901). Zur Genese and Klinische Diagnose der polyzytischen degeneration der Nieren. *Nord. Med. Ark.* **34**, 1–27.

Braasch, W. F. and Schacht, F. W. (1933). Pathological and clinical data concerning polycystic kidney. *Surg. Gynecol. Obstet.* **57**, 467–75.

Brown, R. A. (1951). Polycystic disease of the kidneys and intracranial aneurysms. The etiology and inter-relationship of these conditions: review of recent literature and report of seven cases in which both conditions coexisted. *Glasgow Med. J.* **32**, 333–48.

Bull, P. (1910). Inficierte cystenniere. *Arch. f. Klin. Chir.* **91**, 745–53.

Cairns, H. W. B. (1925). Heredity in polycystic disease of the kidneys. *Quart. J. Med.* **18**, 359–92.

Cannon, J. F. (1947). Hereditary polycystic kidney. *Ann. Intern. Med.* **27**, 610–16.

Carter, C. O. (1974). Polycystic disease presenting in childhood. In *5th Conference on the Clinical Delineation of Birth Defects. Birth Defects Orig. Art. Series* **10**, 16. Liss, New York.

Case Records of the Massachusetts General Hospital (1968). *New Engl. J. Med.* **278**, 899–904.

Chapman, J. R. and Hilson, A. J. W. (1980). Polycystic kidneys and abdominal aortic aneurysms. *Lancet* **1**, 646–7.

Churchill, D. N., Beat, J. C., Morgan, J., Payne, R. H., McManamon, P. J. and Gault, M. H. (1984). Prognosis of adult onset polycystic kidney disease re-evaluated. *Kidney Int.* **26**, 190–3.

Clemmesen, J. (1942). Familiaert malignt hypernephrom en slaegt med hereditaer cystenyre. *Nordisk Med.* **14**, 1472–6.

Crawford, R. H. (1923). Polycystic kidney. *Surg. Gynecol. Obstet.* **36**, 185–8.

Cumming, R. E. (1928). Polycystic kidney disease. *J. Urol.* **19**, 149–79.

Dalgaard, O. Z. (1957). Bilateral polycystic disease of the kidneys. *Acta Med. Scand.* **158**, (Suppl. 328), 1–251.

Danielsen, H., Pedersen, E. B., Nielsen, A. H., Herlevsen, P., Kornerup, H. J. and Posborg, V. (1986). Expansion of extracellular volume in early polycystic kidney disease. *Acta. Med. Scand.* **219**, 399–405.

Darmady, E. M., Offer, J. and Woodhouse, M. A. (1970). Toxic metabolite defect in polycystic disease of the kidney—an hypothesis. *Lancet* **1**, 547–50.

Dausset, J. and Hors, J. (1975). Some contributions of the HL-A complex to the genetics of human disease. *Transplant Rev.* **22**, 44–74.

Davis, J. E. (1925). Congenital polycystic kidneys. *Am. J. Obstet. Gynecol.* **9**, 758–83.

—— (1928). Surgical pathology of malformations in kidneys and ureters. *J. Urol.* **20**, 183–231.

Davis, M. C., Aufleger, M. A., Denney, J. D., Marty, R., Milutinovic, J. and Fialkow, P. J. (1977). Intercostal oblique technique of β-mode ultrasound scanning in polycystic kidney disease. *Med. Ultrasound* **1**, 31.

DeBono, D. P. and Evans, D. B. (1977). The management of polycystic kidney with special reference to dialysis and transplantation. *Quart. J. Med.* **46**, 353–64.

Ditlefsen, E. M. L. and Tonjum, A. M. (1960). Intracranial aneurysms and polycystic kidneys. *Acta. Med. Scand.* **168**, 51–4.

Dunger, R. (1904). Zur Lehre, von der Cystenniere. *Beitr. z. path. Anat. u.z. allg. Path.* **35**, 445–509.

Dyer, P. A., Watters, E. A., Klouda, P. T., Harris, R. and Mallick, N. P. (1982). Absence of linkage between adult polycystic kidney disease and the major histocompatibility system. *Tissue Antigens* **20**, 108–11.

Eulderink, F. and Hogewind, B. L. (1978). Renal cysts in premature children. *Arch. Pathol. Lab. Med.* **102**, 592–5.

Evan, A. P., Gardner, K. D. Jr. and Bernstein, J. (1979). Polyploid and papillary epithelial hyperplasia: a potential cause of ductal obstruction in adult polycystic kidney. *Kidney Int.* **16**, 743–50.

Evans, J. A., Dubilier, W. and Monteith, J. C. (1954). Nephrotomography: a preliminary report. *Am. J. Roetgenol,* **71**, 213–23.

Fellows, R. A., Leonidas, J. C. and Beatty, E. C. Jr. (1976). Radiologic features of 'adult type' polycystic kidney disease in the neonate. *Pediatr. Radiol.* **4**, 87–92.

Fergusson, J. D. (1949). Observations on familial polycystic disease of the kidney. *Proc. R. Soc. Med.* **42**, 806–14.

Fryns, J. P. and van den Berghe, H. (1979). 'Adult' form of polycystic kidney disease in neonates. *Clin. Genet.* **15**, 205–6.

Fuller, C. J. (1929). Familial polycystic disease of the kidneys. *Quart. J. Med.* **22**, 567–74.

Funck-Brentano, J.-L. and Vantelon, J. (1963). Varieties evolutives de la polykystose renale de l'adulte. *Actualities Nephrologiques de l'Hôpital Necker*, pp. 63–77. Flammarion, Paris.

——, —— and Lopez-Alvarez, R. (1964). Les accidents evolutifs de la maladie polykystique des reins. *Presse Méd.* **72**, 1583–8.

Gabow, P. A., Ikle, D. W. and Holmes, J. H. (1984). Polycystic kidney disease: Prospective analysis of nonazotemic patients and family members. *Ann. Intern. Med.* **101**, 238–47.

Gardner, K. D., Jr., Evan, A. P. and Bernstein, J. (1978). Polyps in renal cystic disease. (Letter.) *Lancet* **1**, 878–9.

Gleason, D. C., McAlister, W. H. and Kissane, J. (1967). Cystic disease of the kidneys in children. *Am. J. Roetgenol. Radium Therap. Nucl. Med.* **100**, 135–46.

Halbertsma, L. (1932). Uber einen Klinisch beobachteten Fall erblichen Cystenniere bei 10 järigen Kinde. *Z. f. Kindheilk.* **52**, 145–55.

Hatfield, P. M. and Pfister, R. C. (1972). Adult polycystic disease of the kidneys (Potter type 3). *JAMA* **222**, 1527–31.

Hausman, H. (1940). Polycystic kidney disease. *Am. J. Surg.* **49**, 335–41.

Heggö, O. (1966). A microdisection study of cystic disease of the kidney in adults. *J. Pathol. Bact.* **91**, 311–15.

Higgins, C. C. (1952). Bilateral polycystic kidney disease: review of ninety-four cases. *Arch. Surg.* **65**, 318–29.

Hildebrand (1894). Weiterer Beitrag zur pathologischen anatomie der Nierengeschwülste. *Arch. f. Klin. Chir.* **48**, 343–71.

Hogewind, B. L., Veltkamp, J. J., Koch, C. W. and de Graeff, J. (1980). Genetic counselling for adult polycystic kidney disease. Ultrasound a useful tool in pre-symptomatic diagnosis. *Clin. Genet.* **18**, 168–72.

Igawa, K.-Z. and Miyagishi, T. (1972). The use of scintillation and ultrasonic scanning to disclose polycystic kidneys and liver. *J. Urol.* **108**, 685–8.

Jacobs, C., Brunner, F. P., Chantler, C., Donckerwolcke, R. A., Gurland, H. J., Hathaway, R. A., Selwood, N. H. and Wing, A. J. (1977). Dialysis transplantation nephrology, part I statistical reports. *Proc. Eur. Dialysis and Transplantation Assoc.* **64**, 3–69.

Kaplan, B. S., Rabin, I., Nogrady, M. B. and Drummond, K. N. (1977). Autosomal dominant polycystic renal disease in children. *J. Pediatr.* **90**, 782–3.

Karhunen, P. J. and Tenhu, M. (1986). Adult polycystic liver and kidney diseases are separate entities. *Clin. Genet.* **30**, 29–37.

Kaye, C. and Lewy, P. R. (1974). Congenital appearance of adult-type (autosomal dominant) polycystic kidney disease. *J. Pediatr.* **85**, 807–10.

Kelsey, J. A. and Bowie, J. D. (1977). Gray-scale ultrasonography in the diagnosis of polycystic kidney disease. *Radiology* **122**, 791–5.

Levey, A. S., Pauker, S. G. and Kassirer, J. P. (1983). Occult intracranial aneurysms in polycystic kidney disease. *New Engl. J. Med.* **308**, 986–94.

Loh, J. P., Haller, J. O., Kassner, E. G., Aloni, A. and Glassberg, K. (1977). Dominantly inherited polycystic kidneys in infants: association with hypertrophic pyloric stenosis. *Pediatr. Radiol.* **6**, 27–31.

Lowrie, E. G. and Hampers, C. L. (1981). The success of Medicare's end-stage renal-disease program. *New Engl. J. Med.* **305**, 434–8.

McLean, R. H., Goldstein, J., Conrad, F. U., Rasoulpour, M. and Crawford, B. (1980). Autosomal dominant (adult) polycystic kidney disease in childhood. *Conn. Med.* **44**, 690–2.

McMahon, H. E. (1929). Congenital anomalies of the liver. *Am. J. Pathol.* **5**, 499–508.

Main, D., Mennuti, M. T., Cornfield, D. and Coleman, B. (1983). Prenatal diagnosis of adult polycystic kidney disease. *Lancet* **2**, 337–8.

Marquardt, W. (1936). Zur Kasuistik des familiären Auftretens der Cystennieren. *Der Erbarzt* **3**, 102–3.

Mehrizi, A., Rosenstein, B. J., Pusch, A., Askin, J. A. and Taussig, H. B. (1964). Myocardial infarction and endocardial fibroelastosis in children with polycystic kidneys. *Bull. Johns. Hopkins Hosp.* **115**, 92–8.

Milutinovic, J., Agodoa, L. C. Y., Cutler, R. E. and Striker, G. E. (1980a). Autosomal dominant polycystic kidney disease. Early diagnosis and consideration of pathogenesis. *Am. J. Clin. Pathol.* **73**, 740–7.

——, Fialkow, P. J., Phillips, L. A., Agodoa, L. Y., Bryant, J. I., Denney, J. C. and Rudd, T. G. (1980b). Autosomal dominant polycystic kidney disease: early diagnosis and data for genetic counselling. *Lancet* **1**, 1203–6.

——, ——, Agodoa, L. Y., Phillips, L. A. and Bryant, J. I. (1983). Fertility and pregnancy complications in women with autosomal dominant polycystic kidney disease. *Obstet. Gynaecol.* **61**, 566–70.

——, ——, ——, ——, Rudd, T. G. and Bryant, J. I. (1984). Autosomal dominant polycystic kidney disease: symptoms and clinical findings. *Quart. J. Med.* **53**, 511–22.

Montoliu, J., Torras, A. and Revert, L. (1980). Polycystic kidneys and abdominal aortic aneurysms. *Lancet* **1**, 1133–4.

Noel, L. H., Descamps, B., Jungers, P., Bach, J. F., Busson, M., Guillet, J. and Hors, J. (1976). HLA serotyping in 5 well defined kidney diseases, in HLA and Disease, *INSERM* p. 206.

Oppenheimer, G. D. (1934). Polycystic disease of the kidney. *Ann. Surg.* **100**, 1136–58.

Osathanondh, V. and Potter, E. L. (1964). Pathogenesis of polycystic kidneys. *Arch. Pathol.* **77**, 485–501.

Osler, W. (1902). On heredity in bilateral cystic kidney. *Am. Med.* No. 3, p. 951.

Parsons, F. P., Brunner, F. P., Gurland, H. J., Harlen, H. and Schärer, K. (1972). Combined report on regular dialysis and transplantation in Europe, 11, 1971, *Proc. Eur. Dial. Transplant. Assoc.* **9**, 3–35.

Paus, N. (1914). Cystenniere mit Symptomen von Ruptura renis. *Deut. Z. f. Chir.* **130**, 628–31.

Poinso, R., Monges, H. and Payan, H. (1954). La maladie kystique du foie. *Expansion Scientifique Francaise.*

Poutasse, E. F., Gardner, W. J. and McCormack, L. J. (1954). Polycystic kidney disease and intracranial aneurysm. *JAMA* **154**, 741–4.

Proesmans, W., van Damme, B., Casaer, P. and Marchal, G. (1982). Autosomal dominant polycystic kidney disease in the neonatal period. Association with a cerebral arterio-venous malformation. *Pediatrics.* **70**, 971–5.

Rall, J. E. and Odel, H. M. (1949). Congenital polycystic disease of the kidney. Review of the literature and data on 207 cases. *Am. J. Med. Sci.* **218**, 399–407.

Ratcliffe, P. J., Reeders, S. and Theaker, J. M. (1984). Bleeding oesophageal varices and hepatic dysfunction in adult polycystic kidney disease. *Br. Med. J.* **288**, 1330–1.

Ribbert, M. W. H. (1896). *Die Normale und patholische Physiologic und Anatomie der Niere.* T. G. Fisher & Co, Cassal.

Reeders, S. T., Breuning, M. H., Davies, K. E., Nicholls, R. D., Jarman, A. P., Higgs, D. R., Pearson, P. L. and Weatherall, D. J. (1985). A highly polymorphic DNA marker linked to adult polycystic kidney disease on chromosome 16. *Nature* **317**, 542–4.

——, ——, Corney, G., Jeremiah, S. J., Meera Khan, P., Davies, K. E., Hopkinson, D. A., Pearson, P. L. and Weatherall, D. J. (1986a). Two genetic markers closely linked to adult polcystic kidney disease on chromosome 16. *Br. Med. J.* **292**, 851–3.

——, Zerres, K., Gal, A., Hogenkamp, T., Propping, P., Schmidt, W., Waldherr, R., Dolata, M. M., Davies, K. E. and Weatherall, D. J. (1986b). Prenatal diagnosis of autosomal dominant polycystic kidney disease with a DNA probe. *Lancet* **2**, 6–8.

Rosenfield, A. T., Allen, W. E., Curtis, A. M., Siegel, N. J., Putnam, C. E., Hsia, Y. E. and Taylor, K. J. W. (1977). Gray scale ultrasonography, computerized tomography and nephrotomography in evaulation of polycystic kidney and liver disease. *Urology* **9**, 436–8.

Ross, D. G. and Travers, H. (1975). Infantile presentation of adult-type polycystic kidney disease in a large kindred. *J. Pediatr.* **87**, 760–3.

Sahney, S., Weiss, L. and Levin, N. W. (1982). Genetic counselling in adult polycystic kidney disease. *Am. J. Med. Genet.* **11**, 461–8.

——, Sandler, M. A., Weiss, L., Levin, N. W., Hricak, H. and Madrazo, B. L. (1983). Adult polycystic kidney disease: presymptomatic diagnosis for genetic counselling. *Clin. Nephrol.* **20**, 89–93.

Savera, O. (1946). Zur Erbpathologie der Zystenniere. *Wiener Klin. Wschr.* **58**, 422–6.

Sherwood, T. (1975). Renal masses and ultrasound. *Br. Med. J.* **4**, 682–3.

Shokeir, M. H. K. (1978). Expression of 'adult' polycystic renal disease in the fetus and newborn. *Clin. Genet.* **14**, 61–72.

Simon, H. B. and Thompson, G. J. (1955). Congenital renal polycystic disease. A clinical and therapeutic study of 366 cases. *JAMA* **159**, 657–62.

Steiner, D. R. (1899). Über, grosscystische Degeneration der Nieren und der Leber. *Dtsch. Med. Wsch.* **25**, 677–8.

Stickler, G. B. and Kelalis, P. P. (1975). Polycystic kidney disease: recognition of the 'adult' form (autosomal dominant) in infancy. *Mayo Clin. Proc.* **50**, 547–8.

Takahashi, H., Veyama, Y., Hibino, T., Kuwahara, Y., Suzuki, S., Hioki, K. and Tamaoki, N. (1986). A new mouse model of genetically transmitted polycystic kidney disease. *J. Urol.* **135**, 1280–3.

Thaysen, J. H. and Thomsen, H. S. (1982). Involution of polycystic kidneys during replacement therapy of terminal renal failure. *Acta Med. Scand.* **212**, 389–94.

Virchow, R. (1869). Über hydrops renum cysticus congenitus. *Virchow's Arch. (Pathol. Anat.)* **46**, 506–40.

Ward, J. N., Draper, J. W. and Lavengood, R. W. (1967). A clinical review of polycystic kidney in 53 patients. *J. Urol.* **98**, 48–53.

Werder, A. A., Amos, M. A., Nielsen, A. H. and Wolfe, G. H. (1984). Comparitive effects of germfree and ambient environments on the development of cystic kidney disease in CFWwd mice. *J. Lab. Clin. Med.* **103**, 399–407.

Wobus, R. E. (1918). Congenital polycystic kidney with a report of four cases, occurring in children of the same mother. *Surg. Gynecol. Obstet.* **27**, 423–5.

Wolf, B., Rosenfield, A. T., Taylor, K. J. W., Rosenfield, N., Gottlieb, S. and Hsia, Y. E. (1978). Presymptomatic diagnosis of adult onset polycystic kidney disease by ultrasonography. *Clin. Genet.* **14**, 1–7.

Zerres, K., Weiss, H., Bulla, M. and Roth, B. (1982). Prenatal diagnosis of an early manifestation of autosomal dominant adult-type polycystic kidney disease. *Lancet* **2**, 988.

——, Hansmann, M., Knöpfle, G. and Stephan, M. (1985). Prenatal diagnosis of genetically determined early manifestation of autosomal dominant polycystic kidney disease. *Hum. Genet.* **71**, 368–9.

9.1.4. Hereditary renal cortical microcystic disease

A single family involving a 39-year-old father and all of his three children, two sons and a daughter, has been reported with an asymptomatic renal failure (Melnick *et al.* 1984). All four patients had raised serum urea and uric acid, reduced creatinine clearance, impaired urine-concentrating ability, and a moderate metabolic acidosis. The children had a mild normochromic, normocytic anaemia. There was no proteinuria or haematuria, and no electrolyte disturbance. They were normotensive and there was no retinopathy. Renal biopsies showed microcysts of the renal cortex, some of which contained vestigial glomerular tufts. There is no evidence as to the pathogenesis of this disorder. Inheritance would appear to be autosomal dominant.

Reference

Melnick, S. C., Brewer, D. B. and Oldham, J. S. (1984). Cortical microcystic disease of the kidney with dominant inheritance: a previously undescribed syndrome. *J. Clin. Pathol.* **37**, 494–9.

9.1.5. Medullary sponge kidney

This is a comparatively common radiological diagnosis of dilatation or cyst formation of the medullary collecting tubules, often associated with punctate or linear calcification of the papillae (Fig. 9.3), or even stone formation. It usually has a relatively benign prognosis and is non-progressive (Leonarduzi 1939; Cacchi and Ricci 1949; Ekstom *et al.* 1959; Kuiper 1976). There is some diminution in urine-concentrating

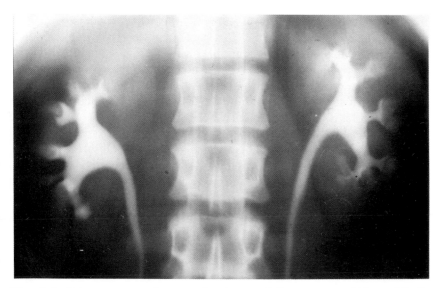

Fig. 9.3. Intravenous pyelogram showing medullary sponge kidney. Kindly provided by Dr R. W. E. Watts.

ability and acidification (Higashihara *et al.* 1984), and in short term response to a potassium load (Green *et al.* 1984). The cause is unknown but it has been regarded as a congenital but non-genetic lesion which is either an asymptomatic coincidental finding or presents with complications such as urolithiasis or renal infection. Abeshouse and Abeshouse (1960) reported five cases and reviewed the pathology. Butler and colleagues (1973) reviewed the subject and presented 33 new cases. There are only rare familial reports, including one of its occurence in a father and his adult daughter (Copping 1967), and another of its occurrence in at least three generations (Kuiper 1971). Nemoy and Forsberg (1968) have observed a case of adult polycystic kidney disease presenting atypically as medullary sponge kidney. Congenital hemihypertrophy has been reported in association with typical sporadic medullary sponge kidney (Harrison and Williams 1971; Sprayregen *et al.* 1971) too often to be purely coincidental.

There have been considerable controversy and semantic confusion over the years regarding familial disorders involving renal medullary lesions. These familial disease differ radically from the benign sporadic medullary sponge kidney just described. As with polycystic kidney disease there appears to be an adult onset dominant form and a juvenile autosomal recessive disorder.

The autosomal dominant disorder has been referred to as medullary sponge kidney or renal medullary cystic disease, with or without the qualifying phrase 'adult onset'. The onset of this disorder is typically in the third to fifth decade, although a range as wide as 8 to 68 years is reported. Death usually ensues 2 to 4 years after diagnosis in the absence of renal dialysis or transplantation. The recessive juvenile disorder, discussed below, has also been termed medullary cystic disease and has for some time been regarded as identical to juvenile nephronophthisis, or hereditary degenerative nephropathy. To add to this confusion the disease in a family with what is probably the adult type has been termed 'progressive hereditary nephropathy'. There is some overlap in age of expression of the adult and juvenile disorders. Onset of juvenile nephronophthisis is between 2 and 14 years and age at death 4 to 20 years. Both disorders, adult and juvenile, present as a progressive nephropathy with little or no proteinuria or haematuria, with refractory anaemia, and cortico-medullary or medullary cysts. Usually the nephropathy is associated with salt loss, not invariable in the adult form; consequently hypertension, if present, is only terminal. The confusion between these two disorders in the literature is exemplified by the paper of Axelsson and Ödlund (1968) who use a family of adult dominant medullary cystic disease to argue for the identity of medullary cystic disease and familial juvenile nephronophthisis. Similarly Chamberlin and coworkers (1977) while accepting the different modes of inheritance, paradoxically regard adult medullary cystic disease and juvenile nephronophthisis as a single entity.

The salt-wasting nature of adult medullary cystic disease led to the first description of this disease as 'renal failure simulating adrenocortical insufficiency' (Thorn *et al.* 1944, 1960). Further reports followed of sporadic cases (Strauss 1962; Gill *et al.* 1969; Snelling *et al.* 1970). Strauss (1962) reviewed 18 cases commenting on this insidious onset, typically in the third or fourth decade (range 8–56 years); anaemia; azotaemia with salt wasting and frequent lack of proteinuria, urinary sediment, or hypertension; association with osteitis fibrosa in childhood or adolescence; and short survival of up to 4 years. One of his patients had an affected twin brother, probably monozygotic; another had an affected brother and a mother who died of 'Bright's disease'. Kliger and Scheer (1976) described impaired renal function or radiological changes in eight out of 12 asymptomatic children of three affected sisters in one family. Gardner and colleagues described two further families (Goldman *et al.* 1966; Gardner 1971) with a similar clinical picture, except that only one member of their second family (family B) had salt wasting. Histologically they described thin cortices with glomerular hyalinization, cortico-medullary or medullary cysts lined by low cuboidal epithelium and an increase in medullary connective tissue. At least one of the families of 'nephronophthisis and medullary cystic disease' reported by Mongeau and Worthen (1967) probably had this adult dominant form of the disease. Some success in treatment by renal transplantation, without subsequent cystic change in the transplanted organ, has been reported (Gardner 1971). The pathogenesis of this disorder, and also of the juvenile form, remains obscure. Experimental studies with rats fed diphenylamine which developed impaired urine-concentrating ability and progressive collecting tubules dilation and sacculation (Thomas *et al.* 1957; Safou *et al.* 1970) suggested a possible nephrotoxic origin for either disease. The similarity of the changes in juvenile nephronophthisis to Balkan nephropathy (Mongeau and Worthen 1967; Hand and Tennant 1968) supports this idea. However, the fact that transplanted kidneys do not become affected in either the adult or juvenile forms (Gardner 1971; Case Records Mass. Gen. Hosp. 1975; Chamberlin *et al.* 1977) provides contrary evidence. Lyon and Hulse (1971) described a recessive gene in the mouse, *kd*, that produces a disease in homozygotes very similar to human nephronophthisis, but no further work appears to have been done with this strain. Pathogenesis is discussed more fully by Strauss (1971).

A number of family studies of the adult form with affected members over several generations confirm its autosomal dominant inheritance. These show transmission from affected fathers to their affected sons and/

or failure to transmit to their daughters, and almost complete penetrance in patients who live long enough (Goldman *et al.* 1966; Gardner 1971; Wrigley *et al.* 1973; Swenson *et al.* 1974). However, although onset is typically in the third to fourth decades there are reports of onset in childhood (Strauss 1962; Snelling *et al.* 1970) or at a later age with slower progression (Wrigley *et al.* 1973; Swenson *et al.* 1974). Occult affection in the mother of two severely affected individuals has also been reported (Whelton *et al.* 1974).

Prenatal diagnosis has not been reported.

References

Abeshouse, B. S. and Abeshouse, G. A. (1960). Sponge kidney: a review of the literature and a report of five cases. *J. Urol.* **84**, 252–67.

Axelsson, U. and Ödlund, B. (1968). Cystic disease of the renal medulla and its possible relation to juvenile nephronophthisis. *Acta Med. Scand.* **183**, 275–80.

Butler, M. R., Devine, H. F. and O'Flynn, J. D. (1973). Medullary sponge kidney: a review of the literature and presentation of 33 cases. *J. Irish Med. Assoc.* **66**, 5–13.

Cacchi, R. and Ricci, V. (1949). Sur une rare maladie kystique multiple des prepamides renales, le 'rein en eponge'. *J. d'Urol.* **55**, 497–519.

Case Records of the Massachusetts Gen. Hosp. (1975). Case 9–1975. *New Engl. J. Med.* **292**, 469–74.

Chamberlin, B. C., Hagge, W. W. and Stickler, G. B. (1977). Juvenile nephronophthisis and medullary cystic disease. *Mayo Clin. Proc.* **52**, 485–91.

Copping, G. A. (1967). Medullary sponge kidney: its occurrence in a father and daughter. *Can. Med. Assoc. J.* **96**, 608–11.

Ekstrom, T., Engfeldt, B., Lagergren, C. and Lindvall, N. (1959). *Medullary sponge kidney.* Almqvist & Wiskell, Stockholm.

Gardner, K. D. (1971). Evolution of clinical signs in adult-onset cystic disease of the renal medulla. *Ann. Intern. Med.* **74**, 47–54.

Gill, G., Pallotta, J., Kashgarion, M., Kessner, D. and Epstein, F. H. (1969). Physiologic studies in renal osteodystrophy treated by subtotal parathyroidectomy. *Am. J. Med.* **46**, 930–40.

Goldman, S. H., Walker, S. R., Merigan, T. C., Gardner, K. D. and Bull, J. M. C. (1966). Hereditary occurrence of cystic disease of the renal medulla. *New Engl. J. Med.* **274**, 984–92.

Green, J., Szylman, P., Sznajder, I. I., Winaver, J. and Better, O. S. (1984). Renal tubular handling of potassium in patients with medullary sponge kidney. A model of renal papillectomy in humans. *Arch. Intern. Med.* **144**, 2201–4.

Handa, S. P. and Tennant, R. (1968). Medullary cystic disease of the kidney: its occurrence in two siblings. *Postgrad. Med. J.* **44**, 792–8.

Harrison, A. R. and Williams, J. P. (1971). Medullary sponge kidney and congenital hemihypertrophy. *Br. J. Urol.* **43**, 552–61.

Higashihara, E., Nutahara, K., Tago, K., Veno, A. and Niijima, R. (1984). Medullary sponge kidney and renal acidification defect. *Kidney Int.* **25**, 453–9.

Kliger, A. S. and Scheer, R. L. (1976). Familial disease of the renal medulla: a study of progeny in a family with medullary cystic disease. *Ann. Intern. Med.* **85**, 190–4.

Kuiper, J. J. (1971). Medullary sponge kidney in three generations. *NY State J. Med.* **71**, 2665–9.

—— (1976). Medulary Sponge Kidney. In *Cystic disease of the kidney* ed. Gardner, K. D. Jr. p. 151. John Wiley, New York.

Leonarduzzi, N. (1939). Reporto peilographico poco commune dilatazione delle vie urinarie intrarenali. *Radiologia Medica (Torino)* **26**, 346.

Lyon, M. F. and Hulse, F. V. (1971). An inherited kidney disease of mice resembling human nephronophthisis. *J. Med. Genet.* **8**, 41–8.

Mongeau, J. G. and Worthen, H. G. (1967). Nephonophthisis and medullary cystic disease. *Am. J. Med.* **43**, 345–55.

Nemoy, N. J. and Forsberg, L. (1968). Polycystic renal disease presenting as medullary sponge kidney. *J. Urol.* **100**, 407–11.

Safouh, M., Crocker, J. F. S. and Vernier, R. L. (1970). Experimental cystic disease of the kidney: sequential, functional and morphologic studies. *Lab. Invest.* **23**, 392–400.

Snelling, C. E., Brown, N. M. and Smythe, C. A. (1970). Medullary sponge kidney in a child. *Can. Med. Assoc. J.* **102**, 518–19.

Sprayregen, S., Strasberg, Z. and Naidich, T. P. (1971). Medullary sponge kidney and congenital total hemihypertrophy. *NY State J. Med.* **73**, 2768–71.

Strauss, M. B. (1962). Clinical and pathological aspects of cystic disease of the renal medulla. An analysis of eighteen cases. *Ann. Intern. Med.* **57**, 373–81.

—— (1971). Medullary cystic disease. In *Diseases of the kidney*, 2nd edn. eds. Strauss, M. B. and Webb, L. G. p. 1259. Little Brown, Boston.

Swenson, R. S., Kempson, R. L. and Friedland, G. W. (1974). Cystic disease of the renal medulla in the elderly. *JAMA* **228**, 1401–4.

Thorn, G. W. Goldfien, A., Suiter, T. B. and Dammin, G. (1960). Hormonal studies in salt-losing nephritis. *Med. Clin. N. Amer.* **44**, 1139–54.

Thomas, J. O., Cox, A. J. and DeEds, F. (1957). Kidney cysts produced by diphenylamine. *Stan. Med. Bull.* **15**, 90–3.

Thorn, G. W., Koepf, G. F. and Clinton, M. (1944). Renal failure simulating adrenocortical insufficiency. *New Engl. J. Med.* **231**, 76–85.

Whelton, A., Ozer, F. L., Bias, W. B., Williams, G. M. and Walker, W. G. (1974). Renal medullary cystic disease: a family study. In *Clinical delineation of birth defects, XVI. Urinary system and others.* ed. Bergsma, D. *Birth Defects Orig. Art. Series.* X (**4**), 154–6.

Wrigley, K. A., Sherman, R. L., Ennis, F. A. and Becker, E. L. (1973). Progressive hereditary nephropathy: a varient of medullary cystic disease. *Arch. Intern. Med.* **131**, 240–4.

9.1.6. Medullary cystic disease (juvenile nephronophthisis) and Jeune's asphyxiating thoracic dystrophy

In 1945 Smith and Graham, in the USA, described a renal disease with medullary cysts. Using this criterion further cases were reported from America, some of which fall into the autosomal dominant adult category discussed above, but others of which were associated with an earlier onset. The disease is readily diagnosed radiologically by nephro-tomography (Spicer *et al.* 1969). Some years later an apparently separate disease without medullary cysts but otherwise similar clinically and histologically, apart from a still earlier onset, was reported from Europe under the names 'familial juvenile nephronophthisis' (Fanconi *et al.* 1951) or 'nephrosclerosis' (Clark 1951). In both diseases one of the earliest clinical manifestations is a urine-concentrating defect with polyuria. The European literature emphasized the familial nature of the disease, consistent with autosomal recessive inheritance (Fanconi *et al.* 1951; Hackzell and Lundmark 1958; Broberger *et al.* 1960; Ivemark *et al.* 1960). Apart from the frequent occurrence of affected sibs, parental consanguinity was also observed (Fanconi *et al.* 1951; Von Sydow and Ranstrom 1962). Renal osteodystrophy has also been reported as a complication (Burke *et al.* 1963).

In 1964 Mangos and colleagues drew the attention of paediatricians to the occurrence of juvenile nephronophthisis in the United States, and suggested that heterozygotes may show impaired urine-concentrating ability. In the same year Winberg suggested that nephronophthisis and medullary cystic disease may be different stages of the same disease. This suggestion was taken up by several other groups (Herdman *et al.* 1967; Mongeau and Worthen 1967; Strauss and Sommers 1967; Pedreira *et al.* 1968). Sworn and Eisinger (1972) actually observed the two disorders in different members of the same sibship with cystic medullary changes only in the eldest sib. Furthermore later American writers have confirmed the familial occurrence of medullary cystic disease with a pattern consistent with autosomal recessive inheritance (Alexander and Campbell 1970). One report suggesting autosomal dominant inheritance of the juvenile form in a family with six out of 12 sibs affected and several affected members of the two preceding generations (Giangiacomo *et al.* 1975) presents good evidence for juvenile medullary cystic disease in the six sibs but only evidence of non-specific renal disease in the earlier generations. This family looks more like recessive medullary cystic disease, especially as there was no renal disease in the parents of the sibs.

Several studies have contributed to the histological picture and to our understanding of the pathogenesis of the juvenile disease. The histology is similar to that in the adult dominant form with glomerular sclerosis, tubular atrophy, and at a later stage medullary cysts (Gibson and Arneil 1972). Several workers have demonstrated that the cysts are found in, or connected to, collecting ducts or tubules, either by microdissection (Sherman *et al.* 1971) or by electron microscopy (Pascal 1973). Giselson and colleagues (1970) demonstrated that the tubular defect antedates glomerular impairment, and Schimke (1975) on the basis of the excessive salt loss suggested that a defect in tubular handling of potassium is the cause of the renal cystic lesion. Pascal (1973) observed excessive basement membrane formation on electron microscopy, and intracytoplasmic vesicles which may be related to an electrolyte transport defect.

Several groups have described skeletal changes in juvenile nephronophthisis (Chakera 1975; Mainzer *et al.* 1970). Robins and coworkers (1976) reviewed these secondary skeletal changes. Shah (1980), who reported three patients with juvenile nephronophthisis and chronic renal failure, pointed out that their skeletal changes were those of Jeune's asphyxyiating thoracic dystrophy. One of his patients with short limbs and thoracic dystrophy had been previously reported by Robins and coworkers (1976), and even earlier by Chakera (1975) without the diagnosis of Jeune's syndrome being made. Whilst typically infants with Jeune's syndrome (Jeune *et al.* 1955) die in infancy, longer survival with renal complications, comprising the changes of juvenile nephronophthisis, is well recognized (Herdman and Langer 1968; Shokeir *et al.* 1971; Bernstein *et al.* 1974; Edelson *et al.* 1974; Gruskin *et al.* 1974; Oberklaid *et al.* 1977).

Donaldson and colleagues (1985) have investigated the relationship between juvenile nephronophthisis and Jeune's syndrome. They studied 14 patients with familial juvenile nephronophthisis, one of whom also had the typical features of Jeune's syndrome. In a review of published series of cases of Jeune's syndrome (Herdman and Langer 1968; Gruskin *et al.* 1971; Shokeir 1971; Bernstein *et al.* 1974; Edelson 1974; Oberklaid *et al.* 1977; Shah 1980) they found that those infants who died from respiratory failure in infancy had autopsy evidence of tubular dilatation, cortical renal cysts, diffuse cystic disease, or cystic dysplasia. Children who survived beyond infancy developed covert or overt renal disease, or died from chronic renal failure with tubular dilatation, glomerular sclerosis, and interstitial nephritis. Several of these authors noted the similarity to nephronophthisis. Donaldson and colleagues believe the renal lesion in older children with Jeune's syndrome to be indistinguishable from that in juvenile nephronophthisis. In conclusion, while nephronophthisis is clearly a component of Jeune's syndrome, and patients with juvenile nephronophthisis may have skeletal changes, their differing clinical presentation leaves little doubt that they are genetically distinct. Indeed since some of the cases quoted above fall into some of the further categories discussed below there is clearly considerable genetic heterogeneity within the group of diseases with familial nephronophthisis. Rayfield and McDonald (1972) confirmed an old suggestion of an association with red hair. As discussed earlier (pp. 463–4) nephronophthisis may be the renal lesion in congenital hepatic fibrosis. It may also be the lesion in the syndrome described by Ivemark discussed below (p. 493), and also in Leber's amaurosis (see p. 493).

There have been numerous other reports of affected sibs (Kobayashi *et al.* 1967; Handa and Tennant 1968; Royer 1968; Gibson and Arneil 1972; Betts and Forrest-Hay 1973; Habib 1974; Kleinknecht *et al.* 1975; Chamberlin *et al.* 1977; Steel *et al.* 1980). Betts and Forrest-Hay (1973) include a concordant monozygotic twin pair. Parental consanguinity has been observed (Bernstein and Gardner 1978; Waldherr *et al.* 1982). Although the familial cases are clearly autosomal recessive some doubt remains regarding the fairly large number of sporadic cases. Whilst many, at least, of these must also be recessive, in the absence of a formal segregation analysis a proportion of non-genetic phenocopies or of fresh mutations of a dominant disorder cannot be excluded.

The disease in the family reported by Collan and colleagues (1977) as hereditary nephronophthisis, which has a life span of three decades, may be distinct from both juvenile nephronophthisis and adult onset medullary renal cystic disease.

References

Alexander, F. and Campbell, S. (1970). Familial uremic medullary cystic disease. *Pediatrics* **45**, 1024–8.

Bernstein, J. and Gardner, K. D. (1978). Familial juvenile nephronophthisis—medullary cystic disease. In *Pediatric renal disease*. Vol. II, ed. Edelmann, C. M. pp. 580–6. Little Brown, Boston.

——, Brough, A. J. and Awen, C. F. (1974). The renal lesion in syndromes of multiple congenital malformations: cerebrohepato-renal syndrome; Jeune's asphyxiating thoracic dystrophy; tuberous sclerosis; Meckel syndrome. *Birth Defects Orig. Art. Ser.* **10**, 35–43.

Betts, P. R. and Forrest-Hay, I. (1973). Juvenile nephronophthisis. *Lancet* **2**, 475–8.

Broberger, O., Winberg, J. and Zetterstrom, R. (1960). Juvenile nephronophthisis. Part I. Genetically determined nephropathy with hypotonic polyuria and azotaemia. *Acta Paediatr.* **49**, 470–9.

Burke, E. C., Stickler, G. B. and Rosevear, J. W. (1963). Renal osteodystrophy in two siblings. *Am. J. Dis. Child.* **105**, 478–86.

Chakera, T. M. H. (1975). Peripheral dysostosis associated with juvenile nephronophthisis. *Br. J. Radiol.* **48**, 765–6.

Chamberlin, B. C., Hagge, N. W. and Stickler, G. B. (1977). Juvenile nephronophthisis and medullary cystic disease. *Mayo Clin. Proc.* **52**, 485–91.

Clark, N. S. (1951). Familial renal insufficiency. *Arch. Dis. Child.* **26**, 351–7.

Collan, Y., Sipponen, P., Haapanen, E., Lindahl, J., Jokinen, E. J. and Hjelt, L. (1977). Hereditary nephronophthisis with a life span of 3 decades—light and electron microscopical, immunohistochemical, clinical and family studies. *Wilhelm Roux. Arch. Develop. Biol.* **3767**, 195–208.

Donaldson, M. D. C., Warner, A. A., Trompeter, R. S., Haycock, G. B. and Chantler, C. (1985). Familial juvenile nephronophthisis, Jeune's syndrome, and associated disorders. *Arch. Dis. Child.* **60**, 426–34.

Edelson, P., Spackman, T. J., Belliveau, R. E. and Mahoney, M. J. (1974). A renal lesion in asphyxiating thoracic dystrophy. *Birth Defects* **10**, 44–50.

Fanconi, G., Hanhart, E., von Albertini, A., Uehlinger, E., Dolivo, G. and Prader, A. (1951). Die familiäre juvenile Nephronophthise. (Die idiopathische Parenchymatöse Schrumpfniere). *Helv. Pediatr. Acta.* **6**, 1–49.

Giangiacomo, J., Monteleone, P. L. and Witzleben, C. L. (1975). Medullary cystic disease vs. nephronophthisis. *JAMA* **232**, 629–31.

Gibson, A. A. M. and Arneil, G. C. (1972). Nephronophthisis: report of 8 cases from Britain. *Arch. Dis. Child.* **47**, 84–9.

Giselson, N., Heingard, D., Holmberg, C-G., Lindberg, L-G., Lindstedt, E., Lindstedt, G. and Schersten, B. (1970). Renal medullary cystic disease or familial juvenile nephronophthisis: a renal tubular disease. *Am. J. Med.* **48**, 174–84.

Gruskin, A. B., Baluarte, H. J., Cote, M. L. and Elfenben, I. B. (1974). The renal disease of thoracic asphyxiant dystrophy. *Birth Defects Orig. Art. Series* **10**, 44–50.

Habib, R. (1974). Nephronophthisis and medullary cystic disease. In *Pediatric nephrology*, Vol. 1, ed. Strauss, J. pp. 393–401. Stratton Intercontinental Medical Book Corp., New York.

Hackzell, G. and Lundmark, C. (1958). Familial juvenile nephronophthisis. *Acta Paediatr.* **47**, 428–40.

Handa, S. P. and Tennant, R. (1968). Medullary cystic disease of the kidney: its occurrence in two siblings. *Postgrad. Med. J.* **44**, 792–8.

Herdman, R. C. and Langer, L. O. (1968). The thoracic asphyxiant dystrophy and renal disease. *Am. J. Dis. Child.* **116**, 192–201.

——, Good, R. A. and Vernier, R. L. (1967). Medullary cystic disease in two siblings. *Am. J. Med.* **43**, 335–44.

Ivemark, B. I., Ljungqvist, A. and Barry, A. (1960). Juvenile nephronophthisis. Part II. A histologic and microangiographic study. *Acta Paediatr.* **49**, 480–7.

Jeune, M., Beraud, C. and Carron, R. (1955). Dystrophie thoracique asphyxiante de caractere familial. *Arch. Fr. Pédiatr.* **12**, 886–91.

Kleinknecht, C., Broyer, M., Bois, E. and Habib, R. (1975). In *Proceedings of the VIth International Congress of Nephrology, Florence, 1975.* p. 658.

Kobayashi, A., Imai, M., Murata, H. *et al.* (1967). Familial juvenile nephronophthisis: report of cases in two siblings. *Acta Paediatr. Jap.* **9**, 1–6.

Mainzer, F., Saldino, R. M., Ozonoff, M. B. and Minagi, H. (1970). Familial nephropathy associated with retinitis pigmentosa, cerebellar ataxia and skeletal abnormalities. *Am. J. Med.* **49**, 556–62.

Mangos, J. A., Opitz, J. M., Lobeck, C. C. and Cookson, D. U. (1964). Familial juvenile nephronophthisis, unrecognised renal disease in United States. *Paediatrica* **34**, 337–45.

Mongeau, J. G. and Worthen, H. G. (1967). Nephronophthisis and medullary cystic disease. *Am. J. Med.* **43**, 345–55.

Oberklaid, F., Danks, D. M., Mayne, V. and Campbell, P. (1977). Asphyxiating thoracic dysplasia. *Arch. Dis. Child.* **52**, 758–65.

Pascal, R. R. (1973). Medullary cystic disease of the kidney: study of a case with scanning and transmission electron microscopy and light microscopy. *Am. J. Clin. Pathol.* **59**, 659–65.

Pedreira, F. A., Marmer, E. L. and Bergstrom, W. H. (1968). Familial juvenile nephronophthisis and medullary cystic disease. *J. Pediatr.* **73**, 77–83.

Rayfield, E. J. and McDonald, F. D. (1972). Red and blonde hair in renal medullary cystic disease. *Arch. Intern. Med.* **130**, 72–5.

Robins, D. G., French, T. A. and Chakera, T. M. H. (1976). Juvenile nephronophthisis associated with skeletal abnormalities and hepatic fibrosis. *Arch. Dis. Child.* **51**, 799–801.

Royer, P. (1968). Hereditary nephronophthisis. In *Nephrology*, Vol. II. eds. Hamburger, J., Richet, G., Crosnier, J., Funck-Bretano, J. L., Antoine, B., Ducrot, H., Mery, J. P. and de Montera, H. pp. 797–802. W.B. Saunders, Philadelphia.

Schimke, R. N. (1975). In *Paediatric nephrology*, eds. Rubin, M. I. and Barratt, T. M. pp. 368–371. Johns Hopkins University Press, Baltimore.

Shah, K. J. (1980). Renal lesion in Jeune's syndrome. *Br. J. Radiol.* **53**, 432–6.

Sherman, F. E., Studnicki, F. M. and Fetterman, G. H. (1971). Renal lesions of familial juvenile nephronophthisis examined by microdissection. *Am. J. Clin. Pathol.* **55**, 391–400.

Shokeir, M. H. K., Houston, C. S. and Awen, C. F. (1971). Asphyxiating thoracic chondrodystrophy: association with renal disease and evidence for possible heterozygous expression. *J. Med. Genet.* **8**, 107–12.

Smith, C. H. and Graham, J. B. (1945). Congenital medullary cysts of the kidneys with severe refractory anaemia. *Am. J. Dis. Child.* **69**, 369–77.

Spicer, R. D., Ogg, C. S., Saxton, H. M. and Cameron, J. S. (1969). Renal medullary cystic disease. *Br. Med. J.* **1**, 824–5.

Steele, B. T., Lirenman, D. S. and Beattie, C. W. (1980). Nephronophthisis. *Am. J. Med.* **68**, 531–8.

Strauss, M. B. and Sommers, S. C. (1967). Medullary cystic disease and familial juvenile nephronophthisis: clinical and pathological identity. *New Engl. J. Med.* **277**, 863–4.

Sworn, M. J. and Eisinger, A. J. (1972). Medullary cystic disease and juvenile nephronophthisis in separate members of the same family. *Arch. Dis. Child.* **47**, 278–81.

Von Sydow, G. and Ranstrom, S. (1962). Familial juvenile nephronophthisis. *Acta Paediatr. Scand.* **51**, 561–74.

Waldherr, R., Lennert, T., Weber, H.-P., Fodisch, H. J. and Scharer, K. (1982). The nephronophthisis complex. *Virchow's Arch. Pathol. Anat.* **394**, 235–54.

Winberg, J. (1964). Re: Congenital cysts. *Am. J. Dis. Child.* **108**, 566.

9.1.7. Atypical nephronophthisis without hypotonic polyuria

In this condition described by Ljunqvist and colleagues (1967), in two unrelated girls, the picture is similar to juvenile nephronophthisis except for lack of salt wasting and polyuria in the early stages, although urine-concentrating ability is impaired. It is not clear that this is in fact a separate disorder.

Reference

Ljunqvist, A., Victorin, L. and Winberg, J. (1967). Atypical nephronopthisis. A clinico-pathologic study of juvenile patients without hypotonic polyuria. *Acta Paediatr. Scand.* **56**, 164–72.

9.1.8. Dominant juvenile nephronophthisis with haematuria and proteinuria

This disorder was reported in a single family with concordant 8-year-old monozygotic male twins (Makker *et al.* 1973). The disease lacked the early features of familial juvenile nephronophthisis and followed a prolonged course with proteinuria and haematuria. The kidneys at the time of renal transplantation showed the typical histology of medullary cystic disease. There was a history of serious chronic renal disease in the mother, her sister, and her mother, and several more distant relatives. These more distant relatives were mostly older adults and their renal disease was not described. It is not clear that it is the same renal disorder throughout the family and the nature and inheritance of that in the twins remains uncertain.

Reference

Makker, S. P., Grupe, W. E., Perrin, E. and Heymann, W. (1973). Identical progression of juvenile hereditary nephronophthisis in monozygotic twins. *J. Pediatr.* **82**, 773–9.

9.1.9. Juvenile nephronophthisis (renal dysplasia) and retinal defect

Families have been reported in which a renal disorder indistinguishable from familial juvenile nephronophthisis occurs in association with a retinal defect. A variety of terms have been used in describing the retinal changes including tapeto-retinal degeneration or retinitis pigmentosa; retinal hypoplasia, aplasia, or dysplasia; and retinal dystrophy. It is not clear from the published descriptions whether these reports are describing the same retinal disorder or distinct disorders. Indeed one report describes variable retinal changes including Leber congenital amaurosis, retinitis pigmentosa, and sector retinitis pigmentosa within the same family (Godel *et al.* 1979). The earliest such report (Senior *et al.* 1961) was of a family in which six out of 13 children had tapeto-retinal degeneration, and at least four, and possibly all six, had nephronophthisis.

Similar accounts of affected sibs or other relatives in single families have appeared since then (Løken *et al.* 1961; Antoine *et al.* 1963; Meier and Hess 1965; Gordillo *et al.* 1967; Herdman *et al.* 1967, Family 1; Sarles *et al.* 1968; Dekarban 1969; Schimke 1969; Bois and Royer 1970; Senior 1973; Kleinknecht *et al.* 1975; Godel *et al.* 1979). In Meier and Hess's family, and also that of Gordillo and colleagues, the parents were first cousins. Also in Meier and Hess's family of six children the renal and retinal changes did not always occur together. They did so in three children, but a fourth child had nephronophthisis alone and another retinitis pigmentosa alone. It has been suggested that the two disorders are segregating independently in this family, but in view of similar findings in several other families since (Gordillo *et al.* 1967; Sarles *et al.* 1968; Schimke 1969; Bois and Royer 1970) it seems more likely to be variable manifestation of a single gene. Schimke's family consisted of two cousins with the full syndrome. One cousin had first-cousin parents, and a sister and the mother of the other cousin both had the retinal dystrophy alone. Bois and Royer reported two affected sibships who were double first cousins with both complete and incomplete forms. In two families there was hepatic fibrosis as well as renal and retinal disorders (Proesmans *et al.* 1975; Delaney *et al.* 1978). The relation if any of these two families, either to those just discussed or to the families discussed earlier with congenital hepatic fibrosis and nephronophthisis, is not clear. Price and Pratt-Johnson (1970) reported a family in which the parents were half-brother and sister. All three of their children had an abnormality of the central ocular fundus with a yellow foveal spot and surrounding pigmentation. An electroretinogram excluded retinitis pigmentosa, and poor dark adaptation in the eldest suggested a disorder of the rods. The two eldest children also had medullary cystic disease. This may be a distinct disorder. Betts and Forrest-Hay (1973) and Steele and coworkers (1980) between them have reported 31 children with juvenile nephronophthisis from 22 families. Ten of these children, from six families, also had retinal dystrophy or degeneration. Even allowing for the probable bias towards selection of children with both defects in their two series, these findings indicate that retinal defect is a common association of juvenile nephronopthisis. The families discussed leave little doubt that the combined defect is inherited in an autosomal recessive manner but with variable expression.

References

Antoine, B., Braun-Vallon, S., d'Anglejeau, G., Perrin, D., Dunod, J. P. and Ryckewaert, A. (1963). Nephropathie familiale avec atteintes osseuses et chorio-retinienne. J. d'Urologie et de Néphrologie, **1-2**, 81–9.
Betts, P. R. and Forrest-Hay, I. (1973). Juvenile nephronophthisis. *Lancet* **2**, 475–8.

Bois, E. and Royer, P. (1970). Association de nephropathie tubulo-interstitialle chronique et de degenerescence tapeto-retinienne. *Arch. Fr. Pédiatr.* **27**, 471–8.

Dekaban, A. S. (1969). Familial occurrence of congenital retinal blindness and developmental renal lesions. *J. Genet. Hum.* **17**, 289–96.

Delaney, V., Mullaney, J. and Bourke, E. (1978). Juvenile nephronophthisis, congenital hepatic fibrosis and retinal hypoplasia in twins. *Quart. J. Med.* **47**, 281–90.

Godel, V., Iaina, A., Nemet, P. and Lazar, M. (1979). Retinal manifestations in familial juvenile nephronophthisis. *Clin. Genet.* **16**, 277–81.

Gordillo, G. P., Alvarez, R. G. and Bessudo, L. (1967). Nefronoptisis juvenil familiar, nefropatia tubulo-intersticial cronica idiopatica, o enfermedad quistica medular. *Bol. Med. Hosp. Infant (Mex.).* **24**, 533–47.

Herdman, R. C., Good, R. A. and Vernier, R. L. (1967). Medullary cystic disease in two siblings. *Am. J. Med.* **43**, 335–44.

Kleinknecht, C., Broyer, M., Bois, F. and Habib, R. (1975). In *Proc. VIth Int. Congr. of Nephrology, Florence, 1975*, p. 658.

Løken, A. C., Hanssen, O., Halvorsen, S. and Jøtster, N. J. (1961). Oculo-renal dysplasia. Sydrome with infantile death from pyelonephritis and retinal dysplasia. *Acta Pediatr. (Uppsala)* **50**, 177.

Meier, D. A. and Hess, J. W. (1965). Familial nephropathy with retinitis pigmentosa. A new oculorenal syndrome in adults. *Am. J. Med.* **39**, 58–69.

Price, J. D. E. and Pratt-Johnson, J. A. (1970). Medullary cystic disease with degeneration. *Can. Med. Assoc. J.* **102**, 165–7.

Proesmans, W., van Damme, B. and Macken, J. (1975). Nephronophthisis and tapetoretinal degeneration associated with liver fibrosis. *Clin. Nephrol.* **3**, 160–4.

Sarles, H. E., Rodin, A. E., Poduska, P. R., Smith, G. H., Fish, J. C. and Remmers, A. R. (1968). Hereditary nephritis, retinitis pigmentosa and chromosomal abnormalities. *Am. J. Med.* **45**, 312–21.

Schimke, R. N. (1969). Hereditary renal-retinal dysplasia. *Ann. Intern. Med.* **70**, 735–44.

Senior, B. (1973). Familial renal–retinal dystrophy. *Am. J. Dis. Child.* **125**, 442–7.

Senior, B., Friedmann, A. I. and Brando, J. L. (1961). Juvenile familial nephropathy with tapetoretinal degeneration. *Am. J. Ophthalmol.* **52**, 625–33.

Steele, B. T., Lirenman, D. S. and Beattie, C. W. (1980). Nephronophthisis. *Am. J. Med.* **68**, 531–8.

9.1.10. Juvenile nephronophthisis, retinitis pigmentosa, and cerebellar ataxia

There have been three families with this triad of abnormalities reported (Fontaine *et al.* 1970; Mainzer *et al.* 1970; Popobic-Rolovic *et al.* 1976). Two out of three sibs were affected in Mainzer and colleagues' family and there were sporadic cases in the other two families. Fontaine and colleagues' patient also showed pyramidal signs and may be distinct from the others. All of these cases are to be distinguished from the ORC syndrome of glomerular nephropathy, tapeto-retinal degradation, and choreoathetosis described in Chapter 7.

References

Fontaine, J-L., Boulesteix, J., Saraux, H., Lasfargues, G., Grenet, P., Nghiem-Minh Dung, Dhermy, P., Roy, C. and Laplane, R. (1970). Nephropathie tubulo-interstitialle de l'enfant avec degenerescence tapetoretinierre. *Arch. Fr. Pédiatr.* **27**, 459–70.
Mainzer, R., Saldino, R. M., Ozonoff, M. B. and Minah, H. (1970). Familial nephropathy associated with retinitis pigmentosa, cerebellar ataxia and skeletal abnormalities. *Am. J. Med.* **49**, 556–62.
Popovic-Rolovic, M., Calic-Persic, N., Bunjevacki, G. and Negovanovic, D. (1976). Juvenile nephronophthisis associated with retinal pigmentary dystrophy, cerebellar ataxia and skeletal abnormalities. *Arch. Dis. Child.* **51**, 801–3.

9.1.11. Polycystic kidney, cataract, and congenital blindness

This combination, in which the polycystic renal disease is of the medullary sponge kidney variety, was first described in a family of five sibs (Fairley *et al.* 1963). Two of the children died at an early age with cystic kidneys and visual defect, one living child has cystic disease and congenital blindness, and the other two sibs have proteinuria. Another family was reported in the same year (Pierson *et al.* 1963), likewise with cystic kidneys, cataracts, and blindness, in two sisters. However, it is doubtful if these two families are instances of identical gene defects as the precise ocular defects are not identical and nor is the type of renal cyst. In Fairley and colleagues family there were large medullary cysts, whereas in Pierson and associates family the renal lesion was microcystic.

References

Fairley, K. F., Leighton, P. W. and Kincaid-Smith, P. (1963). Familial visual defects associated with polycystic kidney and medullary sponge kidney. *Br. Med. J.* **1**, 1060–3.
Pierson, M., Cordier, J., Hervouet, F. and Rauber, G. (1963). Un curieuse association malformative congenitale et familiale atteignant l'oeil et le rein. *J. Genet. Hum.* **12**, 184–213.

9.1.12. Auriculo-polycystic kidney syndrome

Hilson (1957) reported a family in which the propositus (his case 4) had a deformed left ear and a polycystic left kidney. His father had polycystic kidneys and also had a deformed left ear. The father's father and the father's sister both had polycystic kidneys and malformed ears, whereas the brother of the propositus had polycystic kidneys and normal ears. Whether or not this is a distinct syndrome is still unclear.

Reference

Hilson, D. (1957). Malformations of the ears as sign of malformation of the urinary tract. *Br. Med. J.* **2**, 785–9.

9.1.13. Familial dysplasia of kidneys, liver, and pancreas

Cystic dysplasia of the kidneys with bile duct proliferation and increased connective tissue in the portal tracts, and increased pancreatic connective tissue with dilated pancreatic ducts, was described in a girl and her younger brother who both died within 11 weeks of birth (Ivemark *et al.* 1959). This syndrome is not to be confused with that known as the Ivemark syndrome in which there is asplenia and cardiac malformation. A further case of cystic dysplasia of kidneys, liver, and pancreas is mentioned by Adams and colleagues (1974) without details. This disorder must for the present be regarded as possibly autosomal recessive pending the report of further cases.

References

Adams, C. M., Danks, D. M. and Campbell, P. E. (1974). Comments upon the classification of infantile polycystic diseases of the liver and kidney, based upon three-dimensional reconstruction of the liver. *J. Med. Genet.* **11**, 234–43.
Ivemark, B. I., Oldfelt, V. and Zetterström, R. (1959). Familial dysplasia of kidneys, liver and pancreas. A probably genetically determined syndrome. *Acta Paediatr.* **48**, 1–11.

9.1.14. Cystic dysplasia of kidneys and liver, and agenesis of *vermis cerebelli*

There have been several reports of familial partial agenesis of the *vermis cerebelli* (Joubert syndrome) involving sibs and, in some, parental consanguinity (Boltshauser *et al.* 1981). This abnormality was reported in association with cystic dysplasia of the kidneys in four children, including a pair of identical twins by King and others (1984). They also observed features of Leber's amaurosis in their patients and suggested that the two disorders were merely clinical variants of the same autosomal recessive gene defect. Several authors have described cystic kidneys in Leber's amaurosis (Dekaban 1969; Vaizey *et al.* 1977).

References

Bolthauser, E., Herdan, M., Dumermuth, G. and Isler, W. (1981). Joubert syndrome: clinical and polygraphic observations in a further case. *Neuropediatrics* **12**, 181–91.

Dekaban, A. (1969). Hereditary syndrome of congenital retinal blindness (Leber), polycystic kidneys and maldevelopment of the brain. *Am. J. Ophthalmol.* **68**, 1029–37.

King, M. D., Dudgeon, J. and Stephenson, J. B. P. (1984). Joubert's syndrome with retinal dysplasia: neonatal tachypnoea as the clue to a genetic brain-eye malformation. *Arch. Dis. Child.* **59**, 709–18.

Vaizey, M. J., Sanders, M. D., Wybar, K. C. and Wilson, J. (1977). Neurological abnormalitites in congenital amaurosis of Leber. *Arch. Dis. Child.* **52**, 399–402.

9.1.15. Renal dysplasia and asplenia

A curious family has been reported in which features of the syndrome of familial dysplasia of kidneys, liver, and pancreas (Ivemark *et al.* 1959) are combined with those of the asplenia syndrome (Ivemark 1955). The first and second children, male and female, in a family of three children and one spontaneous abortion born to unrelated parents were affected (Crawfurd 1978). Both affected children died within 24 hours of birth with enlarged cystic kidneys, shown in the second child to be grossly dysplastic, a nodular cystic pancreas, and in the second child histological evidence of portal fibrosis and bile duct proliferation. Both had either asplenia or splenic hypoplasia and cardiac anomaly. This must be regarded as another presumptive recessive disorder. Further single case reports of renal dysplasia with hepatic fibrosis, but lacking features of the asplenia syndrome, have appeared (Stroyer and Kissane 1979; Proesmans *et al.* 1986). Stroyer and Kissane's patient, but not that of Proesmans and colleagues, also had pancreatic dysplasia.

References

Crawfurd, M. d'A. (1978). Renal dysplasia and asplenia in two sibs. *Clin. Genet.* **14**, 338–44.

Ivemark, B. I. (1955). Implications of agenesis of the spleen on the pathogenesis of cono-truncus anomalies in childhood: analysis of the heart malformations in spleen agenesis syndrome, with fourteen new cases. *Acta Paediatr.* **44**, (suppl. 104), 1–110.

——, Oldfelt, V. and Zetterström, R. (1959). Familial dysplasia of kidneys, liver and pancreas. A probably genetically determined syndrome. *Acta Paediatr.* **48**, 1–11.

Proesmans, W., Moerman, Ph., Depraetere, M., and Van Damme, R. (1986). Association of bilateral renal dysplasia and congenital hepatic fibrosis. *Int. J. Pediatr. Nephrol.* **7**, 113–16.

Stroyer, D. S. and Kissane, J. M. (1979). Dysplasia of the kidneys, liver and pancreas: report of a variant of Ivemark's syndrome. *Hum. Pathol.* **10**, 228–34.

9.1.16. Meckel–Gruber syndrome

Sibs with microcephaly, occipital encephalocoele, polydactyly, cleft palate, and polycystic kidneys were first reported by Meckel in 1822. Individual and familial case reports followed including a review by Gruber (1934). The essential clinical and pathological features as reviewed by Gruber, and confirmed recently (Seller 1981), are occipital encephalocoele, polycystic kidneys, and death in the perinatal period with the frequent association of a sloping forehead and postaxial polydactyly. More variable features are cleft-lip and palate, eye anomalies, congenital heart defects, microcephaly, talipes, and genital anomalies. Petterson (1983) has undertaken a detailed gross anatomical study of a single case with severe polycystic renal lesions, initially diagnosed clinically as trisomy 13. He compares and contrasts the findings with those in trisomy 13.

Rapola and Salonen (1985) have described the visceral anomalies in 32 autopsied cases from Finland. All of their cases had a central nervous system anomaly, postaxial polydactyly, cystic kidneys, and hepatic portal fibrosis with bile duct proliferation. Males showed severe genital hypoplasia with cryptorchidism, and in over a third of cases epididymal cysts. Just under a third also had pancreatic fibrosis. Spurlock and Taylor (1984) reported an infant with polycystic kidneys and male hermaphroditism. They subsequently accepted (1985) the suggestion of Bernstein and Kissane (1985) that this child had Meckel's syndrome.

The renal lesion comprises cysts of cortex and medulla of varying size and round or square in shape. Maximal dilatation is found in the proximal convoluted tubules, with clustering of cysts around glomeruli. There is extensive dense connective tissue between and surrounding cysts. These appearances somewhat resemble those of adult type polycystic kidney (Potter's type 3) (Cussen and Baxler 1971; Adams *et al.* 1974; Crawfurd *et al.* 1978).

Rapola and Salonen (1985) have given a detailed description of the renal pathology in the study mentioned above. The kidneys were enlarged in 29 out of their 32 cases, grossly in many of them. In all they were cystic with loss of any discernible cortico-medullary boundary. There was a subcapsular zone containing normal glomeruli, some undilated tubules, and minute cysts. This merged into a deeper cortical layer of cysts of 200–600 μm diameter with a tendency to radial elongation. This in turn merged into a still deeper medullary layer with larger cysts up to 1 cm diameter, and intervening smaller cysts, all embedded in an abundant fibrous stroma. Some of the large cysts had a transitional epithelial lining indicating their origin from renal calyces or pelvis, whilst most had a low cuboidal epithelial lining.

Jorgensen (1971) and Adams and colleagues (1974) have undertaken three-dimensional reconstruction of the liver in Meckel's syndrome. The liver shows marked proliferation of bile ducts with only minimal dilatation. Many of the bile ducts are cut longitudinally on histological section and appear to encircle the portal tracts. There is portal fibrosis. Three-dimensional reconstruction shows absence of the main interlobular duct and confirms the presence of concentric rings within the portal tract, joined by radial bile ducts.

Opitz and Howe (1969) proposed that the disorder was inherited in an autosomal recessive manner. This has been amply confirmed by numerous reports of its occurrence in sibs, earlier examples of which were reviewed by Hsia and colleagues (1971), concordance of mono-zygotic twins (Stockard 1921; Hsia *et al.* 1971), and parental con-sanguinity (Kanzow 1859; Tucker *et al.* 1966; Walbaum *et al.* 1967; Fried *et al.* 1971; Crawfurd *et al.* 1978). In most of the cases reported with chromosome analysis no abnormality has been found. In once case an elongated chromosome 3 short arm of uncertain origin was reported, with normal parental karyotypes (Hsia *et al.* 1974).

Prenatal diagnosis on the basis of raised amniotic fluid α-fetoprotein with subsequent termination has been reported in three cases by Seller (1975, 1978). However, Johnson and Holzwarth (1984) monitored three at-risk pregnancies by ultrasonography and α-fetoprotein assay, and failed to diagnose one of two affected fetuses.

References

Adams, C. M., Danks, D. M. and Campbell, P. E. (1974). Comments upon the classification of infantile polycystic diseases of the liver and kidney based upon three dimensional reconstruction of the liver. *J. Med. Genet.* **11**, 234–43.

Bernstein, J. and Kissane, J. M. (1985). Cystic disease of the kidney in newborns. *Hum. Pathol.* **16**, 965.

Crawfurd, M. d'A., Jackson, P. and Kohler, H. G. (1978). Case report: Meckel's syndrome (dysencephalia splanchnocystica) in two Pakistani sibs. *J. Med. Genet.* **15**, 242–5.

Cussen, L. and Baxler, T. J. (1971) quoted by Adams *et al.* (1974) *J. Med. Genet.* **11**, 234–43.

Fried, K., Liban, E., Lurie, M., Friedman, S. and Reisner, S. H. (1971). Polycystic kidneys associated with malformations of the brain, polydactyly and other birth defects in newborn sibs. A lethal syndrome showing the autosomal–recessive pattern of inheritance. *J. Med. Genet.* **8**, 285–90.

Gruber, G. B. (1934). Beitrage zur Frage 'Gekoppetter' Missbildungen (Akrocephalo-syndactylie und Dysencephalia splanchnocystica). *Beitr. Pathol. Anat.* **93**, 459–76.

Hsia, Y. E., Bratu, M. and Herbordt, A. (1971). Genetics of the Meckel syndrome (dysencephalia splanchnocystica). *Pediatrics* **48**, 237–47.

——, Appadorai, V., Breg, W. R. and Howard, R. O. (1974). Chromosomal abnormality (46,XX,3p+) in a case of the Meckel syndrome. *Birth Defects Orig. Art. Series* **10** (8), 19–25.

Johnson, V. P. and Holzwarth, D. R. (1984). Prenatal diagnosis of Meckel syndrome: case reports and literature review. *Am. J. Med. Genet.* **18**, 699–711.

Jorgensen, M. (1971). A case of abnormal intrahepatic bile duct arrangement submitted to three dimensional reconstruction. *Acta Pathol. Microbiol. Scand.*, Section A, **79**, 303–6.

Kanzow, (1859). *Mschr. Geburtshulfe Frauenkrankheiten* **13**, 182. Cited by Theilheber, (1899). Ein Fall von Cystenniere. *Mschr. Geburtsch. Gynäk.* **9**, 496–504.

Meckel, J. F. (1822). Beschreibung zweier, durch sehr ähnliche Bildungsobweichungen ertstellter Geschwister. *Dtsch. Arch. Physiol.* **7**, 99–172.

Opitz, J. M. and Howe, J. J. (1969). The Meckel syndrome (dysencephalia splachnocystica, the Gruber syndrome). In *Congenital Malformation Syndromes. Birth Defects Original Article Series* **5** (2), 167–79.

Pettersen, J. C. (1983). Gross anatomical studies of a newborn with the Meckel syndrome. *Teratology* **28**, 157–64.

Rapola, J. and Salonen, R. (1985). Visceral anomalies in the Meckel syndrome. *Teratology* **31**, 193–201.

Seller, M. J. (1975). Prenatal diagnosis of a neural tube defect: Meckel syndrome. *J. Med. Genet.* **12**, 109–10.

—— (1978). Meckel syndrome and the prenatal diagnosis of neural tube defects. *J. Med. Genet.* **15**, 462–5.

—— (1981). Phenotypic variation in Meckel syndrome. *Clin. Genet.* **20**, 74–7.

Spurlock, R. G. and Taylor, F. M., III (1984). Polycystic kidneys and male hermaphroditism in an infant: a case report and review of the literature. *Hum. Pathol.* **15**, 859–97.

—— and —— (1985). Cystic disease of the kidneys in newborns. *Hum. Pathol.* **16**, 965–6.

Stockard, C. R. (1921). Developmental rate and structural expression: an experimental study of twins, 'double monsters' and single deformities and the interaction among embryonic organs during their origin and development. *Am. J. Anat.* **28**, 115–277.

Tucker, C. C., Finley, S. C., Tucker, E. S. and Finley, W. H. (1966). Oral-facial-digital syndrome with polycystic kidneys and liver. Pathological and cytogenetic studies. *J. Med. Genet.* **3**, 145–7.

Walbaum, R., Dehaene, P. and Duthoit, F. (1967). Polydactylie familiale avec dysplasia neuro-cranienne. *Ann. Génét.* **10**, 39–41.

9.1.17. Oro-facial-digital (OFD) syndrome, type I

This dysmorphic syndrome was first described by Papillon-Leage and Psaume (1954) and by Gorlin and colleagues (1961). The main clinical features are clefts of the jaw and tongue in the region of the lateral incisors and canines, cleft palate and cleft or pseudocleft lip, hamartomas of the tongue, abnormal oral frenulae, dental anomalies, molar and nasal hypoplasia with a broad nasal root, frontal bossing, epicanthic folds, pinnal milia, alopecia, digital anomalies including polydactyly, syndactyly, brachydactyly, and camptodactyly, mental retardation, and familial tremor.

With the single exception of an XXY male (Wahrman *et al.* 1966) patients have all been female. As in addition the sex ratio in affected kindreds is nearer a male:female ratio of 1:2 than 1:1 (Reuss *et al.* 1962), and as there is also an excess of spontaneous abortions in such kindreds it is accepted that inheritance is X linked dominant, lethal in the male. The possible exception among published families is that of Vaillaud and coworkers (1968) who observed 10 affected females in one family consisting of a woman and nine of her granddaughters. These nine granddaughters comprised all the daughters of the grandmother's three unaffected sons. The authors suggested that the OFD gene is on a region of the X chromosome that pairs with the Y and that the Y in the three sons carries a gene that masks expression of the OFD gene on the X. Now that there are a large number of known DNA markers on the X chromosome that have mostly been assigned to fairly narrow regions of the chromosome it should be possible to test this and other hypotheses.

Doege and colleagues (1964) reported a family with 15 affected females including a mother and daughter who both proved, at autopsy, to have bilateral multiple cortical renal cysts, similar to those in adult polycystic kidney disease. The daughter died in renal failure and also had cystic changes in the liver and pancreas. That this may not have been just a chance association is suggested by similar observations in further families with OFD syndrome I. In one instance cystic kidneys were detected on renal arteriography, in a sporadic case in a 48-year-old woman (Harrod *et al.* 1976). In another instance polycystic kidneys were found in at least three members of a family with OFD syndrome I observed by Dr Donnai (1985). One woman in this family, whose daughter is affected and has renal cysts, died in renal failure.

References

Doege, T. C., Thuline, H. C., Priest, J. D., Norby, D. E. and Bryant, J. S. (1964). Studies of a family with the oral facial digital syndrome. *New Engl. J. Med.* **271**, 1073–80.

Donnai, D. (1985). Personal communication.

Gorlin, R. J., Anderson, V. E. and Scott, C. R. (1961). Hypertrophied frenuli, oligophrenia, familial trembling and anomalies of the hand: report of four cases in one family and a *forme fruste* in another. *New Engl. J. Med.* **264**, 486–9.

Harrod, M. J. E., Stokes, J., Peede, L. F. and Goldstein, J. L. (1976). Polycystic kidney disease in a patient with the oro-facial-digital syndrome type I. *Clin. Genet.* **9**, 183–6.

Papillon-Leage, Mme and Psaume, J. (1954). Une malformation hereditaire de la muqueuse buccale brides et freins anormaux: Generalites. *Rev. Stomatol. (Paris)* **55**, 209–27.

Reuss, A. L., Pruzansky, S., Lis, E. F. and Patau, R. (1962). The oral–facial–digital syndrome: a multiple congenital condition of females with associated chromosomal abnormalities. *Pediatrics* **29**, 985–95.

Vaillaud, J. C., Martin, J., Szepetowski, G. and Robert, J. M. (1968). Le syndrome oro-facio-digital: etude clinique et genetique a propos de 10 cas observes dans une meme famille. *Rev. Pédiatr.* **4**, 383–92.

Wahrman, J., Berant, M., Jacobs, J., Aviad, I. and Ben-Hur, N. (1966). The oral-facial-digital syndrome: a male lethal condition in a boy with 47,XXY chromosomes. *Pediatrics* **37**, 812–21.

9.1.18. Ellis–van Creveld syndrome (chondroectodermal dysplasia)

This syndrome was first described by Ellis and van Creveld (1940) with mesomelic dwarfing, polydactyly, and congenital heart defect, especially atrial septal defect. A very large family was studied by McKusick and colleagues (1964) among the Old Order Amish isolate in Pennsylvania, which is highly inbred. Inheritance is clearly autosomal recessive. Mahoney and Hobbins (1977) have suggested that fetoscopy and ultrasound could be used for prenatal diagnosis. Blackburn and Belliveau (1971) described two affected sisters who both died within 3 days of birth. In both autopsy revealed histologically focal dilatation of tubules in both the cortex and medulla. Previous authors have mentioned nephrocalcinosis (Uehlinger 1957) and glomerulosclerosis (Hirokawa and Suzuki 1967) but not tubular dilatation.

References

Blackburn, M. G. and Belliveau, R. E. (1971). Ellis–van Creveld syndrome. *Am. J. Dis. Child.* **122**, 267–70.

Ellis, R. W. B. and van Creveld, S. (1940). A syndrome characterized by ectodermal dysplasia, polydactyly, chondrodysplasia, and congenital morbus cordis. Report of three cases. *Arch. Dis. Child.* **16**, 65–84.

Hirokawa, K. and Suzuki, S. (1967). Ellis–van Creveld syndrome: report of an autopsy case. *Acta Pathol. Jap.* **17**, 139–43.

McKusick, V. A., Egeland, J. A., Eldridge, R. and Krusen, D. E. (1964). Dwarfism in the Amish. I. The Ellis–van Creveld syndrome. *Bull. Johns Hopkins Hosp.* **115**, 306–36.

Mahoney, M. J. and Hobbins, J. C. (1977). Prenatal diagnosis of chondroecto-dermal dysplasia (Ellis–van Creveld syndrome) with fetoscopy and ultrasound. *New Engl. J. Med.* **297**, 258–60.

Uehlinger, E. (1957). Pathologische Anatomie der chondroektodermalen Dysplasie Ellis–van Creveld. *Schweiz. Z. Pathol. Bakt.* **20**, 754–66.

9.1.19. Cornelia de Lange syndrome

This syndrome of severe mental subnormality was described by Cornelia de Lange in 1933 under the title 'typus degenerativus Amstelodamensis'. It is also known as Brachmann–de Lange syndrome. De Lange reported two girls with the disorder. The features apart from mental subnormality are a moderate degree of microcephaly, synophrys, a low hair-line over both the forehead and the back of the neck, long eyelashes, depressed nasal bridge and anteverted nares, low-set ears, broad hands with short tapering fingers, proximally attached thumbs, and clinodactyly (Schlesinger *et al.* 1963; McArthur and Edwards 1967; Pashayan *et al.* 1969; Beck and Mikkelsen 1981). There may be reduction deformities of the arms, often asymetrical (Pashayan *et al.* 1975).

France and colleagues (1969) reported renal hypoplasia, dysplasia, and cystic change in Cornelia de Lange syndrome. However, caution must be exercised in interpreting renal abnormality in de Lange syndrome because renal anomalies are common in trisomy for the distal part of the long arm of chromosome 3, a chromosomal anomaly that resembles de Lange syndrome (Allerdice *et al.* 1975; Wilson *et al.* 1978). Such chromosome 3 duplications, inherited from a parental balanced translocation, may account for some apparently familial cases.

Most cases are sporadic and despite individual reports of chromo-somal abnormality, including 3q duplication, those workers who have analysed series of cases have found no chromosomal abnormality (McArthur & Edwards 1967; Beck and Mikkelsen 1981; Breslau *et al.* 1981). Both dizygotic (Stevenson and Scott 1976) and monozygotic (Carakushansky and Berthier 1976) twin pairs have been reported as discordant. Several groups have reported affected sibs (Borghi *et al.* 1954; Pearce *et al.* 1967) and analyses of large series indicates a sib recurrence risk of 2–5 per cent (Pashayan *et al.* 1969; Beck and Mikkelsen 1981). Pearce and coworkers (1967) also observed two cases with parental consanguinity. These recurrence rates are too low for simple Mendelian inheritance but seem rather high for multifactorial inheritance. The genetics of this disorder remains unresolved.

References

Allerdice, P. W., Browne, N. and Murphy, D. P. (1975). Chromosome 3 duplication q21→qter deletion p25→pter syndrome in children of carriers of a pericentric inversion inv(3) (p25q21). *Am. J. Hum. Genet.* **27**, 699–718.

Beck, B. and Mikkelsen, M. (1981). Chromosomes in the Cornelia de Lange syndrome. *Hum. Genet.* **59**, 271–6.

Borghi, A., Giusti, G. and Bigozzi, U. (1954). Nanismo degenerativo tipo di Amsterdam (typus Amstelodamensis—malattia di Cornelia de Lange): presentazione di un caso e considerazioni di ordine genetico. *Acta Genet. Med. Gemellol.* **3**, 365–72.

Breslau, E. J., Disteche, C., Hall, J. G., Thuline, H. and Cooper, P. (1981). Prometaphase chromosomes in five patients with the Brachmann–de Lange syndrome. *Am. J. Med. Genet.* **10**, 179–86.

Carakushansky, G. and Berthier, C. (1976). The de Lange syndrome in one of twins. *J. Med. Genet.* **13**, 404–6.

France, N. E., Crome, L. and Abraham, J. M. (1969). Pathological features in the de Lange syndrome. *Acta Paediatr. Scand.* **58**, 470–80.

De Lange, C. (1933). Sur un type de degenerescence (typus Amstelodamensis). *Arch. Méd. Enfants* **36**, 713–19.

McArthur, R. G. and Edwards, J. H. (1967). De Lange syndrome: a report of 20 cases. *Can. Med. Assoc. J.* **96**, 1185–98.

Pashayan, H. M., Fraser, F. C. and Pruzansky, S. (1975). Variable limb malformations in the Brachmann–Cornelia de Lange syndrome. *Birth Defects Orig. Art. Series* **11** (5), 147–56.

——, Whelan, D., Guttman, S. and Fraser, F. C. (1969). Variability of the de Lange syndrome: report of 3 cases and genetic analysis of 54 families. *J. Pediatr.* **75**, 853–8.

Pearce, P. M., Pitt, D. B. and Roboz, P. (1967). Six cases of the de Lange's syndrome: parental consanguinity in two. *Med. J. Aust.* **1**, 502–6.

Schlesinger, B., Clayton, B. E., Bodian, M. and Jones, K. V. (1963). Typus degenerativus Amstelodamensis. *Arch. Dis. Child.* **38**, 349–57.

Stevenson, R. E. and Scott, C. I. Jr. (1976). Discordance for Cornelia de Lange syndrome in twins. *J. Med. Genet.* **13**, 402–4.

Wilson, G. N., Hieber, V. C. and Schmickel, R. D. (1978). The association of chromosome 3 duplication and Cornelia de Lange syndrome. *J. Pediatr.* **93**, 783–8.

9.1.20. Acral and renal malformation syndrome

Dieker and Opitz (1969) have described three patients with absence of digits and renal malformations. The renal malformations included renal agenesis, duplication defects, hydronephrosis, and polycystic kidney. The patients were all male and the cases sporadic. Paternal age was increased, 57 years, in one case. The parents were not consanguineous. A further sporadic case has been reported with a paternal age of 44 years (Curran and Curran 1972). These observations suggest that these patients may have a fresh mutation of a gene with autosomal dominant expression. This syndrome should not be confused with that of radial-ray aplasia and renal anomaly, which has been referred to as acro-renal syndrome (see Chapter 10).

Two sisters, born to consanguineous French-Canadian parents, had a split-hand and split-foot deformity, severe mandibular hypoplasia, and renal and genital malformations (Halal *et al.* 1980). This is almost certainly a distinct, probably autosomal recessive, disorder. The mother had a septate uterus and a further living sib a duplex urinary collecting system. If these anomalies represent heterozygous expression then the condition is only incompletely recessive.

References

Curran, A. S. and Curran, J. P. (1972). Associated acral and renal malformations: a new syndrome? *Pediatrics* **49**, 716–52.
Dieker, H. and Opitz, J. M. (1969). Associated acral and renal malformations. *Birth Defects Orig. Art. Series* **5** (3), 68–77.
Halal, F., Desgranges, M.-F., LeDuc, B., Theoret, G. and Bettez, P. (1980). Acro-renal-mandibular syndrome. *Clin. Genet.* **5**, 277–84.

9.2. RENAL DYSPLASIA AND LOWER URINARY TRACT OBSTRUCTION

9.2.1. Cystic dysplastic or multicystic kidneys (Potters' types 2a and 2b)

It is not always realized that cystic dysplasia is the most common type of renal defect in newborn infants with Potter's syndrome. It is associated with irregular kidneys, either enlarged by cysts or hydronephrosis (Potter's type 2a) or small and shrunken or hypoplastic (Potter's type 2b). When bilateral and involving the whole of both kidneys the condition is lethal. When unilateral (multicystic kidney), usually associated with ureteric atresia, or focal (multilocular kidney), it may even be symptomless and is not associated with Potter's syndrome. Associated malformations of other organs are fairly common.

One of the earliest studies of these types of cystic renal defects was that of Ericsson and Ivemark (1958) on renal dysplasia and infection. Although secondary infection is common in dysplastic kidneys, hypertension is not. Chen and colleagues (1985) have recently reported the rare case of hypertension in a neonate with a unilateral multicystic kidney, associated with a high plasma renin. Both blood pressure and renin levels returned to normal following nephrectomy. Hartman and colleagues (1986) described the finding of a Wilms' tumour in a multi-cystic dysplastic kidney. This may have been a case of Perlman's syndrome (see Chapter 12). Ericsson and Ivemark (1958) studied 34 children, radiologically and histologically, presenting with non-lethal urinary tract infection or in other ways. Fifteen were dysplastic, mostly with renal infection and often associated renal malformation. Pathak and Williams (1964) studied 20 cases of unilateral multicystic kidney, 12 of multiple cysts with renal hypoplasia, and seven of multiple cysts with hydronephrosis. The opposite kidney was hydronephritic in 11 and hypoplastic in five cases of unilateral multicystic kidney. This observation highlights the close association between urinary tract developmental anomaly and obstruction discussed earlier. The typical histological appearance of the affected renal tissue (Fig. 9.4) is of cysts of greatly varying size, shape, epithelial lining, and numbers embedded in a parenchyma in which there is greatly increased fibrous connective tissue often of a loose embryonic type. Normal renal structures are absent but small collections of primitive tubules surrounded by whorls of fibrous tissue may be seen. Blood vessels and nerves are often prominent, and even aberrant tissue such as muscle in cyst walls or small islands of cartilage are sometimes present. These various structures form no organized pattern. Unlike adult and infantile polycystic renal disease the liver is not involved in the cystic disease. Several research workers have

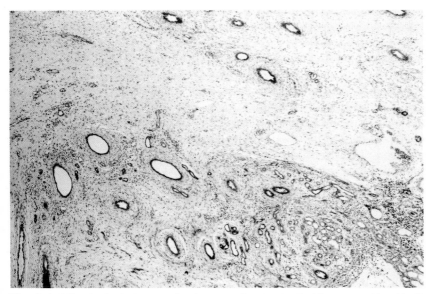

Fig. 9.4. Histological abnormality in a cystic dysplastic kidney ($\times$44). Kindly photographed by the Medical Illustration Department, Clinical Research Centre.

undertaken microdissection studies in renal dysplasia. One of the earliest such studies was on a stillborn fetus with renal dysplasia, absent rectum and small bowel, and a persistent cloaca (Bialestock 1956). Osathanondh and Potter (1964) regard these changes as a developmental one resulting in the secondary obstruction and suggested from their microdissection studies that the normal induction of nephron development by the ampullae of the developing collecting tubules is inhibited, with a failure of branching of the ureteric bud and conversion of terminal ampullae into cysts. Others dispute this interpretation, regarding urethral obstruction as the primary event (Bernstein 1968, 1971; Baert 1978). Potter and Craig (1975) later recognized the primary role of ureteric or urethral obstruction in the pathogenesis of renal dysplasia as well as of more obviously obstructive renal disease. Maizels and Simpson (1983) induced changes similar to human renal dysplasia in chick embryos by culturing renal blastemas *in vitro* so that condensed metanephrogenic mesenchyme was no longer opposed to the ureteric bud. They concluded that they provided evidence for a primary defect of nephron development. This whole topic has already been discussed more fully in the introduction to this chapter.

Risdon (1971a and b) carried out a clinico-pathological study of 107 cases of renal dysplasia, including 76 nephrectomy cases and 41 autopsy cases. The nephrectomy cases he classified under three groups: Group 1 comprised gross renal dysplasia with absence or atresia of the renal pelvis or ureter. Group 2 were cases of segmental renal dysplasia with functional or anatomical abnormality of the ureter leading, despite patency, to urinary stasis or reflux. Many of these involved the upper pole of a duplex kidney drained by an ectopic ureterocoele. There was often an associated pyelonephritis. The affected kidney could be partially cystic, hypoplastic, or hydronephrotic. Group 3 had renal dysplasia associated with obstruction of the lower urinary tract. The dysplasia was usually segmental with some normal renal tissue present. Again associated pyelonephritis was common. These kidneys tended to be hydronephrotic and the most common cause of obstruction was a posterior urethral valve. Risdon's autopsy cases formed part of a series of 121 with congenital renal or lower urinary tract malformation, of which 41 (34 per cent) were dysplastic. Compared with the nephrectomy cases they showed a higher incidence of bilateral involvement and of associated malformations. The most frequent associated malformations were imperforate anus, tracheo-oesophageal fistula with oesophageal atresia, and prune-belly syndrome. Central nervous system malformations were the next most common group. In contrast Pathak and Williams (1964) found cardiovascular anomalies as the commonest associated malformation. In Risdon's autopsy series pyelonephritis was less common than in his nephrectomies, except in lower urinary tract obstruction. The cases could be subdivided into the same three groups as the nephrectomy cases, with severe renal dysplasia due to lower urinary tract obstruction (group 3) associated with hydronephrosis and hydroureters.

Dysplastic kidneys are usually of sporadic occurrence and indeed there is no mention of familial occurrence in the two studies discussed above of Pathak and Williams and of Risdon. Rare instances of renal dysplasia in sibs have been recorded (Cain *et al.* 1974; Pescia *et al.* 1976; Williams and Risdon 1982). The present author has seen a family in which the first and third children, both boys, died in the neonatal period with renal dysplasia. The parents were unrelated but come from villages 15 miles apart in the Punjab. Their first child was born on 12 August 1969 at 32 weeks pregnancy and weighed 4 lb 15 oz (2.24 kg). He developed uraemia and became severely dehydrated with death at 11 days. The second affected boy was born 9 July 1975, a normal girl having been born between the two boys. The second boy was born at 34 weeks and weighed 2.3 kg. He died at 1 day with respiratory difficulties. Both boys at autopsy had hypoplastic kidneys, bilateral hydronephrosis and hydroureters, and hypertrophied bladder. On histological examinations the kidneys from both boys showed gross cystic and dysplastic changes. In the second the prostatic urethra was dilated and there was an atretic obstruction just below the prostate. He also had hyaline membrane disease. Although urethral obstruction was not detected in the first child it must be presumed to have been present during early renal development at least. Whether or not these few isolated instances of affected sibs represent a rare genetic form of renal dysplasia is impossible to say.

The only systematic family study to date has been recently reported in abstract form by Al Saadi and colleagues (1984). They undertook a family history in each case, and physical examination and renal sonography of relatives. They found a second affected sib in only one of 21 families studied, and in that family both affected children had renal dysplasia and posterior urethral valves.

Miranda *et al.* (1972) described a rare syndrome of renal, central nervous, and hepatic anomalies under the rather misleading title of 'familial renal dysplasia', and differentiated the appearance on micro-dissection from that in obstructive renal dysplasia. This syndrome is discussed in Chapter 10. Renal dysplasia is also seen in other inherited disorders discussed above including those described by Ivemark and colleagues (1959) and by Crawfurd (1978). The syndrome of renal dysplasia and Wilms' tumour described by Perlman and colleagues (1973, 1975) and others is discussed in Chapter 12.

Prenatal diagnosis, at 23 weeks gestation, of cystic dysplastic kidneys by ultrasound has been reported (Bartley *et al.* 1977). More recent accounts of ultrasound prenatal diagnosis emphasize the *in utero* evolution of the appearance (D'Alton *et al.* 1986; Hashimoto *et al.* 1986).

References

Al Saadi, A. A., Yoshimoto, M., Bree, R., Farah, J., Chang, C., Sahney, S., Shokeir, M. and Bernstein, J. (1984). A family study of renal dysplasia. *Am. J. Hum. Genet.* **36**, 119S.

Baert, L. (1978). Hereditary polycystic kidney disease (adult form): a microdissection study of two cases at an early stage of the disease. *Kidney Int.* **13**, 579–625.

Bartley, J. A., Golbus, M. S., Filly, R. A. and Hall, B. D. (1977). Prenatal diagnosis of dysplastic kidney disease. *Clin. Genet.* **11**, 375–8.

Bernstein, J. (1968). Developmental abnormalities of renal parenchyma: renal hypoplasia and dysplasia. In *Pathology annual*, ed. Sommers, S. C. pp. 213–47. Appleton-Century-Crofts, New York.

—— (1971). The morphogenesis of renal parenchymal maldevelopment (renal dysplasia). *Pediatr. Clin. N. Am.* **18**, 395–407.

Bialestock, D. (1956). The morphogenesis of renal cysts in the stillborn studied by microdissection technique. *J. Pathol. Bact.* **71**, 51–9.

Cain, D. R., Griggs, D., Lackey, D. A. and Kagon, B. M. (1974). Familial renal agenesis and total dysplasia. *Am. J. Dis. Child.* **128**, 377–80.

Chen, Y.-H., Stapleton, F. B., Roy, S. and Noe, H. N. (1985). Neonatal hypertension from a unilateral multicystic, dysplastic kidney. *J. Urol.* **133**, 664–5.

Crawfurd, M. d'A. (1978). Renal dysplasia and asplenia in two sibs. *Clin. Genet.* **14**, 338–44.

D'Alton, M., Romero, R., Grannum, P., DePalma, L., Jeanty, P. and Hobbins, J. C. (1986). Antenatal diagnosis of renal anomalies with ultrasound. IV. Bilateral multicystic kidney disease. *Am. J. Obstet. Gynecol.* **154**, 532–7.

Ericsson, N. O. and Ivemark, B. I. (1958). Renal dysplasia and pyelonephritis in infants and children. I and II. *Arch. Pathol.* **66**, 255–69.

Hartman, G. E., Smolik, L. M. and Schochat, S. J. (1986). The dilemma of the multicystic dysplastic kidney. *Am. J. Dis. Child.* **140**, 925–8.

Hashimoto, B. E., Filly, R. A. and Callen, P. W. (1986). Multicystic dysplastic kidney in utero: changing appearance on US. *Radiology* **159**, 107–9.

Ivemark, B. I., Oldfelt, V. and Zetterström, R. (1959). Familial dysplasia of kidneys, liver and pancreas. A probably genetically determined syndrome. *Acta Paediatr.* **48**, 1–11.

Maizels, M. and Simpson, S. B., Jr. (1983). Primitive ducts of renal dysplasia induced by culturing ureteral buds denuded of condensed renal mesenchyme. *Science* **219**, 509–10.

Miranda, D., Schinella, R. A. and Finegold, M. J. (1972). Familial renal dysplasia: microdissection studies in siblings with associated central nervous system and hepatic malformations. *Arch. Path.* **93**, 483–91.

Osathanondh, V. and Potter, E. L. (1964). Pathogenesis of polycystic kidneys, Type 2 (multicystic, dysplastic). *Arch. Pathol.* **77**, 474–84.

Pathak, I. G. and Williams, D. I. (1984). Multicystic and cystic dysplastic kidneys. *Br. J. Urol.* **36**, 318–31.

Perlman, M., Goldberg, G. M., Bar-Ziv, J. and Danovitch, G. (1973). Renal hamartomas and nephroblastomatosis with fetal gigantism: a familial syndrome. *J. Paediatr.* **83**, 414–18.

——, Levin, M. and Witters, B. (1975). Syndrome of fetal gigantism, renal hamartomas, and nephroblastomatosis with Wilms' tumor. *Cancer* **35**, 1212–17.

Pescia, G. K., Evans, K. A. and Carter, W. (1976). The risk of recurrence of renal agenesis. Vth Int. Cong. Hum. Genet (abs.), *Excerpta Medica*, p. 94.

Potter, E. L. and Craig, J. M. (1975). *Pathology of the fetus and the infant*, 3rd edn. Year Book Medical Publishers, Chicago.

Risdon, R. A. (1971a). Renal dysplasia: Part I. A clinico-pathological study of 76 cases. *J. Clin. Pathol.* **24**, 57–65.

—— (1971b). Renal dysplasia: Part II. A necropsy study of 41 cases. *J. Clin. Pathol.* **24**, 65–71.

Williams, D. I. and Risdon, R. A. (1982). Hypoplastic, dysplastic and cystic kidneys. Chapter 14 in *Paediatric urology*, 2nd edn. eds. Williams, D. I. and Johnston, J. H. pp. 137–50. Butterworths, London.

9.2.2. Renal cystic disease secondary to early developmental obstruction (Potter type 4)

Osathanondh and Potter (1964) described the results of their micro-dissection studies on kidneys from patients with urethral obstruction but without gross renal pelvic dilatation. These kidneys show numerous small subcapsular cysts on light microscopy (Fig. 9.5). On microdissection these are shown to be formed only within the last one or two generations of nephrons or terminal ends of collecting tubules. They conclude that these changes result from relatively late urethral obstruction in contrast to the more severe dysplastic changes seen in association with earlier, or possibly more severe urethral obstruction.

However, severe renal dysplasia and multiple cortical cysts may occur together in the same patient (Baert 1978). Baert in a microdissection study of seven kidneys from five patients with urethral valve obstruction could find no clear-cut division between Potter's two types of obstructive cystic renal disease, but rather found a continuous spectrum. He concluded that the different findings were purely one of timing of obstruction. Like Potter type 2, type 4 cystic kidneys are usually of sporadic occurrence. However, there have been several reports of posterior urethral valves being observed in twins (Newburger and Davidson 1933; Rolnick 1951) or in sibs (Hasen and Seup Song 1955). Whether these familial observations are due to common environmental factors, multifactorial inheritance, or rare genetic phenocopies is

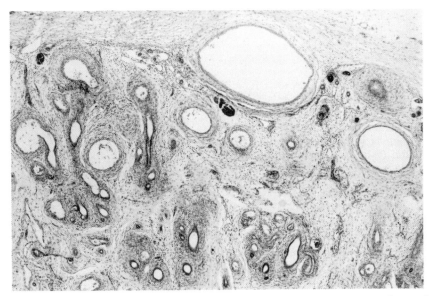

Fig. 9.5. Histological appearance of cortical mycrocystic (Potter type 4) renal cystic disease (×44). Kindly photographed by the Medical Illustration Department, Clinical Research Centre.

unknown. As described elsewhere in this volume similar subcapsular microcysts may be seen in trisomy 13 and other chromosomal anomalies, and also in tuberous sclerosis. In these latter disorders the site of obstruction is presumably more proximal, perhaps even intrarenal. Recently, Halal (1986) has described a lethal syndrome of distal obstructive uropathy with polydactyly in two unrelated male stillborn infants.

References

Baert, L. (1978). Cystic kidneys, renal dysplasia and microdissection data in 5 children with congenital valvular urethral obstruction. *Eur. Urol.* **4**, 382–7.

Halal, F. (1986). Distal obstructive uropathy with polydactyly: a new syndrome? *Am. J. Med. Genet.* **34**, 753–757.

Hasen, H. B. and Seup Song, Y. (1955). Congenital valvular obstruction of the posterior urethra in two brothers. *J. Pediatr.* **47**, 207–15.

Osathanondh, V. and Potter, E. L. (1964). Pathogenesis of polycystic kidneys. Type 4 due to urethral obstruction. *Arch. Pathol.* **77**, 502–9.

Newburger, C. and Davidson, I. (1933). Congenital valves of posterior urethra in twins. *Arch. Pathol.* **16**, 57–62.

Rolnick, H. C. (1951). *The Practice of urology*, Lippincott, Philadelphia.

9.3. SECONDARY TO SYSTEMIC DISORDERS

9.3.1. Tuberous sclerosis

Probably the earliest report of tuberous sclerosis to be published was a description of the autopsy finding of cerebral sclerosis in an infant in a paper by von Recklinghausen (1863) which was cited by Hartdegen (1881), and by Critchley and Earl (1932) in their extensive review of the disease. Bournville (1880) introduced the term 'tuberous sclerosis' for the pathological lesions. Early commentators on the disease, starting with Vogt (1908), regarded it as being characterized by the triad of epilepsy, mental retardation, and the skin lesion adenoma sebaceum. Sherlock (1911) coined the term 'epiloia' for this triad. Later authors recognized that all three features were not necessarily present in any one patient. For example mental retardation is found in only a third of cases (Borberg 1951; Nevin and Pearce 1968) but epilepsy and adenoma sebaceum in over 80 per cent each. Moreover, each of these cardinal features is liable to be absent in very young affected children. It has also been recognized that the expression of the disease is far more diverse than the classical triad (Marshall *et al.* 1959; Scheig and Bornstein 1961; Bundey and Evans 1969; Lagos and Gomez 1969; Bundey *et al.* 1970; Sybert *et al.* 1979). The 'non-classical' features reported include sub-ungal fibromata, retinal phakoma, shagreen or café-au-lait patches and areas of skin depigmentation (white naevi or ash-leaf spots), periventricular calcification as well as sclerosis in the brain, rhabdomyoma of the heart, and renal tumours and cysts. However, café-au-lait patches and white naevi are not specific for tuberous sclerosis (Nicholls 1968; Zaremba 1968). There have been several reports of studies done on large series of cases with reviews of the clinico-pathological features of the disease (Critchley and Earl 1932; Ross and Dickerson 1943; Dawson 1954; Lagos and Gomez 1967; Nevin and Pearce 1968). Lagos and Gomez (1967) reviewed 71 cases seen at the Mayo Clinic between 1935 and 1964. Sixty-two per cent of these were mentally retarded, all with seizures. Adenoma sebaceum was present in 83 per cent, and retinal phakoma in 53 per cent. Over half of their patients had intracranial calcification. Renal tumours were present in all four autopsied patients.

The tumourous lesions in the various tissues are hamartomatous in nature. In the kidneys these take the form of angiomyolipomas. Renal lesions were described in several early studies of the disease (Fisher 1911; Critchley and Earl 1932; Debre *et al.* 1952; Dawson 1954; Osathanondh and Potter 1964). Dawson (1954) found palpable renal tumours in five out of 32 patients, and microscopic renal lesions in each of the five autopsy cases. Critchley and Earl (1932) state that renal tumours are present in 80 per cent of cases at post mortem. Angio-myolipomas of the kidney have been reported in between 40 and 80 per cent of cases of tuberous sclerosis (Chonko *et al.* 1974), and when present are usually multiple and bilateral, and may extensively replace renal parenchyma (Viamonte *et al.* 1966).

Among the diverse 'non-classical' presentations, or later complications, signs, or symptoms due to renal lesions may be seen. Both multiple, and the less common solitary, tumours may bleed and present with pain and shock (MacDougall 1960; Perou and Gray, 1960; Price and Mostofi 1965), or less often with haematuria or merely palpable abdominal masses. The renal lesions are frequently cystic (Herman 1948; LeBrun *et al.* 1955; McQueeney *et al.* 1964), often with clinical and pathological appearances very similar to adult type polycystic kidney disease (Potter type 3) (Pratt-Thomas 1947; Taylor and Genters 1958; Klapproth *et al.* 1959; Engström *et al.* 1962; Osathanondh and Potter 1964; Anderson and Tannen 1969; Cree and Nash 1969; Elkin and Bernstein 1969; Wenzel *et al.* 1970; Chonko *et al.* 1974, cases 2 and 3; Ozer 1974; O'Callaghan *et al.* 1975; Stapleton *et al.* 1980; Cassidy *et al.* 1983; Michel *et al.* 1983), or to Potter type 4 cystic kidneys with cortical microcysts (Simopoulos and Breslow 1968). In some patients the renal lesions have been the only signs of tuberous sclerosis (Klapproth *et al.* 1959; Engstrom *et al.* 1962; Wenzl *et al.* 1970; Chonko *et al.* 1974, case 3; Michel *et al.* 1983). Others have presented at birth or in early infancy with cystic kidneys (Pratt-Thomas 1947; Engstrom *et al.* 1962; Simopoulos and Breslow 1968; Anderson and Tannen 1969; Cree and Nash 1969; Elkin and Berstein 1969; Wenzl *et al.* 1970; Bernstein *et al.* 1974; Ozer 1974; Stapleton *et al.* 1980; Michel *et al.* 1983). Renal tumours may be complicated by intrarenal or intraperitoneal haemorrhage (Herman 1948; MacDougall 1960), or exceptionally by renal failure with uraemia (Scheig and Bornstein 1961; Mirouze *et al.* 1963; Schnitzer 1963; Anderson and Tannen 1969; Jochimsen *et al.* 1969; Chonko *et al.* 1974, case 1). The renal tumours may simulate renal carcinoma (McQueeny *et al.* 1964), although the distinction of tuberous sclerosis from either adult polycystic kidney disease or renal carcinoma can be made by renal arteriography (Viamonte *et al.* 1966; Elkin and Bernstein 1969; Shapiro *et al.* 1984). Chronic renal failure is seldom seen in tuberous sclerosis, probably because most patients with severe renal involvement die from other causes before renal failure can supervene. Nevertheless renal failure has been described on a number of occasions (Kirpicznik 1910; Golji 1961; Mirouze *et al.* 1963; Schnitzer 1963; Anderson and Tannen 1969; Jochimsen *et al.* 1969; Chonko *et al.* 1974). There have even been several reports of patients with tuberous sclerosis with renal involvement either without classic skin lesions, or without central nervous system symptoms, or both (Kofman and Hyland 1959; Scheig and Bernstein 1961; Schnitzer 1963; Price and Mostofi 1965; Anderson and Tannen 1969; Chonko *et al.* 1974). Thus it is important to bear tuberous sclerosis in mind in the differential diagnosis of patients with renal cystic disease, failure or even apparent renal tumour. Such patients, like those at risk of developing tuberous sclerosis through having an affected parent, require a careful clinical examination, using a Wood's lamp if necessary, to exclude adenoma sebaceum, shagreen patches, leaf spots, and subungal fibromata, an ophthalmic examination to exclude retinal phakomata, an ultrasound examination to exclude renal cysts or tumours, and a computed axial tomographic or nuclear magnetic resonance scan of the brain to exclude calcified or sclerotic plaques, especially in a periventricular distribution. Whilst the family history should always be explored it must be remembered that many cases are fresh mutations. An extensive bibliography on renal involvement in tuberous sclerosis has been provided by Chonko and colleagues (1974).

Critchley and Earl (1932) recognized the frequent positive family history, and the liability of '*formes frustes*' to escape diagnosis. Cockayne (1933) pointed out a tendency to dominance in certain families and that in others fresh mutation might be responsible. However, Gunther and Penrose (1935) first clearly established the autosomal dominant pattern of inheritance, from a study of 20 families, and confirmed a high mutation rate which they estimated at 1 in 120 000 to 1 in 60 000 per individual per generation. They also proposed that the wide variation in expression was due to extraneous modifying factors. Later authors, whilst in at least the larger series recognizing the high proportion of sporadic cases which presumably are due to fresh mutation, have confirmed the autosomal dominant inheritance (Moolten 1942; Borberg 1951; Dickerson 1951; Stevenson and Fisher 1956; Marshall *et al.* 1959; Lagos and Gomez 1967; Nevin and Pearce 1968; Zaremba 1968; Bundey and Evans 1969; Bundey *et al.* 1970). Incidence is difficult to estimate because of the variable expression and early death of many children. Dawson (1954) suggested a prevalence in England of 1 in 150 000, and Stevenson and Fisher (1956) gave a similar estimate for Northern Ireland. Nevin and Pearce (1968) estimated 1 in 100 000 for the Oxford Regional Hospital Board's area, and also estimated a live-birth incidence of sporadic cases of about 1 in 50 000, which gives an estimated minimum mutation rate of 10.5 per million genes per generation. Estimates of the proportion of living cases that are sporadic rather than familial also vary. In Nevin and Pearce's Oxford study two-thirds were sporadic, whereas Lagos and Gomez (1967) found only half of their cases to be sporadic, and Gomez (1979) found that the proportion of sporadic cases fell the more carefully the relatives were studied to a minimum of 25 per cent. Bundey and Evans (1969), who reported a family study of 71 cases, put the proportion with fresh mutations as high as 86 per cent. They confirmed the great clinical variability observed by earlier workers. They paid especial attention to the cutaneous manifestations. Sybert and Hall (1979) reported two families in which white naevi were the only manifestation in some members. Without Wood's lamp examination the affected parent would not have been recognized in each of their families. These studies were all undertaken before imaging facilities for brain scanning were widely available. It is now clear that the variable expression led in the past to estimates of mutation frequency and claims of incomplete penetrance that would not now be sustained, either through more careful clinical examination (Sybert and Hall 1979), or through the use of sophisticated imaging techniques (Fleury *et al.* 1979; Cassidy *et al.* 1983). De Groot and colleagues (1981), in an extension of their earlier study (Fleury *et al.* 1979), investigated 95 parents of 48 unrelated patients with a combination of dermatological and ophthalmological methods, and electroencephalogram, skull X-ray, and cranial computerized tomography. They found that nearly a half of their index cases had evidence of an affected parent. Thirteen of their children had one definitely affected parent, but a further 23 parents had one or two questionable signs, mostly white macules. They hope to be able to resolve these uncertain cases by means of electron microscopy of the white macules (Witkiewicz *et al.* 1981). Cassidy and colleagues (1983) also undertook an investigation of parents of patients with tuberous sclerosis. In their case the apparently unaffected parents of 13 patients were investigated by the same methods as Fleury's group but with the addition of renal ultrasound or urography. They detected three previously undiagnosed affected fathers and one mother. Three of these four had skin changes, three had brain calcification, and one had renal cysts. The father with renal cysts also had brain calcification but had no skin or eye manifestations. Six of their index patients also had renal cysts on investigation giving a renal lesion in seven out of 23 probands and affected parents. Nevertheless families still continue to be published in which these appear to be affected sibs with apparently normal parents, indicating incomplete penetrance (Dickerson 1951; Wilson and Carter 1978; Lowry *et al.* 1979; Michel *et al.* 1983). In the cases of Wilson and Carter and of Lowry and colleagues the parents were fully examined clinically, but were reported before computed tomography became available. This must lead to caution in accepting higher estimates of mutation rate, and also in the genetic counselling of at-risk patients. Such caution is reinforced by the failure of several groups to detect any increase in paternal age in sporadic cases (Gunther and Penrose 1935;

Borberg 1951; Nevin and Pearce 1968; Bundey and Evans 1969). Wholly reliable detection of heterozygotes must probably await the development of molecular methods.

In summary, all the available evidence indicates that tuberous sclerosis is inherited in an autosomal dominant manner, probably with a high mutation rate, marked variability of expression, and even occasional failure of penetrance. The pathogenesis of the disease is unknown. Several hypotheses have been put forward to account for the varying pattern of expression of the disease. Lowry and colleagues (1979), reporting a family in which two out of five children, with apparently normal parents had tuberous sclerosis postulated a recessive genocopy or gonadal mosaicism. Although the parents had normal skull X-rays computerized tomography was not available. The authors dismissed non-penetrance rather too readily. Rushton and Shaywitz (1979) described a family in which a boy, his maternal uncle, and great-uncle (the maternal grandfather's brother) all had tuberous sclerosis. The mother and grand-father were clinically unaffected. They postulated the action of a dominant unlinked modifying gene. The idea of modifier genes in tuberous sclerosis is not new (Gunther and Penrose 1935) and is lent support by the frequent observation of similarity in expression within families (Marshall *et al.* 1959; Bundey *et al.* 1970; Michel *et al.* 1983). Gomez (1979) reviewed the Mayo Clinic experience over a period of more than 40 years. Comings (1980) reviewing Gomez's monograph suggested that modification may operate through a mutation of a cell surface protein that is homozygous in the hamartomas but heterozygous in the surrounding tissue. This hypothesis should eventually be testable. An alternative hypothesis that will be testable when DNA analysis of the primary gene mutation is feasible is that the varying expression is in large part due to genetic heterogeneity with different mutations at the tuberous sclerosis locus in different families. Extensive molecular heterogeneity is already emerging for some of the less common mendelian disorders already investigated using DNA probes, such as haemophilia and Lesch–Nyhan disease.

References

Anderson, D. and Tannen, R. L. (1969). Tuberous sclerosis and chronic renal failure. *Am. J. Med.* **47**, 163–8.

Bernstein, J., Brough, A. J. and McAdams, A. J. (1974). The renal lesion in syndromes of multiple congenital malformations—cerebrohepatorenal syndrome; Jeune asphyxiating thoracic dystrophy; tuberous sclerosis; Meckel syndrome. *Birth Defects Orig. Art. Series* **10**(4), 35–43.

Borberg, A. (1951). Clinical and genetic investigations into tuberous sclerosis and Recklinghausen's neurofibromatosis. *Acta Psychiat. Scand.* Suppl. 71.

Bournville, (1880). Contribution a l'etude de l'ioditie. *Arch. Neurol.* **1**, 69–91.

Bundey, S. and Evans, K. (1969). Tuberous sclerosis—a genetic study. *J. Neurol. Neurosurg. Psychiat.* **32**, 591–603.

——, Dutton, G. and Wells, R. S. (1970). Tuberose sclerosis without adenoma sebaceum. *J. Ment. Defic. Res.* **14**, 243–9.

Cassidy, S. B., Pagon, R. A., Pepin, M. and Blumhagen, J. D. (1983). Family studies in tuberous sclerosis: evaluation of apparently unaffected patients. *JAMA* **249**, 1302–4.

Chonko, A. M., Weiss, S. M., Stein, J. H. and Ferris, T. F. (1974). Renal involvement in tuberous sclerosis. *Am. J. Med.* **56**, 124–32.

Cockayne, E. A. (1933). *Inherited abnormalities of the skin and its appendages* p. 291. Oxford University Press, London. [Out of print.]

Comings, D. E. (1980). Review of Gomez's 'Tuberous Sclerosis'. *Am. J. Hum. Genet.* **32**, 285–6.

Cree, J. E. and Nash, F. W. (1969). Tuberous sclerosis with polycystic kidney. *Proc. R. Soc. Med.* **62**, 327.

Critchley, M. and Earl, C. J. C. (1932). Tuberose sclerosis and allied conditions. *Brain* **55**, 311–46.

Dawson, J. (1954). Pulmonary tuberous sclerosis and its relationship to other forms of the disease. *Quart. J. Med.* **23**, 113–45 plus plates 8–15.

Debré, R., Thieffrey, S., Mozziconacci, P., Bargeton, E. and Ramade, J. (1952). La sclerose tubereuse de Bournville chez le nourrison et la petit enfant. *Arch. Fr. Pédiatr.* **9**. 342–82.

De Groot, W. P., Woerdeman, M. J., Witkiewicz, I. M., Fleury, P., Delleman, J. W. and Verbeeten, B. (1981). Tuberous sclerosis. An investigation into the ratio of sporadic versus familial cases. *Br. J. Dermatol.* **104**, 99–100.

Dickerson, W. W. (1951). Familial occurrence of tuberous sclerosis. *Arch. Neurol. (Minneap.)* **65**, 683–702.

Elkin, M. and Bernstein, J. (1969). Cystic disease of the kidney—radiological and pathological considerations. *Clin. Radiol.* **20**, 65–82.

Engström, N., Ljungqvist, A., Persson, B. and Wetterfors, J. (1962). Tuberous sclerosis with a localised angiomatous malformation in the ileum and excessive albumin loss in the lower intestinal tract. Report of a case. *Pediatrics* **30**, 681–95.

Fisher, W. (1911). Die Nierentumouren bei der tuberosen Himsklerose. *Beitr. Pathol. Anat.* **50**, 235.

Fleury, P., De Groot, W. P., Delleman, J. W., Verbeeten, B. and Frankenmolen-Witkiezwicz, I. M. (1979). Tuberous sclerosis: the incidence of sporadic cases versus familial cases. *Brain Dev.* **2**, 107–17.

Golji, H. (1961). Tuberous sclerosis and renal neoplasms. *J. Urol.* **85**, 919–23.

Gomez, M. R. (1979). *Tuberous sclerosis.* Raven Press, New York.

Gunther, M. and Penrose, L. S. (1935). Genetics of epiloia. *J. Genet.* **31**, 413–30.

Hartdegen, A. (1881). Ein Fall von multipler Verhartung des Grosshirns nebst histologisch, eigenartigen harten Geschwulsten der Seitenventrikel ('Glioma gangliocel-lalare') bei einem Neugeborenen. *Arch. f. Psych.* **11**, 171.

Herman, L. (1948). Massive spontaneous haemorrhage into and around parenchymal lesions of the kidney. *J. Urol.* **59**, 544–52.

Jochimsen, P. R., Braunstein, P. M. and Najarian, J. S. (1969). Renal allotransplantation for bilateral renal tumors. *JAMA* **210**, 1721–4.

Kofman, O. and Hyland, H. H. (1959). Tuberous sclerosis in adults with normal intelligence. *Arch. Neurol. Psychiat.* **81**, 43.

Kirpicznik, J. (1910). Ein Fall von tuberoser Sklerose und gleichzeitigen multiplen Nierengeschwulsten. *Virchow's Arch. Pathol. Anat.* **202**, 358–76.

Klapproth, H. J., Poutasse, E. F. and Hazard, J. B. (1959). Renal angiomyolipomas. *Arch. Pathol.* **67**, 400–11.

Lagos, J. C. and Gomez, M. R. (1967). Tuberous sclerosis—reappraisal of a clinical entity. *Mayo Clin. Proc.* **42**, 26–49.

LeBrun, H. I., Kellett, H. S. and MacAlister, C. L. O. (1955). Renal hamartoma. *Br. J. Urol.* **27**, 394–407.

Lowry, R. B., Dunn, H. G. and Paris, R. P. (1979). Inheritance of tuberous sclerosis. *Lancet* **1**, 216.

MacDougall, J. A. (1960). Renal hamartoma causing intraperitoneal haemorrhage. *Br. J. Urol.* **32**, 280–1.

McQueeny, A. J., Dahlen, G. A. and Gebhart, W. F. (1964). Cystic hamartoma (angiomyolipoma) of the kidney simulating renal carcinoma. *J. Urol.* **92**, 98–102.

Marshall, D., Saul, G. B. and Sachs, E. (1959). Tuberous sclerosis: a report of sixteen cases in two family trees revealing genetic dominance. *New Engl. J. Med.* **261**, 1102–5.

Michel, J. M., Diggle, J. H., Brice, J., Mellor, D. H. and Small, P. (1983). Two half-siblings with tuberous sclerosis, polycystic kidneys and hypertension. *Devpt. Med. Child. Neurol.* **25**, 239–44.

Mirouze, J., Barjon, P. and Marty, M. (1963). L'uremie de la maladie de Bournville (a propos de deux observations). *J. Urol. Nephrol.* **69**, 639.

Moolten, S. E. (1942). Hamartial nature of the tuberous sclerosis complex and its bearing on the tumor problem. *Arch. Intern. Med.* **69**, 589.

Nevin, N. C. and Pearce, W. G. (1968). Diagnostic and genetical aspects of tuberous sclerosis. *J. Med. Genet.* **5**, 273–80.

Nicholls, E. M. (1968). Genetic susceptibility and somatic mutation in the production of freckles, birthmarks and moles. *Lancet* **1**, 71–3.

O'Callaghan, T. J., Edwards, J. A., Tobin, M. and Mookerjee, B. K. (1975). Tuberous sclerosis with striking renal involvement in a family. *Arch. Intern. Med.* **135**, 1082–7.

Osathanondh, V. and Potter, E. L. (1964). Pathogenesis of polycystic kidneys type 3 due to multiple abnormalities of development. *Arch. Pathol.* **77**, 485–501.

Ozer, F. L. (1974). Polycystic kidneys as the leading feature of tuberous sclerosis. *Birth Defects Orig. Art. Series* **10**, 160.

Perou, M. L. and Gray, P. T. (1960). Mesenchymal hamartomas of the kidney. *J. Urol.* **83**, 240–61.

Pratt-Thomas, H. R. (1947). Tuberous sclerosis with congenital tumours of the heart and kidney. *Am. J. Pathol.* **23**, 189–99.

Price, E. B. and Mostofi, F. K. (1965). Symptomatic angiomyolipoma of the kidney. *Cancer* **18**, 761–4.

Recklinghausen, V. (1863). *Verhandl. Berl. Gesell. f. Geburtshulfe*, **15**, 75 (cited by Hartdegen, 1881, and by Critchley and Early, 1932).

Ross, A. T. and Dickerson, W. W. (1943). Tuberous sclerosis. *Arch. Neurol. Psychiat.* **50**, 233–57.

Rushton, A. R. and Shaywitz, B. A. (1979). Tuberous sclerosis: a possible modification of phenotypic expression by an unlinked dominant gene. *J. Med. Genet.* **16**, 32–5.

Scheig, R. L. and Bornstein, P. (1961). Tuberous sclerosis in the adult: and unusual case without mental deficiency or epilepsy. *Arch. Intern. Med.* **108**, 789–95.

Schnitzer, B. (1963). Tuberous sclerosis complex. *Arch. Pathol.* **76**, 626–32.

Shapiro, R. A., Skinner, D. G., Stanley, P. and Edelbrock, H. H. (1984). Renal tumors associated with tuberous sclerosis: the case for aggressive surgical management. *J. Urol.* **132**, 1170–4.

Sherlock, E. B. (1911). *The feeble-minded*, Macmillan, London.

Simopoulos, A. P. and Breslow, A. (1968). Tuberous sclerosis in the newborn. *Am. J. Dis. Child.* **14**, 313–16.

Stapleton, F. B., Johnson, D., Kaplan, G. W. and Griswold, W. (1980). The cystic renal lesion in tuberous sclerosis. *J. Pediatr.* **97**, 574–9.

Stevenson, A. C. and Fischer, O. D. (1956). Frequency of epiloia in Northern Ireland. *Br. J. Prev. Soc. Med.* **10**, 134–5.

Sybert, V. P. and Hall, J. G. (1979). Inheritance of tuberous sclerosis. *Lancet* **1**, 783.

Taylor, J. N. and Genters, K. (1958). Renal angiomyolipoma and tuberous sclerosis. *J. Urol.* **79**, 685–96.

Viamonte, M., Rauel, R., Politano, V. and Bridges, B. (1966). Angiographic findings in a patient with tuberous sclerosis. *Am. J. Roentgenol.* **98**, 723–33.

Vogt, H. (1908). Zur Pathologie und Pathologischer Anatomie der verschiedenen Idiotiedformen. II. Tuberose Sklerose. *Monat. f. Psych. u. Neur.* **24**, 106.

Wenzl, J. E., Lagos, J. C. and Albers, D. D. (1970). Tuberous sclerosis presenting as polycystic kidneys and seizures in an infant. *J. Pediatr.* **77**, 673–6.

Wilson, J. and Carter, C. (1978). Genetics of tuberose sclerosis. *Lancet* **1**, 340.

Witkiewicz, I. M., Woerdeman, M. J. and De Groot, W. P. (1981). Tuberous sclerosis. Ultrastructure study of white spots in patients and parents. *Br. J. Derm.* **104**, 100.

Zaremba, J. (1968). Tuberous sclerosis; a clinical and genetical investigation. *J. Ment. Defic. Res.* **12**, 63–80.

9.3.2. Myotonic dystrophy

There is a single report of the association of polycystic kidney disease and myotonic dystrophy (Emery *et al.* 1967). They described a family in which four out of five children had myotonic dystrophy, and three of these four also had polycystic kidneys. The father, aged 70 years, was unaffected and the mother had died age 57 of uraemia but without palpably enlarged kidneys or clinical myotonia. Three other members of the family had myotonic dystrophy without evidence of polycystic kidneys. The association may well be fortuitous with independent segregation of the two traits within the family, especially as there was no histological evidence as to the precise type of renal cysts present, and there have been no further reports of this association.

Reference

Emery, A. E. H., Oleesky, S. and Williams, R. T. (1967). Myotonic dystrophy and polycystic disease of the kidneys. *J. Med. Genet.* **4**, 26–8.

9.3.3. Von Hippel–Lindau's disease

This disorder comprises retinal angiomata, haemangioblastoma of the cerebellum and angiomatous cysts of other viscera, especially the kidneys and pancreas. Renal cysts when present tend to be small cortical cysts. Tumours other than haemangiomas are common such as renal cell carcinomas (q.v.) and, in certain families (Atuk *et al.* 1979) phaeo-chromocytomas. The retinal angiomas were described in the 19th century—the first description, with pathological findings, being that of Collins (1894). However, it is von Hippel's description of the retinal angiomata (1904), together with Lindau's recognition of the association of cerebellar haemangioblastoma and angiomata of abdominal organs (1926), that gave the disease its name. One of the best early descriptions of the disorder was that of Brandt (1921) who reported on his autopsy findings on one of Lindau's two patients. This man had had one eye enucleated. The other contained retinal lesions. He also had cerebellar tumours and tumours of the cauda equina and spinal cord. There were multiple renal cysts and multicentric hypernephroma, and also cysts of the liver and pancreas. Papilloma of the bladder was found, and cystic tumours of both epididymides and metastases in ribs and a vertebra. Metastasis of hypernephroma, unless treated early, is common (Case Records Massachusetts General Hospital 1966), and such tumours are a frequent late development. Fill and colleagues (1979) found hyper-nephromas in 16 out of 42 cases. Several authors have emphasized the value of screening asymptomatic relatives of known patients for early diagnosis and treatment (Melmon and Rosen 1964; Richards *et al.* 1973; Horton *et al.* 1976; Wesolowski *et al.* 1981). The essential histological identity of the retinal, cerebellar, and cord lesions as capillary cavernous haemangiomata, often associated with cyst formation, was confirmed by Silver (1954). Melmon and Rosen (1964) provided an extensive review of the literature up to that time. Simon and Thompson (1955) drew attention to the common finding of renal cysts. Maleck and Greene (1971), in a discussion of all the cases seen at the Mayo Clinic over 35 years, reviewed the urological aspects. Of a total of 22 cases three had renal cell carcinoma, four had renal cysts, five had no renal lesion, and in 10 the renal status was unknown. In all three with renal cell carcinoma the tumours were bilateral. Two of these three cases had been previously

published (Kaplan *et al.* 1961). A recent survey of the clinical and pathological picture of the disease confirms that previously described and
emphasizes that all of the potentially lethal main features are treatable
(Horton *et al.* 1976). Other workers have discussed radiological aspects
of the disease including its renal manifestations (Lee *et al.* 1977; Fill *et
al.* 1979). The latter group studied 221 descendants of a patient with the
disease, of whom 42 were affected. Sixteen of these had renal cell
carcinoma, which was multicentric in 14 and bilateral in 12. Renal cysts
were a common accompaniment of renal tumours and in some cases
small tumours developed within cysts walls. Tumours of more than 2 cm
diameter could be detected by ultrasound. Renal cysts also occurred,
without tumours, in a further 16 cases, varying from solitary cysts to a
polycystic appearance.

There have been many accounts of the familial nature of this disease.
Pratt (1953) was the first to suggest an autosomal dominant inheritance.
Silver (1954) presented a large pedigree covering seven generations with
20 verified cases and eight others with symptoms suggestive of the
disease. It is of interest that two definite and one probable patient in this
family had apparently unaffected parents. Christoferson and colleagues
(1961) specifically recognized the incomplete penetrance and delayed
expression in their large family. Shokeir (1970) in a report on three
families also recognized this incomplete penetrance in one family but
curiously sought to involve autosomal recessive inheritance in another
family with affected cousins. Further large families compatible with autosomal dominant inheritance with variable expression, and often
incomplete penetrance, have been described (Melmon and Rosen 1964;
Maleck and Greene 1971; Richards *et al.* 1973; Horton *et al.* 1976, nine
families; Lee *et al.* 1977; Atuk *et al.* 1979; Fill *et al.* 1979). There is no
difference in severity in males and females and the sex ratio is equal.
There are also sufficient examples of male-to-male transmission to
exclude dominant X-linked inheritance. There has been at least one
report of concordant identical twins (Wesolowski *et al.* 1981).

References

Atuk, N. O., McDonald, T., Wood, T., Carpenter, J. T., Walzak, M. P., Donaldson,
    M., Gillenwater, J. Y., Turner, S. M. and Westfall, V. (1979). Familial pheo-
    chromocytoma, hypercalcemia, and von Hippel–Lindau disease: a ten-year
    study of a large family. *Medicine* **58**, 209–18.
Brandt, R. (1921). Zur Frage der Angiomatosis retinae. *Albrechtv. Graefes Arch.
    Opthalmol.* **106**, 127–65.
Case Records of the Massachusetts General Hospital (1966). *New Engl. J. Med.*
    275, 950–9.

Christoferson, L., Gustafson, M. and Peterson, A. (1961). Von Hippel-Lindau's disease. *JAMA* **178**, 280–2.

Collins, E. T. (1894). Intra-ocular growths. I. Two cases, brother and sister, with peculiar vascular new growth, probably primarily retinal, affecting both eyes. *Trans. Ophthalmol. Soc. UK.* **14**, 141–9.

Fill, W. L., Lamiell, J. M. and Polk, N. O. (1979). The radiographic manifestations of von Hippel–Lindau disease. *Radiology* **133**, 289–95.

Horton, W. A., Wong, V. and Eldridge, R. (1976). Von Hippel–Lindau disease: clinical and pathological manifestations in 9 families with 50 affected members. *Arch. Intern. Med.* **136**, 769–77.

Kaplan, C., Sayre, G. P. and Greene, L. F. (1961). Bilateral nephrogenic carcinomas in Lindau–von Hippel disease. *J. Urol.* **86**, 36–42.

Lee, D. R., Wulfsberg, E. and Kepes, J. J. (1977). Some important radiological aspects of the kidney in Hippel–Lindau syndrome. The value of prospective study in an affected family. *Radiology* **122**, 649–53.

Lindau, A. (1926). Studien über Kleinhirncysten Bau, Pathogenese und Beziehungen zur Angiomatosis Retinae. *Acta Pathol. Microbiol. Scand.* (Suppl. 1), pp. 1–128.

Maleck, R. S. and Greene, L. F. (1971). Urological aspects of Hippel–Lindau syndrome. *J. Urol.* **106**, 800–2.

Melmon, K. L. and Rosen, S. W. (1964). Lindau's disease: review of the literature and study of a large kindred. *Am. J. Med.* **36**, 595–617.

Pratt, R. T. C. (1953). Disease of the nervous system. In *Clinical genetics*, ed. Sorsby, A. p. 303. Butterworth, London.

Richards, R. D., Mebust, W. K. and Shimke, R. N. (1973). A prospective study on von Hippel–Lindau disease. *J. Urol.* **110**, 27–30.

Shokeir, M. H. K. (1970). Von Hippel–Lindau syndrome: a report on three kindreds. *J. Med. Genet.* **7**, 155–7.

Silver, M. L. (1954). Hereditary vascular tumors of the nervous system. *JAMA* **156**, 1053–6.

Simon, H. B. and Thompson, G. J. (1955). Congenital renal cystic disease: clinical and therapeutic study of 366 cases. *JAMA* **159**, 657–62.

Von Hippel, E. (1904). Uber eine sehr seltene Erkraukung der Netzhaut. Klinische Beobachtungen. *Arch. f. Ophthalmol.* **59**, 83–106.

Wesolowski, D. P., Elwood, R. A., Schwab, R. E. and Farah, J. (1981). Hippel–Lindau syndrome in identical twins. *Br. J. Radiol.* **54**, 982–6.

9.3.4. Dandy–Walker syndrome

This syndrome presents early in life as a form of hydrocephalus with bulging occiput. It was thought originally to be due to atresia of the foramina of Luschka and Magendie (Dandy and Blackfan 1914; Taggart and Walker 1942). Benda (1954) considered it to be a developmental anomaly in which the foramina were not necessarily atretic; Hart and coworkers (1972) demonstrated partial or complete cerebellar vermis absence and posterior fossa cyst formation. Radiologically there is thinning and bulging of the bones of the posterior fossa associated with the frequent occurrence clinically of cranial nerve palsies, nystagmus, and ataxia of the trunk.

Benda (1954) reported familial occurrence. Familial occurrence has also been reported by Chemke and associates (1975), and in mono-zygotic twins by Jenkyn and colleagues (1981). It has also been reported in three sibs occurring in association with dysplastic cystic kidneys (D'Agostino *et al.* 1963). Whether or not this is a genuine association, and if so whether it is distinct from the usual Dandy–Walker syndrome, is unclear. These reports of familial occurrence suggests that in some families the anomaly may be inherited in an autosomal recessive manner. However, the great majority of cases are sporadic and genetic hetero-geneity would seem probable, as for example the family of Chemke and associates (1975) with additional anomalies. A very unusual family was reported by Christian and colleagues (1980). Their index case had both the Dandy–Walker and Ellis–van Creveld syndromes, and was homo-zygous for an unusually heterochromatic segment of the long arm of chromosome 9. The child was born to a mentally retarded, short, young mother, probably through an incestuous mating. The mother, her father, and two of her brothers also carried the elongated chromosome 9 hetero-chromatin. One can only speculate on the possible association of any of these abnormalities with genes on chromosome 9.

References

Benda, C. E. (1954). The Dandy–Walker syndrome or the so-called atresia of the foramen of Magendie. *J. Neuropathol. Exp. Neurol.* **13**, 14–29.

Chemke, J., Czernobilsky, B., Mundel, G. and Barishak, Y. R. (1975). A familial syndrome of central nervous system and ocular malformations. *Clin. Genet.* **7**, 1–7.

Christian, J. C., Dexter, R. N., Palmer, C. G. and Muller, J. (1980). A family with three recessive traits and homozygosity for a long 9qh+ chromosome segment. *Am. J. Med. Genet.* **6**, 301–8.

D'Agostino, A. N., Kernohan, J. W. and Brown, J. R. (1963). The Dandy–Walker syndrome. *J. Neuropathol. Exp. Neurol.* **22**, 450–70.

Dandy, W. E. and Blackfan, K. D. (1914). Internal hydrocephalus: an experi-mental, clinical and pathological study. *Am. J. Dis. Child.* **8**, 406–82.

Hart, M. N., Malamud, N. and Ellis, W. G. (1972). The Dandy–Walker syndrome: a clinicopathological study based on 28 cases. *Neurology* **22**, 771–80.

Jenkyn, L. R., Roberts, D. W., Merlis, A. L., Rozycki, A. A. and Nordgren, R. E. (1981). Dandy–Walker malformation in identical twins. *Neurology* **31**, 337–41.

Taggart, J. K. and Walker, A. E. (1942). Congenital atresia of the foramens of Luschka and Magendie. *Arch. Neurol. Psychiat.* **48**, 583–612.

9.3.5. Ehlers–Danlos syndrome

Imahori and colleagues (1969) reported the case of a woman with the severe 'arterial' type of Ehlers–Danlos syndrome (type IV Ehlers–Danlos syndrome). She had had multiple aneurysms and rupture of medium-sized arteries over several years and eventually died aged 42 years from rupture of a splenic artery. An intravenous pyelogram at the age of 31 had demonstrated a cystic left kidney. Autopsy revealed multiple cysts, 0.5–10.0 cm in diameter, in both kidneys.

It remains unclear whether or not this was a coincidental association until further renal studies have been reported in such patients. However, McKusick (1972) has also reported urological abnormalities in Ehlers–Danlos syndrome including haematuria, renal hypoplasia, cortical cysts, and uretero-pelvic obstruction.

Type IV Ehlers–Danlos syndrome is inherited in an autosomal dominant manner in the majority of families (Barabas 1972), although an autosomal recessive form has also been described (Pope *et al.* 1975). There is genetic heterogeneity even among the dominant cases, which may or may not show dilated endoplasmic reticulum (Byers *et al.* 1979). Deficiency of type IV collagen may be common to all forms.

References

Barabas, A. P. (1972). Vascular complications in the Ehlers–Danlos syndrome, with special reference to the 'arterial type' or Sach's syndrome. *J. Cardiovasc. Surg.* **13**, 160–7.

Byers, P. H., Holbrook, K. A., McGillivray, B., MacLeod, P. M. and Lowry, R. B. (1979). Clinical and ultrastructural heterogeneity of type IV Ehlers–Danlos syndrome. *Hum. Genet.* **47**, 141–50.

Imahori, S., Bannerman, R. M., Graf, C. J. and Brennan, J. C. (1969). Ehlers–Danlos syndrome with multiple arterial lesions. *Am. J. Med.* **47**, 967–77.

McKusick, V. A. (1972). *Heritable disorders of connective tissue.* 4th edn. C. V. Mosby, St Louis.

Pope, F. M., Martin, G. R., Lichtenstein, J. R., Penttinen, R., Gerson, B., Rowe, D. W. and McKusick, V. A. (1975). Patients with Ehlers–Danlos syndrome lack type IV collagen. *Proc. Nat. Acad. Sci.* **72**, 1314–16.

9.3.6. Wiedemann–Beckwith syndrome (EMG syndrome)

This syndrome takes its alternative name, EMG from its classical features, namely exomphalos, macroglossia, and gigantism. The gigantism takes the form of generalized overgrowth with high birth weight, stature around the 90th centile, large muscle mass and thick subcutaneous tissue, and visceromegaly. Infants with this syndrome have a tendency to hypoglycaemia. Mental development is variable, ranging from normal through mild to moderate subnormality. Other prominent features include the exomphalos and macroglossia of the EMG title, linear indentations of the ear lobes, rather staring eyes with relative hypoplasia of the lower rim of the orbit, and neonatal polycythaemia. The disorder was first described by Wiedemann (1964, 1969, 1973) and by Beckwith (1969). Among the numerous subsequent papers are reviews by Irving (1967), Filippi and McKusick (1970) and Pettenati and colleagues (1986). Beckwith (1969) pointed out the large kidneys and medullary cystic dysplasia that comprises the renal manifestations. Such renal abnormalities are commonly found whenever looked for, and were, for example, present in all 15 of the patients investigated for this by Pettenati and colleagues.

Patients with Wiedemann–Beckwith syndrome are liable to develop embryonal tumours including Wilms' tumour, rhabdomyosarcoma, hepatoblastoma, and adrenal adenoma or carcinoma (Reddy *et al.* 1972; Sotelo-Avila and Gooch 1976; Sotelo-Avila *et al.* 1980), and may develop more than one type of tumour simultaneously (Riedel 1952; Muller *et al.* 1978). The loss of heterozygosity for loci on the chromosome 11 short arm, due to mitotic events, in Wilms' tumour is discussed in Chapter 12 on renal tract neoplasia. Recently, Koufos and colleagues (1985) have demonstrated similar loss of heterozygosity for 11p loci in hepatoblastomas and rhabdomyosarcomas from patients who were constitutionally heterozygous. The authors propose that the liability of patients with Wiedemann–Beckwith syndrome to develop several different embryonal tumours and their own evidence, and that of others, for loss of heterozygosity for loci on chromosome 11p in at least three such tumour types suggest a common pathogenetic mechanism for these tumours.

Although the great majority of cases are of sporadic occurrence Wiedemann (1964), Irving (1967), and several others have reported affected sibs or cousins. Best and Hoekstra (1981) reported a mother, her brother, and two of her children by different fathers, all of whom were affected. They concluded that inheritance was autosomal dominant with variable expression, a view that is now generally accepted. A recent study of five families provides further evidence for autosomal dominant inheritance with variable expression (Niikawa *et al.* 1986); and Pettenati and colleagues (1986) found familial occurrence of at least some of the classic features in 9 out of 19 families. However, it may be that at least some cases have a more complex origin in the light of a report of discordant monozygotic twins (Bose *et al.* 1985). It is important in apparently sporadic cases to distinguish presumed fresh mutation from a failure of penetrance in a parent. Recent studies suggest, on the basis of a chromosome duplication or deletion, the assignment of the gene for Wiedemann–Beckwith syndrome to 11p13–11p15 (Waziri *et al.* 1983; Turleau *et al.* 1984; Schmutz 1986), although by no means all cases have any detectable abnormality of this chromosome (Nakagome *et al.* 1984; Pettenati *et al.* 1986).

Winter and associates (1986) have reported prenatal diagnosis of Wiedemann–Beckwith syndrome.

References

Beckwith, J. B. (1969). Macroglossia, omphalocele, adrenal cytomegaly, gigantism and hyperplastic visceromegaly. *Birth Defects Orig. Art. Series* **5**(2), 188–96.

Best, L. G. and Hoekstra, R. E. (1981). Wiedemann–Beckwith syndrome: autosomal dominant inheritance in a family. *Am. J. Med. Genet.* **9**, 291–9.

Bose, B., Wilkie, R. A., Madlom, M., Forsyth, J. S. and Faed, M. J. W. (1985). Wiedemann–Beckwith syndrome in one of monozygotic twins. *Arch. Dis. Child.* **60**, 1191–2.

Filippi, G. and McKusick, V. A. (1970). The Beckwith–Wiedemann syndrome. *Medicine* **49**, 279–98.

Irving, I. M. (1967). Exomphalos with macroglossia: a study of 11 cases. *J. Pediatr. Surg.* **2**, 499–507.

Koufos, A., Hansen, M. F., Copeland, N. G., Jenkins, N. A., Lampkin, B. C. and Cavenee, W. K. (1985). Loss of heterozygosity in three embryonal tumours suggests a common pathogenetic mechanism. *Nature* **316**, 330–4.

Muller, S., Gadner, H., Weber, B., Vogel, M. and Riehm, H. (1978). Wilms' tumours and adrenocortical carcinoma with hemi-hypertrophy and hamartomas. *Eur. J. Pediatr.* **127**, 219–26.

Nakagome, Y., Ise, T., Sakurai, M., Nakajo, T., Odamato, E., Takano, T., Nakahuri, T., Tsuchida, Y., Nagahara, N., Takada, Y., Ohsawa, Y., Sawaguchi, S., Toyosaka, A., Kobayashi, N., Matsunaga, E. and Saito, S. (1984). High resolution studies in patients with aniridia-Wilms' tumor association, Wilms' tumor or related congenital abnormalities. *Hum. Genet.* **67**, 245–8.

Niikawa, N., Ishikiriyama, S., Takahashi, S., Inagawa, A., Tonoki, H., Ohta, Y., Hase, N., Kamei, T. and Kaji, T. (1986). The Wiedemann–Beckwith syndrome: pedigree studies on five families with evidence for autosomal dominant inheritance with variable expressivity. *Am. J. Med. Genet.* **24**, 41–55.

Pettenati, M. J., Haines, J. L., Higgins, R. R., Wappner, R. S., Palmer, C. G. and Weaver, D. D. (1986). Wiedemann–Beckwith syndrome: presentation of clinical and cytogenetic data on 22 new cases and review of the literature. *Hum. Genet.* **74**, 143–54.

Reddy, J. K., Schimke, R. N., Chang, C. H. J., Svoboda, D. J., Slaven, J. and Therou, L. (1972). Beckwith–Wiedemann syndrome, Wilms' tumor, cardiac hamartoma, persistent visceromegaly, and glomerulogenesis in a 2-year old boy. *Arch. Pathol.* **94**, 523–32.

Riedel, H. A. (1952). Adrenogenital syndrome in a male child due to adrenocortical tumor: report of a case with hemihypertrophy and subsequent development of embryoma (Wilms' tumor). *Pediatrics* **10**, 19–27.

Schumtz, S. M. (1986). Deletion of chromosome 11 (p 11 → p 13) in a patient with Beckwith–Wiedemann syndrome. *Clin. Genet.* **30**, 154–6.

Sotelo-Avila, C. and Gooch, W. M. (1976). Neoplasms associated with the Beckwith–Wiedemann syndrome. *Perspect. Pediatr. Pathol.* **3**, 255–72.

——, Gonzalez-Crussi, F. and Fowler, J. W. (1980). Complete and incomplete forms of Beckwith–Wiedemann syndrome: their oncogenic potential. *J. Pediatr.* **96**, 47–50.

Turleau, C., De Grouchy, J., Chavin–Colin, F., Martelli, H., Voyer, M. and Chalas, R. (1984). Trisomy 11p15 and Beckwith Wiedemann syndrome, a report of two cases. *Hum. Genet.* **67**, 219–21.

Waziri, M., Patel, S. R., Hanson, J. W. and Bartley, J. A. (1983). Abnormality of chromosome 11 in patients with features of Beckwith–Wiedemann syndrome. *J. Pediatr.* **102**, 873–6.

Wiedemann, H.-R. (1964). Complexe malformatif familial avec hernie ombicale et macroglossie—un 'syndrome nouveau'? *J. Genet. Hum.* **13**, 223–32.

—— (1969). Das E.M.G.-syndrome: Exomphalos, Makroglossie, Gigantismus und Kohlenhydrat-stoffwechselstoerung. *Z. Kinderheilk.* **106**, 171–85.

—— (1973). Exomphalos–Macroglossie–Gigantisimus Syndrome. *Z. Kinderheilk.* **115**, 193.

Winter, S. C., Curry, C. J. R., Smith, J. C., Kassel, S., Miller, M. and Andrea, J. (1986). Prenatal diagnosis of the Beckwith–Wiedemann syndrome. *Am. J. Med. Genet.* **24**, 137–41.

10. Primary renal tract malformations

Renal tract malformations in chromosomal disorders have been discussed in Chapter 3. Developmental defect may also play a part in the aetiology of renal dysplasia as discussed in Chapter 9. Indeed renal dysplasia and renal agenesis may occur in the same family, or even on opposite sides in the same individual. However, this chapter is devoted to primary malformations of the kidney and lower urinary tract not forming part of the multiple anomaly syndromes discussed elsewhere in this monograph. Apart from specific recognizable syndromes associated malformations of the lower genito-urinary tract are common in patients with renal malformation, and even in non-genito-urinary tract malformation associated upper or lower urinary tract malformations are far from rare. Robertson and colleagues (1986) have refuted one previously suggested association of supernumerary nipples and renal anomalies in black children.

Most such malformations are of unknown aetiology, not being associated with any known teratogen, nor being simply inherited. The overall incidence of urinary tract malformations, excluding hypospadias, is about 3 per 1000 births (Leck *et al.* 1968). However, many do show an increased incidence in close relatives of index cases compared with that in the general population. This suggests that a multifactorial genetic predisposition may play a role in their causation, and necessitates the collection of adequate family data to provide a sound basis for genetic counselling. Carter (1984) has provided a brief recent review of the genetics of urinary tract malformation in one of his last publications. However, the assumption of a multifactorial mechanism for the genetic determination of these malformations may be an oversimplification, as evidenced by the high (3.5 per cent) incidence of renal agenesis in the sibs of index cases (Carter *et al.* 1979). Barakat and colleagues (1986) have produced a tabulated review of genetic disorders with urogenital anomalies.

Many of the more serious urinary tract malformations are detectable prenatally by fetal diagnostic ultrasound (Kaffe *et al.* 1977a and b; Gruenewald *et al.* 1984; Hobbins *et al.* 1984; Kullendorf *et al.* 1984; Quinlan *et al.* 1986). Unfortunately the availability of this diagnostic facility is limited, in contrast to the now general availability of the simpler obstetric ultrasound. Mothers known to be at increased risk of having a fetus with one of the more serious urinary tract malformations should be offered fetal diagnostic ultrasound, when appropriate, as a reassurance; or if urinary tract abnormality is detected to permit termination where this is lethal, or in some other cases the institution of early postnatal or even prenatal treatment (Hobbins *et al.* 1984; Turnock and Shawis 1984). Most mothers are prepared to travel some distance to one of the few units undertaking this investigation.

Stephens (1983) has written a monograph on urinary tract malformations which contains material of interest to the geneticist, especially in the appendices.

References

Barakat, A. Y., Seikaly, M. G. and der Kaloustian, V. M. (1986). Urogenital abnormalities in genetic disease. *J. Urol.* **136**, 778–85.

Carter, C. O. (1984). The genetics of urinary tract malformations. *J. Genet. Hum.* **32**, 23–9.

——, Evans, K. and Pescia, G. (1979). A family study of renal agenesis. *J. Med. Genet.* **16**, 176–88.

Gruenewald, S. M., Crocker, E. F., Walker, A. G. and Trudinger, B. J. (1984). Antenatal diagnosis of urinary tract abnormalities: correlation of ultrasound appearance with postnatal diagnosis. *Am. J. Obstet. Gynecol.* **148**, 278–83.

Hobbins, J. C., Romero, R., Grannum, P., Berkovitz, R. L., Cullen, M. and Mahoney, M. (1984). Antenatal diagnosis of renal anomalies with ultrasound. I. Obstructive uropathy. *Am. J. Obstet. Gynecol.* **148**, 868–77.

Kaffe, S., Godmilow, L., Walker, B. and Hirschhorn, K. (1977a). Prenatal diagnosis of bilateral renal agenesis. *Obstet. Gynecol.* **49**, 478–80.

——, Rose, J. S., Godmilow, L., Walker, B. A., Kerenyi, T., Beratis, N., Reyes, P. and Hirschhorn, K. (1977b). Prenatal diagnosis of renal anomalies. *Am. J. Med. Genet.* **1**, 241–51.

Kullendorf, C. M., Larsson, L. T. and Jörgensen, C. (1984). The advantage of antenatal diagnosis of intestinal and urinary tract malformations. *Br. J. Obstet. Gynaecol.* **91**, 144–7.

Leck, I., Record, R. G., McKeown, T. and Edwards, J. H. (1968). The incidence of malformations in Birmingham, England, 1950–1959. *Teratology* **1**, 263–80.

Quinlan, R. W., Cruz, A. C. and Huddleston, J. F. (1968). Sonographic details of fetal urinary-tract anomalies. *Obstet. Gynecol.* **67**, 558–65.

Robertson, A., Sale, P. and Sathyanarayan, P. A.-C. (1986). Lack of association of supernumerary nipples with renal anomalies in black infants. *J. Pediatr.* **109**, 502–3.

Stephens, F. D. (1983). *Congenital malformations of the urinary tract.* Praeger, New York.

Turnock, R. R. and Shawis, R. (1984). Management of fetal urinary tract anomalies detected by prenatal ultrasonograhy. *Arch. Dis. Child.* **59**, 962–5.

10.1. RENAL

10.1.1. Renal agenesis and hypoplasia

Renal agenesis, which in its bilateral form is inevitably lethal in the prenatal period, is compatible in its unilateral form with entirely normal life. Nevertheless, although many cases are detected coincidentally, renal disease in the solitary kidney is common—in 67 per cent of patients in Dees' (1960) series, and about half of Holmes' (1972) series. Renal hypoplasia too is often associated with disease and urosurgeons used to recommend removal of solitary hypoplastic kidneys, although they probably did not always distinguish hypoplastic from small dysplastic kidneys (Burkland 1954). Renal agenesis is probably the most extensively studied of the urinary tract malformations and provides a valid model of the problems that arise in attempting to analyse the role of genetic factors in the causation of this group of developmental errors.

Renal agenesis may be classified in several different ways: unilateral or bilateral, with or without ureteric remnants, isolated or associated with other malformations. It has been suggested at one time or another that each of these distinctions was aetiologically significant (Potter 1965; Buchta *et al.* 1973), and yet within each classification each type may occur within the same family. A single family may have both unilateral and bilateral cases, or affected individuals with or without ureteric remnants. Agenesis of one kidney may be associated with dysplasia of the other kidney in the same individual, or in other members of the same family. Horseshoe and duplex kidney may also occur in other family members. This wide spectrum of expression within families makes genetic classification on phenotypic criteria very difficult.

Renal agenesis may be associated with genital, hindgut, or caudal skeletal defects (Ashley and Mostofi 1960), including as an extreme form sirenomelia, discussed below. This cluster of caudal anomalies was termed the syndrome of caudal regression by Duhamel (1961), while Buchta and colleagues (1973) used the phrase 'single developmental field effect', in either case implying a developmental defect due to damage to, or an error in development of, tissues derived from specific caudal somites. This picture of overlapping anomalies does not imply a single aetiology, as the urogenital tract and related structures have only a limited spectrum of responses to teratogenic factors, and it undoubtedly masks a great deal of genetic as well as environmental heterogeneity. Renal agenesis may also occur in association with malformations of non-caudal structures, that is, as part of a true multiple anomaly sydrome. Some such syndromes are known to be genetically determined and for others the aetiology is unknown.

Experimental studies have indicated possibilities for the origin of urogenital malformations but do not indicate whether any analogous mechanism operates in naturally occurring malformations in humans. For example Boyden (1927) showed that experimental obstruction of the mesonephric ducts results in renal agenesis, and Wolff (1936, 1948) produced varying anomalies within the spectrum of caudal regression by irradiating caudal somites. Animal models, such as the sirenomelic mutation (sr) in the mouse, are probably not particularly helpful because of the extraordinary diversity in the development of the urogenital system in different mammalian species.

Clinically bilateral renal agenesis is characterized by Potter's syndrome of flattened facies with epicanthus and long low-set ears, spade-like hands, talipes, and pulmonary hypoplasia (Potter 1946a and b). Death is from pulmonary insufficiency in the perinatal period or renal insufficiency within the first 2 weeks (Potter 1972). The hypothesis that the non-renal features of Potter's syndrome are due to oligohydramnios has been amply confirmed, both experimentally (Bain and Scott 1960; De Myer and Baird 1969) and clinically (Ratten *et al.* 1973; Fantel and Shepard 1975), despite occasional claims of its occurrence in the absence of oligohydramnios (Sylvester and Hughes 1954). Museles and colleagues (1971) have shown that unilateral renal agenesis, horeshoe kidney, and other renal anomalies can often be detected at birth by careful abdominal palpation.

Several groups have undertaken cytogenetic studies in patients with renal agenesis and detected no abnormality (Passarge and Sutherland 1965; Court-Brown *et al.* 1966; Scott and Bain 1966). Others have noted a normal femal karyotype, 46,XX, in patients with some degree of masculinization as part of an associated genital anomaly (Frazer 1966; Schlegel *et al.* 1966a and b).

Various estimates of the frequency of bilateral renal agenesis have been published. Potter (1946b) gave a figure of 0.3 per thousand births, while Leck and colleagues (1968) in their survey of malformations in Birmingham for the 1950–1959 decade put it at 0.39 per thousand births. Butler and Alberman (1969) in the more widely based British Perinatal Mortality survey obtained a lower figure, 0.13 per thousand live births, and the most recent estimate for England and Wales for 1974–77, at 0.12 per thousand (Carter and Evans 1981) is similar. Unilateral renal agenesis is more common than bilateral, both Warkany (1971b) and Museles and associates (1971) giving figures of 1 in 600 for the former. An ultrasound survey of 682 adults found a prevalence of unilateral agenesis of 3 per thousand (Roodhooft *et al.* 1984).

Despite the fact that the great majority of cases are of sporadic occurrence there has long been a suspicion that genetic factors were involved, first voiced by Almolsch (1937). The limited number of twin pairs reported lend some support to a genetic component in the aetiology. Davidson and Ross (1954) mentioned that there were six discordant twin pairs in the literature without giving references or stating their zygosity. These may have included the discordant monozygotic pair of male twins of Levin (1952). Leaving aside Davidson and Ross' unidentified twins the published twin pairs, excluding those with sirenomelia, are given in Table 10.1 from which it emerges that out of seven known monozygotic pairs two were partially and two fully concordant. Unfortunately there have been no definately dizygotic pairs reported so that comparison of monozygotic to dizygotic concordance is not possible.

Familial occurrence has been reported with much greater frequency, the earliest example being one of affected brothers (Madisson 1934). Several subsequent reports have likewise been of affected sibs, and in at least the more recent reports parents have been investigated to exclude unilateral involvement (Baron 1954; Arends 1957; Rosenfeld 1959; Gorvoy et al. 1962; Morillo-Cucci et al. 1971; Rizza and Downing 1971; Buchta et al. 1973; Whitehouse and Mountrose 1973, two separate sib pairs plus two further pairs of sibs in one family; Cain et al. 1974; Hack et al. 1974; Fitch 1977; Schinzel et al. 1978). In only the last of these is parental consanguinity recorded. In Carter and coworkers' study (1979) four out of 92 (4.34. per cent) brothers and three out of 107 (2.80 per

Table 10.1. *Twin pairs with bilateral renal agenesis in propositus*

Reference	Zygosity	Sex	Concordant or discordant
Levin (1952)	MZ	M	Disc.
Waardenburg (1952)	MZ	—	Conc.
Bain and Scott (1960)	—	—	Disc.
Pasquier et al. (1971)	—	—	Disc.
Mauer et al. (1974)	MZ (MA)	—	One bilateral, other unilateral
Carter et al. (1979)	MZ (MC)	M	One bilateral, other unilateral
	MZ (MA and MC)	M	Disc.
	MZ	M	Disc.
	—	M	Disc.
	—	M	Disc.
Yates et al. (1984)	MZ (MC)	F	Conc.

Abbreviations: MZ=monozygotic, MA=monoamniotic, MC=monochorionic, M=male, F=female, Conc.=concordant, Disc.=discordant.

cent) sisters also had renal agenesis, a combined incidence of 7/199 (3.52 per cent) for all sibs. Two sporadic cases only in their series had consanguineous parents. Their bilateral index patients had 705 first cousins of whom none were known to be affected.

There have also been several reports of renal agenesis in two or three generations of a family usually in direct line of descent and affecting both sexes (Buchta *et al.* 1973; Kohn and Borns 1973; Perlman *et al.* 1976; Zonana *et al.* 1976; McPherson 1982; Monn and Nordshus 1984). Bound (1943) observed unilateral renal agenesis in a boy and his maternal great uncle. Several of these authors have been tempted to invoke a single autosomal gene with dominant inheritance for unilateral and bilateral renal agenesis, for example Kohn and Borns (1973), whereas others have suggested recessive inheritance (Hack *et al.* 1974). More recent authors, impressed by the further association with renal dysplasia, have used the terms 'renal adysplasia', originally introduced by Buchta and colleagues (1973), or 'urogenital adysplasia', often prefixed 'hereditary' (Schimke and King 1980; Monn and Nordshus 1984). In Carter and colleagues' (1979) study only one parent of 108 index patients with bilateral renal agenesis was affected. This was a father who had bilateral renal hypoplasia two of whose three children had bilateral agenesis.

A single family has been reported compatible with X-linked inheritance in which two out of three brothers and their male cousin had bilateral renal agenesis (Pashayan *et al.* 1977). The mothers of the brothers and of the cousin were sisters, and the authors postulate X linkage which obviously cannot be excluded.

Interest in the possible genetic origin of renal agenesis goes back at least to Almolsch (1937) but the first serious discussion of the question was that of Holmes (1972) who suggested a genetic basis for unilateral agenesis. Both Fitch (1977) and Shokeir (1978) have pointed out the frequent association of unilateral and bilateral renal agenesis in the same family and have argued that either may be variable forms of expression of the same gene with autosomal dominant inheritance. Shokeir (1978) suggests that the well-known excess in males is due to a sex-limited factor. Fitch (1977), like Pinsky (1974) earlier, argues for genetic heterogeneity, with both genetically and non-genetically determined cases.

The only systematic study so far is that of Carter and associates (1979) who considered that the available data did not permit any conclusions regarding the type of inheritance. They suggested that the overall sib incidence of bilateral index cases, of 3.5 per cent observed by them is too high for a simple polygenic mechanism, as postulated earlier by Buchta and colleagues (1973). They accepted that their material may be genetically heterogeneous but pointed out that they have no evidence for this, apart from one case that they may have had the recessive cryptoph-thalmos syndrome. Their data with no family with more than two affected sibs and no excess of parental consanguinity do not support recessive inheritance for the majority of cases. Still less do their data support auto-somal dominance or X linkage as the usual mode of inheritance. It must be remembered that the Carter study was undertaken before ultrasound imaging of the renal tract had become widely available. They may have substantially underestimated the incidence of unilateral agenesis and other occult renal malformations among the relatives of their index cases, as recognized by Carter (1984). An early study of apparently normal relatives using nephrosonography revealed that two out of four sibs of one patient with unilateral renal agenesis and dysplasia in the other kidney also had unilteral agenesis and that their father had duplication of his left collecting system (Zonana *et al.* 1976). Similarly Roodhooft and colleagues (1984) in a grey-scale ultrasonographic study of the first-degree relatives of 41 patients with bilateral renal agenesis, severe dysgenesis, or mixed unilateral agenesis and contralateral dysgensis found asymptomatic renal malformations in 10 out of 111 (9 per cent). Half of these affected relatives has unilateral renal agenesis compared with only 0.3 per cent among 682 adult control subjects. The incidence of unilateral renal agenesis did not differ significantly between parents and sibs. Their observations would support a multifactorial origin of renal agenesis. Any new systematic study that also examines at least the available first-degree relatives using ultrasound might further clarify the genetics of this malformation. Meanwhile the 3.5–4.5 per cent sib incidence, found by Carter's and by Roodhooft's two groups, should be used for genetic counselling purposes provided renal malformation has been excluded in the parents by ultrasound. The mothers should also be offered ultrasound in pregnancy for prenatal diagnosis (Romero *et al.* 1985). Various workers have speculated on the potential of α-fetoprotein in prenatal diagnosis of renal agenesis. Ainbender and Brown (1976) found a normal level of serum α-fetoprotein in two neonates with renal agenesis compared with normal term infants, and Seller and Berry (1978) confirmed that the amniotic fluid α-fetoprotein was normal at amniocentesis in two pregnancies with an affected fetus. However, Balfour and Laurence (1980) reported raised maternal serum α-fetoprotein in two other pregnancies with affected infants. In both amniocentesis failed, presumably due to oligohydramnios. Hence it is not yet possible to draw any conclusion about the value of α-fetoprotein for prenatal diagnosis.

A hint that environmental factors may play a role in at least some cases of renal malformation comes from the report of a cluster of four cases with similar fetal malformations detected by ultrasound over a period of

18 days at one hospital. The malformation involved the alimentary and urinary tracts with latter including renal agenesis, hypoplasia, and dysplasia (Bennet 1982). Further evidence for environmental induction of renal agenesis and other urinary tract malformations comes from observations on infants born to mothers exposed during early pregnancy to potential teratogens. Polycystic kidney, unilateral renal agenesis and duplication defects have been reported in the congenital rubella syndrome (Menser *et al.* 1967). Similarly unilateral renal agenesis, rotational anomalies, hydronephrosis, duplication defects, and horseshoe kidney have all been described in thalidomide embryopathy (Warkany 1971a). Unilateral renal agenesis has also been recorded in infants whose mothers have been under anticonvulsant therapy, as in the fetal tri-methadione syndrome (Zachai *et al.* 1975). Finally renal hypoplasia, duplication defects, and horseshoe kidney have been reported in the fetal alcohol syndrome (Qazi *et al.* 1979), and also impaired renal acidification (Assadi and Ziai 1985). However, a recent report of a 10-year follow up of 11 patients with fetal alcohol syndrome makes no mention of renal abnormalities in any of them (Streissguth *et al.* 1985). But even if these associations are accepted as being genuine they do not necessarily indicate the involvement of unknown environmental factors in cases without known exposure to any teratogen.

References

Ainbender, E. and Brown, E. (1976). Bilateral renal agenesis and serum αfeto-protein (letter). *Lancet* **1**, 99.

Almolsch, A. L. (1937). Bilateral metanephric agenesis. *J. Urol.* **38**, 360–70.

Arends, N. W. (1957). Bilateral renal agencies in siblings. *J. Am. Osteopath. Assoc.* **56**, 681–4.

Ashley, D. J. and Mostofi, F. K. (1960). Renal agenesis and dysgenesis. *J. Urol.* **82**, 211–30.

Assadi, F. K. and Ziai, M. (1985). Impaired renal acidification in infants with fetal alcohol syndrome. *Pediatr. Res.* **19**, 850–3.

Bain, A. D. and Scott, J. S. (1960). Renal agenesis and severe urinary tract dysplasia, a review of 50 cases with particular reference to the associated abnormalities. *Br. Med. J.* **1**, 841–6.

Balfour, R. P. and Laurence, K. M. (1980). Raised serum AFP levels and fetal renal agenesis. *Lancet* **1**, 317.

Baron, C. (1954). Bilateral agenesis of the kidney in two consecutive infants. *Am. J. Obstet. Gynecol.* **67**, 667–70.

Bennett, M. J. (1982). Cluster of uncommon fetal abnormalities. *Lancet* **1**, 1360–1.

Bound, J. P. (1943). Two cases of congenital absence of one kidney in the same family. *Br. Med. J.* **2**, 747.

Boyden, E. A. (1927). Experimental obstruction of the mesonephric ducts. *Proc. Soc. Exp. Biol. Med.* **24**, 572–6.

Buchta, R. M., Visekul, C., Gilbert, E. F., Sarto, G. E. and Optiz, J. M. (1973). Familial bilateral renal agenesis and hereditary renal dysplasia. *Z. Kinderheilk.* **115**, 111–29.

Burkland, C. E. (1954). Clinical considerations in aplasia, hypoplasia and atrophy of the kidney. *J. Urol.* **71**, 1–13.

Butler, N. and Alberman, E. (1969). *Perinatal problems.* The second report of the British Perinatal Mortality survey. Churchill Livingstone, London.

Cain, D. R., Griggs, D., Lackey, D. A. and Kagan, B. M. (1974). Familial renal agenesis and total dysplasia. *Am. J. Dis. Child.* **128**, 377–80.

Carter, C. O. (1984). The genetics of urinary tract malformations. *J. Génét. Hum.* **32**, 23–9.

—— and Evans, K. (1981). Birth frequency of renal agenesis. *J. Med. Genet.* **18**, 158–9.

——, —— and Pescia, G. (1979). A family study of renal agenesis. *J. Med. Genet.* **16**, 176–88.

Court-Brown, W. M., Jacobs, P. A. and Stewart, A. L. (1966). Anti-mongolism (letter). *Lancet* **1**, 497.

Davidson, W. M. and Ross, G. I. M. (1954). Bilateral absence of kidneys and related congenital abnormalities. *J. Pathol. Bact.* **68**, 459–74.

Dees, J. E. (1960). Prognosis of the solitary kidney. *J.Urol.* **83**, 550–2.

DeMyer, W. and Baird, I. (1969). Mortality and skeletal malformations from amniocentesis and oligohydramnios in rats; cleft palate, club foot, microstomia adactyly. *Teratology* **2**, 33–7.

Duhamel, B. (1961). From the mermaid to anal imperforation: the syndrome of caudal regression. *Arch. Dis. Child.* **36**, 152–5.

Fantel, A. G. and Shepard, T. H. (1975). Potter syndrome: Non-renal features induced by oligoamnios. *Am. J. Dis. Child.* **129**, 1346.

Fitch, N. (1977). Heterogeneity of bilateral renal agenesis. *Can. Med. Assoc. J.* **116**, 381–2.

Frazer, G. R. (1966). XX chromosomes and renal agenesis (letter). *Lancet* **1**, 1427.

Gorvoy, J. D., Smulewicz, J. and Rothfeld, S. H. (1962). Unilateral renal agenesis in two siblings: case report. *Pediatrics* **29**, 270–3.

Hack, M., Jaffe, J., Blankstein, J., Goodman, R. M. and Brish, M. (1974). Familial aggregation in bilateral renal agenesis. *Clin. Genet.* **5**, 173–7.

Holmes, L. B. (1972). Unilateral renal agenesis: common, serious, hereditary. *Paediatr. Res.* **6**, 419.

Kohn, G. and Borns, P. F. (1973). The association of bilateral and unilateral renal aplasia in the same family. *J. Pediatr.* **83**, 95–7.

Leck, I., Record, R. G., McKeown, T. and Edwards, J. H. (1968). The incidence of malformations in Birmingham, England, 1950–1959. *Teratology* **1**, 263–80.

Levin, H. (1952). Bilateral renal agenesis. *J. Urol.* **67**, 86–91.

McPherson, E. (1982). Unilateral and bilateral renal agenesis: implications for genetic counselling. *Am. J. Hum. Genet.* **34**, 101A.

Madisson, H. (1934). Uber das Fehlen beider Nieren (Aplasia renum bilateralis). *Zentralbl. f. Allgemeine Pathol. und Patholog. Anat.* **60**, 1–8.

Mauer, S. M., Dobrin, R. S. and Vernier, R. L. (1974). Unilateral and bilateral renal agenesis in monoamniotic twins. *J. Pediatr.* **84**, 236–8.

Menser, M., Roberston, S. E. J., Dorman, D. C., Gillespie, A. M. and Murphy, A. M. (1967). Renal lesions in congenital rubella. *Pediatrics* **40**, 901–4.

Monn, E. and Nordshus, T. (1984). Hereditary renal adysplasia. *Acta. Paediatr. Scand.* **73**, 278–80.

Morillo-Cucci, G., Simpson, J. L., Halsey, H. and German, J. (1971). Two sibs with bilateral renal agenesis. *Birth Defects Orig. Art. Series.* **10**(4) 169–70. Nat. Found. March of Dimes, NY.

Museles, M., Gaudry, C. L. and Bason, W. M. (1971). Renal anomalies in the newborn found by deep palpation. *Pediatrics* **47**, 97–100.

Pashayan, H. M., Dowd, T. and Nigro, A. V. (1977). Bilateral absence of the kidneys and ureters. Three cases reported in one family. *J. Med. Genet.* **14**, 205–9.

Pasquier, B., Caouderc, P., Bost, M. and Rambaud, P. (1971). Syndrome de Potter et polykysptose renal du nouveau-ne. *Sem.-Hôp. de Paris* **47**, 2779–88.

Passarge, E. and Sutherland, J. B. (1965) Potter's syndrome: chromosome analysis of 3 cases with Potter's syndrome or related syndromes. *Am. J. Dis. Child.* **109**, 80–3.

Perlman, M., Williams, J. and Ornoy, A. (1976). Familial ureteric bud anomalies. *J. Med. Genet.* **13**, 161–2.

Pinsky, L. (1974). A community of malformation syndromes involving the Müllerian ducts, distal extremities, urinary tract and ears. *Teratology* **9**, 65–79.

Potter, E. L. (1946a). Facial characteristics of infants with bilateral renal agenesis. *Am. J. Obstet. Gynecol.* **51**, 885–8.

—— (1946b). Bilateral renal agenesis. *J. Pediatr.* **29**, 68–76.

—— (1965). Bilateral absence of ureter and kidney. *Obstet. Gynecol.* **25**, 3–12.

—— (1972). Extrinsic abnormalities of the kidney. In *Normal and abnormal development of the kidneys*, pp. 85–102. Year Book Medical Publishers, Chicago.

Qazi, Q., Masakawa, A., Milman, D., McGann, B., Chua, A. and Haller, J. (1979). Renal anomalies in fetal alcohol syndrome. *Pediatrics* **63**, 886–9.

Ratten, G. J., Beischer, N. A. and Fortune, D. W. (1973). Obstetric complications when the fetus has Potter's syndrome. I. Clinical considerations. *Am. J. Obstet. Gynecol.* **115**, 890–6.

Rizza, J. M. and Downing, S. E. (1971). Bilateral renal agenesis in two female siblings. *Am. J. Dis. Child.* **121**, 60–3.

Romero, R., Cullen, M., Grannum, P., Jeanty, P. E., Reece, A., Venus, I. and Hobbins, J.C. (1985). Antenatal diagnosis of renal anomalies with ultrasound. III. Bilateral renal agenesis. *Am. J. Obstet. Gynecol.* **151**, 38–43.

Roodhooft, A. M., Birnholz, J. C. and Holmes, L. B. (1984). Familial nature of congenital absence and severe dysgenesis of both kidneys. *New Engl. J. Med.* **310**, 1341–5.

Rosenfeld, L. (1959). Renal agenesis. *JAMA.* **170**, 1247–8.

Schimke, R. N. and King, C. R. (1980). Hereditary urogenital adysplasia. *Clin. Genet.* **18**, 417–20.

Schinzel, A., Homberger, C. and Sigrist, T. (1978). Bilateral renal agenesis in 2 male sibs born to consanguineous parents. *J. Med. Genet.* **15**, 314–16.

Schlegel, R. J., Aspillaga, M. J., Neu, R. L., Leao, J. C. and Gardner, L. I. (1966a). XX chromosomes and renal agenesis (letter). *Lancet* **1**, 820.

——, ——, ——, Carneiro-Leao, J. and Gardner, L. I. (1986b). An XX sex chromosome complement in an infant having male-type external genitals, renal agenesis and other anomalies. *J. Pediatr.* **69**, 812–14.

Scott, J. S. and Bain, A. D. (1966). XX chromosomes and renal agenesis. (letter). *Lancet* 1, 1035–6.

Seller, M. J. and Berry, A. C. (1978). Amniotic-fluid alphafetoprotein and fetal renal agenesis. (letter). *Lancet* 1, 660.

Shokeir, M. H. K. (1978). Aplasia of the Müllerian system: evidence for probable sex-linked autosomal dominant inheritance. *Birth Defects Orig. Art. Series.* 14, (6C), 147–65.

Streissguth, A. P., Clarren, S. K. and Jones, K. L. (1985). Natural history of the fetal alcohol syndrome: a 10-year follow-up of eleven patients. *Lancet* 2, 85–91.

Sylvester, P. E. and Hughes, D. R. (1954). Congenital absence of both kidneys: a report of four cases. *Br. Med. J.* 1, 77–9.

Waardenburg, P. J. (1952). Einseitige Aplasie der Neiren und ihrer Abfuhrwege bei beiden eineiigen Zwillingspaarlingen. *Acta Genet. Med. Gemellol. (Roma)* 1, 317–20.

Warkany, J. (1971a). *Congenital malformations. Notes and comments.* p. 92. Year Book Medical Publishers, Chicago.

—— (1971b). *Congenital malformations. Notes and comments,* pp. 1037–73. Year Book Medical Publishers, Chicago.

Whitehouse, W. and Mountrose, U. (1973). Renal agenesis in non-twin siblings. *Am. J. Obstet. Gynecol.* 116, 880–2.

Wolff, E. (1936). Les bases de la tératogénese expérimental des vertebrés amniotes d'apres les résultats de méthodes directes. *Arch. Anat. (Strasb.)* 22, 1–375.

—— (1948). La science des monstres. Gallimand, Paris.

Yates, J. R. W., Mortimer, G., Connor, J. M. and Duke, J. E. (1984). Concordant monozygotic twins with bilateral renal agenesis. *J. Med. Genet.* 21, 66–7.

Zachai, E., Mellman, W. J., Neiderer, B. and Hanson, J. (1975). The fetal trimethadione syndrome. *J. Pediatr.* 87, 280–4.

Zonana, J., Rimoin, D. L., Hollister, D. W., Lachman, R. S., Sarti, D. A. and Kaback, M. M. (1976). Renal agenesis—a genetic disorder? Pediatr. Res. 10, 420.

Oligomeganephronic renal hypoplasia

A rare syndrome of oligomeganephronic renal hypoplasia was described by Royer and colleagues (1962). Some 40 cases, all sporadic, have subsequently been reported (Zollinger and Milhatsch 1978). The affected children develop polyuria and dehydration within the first few hours to weeks of life. Anaemia, growth retardation, and uraemic renal failure ensue with eventual early death. The kidneys are small and on histological examination the number of nephrons is greatly reduced but those that are present are greatly enlarged. There is no dysplasia. An ultrastructural study on a single case has recently been reported (Janin-Mercier *et al.* 1985). There has been a single recent report of familial occurrence in a girl and her brother, born to unrelated parents (Moerman *et al.* 1984). This disorder must not be confused with the rare simple renal hypoplasia in which the nephrons are also reduced in number but are of normal size.

References

Janin-Mercier, A., Palcoux, J. B., Gubler, M. C., de Latour, M., Dalens, H. and Fonck, Y. (1985). Oligomeganephronic renal hypoplasia with tapetoretinal degeneration. Report of one case with ultrastructural study of the renal biopsy. *Virchow's Arch. (Pathol. Anat.)* **407**, 477–83.

Moerman, P. H., van Damme, B., Proesmans, W., Devlieger, H., Goddeeris, P. and Lauweryns, J. (1984). Oligomeganephronic renal hypoplasia in two siblings. *J. Pediatr.* **105**, 75–7.

Royer, P., Habib, R., Mathieu, H. and Courtecuisse, V. (1962). Bilateral congenital renal hypoplasia with reduction in number and hypertrophy of the nephrons in children. *Ann. Pediatr.* **9**, 133–46.

Zollinger, H. V. and Mihatsch, M. J. (1978). *Renal pathology in biopsy.* Springer-Verlag, New York.

Renal agenesis with associated malformations

The two most common groups of malformations seen in association with renal agenesis are those involving either the genital tract or the ear. These two types of associated malformation have even been reported as occurring together in the same individual, as in the family originally reported by Schmidt and colleagues (1952) and restudied by Winter and others (1968). In that family four out of seven sisters had bilateral or unilateral renal agenesis or hypoplasia. Three of these four also had vaginal atresia and two had abnormalities of the otic ossicles. Melnick (1980) subsequently termed this disorder oto-renal genital syndrome. Pinsky (1974) reviewed this combined association, along with another common associated malformation, that of the distal extremities. He pointed out that abnormalities of the müllerian ducts, distal extremities, ears, and urinary tract occur in varying combinations in no less than six specific syndromes: the hand–foot–uterus syndrome (Stern *et al.* 1970), camptobrachydactyly (Edwards and Gale 1972), vaginal atresia (hydrometrocolpos)–polydactyly syndrome (McKusick *et al.* 1964; McKusick 1971), the syndrome of Rüdiger and others (1971), oto-renal genital syndrome (Schmidt *et al.* 1952; Winter *et al.* 1968), and the cryptophthalmos syndrome (Fraser 1962, 1966).

To these six syndromes may be added two possible further syndromes. The first was described by von Voss and colleagues (1979) and termed the DK-phocomelia syndrome by Cherstvoy and associates (1980). Both groups described a single patient, female in the first case and male in the second. Both had major malformations of the brain, including encephalocele, and of the upper limbs and thrombocytopenia. In the first case there was vaginal atresia and uterine hypoplasia with a minor urinary tract anomaly, the ureters crossing the lower poles of the kidneys. In the second case there was penile hyperplasia and agenesis of kidneys and ureters. The karyotype in the second patient was 46,XY. The final syndrome in this group was defined by Donnai and colleagues (1986) on the basis of three unrelated cases of their own and five cases in the litera- ture, including two sib pairs, reviewed in detail (Kohler 1983, Rutledge *et al.* 1984). They also considered eight further reported patients probably to have the same syndrome (Lowry *et al.* 1968; Pfeiffer 1969; Patterson *et al.* 1983; Zizka *et al.* 1983; Greene *et al.* 1984; Lipson and Hayes 1984). The main features of this lethal multiple congenital anomaly syndrome are postaxial polydactyly of hands and/or feet, micrognathia, hypoplasia of tongue, low-set malformed ears, congenital heart defects, unilobular lungs, renal hypoplasia, intestinal aganglionosis, mild limb shortening and sex reversal in males, with female or ambiguous external genitalia in patients with testes and a 46,XY karyotype. They propose the name Lowry, Miller, MacLean syndrome as these authors gave the earliest description. However, Donnai, Young and their colleagues are the first to define this syndrome properly and the eponym Donnai, Young syndrome might be better justified.

These eight syndromes are listed in Table 10.2.

This combined association of malformations was further discussed by Duncan and associates (1979) on the basis of two cases of their own and a review of 28 other cases in the literature. They attributed this constella- tion of anomalies to some alteration of the blastemas of the cervico- thoracic somites and the pronephric ducts. All but one of the 30 cases they reviewed had müllerian duct aplasia or dysplasia, 26 had renal agenesis and/or ectopy and 24 had anomalous vertebrae involving the fifth cervical to first thoracic vertebra or other cervicothoracic somite anomalies. They found no reports of chromosomal anomalies, nor of familial occurrence, suggesting some unidentified mechanism of acquired teratogenesis. They termed this constellation of anomalies the 'MURCS association' referring to müllerian duct aplasia–renal aplasia–cervico- thoracic dysplasia. A patient with an extended MURCS association including cleft lip, vascular anomaly, and cerebellar cyst has recently been reported (Greene *et al.* 1986). A variant of this malformation constellation is the association of renal agenesis, polydactyly, vertebral anomaly and imperforate anus (Carpentier and Potter 1959). In one patient with this combination the grandmother had vertebral anomalies and a hypoplastic thumb (Say *et al.* 1971).

Müllerian duct anomalies, such as absent vagina and/or uterus, as for example in the Mayer–Rokitansky syndrome of absent vagina, are very common in association with renal agenesis (Almoslch 1937; Bryan *et al.*

Table 10.2. *Syndromes with urinary and genital tract, ear, and distal extremity malformation (after Pinsky 1974)*

Syndrome	Urinary tract anomaly	Genital tract anomaly	Distal extremity anomaly	Ear anomaly	Inheritance
Hand–foot–uterus syndrome	—	Uterine duplication	Short and fused metacarpals and metatarsals	—	AD
Vaginal atresia–polydactyly syndrome	Double ureter, ureteral stenosis, polycystic kidney	Vaginal atresia	Polydactyly	—	AR
Camptobrachydactyly	Urinary incontinence (? bladder neck dysmorphism)	Septate vagina	Brachypolydactyly	—	AD
Syndrome of Rudiger et al.	Uretero-vesical junction stenosis	Bicornuate uterus	Brachydactyly	Lack of pinna cartilage	?AR
Oto-renal genital syndrome	Renal agenesis	Vaginal atresia	Clinodactyly	External and middle ear anomalies	AR
Cryptophthalmos syndrome	Renal agenesis	Vaginal atresia and bicornuate uterus	Syndactyly	External and middle ear anomalies	AR
DK–phocomelia–thrombocytopenia syndrome	Renal agenesis or ureteral malposition	Vaginal atresia and uterine hypoplasia or penile hyperplasia	Phocomelia or other major limb malformation	—	Sporadic
Domnai–Young syndrome	Renal hypoplasia	Sex reversal in males	Postaxial polydactyly	Low set and malformed	AR

Abbreviations: AD = autosomal dominant, AR = autosomal recessive.

1949; Griffin *et al.* 1976; Tarry *et al.* 1986). Tarry and colleagues propose a classification of müllerian and ovarian anomalies graded MO-M4 according to severity. Their classification could usefully be extended to include renal anomalies similarly graded: RO normal, R1 vesicoureteral reflux, R2 hydronephrosis or renal dysplasia, R3 unilateral ureteric agenesis, and R4 unilateral renal agenesis. They may even extend to female hermaphroditism with masculinization of external genitalia (Siegel, 1944; Perloff *et al.* 1953; Broster 1956; Carpentier and Potter 1959; Franks and Northcutt 1963; Berger and Klempman 1965; Schlegel *et al.* 1966), all reports of which have been of sporadic cases. Wiersma and coworkers (1976) estimated that major or minor genital anomalies are present in as many as 70 per cent of patients with unilateral renal agenesis. Buchta and colleagues (1973) reported two families in which renal adysplasia and müllerian abnormalities occurred in two (family D) or four generations (family E). The association of renal agenesis and müllerian abnormalities has been reported by others (Kohn and Borns 1973; Griffin *et al.* 1976; Schimke and King 1980); and in some cases the müllerian anomaly has been uterus didelphys (Miyazaki *et al.* 1986) or unicornuate uterus (Sayer and O'Reilly 1986). Schimke and King (1980) reported a family with renal agenesis, or dysplasia, and uterine anomaly transmitted through three generations. They introduced the term 'hereditary urogenital adysplasia'. Holmes (1972) in a discussion of the genetics of unilateral renal agenesis noted that half of a series of 60 affected children had associated congenital malformations, mainly müllerian. He divided these into four types: absence of half of the bladder trigone with its ureter, and ipsilateral absence of testes or ovary, uterus, and in some cases vagina, seen in 19 cases; imperforate anus, vertebral and preaxial forearm anomaly, with or without further skeletal anomalies of leg and pelvis in six cases; cloacal exstrophy and skeletal defects in two cases; and persistence of uterus and vagina in a male. Holmes' imperforate anus and skeletal anomaly group corresponds to the similar group described by Carpentier and Potter (1959) and to the possibly hereditary case of Say and colleagues (1971). Recently two new families have been reported with combined renal agenesis and dysplasia and müllerian abnormalities in some of the affected members, in two generations of each family (Biedel *et al.* 1984). The authors argue for autosomal dominant inheritance in their own families and those of Schimke and King (1980), Kohn and Borns (1973), and Buchta and colleagues (1973) (families D and E).

Associated anomalies of the male genital tract, especially the seminal vesicle, may also be seen. Fuselier and Peters (1976) reported a case of seminal vesicle cyst with ipsilateral renal agenesis, and reviewed 19 similar cases. Gravgaard and others (1978) described a man with a double vas deferens opening into the seminal vesicle and ipsilateral renal agenesis. Until an operation specimen was examined histologically this had simulated an ectopic ureter. Knudsen and colleagues (1979) reported a remarkable family in which a brother and sister both had renal agenesis, associated in him with an ipsilateral seminal vesicle cyst and in her with the embryologically analgous Gartner's duct cyst, and a bicornuate uterus. Others have reported renal agenesis in males associated with absence of the vas deferens (Ochsner *et al.* 1972; Cain *et al.* 1974). The Kallman syndrome of hypogonadotrophic hypogonadism and anosmia or hyposmia predominantly in males, with or without central facial clefting, has been reported in families showing autosomal dominant, autosomal recessive and X-linked recessive inheritance (see McKusick 1983). In at least one family with the X-linked form there was also unilateral renal agenesis (Wegenke *et al.* 1975). Two brothers and their male double first cousin were affected and there were minor features in the female carriers.

Hilson (1957) reviewed the association of ear malformation with renal agenesis and other urinary tract malformations noting that bat ears and other malformations of the external ear were often present in familial cases. A more recent review, confirming the non-syndromic association of ear and renal malformations and delineating several syndromes of ear dysplasia and renal adysplasia, is that of Melnick (1980). He recognizes three main syndrome groups in which external ear malformations, with or without middle ear defects, are a consistent component; an oto-mandibular group, branchio-oto-dysplasia and a third group that includes renal malformation—the ear dysplasia–renal adysplasia group. The different syndromes within this last group specifically associated with renal aplasia or hypoplasia are listed in Table 10.3, compiled from Melnick's and more recent papers.

Branchio-oto-renal dysplasia or syndrome was probably present in two of the families described by Hilson (1957). The family reported by Martins (1961) probably also had this syndrome, but the first clear definition was that of Melnick and colleagues (1975, 1976) in a family in which the father and a son and two daughters, out of six living children, had a mixed hearing loss with a Mondini cochlear malformation (hypoplasia of the cochlear apex) and stapes fixation, cup-shaped pinnae, pre-auricular sinuses and branchial cleft fistulae, and renal hypoplasia with dysplasia. Reports of further families followed rapidly (Fitch and Srolovitz 1976; Fraser *et al.* 1978; Melnick *et al.* 1978; Cremers and Fikkers-van Noord 1980; Cremers *et al.* 1981; Carmi *et al.* 1983). Widdershoven and coworkers (1983) studied 16 patients all of whom had renal tact malformations on urography, which may include mega-cystis and microcolon. Nevertheless there is considerable variation in

Table 10.3. *Syndromes of ear malformation and renal adysplasia*

Syndrome	Ear defect	Renal defect	Mode of inheritance
1. Oto-renal syndrome	Preauricular pits	Hypoplasia and nephritis	AD
2. Branchio-oto-renal syndrome	Cupped pinnae, preauricular sinuses and mixed hearing loss with Mondini cochlear malformation and fixed stapes	Aplasia, dysplasia and pelvi-ureteric duplication defects	AD
3. Auricular–renal adysplasia–hypospadias syndrome	'Bat ears' or Potter's facies ears	Bilateral or unilateral renal agenesis, and hypospadias	AD
4. Oto-renal genital syndrome	Low-set, lop ears, external auditory meatal atresia, otic ossicle abnormalities with conductive hearing loss	Bilateral or unilateral renal agenesis or hypoplasia and vaginal atresia	AR
5. Polydactyly, cleft-lip, hamartoma, renal, deafness, retardation syndrome	Moderate conductive hearing loss	Bilateral or unilateral renal agenesis	AR

Abbreviations: AD = autosomal dominant, AR = autosomal recessive expression in this syndrome and it remains unsettled as to whether branchio-oto syndrome without renal anomaly is a distinct disorder, as Melnick and associates (1978) believe, or is merely part of the range of expression of branchio-oto-renal syndrome, as Cremers and Fikkers-van Noord (1980) maintain. Heimler and Lieber (1986) have reported a family that supports the latter view. Oto-branchial anomalies were associated with a wide range of upper or lower tract abnormalities, or none at all, in different members of the family. Fraser and colleagues (1980) concluded that the syndrome is more common that is generally recognized. They studied over 400 children in Montreal schools for the deaf and found 19 with preauricular pits, and confirmed the diagnosis of branchio-oto-renal syndrome in four out of nine families that agreed to family investigations, including audiograms and pyelography. They estimated that 6 per cent of heterozygotes have severe renal dysplasia and that a preauricular pit at birth indicates a 1 in 200 chance of severe hearing loss. What is undoubted from all of these studies is that inheritance is autosomal dominant. Although it has not yet been reported the more severe renal abnormalities should be detectable by prenatal diagnostic ultrasound.

Auriculo-renal adysplasia–hypospadias syndrome is a private syndrome present in one of Hilson's (1957) families (his case 3) in which the propositus had bilateral renal agenesis resulting in neonatal death. He also had hypospadias and the deformed ears of Potter's syndrome. His father had hypospadias and bat ears, the father's sister had four children of whom one had unilateral renal agenesis and two had hypospadias with unilateral bat ear. The paternal grandmother was said to have had polycystic kidney disease.

Oto-renal syndrome is also a private syndrome in which nephritis was present in a six-generation family involving a male in the first generation, six of his grandchildren, and eight of their descendants spread over a further three generations (Lachiewicz *et al.* 1985). Renal disease was more severe in males. Eight of the nephritic patients developed proteinuria at a young age. Nephrectomy from one showed simple renal hypoplasia with glomerulomegaly, segmental sclerosis, and hyalinosis. Others had chronic tubular changes and interstitial nephritis, and one patient had small remnants of nephroblastomatosis.

Of the 15 patients with nephritis 12 had preauricular pits and another 10 family members not known to have nephritis also had preauricular pits. Audiograms were normal. The authors, who claim that there is a significant association of nephritis and preauricular pits in this family, suggested that the two clinical abnormalities were due either to the same gene or to genetically linked genes. Penetrance, on the assumption of autosomal dominance, was 80 per cent for renal disease and 85 per cent for preauricular pits.

Oto-renal genital syndrome is the syndrome first described in the family already mentioned by Schmidt and colleagues (1952), but more fully described by Winter and others (1968). In that family vaginal atresia, unilateral or bilateral renal agenesis, or hypoplasia and anomalies of the otic ossicles were found in varying combinations in four sisters. A possible futher family with this syndrome was described by Turner (1970). The proposita had a right renal agenesis, vaginal atresia and mild hearing loss with a narrow external auditory meatus. A sib had died in the neonatal period with a history suggestive of renal agenesis, and another sib also had narrow external auditory canals, and a possibly unrelated hydrocephalus.

Polydactyly, cleft-lip, hamartoma, renal, deafness, retardation syndrome is another private syndrome reported by Mattei and Ayme (1983) in three male sibs. The propositus had unilateral renal agenesis shown on intravenous pyelography, preaxial polydactyly of the feet, median cleft-lip, short philtrum, and fatty hamartomas of the tongue. He was severely mentally and growth retarded and had bilateral moderate conductive hearing loss. Male monozygotic twin brothers of the propositus had died in the neonatal period 4 years earlier, and both had had polydactyly of the hands and feet and severe bilateral renal hypoplasia with cystic change. This disorder is presumably either autosomal, or X linked recessive.

Ocular abnormalities are a less common association with renal agenesis. Brief mention has already been made of the cryptophthalmos syndrome first described by G. R. Fraser (1962, 1966) in two separate families. In each family two sisters had varying combinations of cryptophthalmos, aplasia or malformation of the lacrimal ducts, middle and outer ear malformations, hypertelorism with cleavage along the mid-plane of the nares and tongue and a high palate, laryngeal stenosis, syndactyly, displaced umbilicus and nipples, renal agenesis or dysplasia, vaginal atresia, labial fusion, malformed fallopian tubes, and bicornuate uterus with wide separation of the symphysis pubis. Bilateral, or in one case unilateral, renal agenesis was found in eight of nine sibs of index cases studied by Thomas and colleagues (1986), and all seven of their index cases had bilateral renal agenesis. Gonadal dysgenesis with *in situ* gonadoblastoma has recently been reported in one case (Greenberg *et al.* 1986). Further families have been reported, in some of which there has been parental consanguinity (Gupta and Saxena 1962; Francois 1969; Ide and Wollschaeger 1969; Azevedo *et al.* 1973, Varnek 1978), or multiple affected sibs (Burn and Marwood 1982; Hancheng 1986; Thomas *et al.* 1986), confirming an autosomal recessive mode of inheritance. Mortimer and associates (1985) reported monozygotic twins concordant for Fraser syndrome, without cryptophthalmos but with bilateral renal agenesis. Duke-Elder (1963) reviewed the older literature on cryptophthalmos and its frequent association with other malformations. Brownstein and others (1976) reported the association of bilateral renal agenesis with a different complex of ocular abnormalities in a single case. These included the absence of keratocytes in the inner central corneal stroma, cataract with retention of cell nuclei in the lens nucleus, hypoplasia of the ganglion cell and nerve fibre layers of the retina, and lack of nerve bundles in the optic nerve. Microphthalmos and persistent pupillary membrane may have been due to prematurity. It should be noted that isolated cryptophthalmos is genetically distinct, being inherited in an autosomal dominant manner.

Renal agenesis or ectopia may occur in association with müllerian anomalies in the Klippel–Feil syndrome, and some such reported families are suggestive of autosomal dominant inheritance (Park *et al.* 1971; Ramsey and Bliznak 1971; Baird and Lowry 1974; Duncan 1977; Duncan *et al.* 1979).

Sommer and colleagues (1974) reported a brother and sister with partial aniridia, congenital glaucoma, telecanthus, frontal bossing, mental subnormality, and unilateral renal agenesis.

Other familial malformations rarely associated with renal agenesis or dysplasia include hepatic and central nervous system malformation (Miranda *et al.* 1972), and the neurofacial digito-renal syndrome (Freire-Maia *et al.* 1982). The former syndrome was observed in two families—a brother and sister in the first, and two brothers in the second. In both the renal lesion was bilateral dysplasia, but the appearance on microdissection differed, with irregular branching of collecting ducts with segmental variation in calibre in the first family but uniform collecting ducts terminating in ampullary cysts in the second. This suggests possible genetic heterogeneity. The latter syndrome (NFDR syndrome) was present in two brothers with mental subnormality, abnormal electroencephalogram without seizures, a bifid nose, prominent forehead, malformed pinnae, short stature, and triphalangeal thumbs. One brother had unilateral renal agenesis. Renal agenesis, hypoplasia, ectopia, or horseshoe kidney may occur as part of the spectrum of malformations that are seen in Fanconi's pancytopenia, an autosomal recessive disorder (McDonald and Goldshmidt 1959). Unilateral renal agenesis and hydronephrosis have been reported in the autosomal dominant multiple lentigenes syndrome (Swanson *et al.* 1971), renal agenesis alone in the 17p13 deletion Miller–Diecker or lissencephaly syndrome (Miller 1963; Dobyns *et al.* 1983) described in Chapter 3, unilateral or bilateral renal agenesis, renal dysplasia, and hydroureter in the X-linked recessive Lenz microphthalmia (Gorlin *et al.* 1976), and unilateral renal and testicular agenesis in Darier's disease (Matsuoka *et al.* 1985).

A family with a curious combination of torticollis, spontaneous keloids, pigmented naevi, cryptorchidism, infertility, and renal abnormalities in males has been reported (Goeminne 1968). One male with the full syndrome also had a basal cell epithelioma. The renal abnormalities comprised renal hypoplasia and chronic pyelonephritis but were only present in two out of six affected males. There was also considerable variation in expression of the other features apart from the torticollis. The pedigree was consistent with incomplete X-linked dominant inheritance. Zuffardi and Fraccaro (1982) subsequently assigned the gene locus for this rare syndrome to Xq28, distal to G6PD.

References

Almolsch, A. L. (1937). Bilateral metanephric agenesis. *J. Urol.* **38**, 360–70.

Azevedo, E. S., Biondi, J. and Ramalho, L. M. (1973). Cryptophthalmos in two families from Bahia, Brazil. *J. Med. Genet.* **10**, 389–92.

Baird, P. A. and Lowry, R. B. (1974). Absent vagina and the Klippel–Feil anomaly. *Am. J. Obstet. Gynecol.* **118**, 290–1.

Berger, G. M. and Klempman, S. (1965). A case of female hermaphroditism with associated congenital defects: review of some aetiologic problems. *S. Afr. Med. J.* **39**, 23–6.

Biedel, C. W., Pagon, R. A. and Zapata, J. O. (1984). Müllerian anomalies and renal agenesis: autosomal dominant urogenital adysplasia. *J. Pediatr.* **104**, 861–4.

Broster, L. R. (1956). A form of intersexuality. *Br. Med. J.* **1**, 149–51.

Brownstein, S., Kirkham, T. H. and Kalousek, D. K. (1976). Bilateral renal agenesis with multiple congenital ocular anomalies. *Am. J. Ophthalmol.* **82**, 770–4.

Bryan, A. L., Nigro, J. A. and Counseller, V. S. (1949). One hundred cases of congenital absence of the vagina. *Surg. Gynecol. Obstet.* **88**, 79–86.

Buchta, R. M., Visekul, C., Gilbert, E. F., Sarto, G. E. and Opitz, J. M. (1973). Familial bilateral renal agenesis and hereditary renal adysplasia. *Z. Kinderheilk.* **115**, 111–29.

Burn, J. and Marwood, R. P. (1982). Fraser syndrome presenting as bilateral renal agenesis in three sibs. *J. Med. Genet.* **19**, 360–1.

Cain, D. R., Griggs, D., Lackey, D. A. and Kagan, B. M. (1974). Familial renal agenesis and total dysplasia. *Am. J. Dis. Child.* **128**, 377–80.

Carmi, R., Binshtock, M., Abeliovich, D. and Bar-Ziv, J. (1983). The branchio-oto-renal (BOR) syndrome: report of bilateral renal agenesis in three sibs. *Am. J. Med. Genet.* **14**, 625–7.

Carpentier, P. J. and Potter, E. L. (1959). Nuclear sex and genital malformation in 48 cases of renal agenesis, with special reference to non-specific female pseudohermaphroditism. *Am. J. Obstet. Gynecol.* **78**, 235–58.

Cherstvoy, E., Lazjuk, G., Lurie, I., Ostrovskaya, T. and Shved, I. (1980). Syndrome of multiple congenital malformations including phocomelia, thrombocytopenia, encephalocele, and urogenital abnormalities. *Lancet* **2**, 485.

Cremers, C. W. R. J. and Fikkers-van Noord, M. (1980). The earpits–deafness syndrome: clinical and genetic aspects. *Int. J. Pediatr. Otorhinolaryngol.* **2**, 309–22.

——, Thijssen, H. O. M., Fischer, A. J. E. M. and Marres, E. H. M. A. (1981). Otological aspects of the earpit–deafness syndrome. *ORL* **43**, 223–39.

Dobyns, W. B., Stratton, R. F., Parke, J. T., Greenberg, F., Nussbaum, R. L. and Ledbetter, D. H. (1983). The Miller–Diecker syndrome: lissencephaly and monosomy 17p. *J. Pediatr.* **102**, 552–8.

Donnai, D., Young, I. D., Owen, W. G., Clark, S. A., Miller, P. F. W. and Knox, W. F. (1986). The lethal multiple congenital anomaly syndrome of polydactyly, sex reversal, renal hypoplasia and unilobular lungs. *J. Med. Genet.* **23**, 64–71.

Duke-Elder, S. (1963). *System of ophthalmology, normal and abnormal development*, Vol. 3, Part 2. pp. 829–34. C. V. Mosby, St Louis.

Duncan, P. A. (1977). Embryologic pathogenesis of renal agenesis associated with cervical vertebral anomalies (Klippel–Feil phenotype). *Birth Defects Orig. Art. Series* **13** (30), 91–101.

——, Shapiro, L. R., Stagel, J. J., Klein, R. M. and Addonizio, J. C. (1979). The MURCS association: Müllerian duct aplasia, renal aplasia, and cervicothoracic somite dysplasia. *J. Pediatr.* **95**, 399–402.

Edwards, J. A. and Gale, R. P. (1972). Camptobrachydactyly: a new autosomal dominant trait with two probable homozygotes. *Am. J. Hum. Genet.* **24**, 464–74.

Fitch, N. and Srolovitz, H. (1976). Severe renal dysplasia produced by a dominant gene. *Am. J. Dis. Child.* **130**, 1356–7.

Francois, J. (1969). Syndrome malformatif avec cryptophthalmos. *Acta Genet. Med. Gemellol.* **18**, 18–50.

Franks, R. C. and Northcutt, R. (1963). Female pseudohermaphroditism and renal anomalies. *Am. J. Dis. Child.* **105**, 490–6.

Fraser, F. C., Ling, D., Clogg, D. and Nogrady, B. (1978). Genetic aspects of the BOR syndrome-branchial fistulas, ear pits, hearing loss and renal anomalies. *Am. J. Med. Genet.* **2**, 241–52.

——, Sproule, J. R. and Halal, F. (1980). Frequency of the branchio-oto-renal (BOR) syndrome in children with profound hearing loss. *Am. J. Med. Genet.* **7**, 341–9.

Fraser, G. R. (1962). Our genetical load. A review of some aspects of genetical variation. *Ann. Hum. Genet.* **25**, 387–415.

—— (1966). XX chromosomes and renal agenesis. *Lancet* **1**, 1427.

Freire-Maia, N., Pinheiro, M. and Opitz, J. M. (1982). The neurofaciodigito-renal (NFDR) syndrome. *Am. J. Med. Genet.* **11**, 329–36.

Fuselier, H. A. Jr. and Peters, D. H. (1976). Cyst of seminal vesicle with ipsilateral renal agenesis and ectopic ureter: case report. *J. Urol.* **116**, 833–5.

Goeminne, L. (1968). A new probably X-linked inherited syndrome: congenital torticollis, multiple keloids, cryptorchidism and renal dysplasia. *Acta Genet. Med. Gemellol.* **17**, 439–67.

Gorlin, R. J., Pinborg, J. J. and Cohen, M. M. (1976). *Syndromes of the head and neck*, 2nd edn. McGraw-Hill, New York.

Gravgaard, E., Farsdale, L. and Moller, S. M. (1978). Double vas deferens and epididymis associated with ipsilateral renal agenesis simulating ectopic ureter opening into the seminal vesicle. *Scand. J. Urol. Nephrol.* **12**, 85–7.

Greenberg, F., Keenan, B., De Yanis, V. and Finegold, M. (1986). Gonadal dysgenesis and gonadoblastoma *in situ* in a female with Fraser (cryptophthalmos) syndrome. *J. Pediatr.* **108**, 952–4.

Greene, C., Pitts, W. Rosenfeld, R. and Luzzatti, L. (1984). Smith–Lemli–Opitz syndrome in two 46,XY infants with female external genitalia. *Clin. Genet.* **25**, 366–72.

Greene, R. A., Bloch, M. J., Huff, D. S. and Iozzo, R. V. (1986). MURCS association with additional congenital anomalies. *Hum. Pathol.* **17**, 88–91.

Griffin, , J. E., Edwards, C., Madden, J. D., Harrod, M. J. and Wilson, J. D. (1976). Congenital absence of the vagina: the Mayer–Rokitansky–Kuster–Hauser syndrome. *Ann. Intern. Med.* **85**, 224–36.

Gupta, S. P. and Saxena, R. C. (1962). Cryptophthalmos. *Br. J. Ophthalmol.* **46**, 629–32.

Hancheng, Z. (1986). Cryptophthalmos: a report on three sibling cases. *Br. J. Ophthalmol.* **70**, 72–4.

Heimler, A. and Lieber, E. (1986). Branchio-oto-renal syndrome: reduced penetrance and variable expressivity in four generations of a large kindred. *Am. J. Med. Genet.* **25**, 15–27.

Hilson, D. (1957). Malformations of ears as sign of malformation of the genito-urinary tract. *Br. Med. J.* **2**, 785–9.

Holmes, L. B. (1972). Unilateral renal agenesis: common, serious, ? hereditary. *Pediatr. Res.* **6**, 419.

Ide, C. H. and Wollschlaeger, P. B. (1969). Multiple congenital abnormalities associated with cryptophthalmia. *Arch. Ophthalmol.* **81**, 638–44.

Knudsen, J. B., Brun, B. and Emus, H. C. (1979). Familial renal agenesis: seminal vesicle cyst and vaginal cyst with bicornuate uterus in siblings. *Scand. J. Urol. Nephrol.* **13**, 109–12.

Kohler, H. G. (1983). Brief clinical report: familial neonatally lethal syndrome of hypoplastic left heart, absent pulmonary lobation, polydactyly and talipes, probably Smith–Lemli–Opitz syndrome. *Am. J. Med. Genet.* **14**, 423–8.

Kohn, G. and Borns, P. F. (1973). The association of bilateral and unilateral renal aplasia in the same family. *J. Pediatr.* **83**, 95–7.

Lachiewicz, A. M., Sibley, R. and Michael, A. F. (1985). Hereditary renal disease and preauricular pits: report of a kindred. *J. Pediatr.* **106**, 948–50.

Lipson, A. and Hayes, A. (1984). Smith–Lemli–Opitz syndrome and Hirschsprung disease. *J. Pediatr.* **105**, 177.

Lowry, R. B., Miller, J. R. and MacLean, J. R. (1968). Micrognathia, polydactyly and cleft-palate. *J. Pediatr.* **72**, 859–61.

McDonald, R. and Goldshmidt, B. (1959). Pancytopenia with congenital defects (Fanconis' anaemia). *Arch. Dis. Child.* **34**, 367–72.

McKusick, V. A. (1971). Transverse vaginal septum (hydrometrocolpos). *Birth Defects Orig. Art. Series.* **7**, 326.

—— (1983). *Mendelian inheritance in man*, 6th edn. pp. 317, 792 and 1063–4. Johns Hopkins Univ. Press, Baltimore.

——, Bauer, R. L., Koop, C. E. and Scott, R. B. (1964). Hydrometrocolpos as a simply inherited malformation. *JAMA* **189**, 813–16.

Martins, A. G. (1961). Lateral cervical and preauricular sinuses: their transmission as dominant characters. *Br. Med. J.* **2**, 255–6.

Matsuoka, L. Y., Wortsman, J. and McConnache, P. (1985). Renal and testicular agenesis in a patient with Darier's disease. *Am. J. Med.* **78**, 873–7.

Mattei, J.-F. and Ayme, S. (1983). Syndrome of polydactyly, cleft lip, lingual hamartomas, renal hypoplasia, hearing loss, and psychomotor retardation: variant of the Mohr syndrome or a new syndrome. *J. Med. Genet.* **20**, 433–5.

Melnick, M. (1980). Hereditary hearing loss and ear dysplasia–renal adysplasia syndromes: syndrome delineation and possible pathogenesis. *Birth Defects Orig. Art. Series* **16** (7), 59–72.

——, Bixler, D., Silk, K., Yune, H. and Nance, W. E. (1975). Autosomal dominant branchio-oto-renal dysplasia. *Birth Defects Orig. Art. Series* **11** (5), 121–8.

——, ——, Nance, W. E., Silk, K. and Yune, H. (1976). Familial branchio-oto-renal dysplasia: a new addition to the branchial arch syndromes. *Clin. Genet.* **9**, 25–34.

——, Hodes, M. E., Nance, W. E., Yune, H. and Sweeney, A. (1978). Branchio-oto-renal dysplasia and branchio-oto-dysplasia: two distinct autosomal dominant disorders. *Clin. Genet.* **13**, 425–42.

Miller, J. Q. (1963). Lissencephaly in two siblings. *Neurology* **13**, 841–50.

Miranda, D., Schinella, R. A. and Finegold, M. J. (1972). Familial renal dysplasia: microdissection studies in siblings with associated central nervous system and hepatic malformations. *Arch. Pathol.* **93**, 483–91.

Miyazaki, Y., Ebisuno, S., Uekado, Y., Ogawa, T., Senzaki, A. and Ohkawa, T. (1986). Uterus didelphys with unilateral imperforate vagina and ipsilateral renal agenesis. *J. Urol.* **135**, 107–9.

Mortimer, G., McEwan, H. P. and Yates, J. R. W. (1985). Fraser syndrome presenting as monozygotic twins with bilateral renal agenesis. *J. Med. Genet.* **22**, 76–8.

Ochsner, M. G., Brannan, W. and Goodier, E. H. (1972). Absent vas deferens associated with renal agenesis. *JAMA* **222**, 1055–6.

Park, I. J., Jones, H. W. Jr., Nager, G. T., Chen, S. C. A. and Hussels, I. E. (1971). A new syndrome in two unrelated females: Klippel–Feil deformity, conductive deafness and absent vagina. *Birth Defects Orig. Art. Series* **8** (6), 311–17.

Patterson, K., Toomey, K. E. and Chandra, R. A. (1983). Hirschsprung disease in a 46,XY phenotypic infant girl with Smith–Lemli–Opitz syndrome. *J. Pediatr.* **103**, 425–7.

Perloff, W. H., Conger, K. B. and Levy, L. M. (1953). Female pseudohermaphroditism: a description of two unusual cases. *J. Clin. Endocrinol.* **13**, 783–90.

Pfeiffer, R. A. (1969). Associated deformities of the head and hands. *Birth Defects* **5** (3), 18–34.

Pinsky, L. (1974). A community of malformation syndromes involving the Müllerian ducts, distal extremities, urinary tract and ears. *Teratology* **9**, 65–79.

Ramsey, J. and Bliznak, J. (1971). Klippel–Feil syndrome with renal agenesis and other anomalies. *Am. J. Roentgenol.* **113**, 460–3.

Rüdiger, R. A., Schmidt, W., Loose, D. A. and Passarge, E. (1971). Severe developmental failure with coarse facial features, distal limb hypoplasia, thickened palmar creases, bifid uvula and ureteral stenosis: a previously unidentified familial disorder with lethal outcome. *J. Pediatr.* **79**, 977–81.

Rutledge, J. C., Friedman, J. M., Harrod, M. J. E., Currarino, G., Wright, C. G., Pinckney, L. and Chen, H. (1984). A 'new' lethal multiple congenital anomaly syndrome: joint contractures, cerebellar hypoplasia, renal hypoplasia, urogenital anomalies, tongue cysts, shortness of limbs, eye abnormalities, defect of the heart, gallbladder agenesis and ear malformations. *Am. J. Med. Genet.* **19**, 255–64.

Say, B., Balci, S., Pirnar, T. and Hicsonmez, A. (1971). Imperforate anus/poly-dactyly/vertebral anomalies syndrome: a hereditary trait? *J. Pediatr.* **79**, 1033–4.

Sayer, T. and O'Reilly, P. H. (1986). Bicornuate and unicorunuate uterus associ-ated with unilateral renal aplasia and abnormal solitary kidneys: report of 3 cases. *J. Urol.* **135**, 110–11.

Schimke, R. N. and King, C. R. (1980). Hereditary urogenital adysplasia. *Clin. Genet.* **18**, 417–20.

Schlegel, R. J., Aspillaga, M. J., Neu, R. L., Carneiro-Leao, J. and Gardner, L. I. (1966). An XX sex chromosome complement in an infant having male-type external genitals, renal agenesis and other anomalies. *J. Pediatr.* **69**, 812.

Schmidt, E. C. H., Hartley, A. A. and Bower, R. (1952). Renal aplasia in sisters. *Arch. Pathol.* **54**, 403–6.

Siegel, I. (1944). A case of pseudohermaphrodismus feminus externus with uterus didelphys, imperforate anus and vagina. *Am. J. Obstet. Gynecol.* **47**, 705–6.

Sommer, A., Rathbun, M. A. and Battles, M. L. (1974). A syndrome of partial aniridia, unilateral renal agenesis and mild psychomotor retardation in siblings. *J. Pediatr.* **85**, 870–2.

Stern, A. M., Gall, J. C., Perry, B. L., Stimson, C. W., Weitkamp, L. R. and Poznanski, A. K. (1970). The hand–foot–uterus syndrome. *J. Pediatr.* **77**, 109–16.

Swanson, S. L., Santen, R. J. and Smith, D. W. (1971). Multiple lentigenes syndrome: new findings of hypogonadotrophism, hyposmia and unilateral renal agenesis. *J. Pediatr.* **78**, 1037–9.

Tarry, W. F., Duckett, J. W. and Stephens, F. D. (1986). The Mayer–Rokitansky syndrome: pathogenesis, classification and management. *J. Urol.* **136**, 648–52.

Thomas, I. T., Frias, J. L., Felix, V., Sanchez de Leon, L., Helnondez, R. A. and Jones, M. C. (1986). Isolated and syndromic cryptophthalmos. *Am. J. Med. Genet.* **25**, 85–98.

Turner, G. (1970). A second family with renal, vaginal, and middle ear anomalies. *J. Pediatr.* **76**, 641.

Varnek, L. (1978). Cryptophthalmos, dyscephaly, syndactyly and renal aplasia. *Acta ophthalmol.* **56**, 302–13.

von Voss, H., Kramer, H., Gobel, V. and Kemperdick, H. (1979). *Klinische Genetik in der Pädiatrie*, Kiel, p. 70. Georg Thieme, Stuttgart.

Winter, J. S. D., Kohn, G., Mellman, W. J. and Wagner, S. (1968). A familial syndrome of renal, genital and middle ear anomalies. *J. Pediatr.* **72**, 88–93.

Wegenke, J. D., Uehling, D. T., Wear, J. B., Gordon, E. S., Bargman, J. G., Deacon, J. S. R., Herrmann, J. P. R. and Opitz, J. M. (1975). Familial Kallmann syndrome with unilateral renal aplasia. *Clin. Genet.* **7**, 368–81.

Widdershoven, J., Monnens, L., Assmann, K. and Cremers, C. (1983). Renal disorders in the branchio-oto-renal syndrome. *Helv. Paediatr. Acta* **38**, 513–22.

Wiersma, A. F., Peterson, L. F. and Justema, E. J. (1976). Uterine anomalies associated with unilateral renal agenesis. *Obstet. Gynecol.* **47**, 654–7.

Zizka, J., Maresora, J., Kerekes, Z., Nozicka, Z., Juttnerova, V. and Balicek, P. (1983). Intestinal aganglionosis in the Smith–Lemli–Opitz syndrome. *Acta Paediatr. Scand.* **72**, 141–3.

Zuffardi, O. and Fraccaro, M. (1982). Gene mapping and serendipity. The locus for torticollis, keloids, cryptorchidism and renal dysplasia (31430 McKusick) is at Xq28, distal to the G6PD locus *Hum. Genet.* **62**, 280.

Sirenomelia (sympodia or mermaid fetus), and caudal regression

Sirenomelia is another disorder in which renal agenesis, or severe renal hypoplasia, is associated with other malformations. These include imperforate anus, sacral agenesis and variable degrees of fusion of the lower limbs, and a single umbilical artery. In a minority of cases malformations of the upper half of the body are also present, as for example asplenia, diaphragmatic agenesis, cardiac defect, and oesophageal atresia or tracheo-oesophageal fistula. The great majority of cases are male (Hendry and Kohler 1956).

This striking malformation has been recognized for several centuries. One of the earliest factual descriptions, that of Hartmann (1691), was preceded by more fanciful descriptions which undoubtedly owed much to the mermaid or siren myths.

The degree of lower limb fusion distally determines the type of symmelia present, that is, sympus dipus with two feet, monopus with one foot, or apus without a foot and with the fused limb ending in a stump or single toe (Förster 1865). The long bones of the lower limb may or may not be fused within the single limb, which is in either case rotated through 180°.

The urinary tract lesion in the majority of cases is a bilateral renal agenesis with a consequent oligohydramnios, Potter's facies, and perinatal death. That oligohydramnios in sirenomelia is secondary to renal aplasia and is not the primary cause of the malformation is clear from the observation of exceptional cases without oligohydramnios or Potter's facies (Hendry and Kohler 1956; Crawfurd *et al.* 1966). Rudimentary kidneys have been reported (Bearn 1960; Crawfurd *et al.* 1966; Malkasian *et al.* 1969; Sun *et al.* 1986). Unique findings are a horseshoe kidney (Hendry and Kohler 1956), large cystic kidneys (David and Fein 1974), and normal kidneys but extroversion of the bladder (Crawfurd *et al.* 1985).

Despite some 350 cases having been reported (Crawfurd *et al.* 1985) the anomaly is comparatively rare. The incidence has been variously estimated at 1 in 60 000 live births (Crawfurd *et al.* 1966) or 1 in 47 000 total births (Stevenson *et al.* 1966).

Sirenomelia is generally regarded as one extreme of a spectrum of developmental anomalies affecting the caudal end of the embryo (Duhamel 1961). The concept of some teratogenic influence on the caudal embryo is supported by experimental studies in which irradiation of caudal somites of chicks results in lesions similar to human sireno-melia (Wolff 1936, 1948; Gloor and Schinz 1950). However, there is little evidence as to the nature of the teratogenic mechanism in human cases. Normal karyotypes have been found where chromosomal analysis has been performed (Passarge and Sutherland 1965; Crawfurd *et al.* 1966; Malkasian *et al.* 1969). There is no significant evidence either of maternal radiation exposure or of maternal viral infection in the first trimester. There have been only a very few instances of maternal drug exposure, as for example the suggestion of vitamin A teratogenesis in a case of partial sirenomelia (Von Lennep *et al.* 1985).

There is evidence of both multifactorial predisposition to sirenomelia in specific strains of mice (Gluecksohn-Schoenheimer and Dunn 1945), and of a specific recessive mutation (sr) in mice producing sirenomelia in homozygotes (Hornbeek 1970; Hornbeek and Schreiner 1973). There is no comparable evidence for a genetic basis for human sirenomelia. Crawfurd and colleagues (1985) could find no report of affected sibs who were not either definite or possible monozygotic twins. They also found that among monozygotic twins only a minority, three out of 12 pairs, show partial or complete concordance. This excludes a single abnormal gene as the cause of most human cases. The one striking observation regarding human sirenomelia is the high proportion of affected infants that are one of a monozygotic twin pair (Stevenson *et al.* 1966; Davies *et al.* 1971), especially monoamniotic (Crawfurd *et al.* 1985). Kohler (1972) has pointed out the rarity of monoamniotic twinning, one in 30 000 to 40 000 pregnancies. The idea that mono-zygotic twinning, acting through a variety of possible mechanisms, may play a role in the causation of sirenomelia has been advanced by several groups (Davies *et al.* 1971; Smith *et al.* 1976; Crawfurd *et al.* 1985).

Apart from sirenomelia less extreme forms of caudal regression may also occur in association with renal and other malformations. Sisk and colleagues (1978) reported two unrelated cases of infants with micro-cephaly, agenesis of the lower spine, foot deformities, and urological and other malformations. The urological defects in the first child were bilateral ureteric calyces and a left vesico-ureteric reflux, and in the second child bilateral uretero-vesical junction stenosis. The sporadic occurrence of the caudal regression anomaly in association with maternal diabetes is well recognized (Passarge and Lenz 1966), but there is at least one report of this association occurring in sibs (Stewart and Stoll 1979). They reported a brother and sister both affected and both with urinary tract malformations. These authors, and others, have reported normal karyotypes in caudal regression syndrome. An exception to this general rule is the case reported by Jensen and Hansen (1981) in which a male infant had severe caudal regression syndrome with total absence of kidney, ureter, bladder, and external genitalia. Chromosomal analysis revealed the presence of an extra bisatellited minute chromosome in 53 out of 63 cells examined, probably at least mainly derived from chromosome 22. The authors suggested that the chromosome abnormality was causal but accepted that it might be merely coincidental.

References

Bearn, J. G. (1960). The association of sirenomelia with Potter's syndrome. *Arch. Dis. Child.* **35**, 254–8.

Crawfurd, M. d'A., Ismail, S. R. and Wigglesworth, J. S. (1966). A monopodal sireniform monster with dermatoglyphic and cytogenetic studies. *J. Med. Genet.* **3**, 212–16.

——, Keeling, J. W. and Kohler, H. G. (1985). Sirenomelia: a report of four cases (unpublished observations).

David, M. P. and Fein, A. (1974). Sirenomelia. Report of a case with thoughts on the teratogenic mechanism. *Obstet. Gynecol.* **44**, 91–8.

Davies, J., Chazen, E. and Nance, W. E. (1971). Symmelia in one of monozygotic twins. *Teratology* **4**, 367–78.

Duhamel, B. (1961). From the mermaid to anal imperforation: the syndrome of caudal regression. *Arch. Dis. Child.* **36**, 152–5.

Förster, A. (1865). Die Missbildungen des Menschen systematisch Dangest ellt, 2nd edn. Mauke, Jena.

Gloor, H. and Schinz, H. R. (1950). Kurze Einführung in die allgemeine Missbildungslehre. *Dtsch. Med. Wschr.* **75**, 911–18.

Gluecksohn-Schoenheimer, S. and Dunn, L. C. (1945). Sirens aprosopi and intestinal abnormalities in the house mouse. *Anat. Rec.* **92**, 201–13.

Hartmann, Ph. J. (1691). Anatome monstri. *Ephem. Acad. Nature Curios. Decuria II, Annus X. Observ.* 162.

Hendry, H. W. and Kohler, H. G. (1956). Sirenomelia ('Mermaid'). *J. Obstet. Gynaecol. Br. Emp.* **63**, 865–70.

Hornbeek, F. K. (1970). A gene producing symmelia in the mouse. *Teratology* **3**, 7–10.

—— and Schreiner, C. (1973). Abnormal segregation and sex ratio and reduced litter size associated with siren phenotype in mice. *Teratology* **7**, 195–8.

Jensen, P. K. A. and Hansen, P. (1981). A bisatellited marker chromosome in an infant with the caudal regression anomalad. *Clin. Genet.* **19**, 126–9.

Kohler, H. G. (1972). An unusual case of sirenomelia. *Teratology* **6**, 295–301.

Malkasian, G. D. Jr., Sayre, G. P. and Titus, J. L. (1969). Sympus apus. *Obstet. Gynecol.* **33**, 715–20.

Passarge, E. and Lenz, W. (1966). Syndrome of caudal regression in infants of diabetic mothers: observations of further cases. *Pediatrics* **37**, 672–5.

—— and Sutherland, J. M. (1965). Potter's syndrome. *Am. J. Dis. Child.* **109**, 80–4.

Sisk, C. J., Hodes, M. E. and Weaver, D. W. (1978). Microcephaly and the caudal regression anomalad. In *Annual review of birth defects, 1977, Part B, Recent advances and new syndromes*, eds. Summitt, R. L. and Bergsma, D. *Birth Defects Orig. Art. Series* **14** (6B), pp. 379–80.

Smith, D. W., Bartlett, C. and Harrah, L. M. (1976). Monozygotic twinning and the Duhamel anomalad (imperforate anus to sirenomelia): a non-random association between two aberrations in morphogenesis. *Birth Defects Orig. Art. Series* **12**, 53–63.

Stevenson, A. C., Johnston, H. A., Golding, D. R. and Stewart, M. I. P. (1966). Congenital malformations. A report of the study of a series of consecutive births in 24 centres. *Bull. WHO* **34** (Suppl.) 1–127.

Stewart, J. M. and Stoll, S. (1979). Familial caudal regression anomalad and maternal diabetes. *J. Med. Genet.* **16**, 17–20.

Sun, C.-C. J., Raffel, L. J., Wright, L. L. and Mergner, W. J. (1986). Immature renal tissue in colonic wall of a patient with cardial regression syndrome. *Arch. Path. Lab. Med.* **110**, 653–5.

Von Lennep, E., El Khazen, N., de Pierreux, G., Amy, J. J., Rodesch, F. and van Regemorter, N. (1985). A case of partial sirenomelia and possible vitamin A teratogenesis. *Prenatal Diagnosis* **5**, 35–40.

Wolff, E. (1936). Les bases de la tératogénese expérimentale des vertebrés amniotes, d'apres les resultats de methodes directes. *Arch. Anat. (Strasb.)* **22**, 1–375.

—— (1948). *La science des monstres.* Gallimand, Paris.

10.1.2. Fused kidneys

Fusion of the two kidneys at one or other pole, horseshoe kidney, is a well-recognized renal malformation. Estimates of its incidence vary from about 1 in 400 to 1 in 1000. Walters and Priestley (1932) give an incidence of 1 in 1000; Bell (1950), in a large post-mortem series, 1 in 500; and Glenn (1959) 1 in 400. In the great majority of cases it is the lower poles which fuse, but rarely the upper poles fuse to give an inverted horseshoe or there is total fusion. Symptoms, when present, are usually related either to hypertension or to obstruction of the ureters as they cross the bridge of renal tissue. A common association of fused kidney is multiple and anomalous renal arteries (Robertson *et al.* 1967). Males predominate over females, as for example in Dajani's (1966) series of 29 cases with 24 males to five females. Reference has already been made in Chapter 3 to the frequent occurrence of horseshoe kidney in Turner's syndrome, and instances of Turner's syndrome are likely to be found among female cases in any large series, as for example a single case in Dajani's series and three in Boatman and colleagues' (1972) consecutive series. They found that other congenital malformations were also frequently present. They observed 51 anomalies in 32 patients, one-third of their total series of 96. These included, in addition to the Turner's syndrome cases, 16 other urogenital anomalies, 11 musculo-skeletal defects, 10 cardiovascular and 7 neural tube defects including three meningomyeloceles, five gastrointestinal anomalies, and two cases of trisomy 18.

In the great majority of cases there is no family history of fused kidneys. However, it must be remembered that without extensive family investigation symptomless renal fusion in close relatives would not be recognized. Bridge (1960) recorded monozygotic twins, one with horseshoe kidney and the other with a crossed ectopic kidney, suggesting that ectopia is of similar pathogenesis to fused kidney. Discordance for horseshoe kidney in monozygotic twins has been reported by Leiter (1972) and Kalra and coworkers (1985). Robertson (1968) studied 100 relatives of a patient with a horseshoe kidney. There were no further cases of fused kidney identified, even among seven relatives found to be hypertensive and subjected to renal angiography. However, 18 relatives were also hypertensive, and all but one of those who underwent angiography had renal arterial anomalies. Perlman and colleagues (1976) described a family in which a woman had a right double kidney, her daughter had left agenesis and her son a horseshoe kidney. George (1981) described a family in which a father had polycystic kidneys leading to renal failure. One son had a horseshoe kidney, and another son had loin pain and microscopic haematuria with no cysts seen on a renal biopsy.

The only report of the familial occurrence of horseshoe kidney, without associated duplication defects and not forming part of a multiple malformation syndrome, found in the literature is that of David (1974). He reported a boy and his two sisters, one of whom also had a meningomyelocoele, all with horseshoe kidney. The mother had malrotation of her left kidney but no fusion. Horseshoe kidney, with renal cysts and hydronephrosis, has also been reported in sporadic myelomeningocoele (Cameron 1956). On the basis of these few reports it would appear that genetic factors probably do not play a major role in the aetiology of fused kidneys. A final verdict on this must await a careful family study using ultrasound to investigate all close relatives.

There is at least one dysmorphic syndrome, facio-cardio-renal syndrome, in which horseshoe kidneys are a regular feature. A single family has been reported in which two brothers and a sister with severe mental subnormality had a characteristic facial appearance of large chin, open mouth and broad nasal bridge, cardiac enlargement with conduction defects and endocardial fibroelastosis, and horseshoe kidneys (Eastman and Bixler 1977). Horseshoe kidney and hydronephrosis are occasional autopsy findings in infants with thanatophoric dwarfism. This disorder, which is genetically heterogeneous (Sillence *et al.* 1978), is probably the most commonly met type of lethal skeletal dysplasia of the newborn. Horseshoe kidney has also been reported in the oro-cranial-digital syndrome (Juberg and Hayward 1969), and along with hypospadias and renal cysts in Robert's syndrome (Freeman *et al.* 1974).

Cook and Stephens (1977) have drawn attention to the similar origin of fused and ectopic kidneys. Fused ectopic kidneys may both be on the right or the left with the two ureters both on the same side as the two kidneys. Alternatively one kidney may be served by a contralateral ureter, and when this is the lower kidney the ipsilateral ureter from the upper kidney must cross over it, usually behind it. There are no reported genetic studies of renal ectopia, other than a report of monochorionic diamniotic identical twins concordant for fused ectopic kidneys on the right side of the abdomen (Greenberg and Nelsen 1971).

A single family has been reported in which a father had unilateral renal agenesis and his two sons both had a crossed ectopic kidney. All three also had radial ray aplasia, defining a radial ray alplasia, renal anomaly syndrome (Sofer *et al.* 1983; Meizner *et al.* 1986). The second affected male child was diagnosed prenatally and the pregnancy terminated.

References

Bell, E. T. (1950). *Renal diseases*, 2nd edn. p. 79. Lea & Febiger, Philadelphia.

Boatman, D. L., Kolln, C. P. and Flocks, R. H. (1972). Congenital anomalies associated with horseshoe kidney. *J. Urol.* **107**, 205–7.

Bridge, R. A. C. (1960). Horseshoe kidneys in identical twins. *Br. J. Urol.* **32**, 32–3.

Cameron, A. H. (1956). The spinal cord lesion in spina bifida cystica. *Lancet* **2**, 171–4.

Cook, W. A. and Stephens, F. D. (1977). Fused kidneys: morphologic study and theory of embryogenesis. In *Urinary system malformations in children*, eds. Bergsma, D. and Duckett, J. W. *Birth Defects Orig. Art. Series* **13**(5), 327–40.

Dajani, A. M. (1966). Horseshoe kidney: a review of 29 cases. *Br. J. Urol.* **38**, 388–402.

David, R. S. (1974). Horseshoe kidney: a report of one family. *Br. Med. J.* **4**, 571–2.

Eastman, J. R. and Bixler, D. (1977). Facio-cardio-renal syndrome: a newly delineated recessive disorder. *Clin. Genet.* **11**, 424–30.

Freeman, M. V. R., Williams, D. W., Schimke, R. N., Temtamy, F. A., Vachier, E. and German, J. (1974). *The Robert's syndrome. Clin. Genet.* **5**, 1–16.

Glenn, J. F. (1959). Analysis of 51 patients with horseshoe kidney. *New Engl. J. Med.* **261**, 684–7.

George, C. R. P. (1981). Familial association of polycystic kidneys, horseshoe kidney and loin-pain–haematuria syndrome (letter). *J. R. Soc. Med.* **77**, 77–8.

Greenberg, L. W. and Nelsen, C. E. (1971). Crossed fused ectopia of the kidneys in twins. *Am. J. Dis. Child.* **122**, 175–6.

Juberg, R. C. and Hayward, J. R. (1969). A new familial syndrome of oral, cranial and digital anomalies. *J. Pediatr.* **74**, 755–62.

Kalra, D., Broomhall, J. and Williams, J. (1985). Horseshoe kidney in one of identical twin girls. *J. Urol.* **134**, 113.

Leiter, E. (1972). Horseshoe kidney in monozygotic twins. *J. Urol.* **108**, 683–4.

Meizner, I., Bar-Ziv, J., Bark, Y. and Abeliovich, D. (1986). Prenatal ultrasonic diagnosis of radial-ray aplasia and renal anomalies (acro-renal syndrome). *Prenatal Diagnosis* **6**, 223–5.

Perlman, M., Williams, J. and Ornoy, A. (1976). Familial ureteric bud anomalies. *J. Med. Genet.* **13**, 161–3.

Robertson, P. W. (1968). Horseshoe kidney, renal arterial anomalies, and hypertension: a study of one family. *Br. Med. J.* **2**, 793–7.

——, Hull, D. H., Klidjian, A. and Dyson, M. L. (1967). Renal artery anomalies and hypertension in a study of 340 patients. *Am. Heart J.* **73**, 296–307.

Sillence, D. O., Rimoin, D. L. and Lachman, R. S. (1978). Neonatal dwarfism. *Pediatr. Clin. N. Am.* **25**, 453–83.

Sofer, S., Bar-Ziv, J. and Abeliovich, D. (1983). Radial ray aplasia and renal anomalies in a father and son. A new syndrome. *Am. J. Med. Genet.* **14**, 151–7.

Walters, W. and Priestley, J. B. (1932). Horseshoe kidney—a review of 68 surgical cases. *J. Urol.* **28**, 271–7.

10.1.3. Congenital hydronephrosis

Congenital hydronephrosis may be unilateral or bilateral and may or may not be associated with hydroureter. Bilateral hydronephrosis and hydroureter is generally assumed to be due to lower urinary tract obstruction, which can often but not always be demonstrated. It is usually associated with urethral, or bladder neck, obstruction. Hydronephrosis with hydroureters due to bladder neck obstruction was reported as occurring in two brothers (Finkle *et al.* 1956). Simpson and German (1970) reported familial bladder neck obstruction in sibs in three families, and in two or three generations in two further families. However, Reule and Ansell (1967) observed discordance for hydronephrosis with bladder neck stenosis in a monozygotic twin pair. Urethral stenosis and prune-belly syndrome are discussed later in this chapter.

Similar findings have been reported in a brother and sister with a multiple anomaly syndrome including distal limb hypoplasia, coarse facial features, and severe developmental failure (Rudiger *et al.* 1971). However, two sisters with a similar syndrome lacked the urinary tract anomalies (Fryns *et al.* 1979).

Hydronephrosis without hydroureter, and in the absence of renal stones or inflammatory stenosis of the upper ureter, is thought to be due to pelvi-ureteric obstruction. The cause or causes of such obstruction are still unclear despite many possible mechanisms that have been postulated in earlier studies. Many early workers demonstrated aberrant renal vessels crossing behind the pelvi-ureteric junction, usually an artery to the lower pole of the kidney in a high proportion of their cases. Henline (1935) for example observed such aberrant vessels in 29 out of 66 cases of uretero-pelvic obstruction, and Soley (1946) in seven out of 19 cases in children. Atwell has postulated that pelvi-ureteric junction hydronephrosis is aetiologically related to pelvicalicial duplication, paraureteric diverticula and vesico-ureteral reflux on the basis of increased frequencies of these disorders among the close relatives of patients with paraureteric diverticula (Atwell and Allen 1980) or pelvi-ureteric junction hydronephrosis (Atwell 1985).

Aaron and Robbins (1948), in what was probably the earliest report of the familial occurrence of this type of hydronephrosis, described two brothers with unilateral hydronephrosis without hydroureter. One involved the right and the other the left kidney. In both an aberrant renal artery supplying the lower pole of the affected kidney was seen at operation and assumed to be the cause. Several similar reports followed. Cannon (1954) observed unilateral hydronephrosis in five males in three generations of a single family. Raffle (1955) made a similar observation in four members of a family over two generations, but with apparent skipping of the parent of the youngest. At least one of his patients had an aberrant vessel. Jewell and Buchert (1962) described four definite and one possible further case in three or four generations of a family. Two of these patients had aberrant vessels, but another had a kinked pelvi-uretic junction. Martin and Goodwin (1968) also observed familial hydronephrosis; however, in their family this was unilateral in two cousins but bilateral in the brother of one of them. The latter patient had an aberrant renal artery on one side only. Lenz (1968) observed familial hydronephrosis without hydroureter in association with duplication of the collecting system.

Simpson and German (1970) reported seven families with multiple urinary tract anomalies, mostly obstructive uropathy, of which one involved pelvi-ureteric obstruction in three sibs and their grandmother. Grosse and colleagues (1973) described a family with bilateral hydronephrosis in a mother and her two sons. One son had a horseshoe kidney without any obvious cause for pelvi-ureteric obstruction. The mother and her other son had fibrous bands at the pelvi-ureteric junction that may have been either primary or secondary to local inflammation. Grosse and colleagues question the usual assumption that aberrant renal arteries when present are a cause of obstruction.

Grosse's view receives support from the study of Antonakopoulos and associates (1985) who demonstrated by light microscopy the presence of an abnormal muscle arrangement at the pelvi-ureteric junction in 18 out of 26 cases with pelvi-ureteric obstruction hydronephrosis. The muscle bundles were arranged into an outer circular and inner longitudinal layer instead of in the usual interwoven pattern present in all 17 of their control cases. They made no reference to whether or not any of their cases were familial so no conclusions can be drawn in that respect.

The few familial reports discussed above may represent a rare form of congenital hydronephrosis due to one or more single genes with dominant inheritance of one or more primary mechanisms of pelvi-ureteric obstruction, but they provide insuffient evidence to establish any case for this.

There has been a single report of ultrasound prenatal diagnosis of congenital hydronephrosis (McCormack *et al.* 1981, 1982), and one report of failure to detect hydronephrosis when present (Wlalimiroff *et al.* 1985).

Congenital hydronephrosis has been reported in a wide variety of malformation syndromes, some of which have been mentioned in earlier sections. It has also been reported as an occasional finding in several other syndromes. The Johanson–Blizzard syndrome consists of hypoplasia of the alae nasae, congenital deafness, hypothyroidism, growth retardation, malabsorption associated with pancreatic achylia, absent permanent teeth, midline scalp defects, and mental retardation (Johanson and Blizzard 1971; Park *et al.* 1972). This group studied three patients all of whom had genital anomalies and hydronephrosis or caliectasis. Two patients had an imperforate anus. Inheritance is autosomal recessive (Mardini *et al.* 1978; Schussheim *et al.* 1976; Day and Israel 1978). Uretero-pelvic junction obstruction has been reported in the Russel–Silver syndrome (Haslam *et al.* 1973). Hydronephrosis and hydroureter may occur in the syndrome of congenital lipodystrophic diabetes with acanthosis nigricans (Reed *et al.* 1965), and hydronephrosis and polycystic kidney in the ectromelia–ichthyosis syndrome (Cullen *et al.* 1969). Apparent autosomal dominant inheritance of hydronephrosis and hydroureter with urethral valves, and a peculiar facial expression with inappropriate smiling and crying, occurs in the Ochoa syndrome (Elejalde 1979). This combination was seen in seven children from three unrelated families. Three affected males were also cryptorchid. Urogenital anomalies, including hydronephrosis and hydroureter due to urethral atresia, also form part of the syndrome of spondylocostal dysostosis with anal atresia and urogenital anomalies (Casamassina *et al.* 1981). These authors described this syndrome in two brothers in an inbred Mennonite family. The karyotype was normal. This is presumably an autosomal recessive disorder.

Either hydronephrosis and hydroureter due to urethral atresia, or ureteric stenosis with cystic renal dysplasia, have been described in the sporadic syndrome of female hermaphroditism with anorectal, müllerian duct and urinary tract malformations (Wenstrup and Pagon 1985). These authors described four infants all of whom had imperforate anus, a phallus with or without a urethral meatus, uterine and vaginal abnormalities, and normal ovaries as well as the urinary tract anomalies.

Hydronephrosis and hydroureter were present in a brother and sister with a complex syndrome of midface retraction (Schinzel and Giedion 1978). The other features of this syndrome include severe midface retraction with a saddle nose with short bridge, upturned tip of nose, and choanal atresia; prominent forehead and wide cranial sutures and fontanelles, hypertrichosis, congenital heart defect, moderate mesomelic limb shortening and hypoplasia of middle and terminal phalanges, and genital anomalies. There is physical and mental retardation. Seizures with abnormal electroencephalographic records and recurrent apnoeic episodes are common. There is also delayed dental eruption. Donnai and Harris (1979) reported a case of Schinzel–Giedion syndrome with most of the above features but without hydronephrosis. However, other patients with the syndrome have been described with hydronephrosis. Inheritance is probably autosomal recessive. There has been a single case report of a left hydronephrosis with a normal micturating cystourethrogram in a boy with cerebral gigantism, or Sotos syndrome (Adam *et al.* 1986). Unilateral hydronephrosis has been reported on two occasions in patients with autosomal recessive Warburg (HARD±E) syndrome of hydrocephalus, agyria, retinal dysplasia with or without encephalocele (Yanoff *et al.* 1978; Attia *et al.* 1986). Attia and colleagues' patient also had contralateral foci of renal dysplasia.

References

Aaron, G. and Robbins, M. A. (1948). Hydronephrosis due to aberrant vessels: remarkable familial incidence with report of cases. *J. Urol.* **60**, 702–5.

Adam, K. A. R., Frayh, A. R. S. A., Sharma, A. and Taha, S. A. (1986). Cerebral gigantism with hydronephrosis: a case report. *Clin. Genet.* **29**, 178–80.

Antonakopoulos, G. N., Fuggle, W. J., Newman, J., Considine, J. and O'Brien, J. M. (1985). Idiopathic hydronephrosis: light microscopic features and pathogenesis. *Arch. Pathol. Lab. Med.* **109**, 1097–101.

Attia, M. F. D., Burn, J., McCarthy, J. H., Purohit, D. P. and Milligan, D. W. A. (1986). Warburg (HARD±E) syndrome without retinal dysplasia: case report and review. *Br. J. Ophthalmol.* **70**, 742–7.

Atwell, J. D. (1985). Familial pelviureteric junction hydronephrosis and its association with a duplex pelvicaliceal system and vesicoureteric reflux. A family study. *Br. J. Urol.* **57**, 365–9.

—— and Allen, N. H. (1980). The interrelationship between paraureteric diverticula, vesicoureteral reflux and duplication of the pelvicalicial collecting system: a family study. *Br. J. Urol.* **52**, 269–73.

Cannon, J. F. (1954). Hereditary unilateral hydronephrosis. *Ann. Intern. Med.* **41**, 1054–60.

Casamassima, A. C., Morton, C. C., Nance, W. E., Kodroff, M., Caldwell, R., Kelly, T. and Wolf, B. (1981). Spondylocostal dysostosis associated with anal and urogenital anomalies in a Mennonite sibship. *Am. J. Med. Genet.* **8**, 117–27.

Cullen, S. I., Harris, D. E., Carter, C. H. and Reed, W. B. (1969). Congenital unilateral ichthyosiform erythroderma. *Arch. Dermatol.* **99**, 724–29.

Day, D. W. and Israel, J. N. (1978). Johanson–Blizzard syndrome. *Birth Defects Orig. Art. Series* **14**(6B), 275–87.

Donnai, D. and Harris, R. (1979). A further case of a new syndrome including midface retraction, hypertrichosis, and skeletal anomalies. *J. Med. Genet.* **16**, 483–6.

Elejalde, B. R. (1979). Genetic and diagnostic considerations in three families with abnormalities of facial expression and congenital urinary obstruction: 'The Ochoa Syndrome'. *Am. J. Med. Genet.* **3**, 97–108.

Finkle, A. L., McPhee, V. C. and Van der Reis, L. (1956). Congenital bladder neck obstruction in male siblings. *Calif. Med.* **85**, 260–4.

Fryns, J. P., Moerman, F., Goddeeris, P., Bossuyt, C. and Van der Berghe, H. (1979). A new lethal syndrome with cloudy corneae, diaphragmatic defects and distal limb deformities. *Hum. Genet.* **50**, 65–70.

Grosse, F. R., Kaveggia, L. and Opitz, J. M. (1973). Familial hydronephrosis. *Z. Kinderheilk.* **114**, 313–22.

Haslam, R. H. A., Berman, W. and Heller, R. M. (1973). Renal abnormalities in the Russel–Silver syndrome. *Pediatrics* **51**, 216–22.

Henline, R. B. (1935). The causes and treatment of non calculous ureteropelvic obstruction. *J. Urol.* **34**, 584–607.

Jewell, J. H. and Buchert, W. I. (1962). Unilateral hereditary hydronephrosis: a report of four cases in three successive generations. *J. Urol.* **88**, 129–36.

Johanson, A. and Blizzard, R. (1971). A syndrome of congenital aplasia of the alae nasi, deafness, hypothyroidism, dwarfism, absent permanent teeth and malabsorption. *J. Pediatr.* **79**, 982–7.

Lenz, W. (1968). Harnorgane. In *Kurzes Handbüch in fünf Banden*. Vol. 3, (ed. P. E. Becker), pp. 253–87. G. Thieme-Verlag, Stuttgart.

McCormack, M. K. (1982). Prenatal detection of the autosomal dominant type of congenital hydronephrosis by ultrasonography. *Prenatal Diagnosis* **2**, 157–61.

——, D'Aguillo, A. and Scully, J. (1981). Autosomal dominant congenital hydronephrosis (CH): prenatal diagnosis of ultrasound (abs.). *Am. J. Med. Genet.* **33**, 85A.

Mardini, M. K., Ghandour, M., Sakati, N. A. and Nyhan, W. L. (1978). Johanson-Blizzard syndrome in a large inbred kindred with three involved members. *Clin. Genet.* **14**, 247–50.

Martin, D. C. and Goodwin, W. E. (1968). Hereditary and familial aspects of some common urologic problems. *Urology Digest* **7**, 11–17.

Park, I. J., Johanson, A., Jones, H. W. and Blizzard, R. (1972). Special female hermaphroditism associated with multiple disorders. *Obstet. Gynecol.* **39**, 100–6.

Raffle, R. B. (1955). Familial hydronephrosis. *Br. Med. J.* **1**, 580–2.

Reed, W. B., Dexter, R., Corley, C. and Fish, C. (1965). Congenital lipodystrophic diabetes with acanthosis nigricans. *Arch. Dermatol.* **91**, 326–34.

Reule, G. R. and Ansell, J. S. (1967). Discordant occurrence of genito-urinary defects in monozygotic twins. *J. Urol.* **97**, 1078–81.

Rudiger, R. A., Schmidt, W., Loose, D. A. and Passarge, E. (1971). Severe developmental failure with coarse facial features, distal limb hypoplasia, thickened palmar creases, bifid uvula, and ureteral stenosis: a previously unidentified familial disorder with lethal outcome. *J. Pediatr.* **79**, 977–87.

Schinzel, A. and Giedion, A. (1978). A syndrome of severe midface retraction, multiple skull anomalies, clubfeet and cardiac and renal malformations in sibs. *Am. J. Med. Genet.* **1**, 361–75.

Schussheim, A., Choi, S. J. and Silverberg, M. (1976). Exocrine pancreatic insufficiency with congenital anomalies. *J. Pediatr.* **89**, 782–4.

Simpson, J. L. and German, J. (1970). Familial urinary tract anomalies (letter). *JAMA* **212**, 2264–5.

Soley, P. J. (1946). Ureteropelvic obstruction in children. Incidence and etiology. *J. Urol.* **55**, 46–51.

Wenstrup, R. J. and Pagon, R. A. (1985). Female pseudohermaphroditism with anorectal, Müllerian duct, and urinary tract malformations: report of four cases. *J. Pediatr.* **107**, 751–4.

Wladimiroff, J. W., Beemer, F. A., Scholtmeyer, R. J., Stewart, P. A., Spritzer, R. and Wolff, E. D. (1985). Failure to detect fetal obstructive uropathy by second trimester ultrasound. *Prenatal Diagnosis* **5**, 41–6.

Yanoff, M., Rorke, L. B. and Allman, M. I. (1978). Bilateral optic system aplasia with relatively normal eyes. *Arch. Ophthalmol.* **96**, 97–101.

10.2. URETER AND BLADDER

10.2.1. Megacystis, megaloureter, and double ureter

The association of megacystis with megaduodenum or intestinal pseudo-obstruction was first described by Law and Ten Eyck (1962) in a family in which they observed nine affected individuals, including male-to-male transmission. Megacystis, with non-obstructive vesico-ureteral reflux, was also reported in another family suggestive of autosomal dominant inheritance, but without mention of megaduodenum (Tobenkin 1964). Subsequent reports have confirmed the association of megacystis and megaduodenum in a syndrome with autosomal dominant inheritance (Newton 1968; Schuffler and Pope 1977; Faulk *et al.* 1978). Both Schuffler and Pope, and Faulk and colleagues described a visceral myopathy as the pathogenesis of this disorder. Intestinal pseudo-obstruction may occur as a complication of progressive systemic sclerosis or other diseases affecting the gut, or as a visceral neuropathy unassociated with megacystis or vesico-ureteral reflux, as well as with visceral myopathy (Anuras *et al.* 1981; Schuffler *et al.* 1981). The megacystis–microcolon–intestinal hypoperistalsis syndrome is a distinct sporadic disorder not associated with urinary tract abnormality (Krook 1980).

One of the earliest observations of the familial occurrence of hydro-nephrosis with megaloureters was that of Mackay (1945). He described three affected sibs with a suggestive history in earlier generations.

Whether or not this anomaly is distinct from hydronephrosis and hydroureter secondary to lower urinary tract obstruction is open to question.

Ureterocoele has been reported as occurring in identical twins (Riba 1936).

Duplication of the collecting system was also present in one family with congenital hydronephrosis discussed above (Lenz 1968). Earlier reports of the familial occurrence of double collecting systems include those of Ritter (1935), Frissel (1942), Rossle (1942), Girsh and Karpinski (1956), Burkland (1958), and Dietel (1964). Girsh and Karpinski reported a mother and her two daughters all with unilateral incomplete double ureter, pelvis, and kidney. Simpson and German (1970) include a family in which two sisters had duplication of a kidney and ureter. Atwell and colleagues (1974) argue from the family reported by them for autosomal dominant inheritance of duplication defects. The lack of specificity of ureteric bud anomalies is born out by the family reported by Perlman and others (1976). A mother had a right double kidney and collecting system, her daughter a left renal agenesis, and her son a horseshoe kidney. Duplication defects may even involve the bladder as in the patient reported by Ramsay (1984) who in addition to bilateral duplex kidneys and ureters also had a septum separating anterior and posterior bladder cavities. They may also be associated with uterine malformation, as in identical twins concordant for uterus didelphys and bilateral duplex kidneys and ureters (Daw and Toon 1985). As with the malformations already discussed, this small number of reports of familial occurrence of duplication defects of the urinary system does not provide sufficient evidence to establish a case for a monogenic determination of even a minority of cases, or even a strong case for polygenic determination.

However, multiple congenital anomaly syndromes including urinary tract duplication present a different story. Nillson (1960) reported a family with multiple ureteric bud anomalies associated with Fanconi's anaemia. This may of course have been a coincidental association as there have been no subsequent similar reports. Fraser and associates (1983) have described two families with a syndrome comprising bilateral sensorineural hearing loss, preauricular pits or tags or ear malformation, and either unilateral or bilateral urinary tract duplication. These abnormalities were present in at least three individuals in two generations in the first family, and at least six individuals in three generations in the second family. The parents of one affected girl, whose mother was also affected, were second cousins, and there is at least one unequivocal example of an affected father and son in this family. If sensorineural hearing loss alone is accepted as indicative of the disorder then there is

)ne further example of male-to-male transmission, and one of non-
)enetrance in a mother, in this family. These two families appear to have
a distinct disorder from branchio-oto-renal (BOR) syndrome in which
here is renal hypoplasia. The authors suggest the name branchio-oto-
ureteral (BOU) syndrome. The pattern of transmission suggests auto-
,omal dominant inheritance. A curious association of inguinal hernia (17
)ut of 229 male patients) and genito-urinary tract anomalies, including
duplex kidney (12 out of 282 patients), with Perthe's disease has been
eported. There was a smaller increase, about 2 per cent, in genito-
urinary anomalies among parents of the index cases, with a duplication
defect in three out of 11 parents with urinary tract abnormalities
Catterall *et al.* 1971). There is no evidence that this association is geneti-
ally determined.

References

\nuras, S., Shaw, A. and Christensen, J. (1981). The familial syndromes of
intestinal pseudoobstruction. *Am. J. Hum. Genet.* **33**, 584–91.

\twell, J. D., Cook, P. L., Howell, C. J., Hyde, I. and Parker, B. C. (1974).
Familial incidence of bifid and double ureters. *Arch. Dis. Childh.* **49**, 390–3.

3urkland, C. E. (1958). The significance of genetic and environmental factors in
urogenital disease. *J. Urol.* **79**, 532–48.

Catterall, A., Lloyd Roberts, G. C. and Wynn-Davies, R. (1971). Association of
Perthe's disease with congenital anomalies of genitourinary tract and inguinal
region. *Lancet* **1**, 996–7.

)aw, E. and Toon, P. (1985). Identical twins with uterus didelphys and duplex
kidneys. *Postgrad. Med. J.* **61**, 269–70.

)ietel, H. (1964). Cited in Lenz, W. (1964). *Humangenetik*, Vol. 3, part 1, ed.
Becker, B. E. Georg Thieme, Stuttgart.

'aulk, D. L., Anuras, S., Gardner, G. D., Mitros, F. A., Summers, R. W. and
Christensen, J. (1978). A familial visceral myopathy. *Ann. Intern. Med.* **89**,
600–6.

'raser, F. C., Ayme, S., Halal, F. and Sproule, J. (1983). Autosomal dominant
duplication of the renal collecting system, hearing loss, and external ear
anomalies: a new syndrome. *Am. J. Med. Genet.* **14**, 473–8.

'rissel, E. (1942). Missbildungen der harnwege mit familiaren auftreten von
doppelureter bei kindern. *Acta Paediatr. Scand.* **29**, 418–32.

3irsh, L. S. and Karpinski, F. E. (1956). Urinary-tract malformations: their
familial occurrence with special reference to double pelvis and double kidney.
New Engl. J. Med. **254**, 854–5.

Krook, P. M. (1980). Megacystis–microcolon–intestinal hypoperistalsis syndrome
in a male infant. *Radiol.* **136**, 649–50.

_aw, D. H. and Ten Eyck, E. A. (1962). Familial megaduodenum and megacystis.
Am. J. Med. **33**, 911–22.

_enz, W. (1968). Harnorgane, In *Ein Kurzes Handbuch in Fünf Banden*, Vol. 3.
ed. Becker, P. E. pp. 253–87. Georg Thieme-Verlag, Stuttgart.

MacKay, H. (1945). Congenital bilateral megaloureters with hydronephrosis. A remarkable family history. *Proc. Roy. Soc. Med.* **38**, 567–68.

Newton, W. T. (1968). Radical enterectomy for hereditary megaduodenum. *Arch Surg.* **96**, 549–53.

Nillson, L. R. (1960). Chronic pancytopenia with multiple congenital anomalies (Fanconi's anaemia). *Acta Paediatr. Scand.* **49**, 518–29.

Perlman, M., Williams, J. and Ornoy, A. (1976). Familial ureteric bud anomalies *J. Med. Genet.* **13**, 161–3.

Ramsay, J. W. A. (1984). Multiple congenital defects of the urinary tract. *J. R Soc. Med.* **77**, 889–91.

Riba, L. B. (1936). Ureterocele: with case reports of bilateral ureterocele in identical twins. *Br. J. Urol.* **8**, 119–31.

Ritter, A. (1935). Veverbung von Ureter und Nierenbecken-anomalien und ihre klinische Bedeutung. *Helv. Med. Acta* **2**, 169–73.

Rossle, R. (1942). Weitere Beobachtungen uber Sektionsbefunde bei Blutsver wandten. *Arch. f. Pathol. Anat.* **308**, 495–507.

Schuffler, M. D. and Pope, C. III. (1977). Studies of idiopathic intestinal pseudoobstruction. II. Hereditary hollow visceral myopathy: family studies *Gastroenterology* **73**, 339–44.

——, Rohrmann, C. A., Chaffee, R. G., Brand, D. L., Delaney, J. H. and Young J. H. (1981). Chronic intestinal pseudoobstruction: a report of 27 cases and review of the literature. *Medicine* **60**, 173–96.

Simpson, J. L. and German, J. (1970). Familial urinary tract anomalies (letter) *JAMA* **212**, 2264–5.

Tobenkin, M. I. (1964). Hereditary vesicoureteral reflux. *Sth. Med. J.* **57**, 139–47.

10.2.2. The exstrophy–epispadias complex and other vesical anomalies

Exstrophy and agenesis of the bladder, bladder diverticula, and bladder malformations are all rare anomalies of mostly sporadic occurrence.

Agenesis of the bladder has been estimated to have a birth incidenc of 1 in 600 000 (Glenn 1959). Raafat and associates (1982) hav reported a small cluster of three cases occurring within a 4-month perio in east London, all associated with hydrops and death *in utero*. There do not seem to have been any reports of familial cases.

Bladder diverticula are usually asymptomatic. They may be secondar to obstruction of the bladder outlet, or occur as part of multiple anomal syndromes. They have for example been described in patients wit Menkes' syndrome (Harcke *et al.* 1977), Williams syndrome (Babbitt *et al.* 1979) in which renal artery stenosis (Chantler *et al.* 1966) an nephrocalcinosis (Burn 1986) have also been reported, Ehlers–Danlo syndrome or cutus laxa (Goltz and Hult 1965; Agha *et al.* 1978), prune belly syndrome (Duckett 1976) and the Patterson pseudoleprechaunis syndrome (Patterson and Watkins 1962; Patterson 1969; McKusic

1972; David *et al.* 1981). Many are of idiopathic origin. There appears to be only a single case report of familial occurrence, associated with bladder outlet obstruction, involving a 47-year-old man, his brothers with a son of one of them, their father, and probably their grandfather (Hofmann *et al.* 1984). No females were affected or transmitted the defect in their family. The authors propose autosomal dominant inheritance with sex limitation to the male. Congenital urethral diverticula are rare. A single case report describes an anterior urethral diverticulum associated with bilateral urinomas and dysplastic kidneys (Sirota *et al.* 1986).

A variety of urogenital defects are associated with a lower abdominal wall midline defect in what is termed the exstrophy–epispadias complex. In its mildest form this results in epispadias, and in more severe forms partial or complete bladder exstrophy. In the most severe form there is a cloacal exstrophy. Bladder exstrophy has a live-birth incidence of about 1 in 10 000 to 1 in 40 000 (Rickham 1961; Leck *et al.* 1968), with the higher figures being more likely.

Several authors have published series of cases in which there have been a few instances of familial occurrence. In one of the earliest such studies Uson and coworkers (1959) observed concordance in male monozygotic twins. Reule and Ansell (1967) reported a discordant monozygotic twin pair. Higgins (1962) reported a series of 138 cases and observed two affected sib and two twin pairs. Two affected brothers were noted in a series of 80 cases (Williams and Savage 1966). Chisholm and McParland (1979) noted two affected sib pairs among 137 cases, and also found a normal chromosome constitution in 35 of their patients. However, in a family study involving 102 index patients with bladder or cloacal extrophy Ives and colleagues (1980) found no recurrence among 162 sibs. They suggest that the recurrence risk for sibs is less than 1 per cent. A more recent family study (Shapiro *et al.* 1984) found exstrophy and/or epispadias in three out of 215 children of index patients, in all of five male monozygotic cotwins but only one of three female monozygotic cotwins. Five dizygotic twin pairs were discordant. Data on sibs were not obtained. This study may have overrepresented affected relatives, having been based on a questionnaire sent to 92 paediatric urologists combined with a literature review. It does suggest that the risk for male relatives is higher than for females. Despite the slightly higher risk for children reported by Shapiro and colleagues it would still seem reasonable to use a 1 per cent sib or child risk for genetic counselling purposes.

Prenatal diagnosis by ultrasound should be feasible (Campbell and Pearce 1983), and maternal serum or amniotic fluid α-fetoprotein was found to be raised in a case of exstrophy of the cloaca (Gosden and Brock 1981).

Exstrophy may also occur as part of a wider malformation complex involving exomphalos, imperforate anus, and spinal defects (OEIS complex) (Carey *et al.* 1978), or in association with renal agenesis or hypoplasia in the syndrome of gross body wall defect with limb reduction anomalies (Pagon *et al.* 1979).

Gundrum (1922) described familial bladder atony involving eight males and one female in three generations of a family, with apparent autosomal dominant inheritance.

References

Agha, A., Sakati, N. O., Higginbottom, M. C., Jones, K. L., Bay, C. and Nyhan, W. L. (1978). Two forms of cutis laxa presenting in the newborn period. *Acta Paediatr. Scand.* **67**, 775–80.

Babbit, D. P., Dobbs, J. and Baedecker, R. A. (1979). Multiple bladder diverticula in Williams 'Elfin-Facies' syndrome. *Pediatr. Radiol.* **8**, 29–31.

Burn, J. (1986). Williams syndrome. *J. Med. Genet.* **23**, 389–95.

Campbell, S. and Pearce, J. M. (1983). The prenatal diagnosis of fetal structural anomalies by ultrasound. *Clin. Obstet. Gynaecol.* **10**, 475–506.

Carey, J. C., Greenbaum, B. and Hall, B. D. (1978). The OEIS complex (omphalocele, exstrophy, imperforate anus spinal defects). *Birth Defects Orig. Art. Series* **14** (6B), 253–63.

Chantler, C., Davies, D. H. and Joseph, M. C. (1966). Cardiovascular and other associations of infantile hyperglycaemia. *Guy's Hosp. Rep.* **115**, 221–41.

Chisholm, T. C. and McParland, F. A. (1979). In *Pediatric surgery*, 3rd end., vol. 2. eds. Ravitch, M. M., Welch, K. J., Benson, C. D., Aberdeen, O. and Randolph J. G. p. 1239. Year Book Medical Publishers, Chicago.

David, T. J., Webb, B. W. and Gordon, I. R. S. (1981). The Patterson syndrome, leprechaunism and pseudoleprechaunism. *J. Med. Genet.* **18**, 294–8.

Duckett, J. W. (1976). The prune-belly syndrome. Chapter 16 in *Clinical pediatric urology*, eds. Kelais, P. P., King, L. R. and Belman, A. B. pp. 615–35. W.B. Saunders, Philadelphia.

Glenn, J. F. (1959). Agenesis of the bladder. *JAMA* **169**, 2016–17.

Goltz, R. W. and Hult, A. M. (1965). Generalized elastolysis (cutis laxa) and Ehlers–Danlos syndrome (cutis hyperelastica): a comparative clinical and laboratorial study. *S. Med. J.* **58**, 848–54.

Gosden, C. and Brock, D. J. H. (1981). The prenatal diagnosis of exstrophy of the cloaca. *Am. J. Med. Genet.* **8**, 95–109.

Gundrum, F. F. (1922). Familial bladder atony. *JAMA* **78**, 411–12.

Harcke, H. T., Capitanio, M. A., Grover, W. D. and Valdes-Dapena, M. (1977). Bladder diverticula and Menkes' syndrome. *Radiology* **124**, 459–61.

Higgins, C. C. (1962). Exstrophy of the bladder: report of 158 cases. *Am. Surg.* **28**, 99–102.

Hofmann, R., Hegemann, M., Mauermayer, W. and Endres, M. (1984). Hereditary autosomal dominant form of bladder diverticula in male patients. *J. Urol.* **131**, 338–9.

Ives, E., Coffey, R. and Carter, C. O. (1980). A family study of bladder exstrophy. *J. Med. Genet.* **17**, 139–41.

Leck, I., Record, R. G., McKeown, T. and Edwards, J. H. (1968). The incidence of malformations in Birmingham, England 1950–1959. *Teratology* **1**, 263–80.

McKusick, V. A. (1972). Patterson's leprechaunoid syndrome. In *Heritable disorders of connective tissue,* 4th edn. pp. 376–7. C. V. Mosby, St. Louis.

Pagon, R. A., Stephens, T. D., McGillivray, B. C., Siebert, J. R., Wright, V. J., Hsu, L. L., Poland, B. J., Emanuel, I. and Hall, J. G. (1979). Body wall defects with reduction limb anomalies: a report of fifteen cases. *Birth Defects Orig. Art. Series.* **15** (5A), 171–85.

Patterson, J. H. (1969). Presentation of a patient with leprechaunism. The clinical delineation of birth defects. IV. Skeletal dysplasias. *Birth Defects Orig. Art. Series.* **5**(4), 117–21.

—— and Watkins, W. L. (1962). Lephrechaunism in a male infant. *J. Pediatr.* **60**, 730–9.

Raafat, F., Butler, L. J. and Mahoney, M. (1982). Cluster of uncommon fetal abnormalities. *Lancet* **2**, 270.

Reule, G. R. and Ansell, J. S. (1967). Discordant occurrence of genitourinary defects in monozygotic twins. *J. Urol.* **97**, 1078–81.

Rickham, P. P. (1961). The incidence and treatment of ectopia vesicae. *Proc. R. Soc. Med.* **54**, 389–92.

Shapiro, E., Lepor, H. and Jeffs, R. D. (1984). The inheritance of the exstrophy-epispadias complex. *J. Urol.* **132**, 308–10.

Sirota, L., Katz, R., Samuel, N. Bar-Ziv, J. and Dulitzky, F. (1986). Congenital anterior urethral diverticulum associated with bilateral urinomas and dysplastic kidneys. *Helv. Paediatr.* **41**, 353–7.

Uson, A. C., Lattimer, J. K. and Melicow, M. M. (1959). Types of exstrophy of urinary bladder and concomitant malformations. A report based on 82 cases. *Pediatrics* **23**, 927–33.

Williams, D. I. and Savage, J. (1966). Reconstruction of the exstrophied bladder. *Br. J. Surg.* **53**, 169–73.

10.2.3. Prune-belly syndrome

This syndrome, which has an incidence in Caucasian populations of about 1 in 30 000 live births (Baird and MacDonald 1981), is characterized by an absence or hypoplasia of the anterior abdominal wall musculature producing a thin protruding abdominal wall through which the intestinal pattern, and sometimes a distended bladder, are visible. The frequently wrinkled appearance of this thin abdominal wall in the infant led William Osler (1901) to name the defect 'prune-belly' syndrome. In addition there are usually urinary tract anomalies of greatly varying severity, commonly associated with urethral obstruction in the more severe cases, and cryptorchidism. The vast majority of cases are male (Williams and Burkholder 1967) and in the rare femal occurrences the urinary tract anomalies are nearly always mild. The three main features of abdominal wall defect, urinary tract anomaly, and cryptor-chidism have led to the alternative name of 'triad syndrome'. A variety of associated malformation have been reported of which the most common are club feet, hip dysplasia, and pulmonary hypoplasia (Geary *et al.* 1986). Others include microcephaly, gastroschisis or omphalocoele, congenital heart defects, and imperforate anus. Urinary tract anomalies vary from mild vesico-ureteral reflux without anatomical abnormality, through combined hydronephrosis, hydroureter, and megacystis with posterior urethral valves to lethal bilateral renal dysplasia (Pagon *et al.* 1979). The morphological defects and the embryopathogenesis of prune-belly syndrome have recently been reviewed by Stephens (1983). A curious case of unilateral prune belly triad was described by Texter and Murphy (1968).

The earliest description of the abdominal wall defects appeared in the early 19th century (Frohlich 1839) and of the complete triad at the end of that century (Parker 1895). Further papers appeared over the first six decades of this century (Fletcher 1928; Kohn 1935; Roberts 1956; Nunn and Stephens 1961), but the bulk of papers have been published over the last 20 odd years. Many reports have dealt with the problems of conservative or surgical management, the best response to operative correction being obtained in the later onset cases (Woodhouse *et al.* 1982).

Many hypotheses have been proposed regarding the aetiology and pathogenesis of this disorder. Certainly no one aetiology can account for all cases as the observation of chromosomal abnormalities in a minority, Turner's syndrome (Pagon *et al.* 1979; Adeyokunnu and Familusi 1982), trisomy for chromosome 18 (Garlinger and Ott 1974), and trisomy for an unidentified fragment (Qazi *et al.* 1973) or mosaic monosomy 16 (Harley *et al.* 1972) confirm heterogeneity.

One hypothesis postulates a primary mesodermal defect (Ives 1974; Willert *et al.* 1978; Weber *et al.* 1978) to account for the varied structures involved. However, this does not explain the male preponder-ance, nor the fact that testes, although undescended, are usually normal. Afifi and colleagues (1972), who demonstrated myopathic changes in residual rectus abdominis muscle, proposed a primary myopathy but there is no good reason to assume that myopathic changes limited to one muscle group are primary, nor will they account for the features of the disorder unrelated to the abdominal wall. A third hypothesis, proposed by King and Prescott (1978) and by Pagon and colleagues (1979), is that the syndrome is secondary to urethral obstruction, to which the male is more liable, with the abdominal wall defect being secondary to the increased intra-abdominal pressure of the distended bladder. The main difficulties with this idea are the fact that urethral obstruction cannot be demonstrated in all cases, and seems especially unlikely in many milder cases, the presence of abdominal wall defect in cases with a persistent patent urachus, and the absence of prune-belly syndrome in many cases of urethral obstruction with urinary tract anomaly. Nevertheless this hypothesis has received support from several recent papers (Burton and Dillard 1984; Moerman *et al.* 1984; Nakayama *et al.* 1984), and despite unexplained aspects seems to fit the observations best to date.

Whatever the pathogenesis a genetic basis for the disorder has to be considered. The major difficulties with any genetic hypothesis covering the majority of cases are the observations that the great majority are sporadic, for example none of the 47 cases of Woodhouse and colleagues (1982) were familial, the fact that five pairs of monozygotic twins have been reported as being discordant (Ives 1974) in contrast to only two concordant like-sex pairs (Sladezyk 1967; Petersen *et al.* 1972), and that there have been only two reports of parental consanguinity (Fletcher 1928; Afifi *et al.* 1972).

Clearly the majority of cases cannot be primarily genetic and their aetiology and pathogenesis remain unknown. Nevertheless, the number of reports of familial cases is large enough to postulate that at least a few cases may be genocopies of the more common non-genetic form.

The male preponderance led Williams and Burkholder (1967) and Burke and coworkers (1969) to favour X-linked recessive inheritance. However, this male preponderance, with mainly mild forms in females, is more likely to be due to sex influence than to sex linkage in view of one of the cases described by Rogers and Ostrow (1973). Their patient had ambiguous genitalia with a uterus and ovaries and an XX karyotype, but had left renal dysplasia with dilated ureters and bladder.

Possible autosomal recessive inheritance in some cases is supported by a number of families with affected sibs and also by the rare parental consanguinity already mentioned. Concordant like-sex twins have also been reported twice (Sladezyk 1967; Peterson *et al.* 1972), although as already mentioned there have been more examples of monozygotic twin discordance. Affected cousins of proposita have been noted by three groups (Sladezyk 1967; Garlinger and Ott 1974; Adeyokunnu and Familusi 1982), which would be expected for a common recessive disorder but not for a rare one. This suggests that the observation of affected cousins is more likely to be due to polygenic predisposition. Affected sibs have been recorded in eight families (Kohn 1935; Grenet *et al.* 1972; Harley *et al.* 1972; Bronzini and Moscatelli 1973; Garlinger and Ott 1974; Welling *et al.* 1975; Riccardi and Grum 1977; Adeyokunnu and Familusi 1982). The sib pair observed by Adeyokunnu and Familusi are unusual in that it comprises a boy and his sister with Turner's syndrome. They also comment on a high incidence in Nigeria,

24 cases seen by them over 8 years. To these eight sib pairs may be added one further pair born to a woman seen by the present author, of interest because it demonstrates prenatal diagnosis of the lethal form. The patient had had a previous normal daughter. An ultrasound prenatal diagnosis of prune-belly syndrome was made at King's College Hospital in the succeeding two pregnancies, leading to termination of pregnancy at 26 and 20 weeks respectively. On both occasions the fetus was confirmed as having a prune belly and small cystic kidneys with calyceal dilatation, dilated ureters and hypertrophied bladder, and high positioned testes. On the first occasion the fetus was too macerated for histological examination but in the second fetus cystic dysplasia of the kidneys was confirmed on histology. In neither fetus was a urethral obstruction demonstrated. The parents are unrelated. Third-trimester ultrasound prenatal diagnosis has been reported previously (Garrett *et al.* 1975; Okulski 1977; Bovicelli *et al.* 1980).

As over 300 cases have been recorded the above observations clearly do not indicate a single gene origin for the majority of cases. Whilst an autosomal recessive genocopy, or a dominant fresh mutation, cannot be excluded for a minority of cases other explanations seem more likely. The most plausible of these must be polygenic predisposition and the suggestion of Riccardi and Grum (1973) of a two-step mutational process involving either a premutation followed by a second mutation at the same locus, or two mutations at separate loci, with sex-limited expression. It may be that a more systematic family study of a series of cases than has been done so far may provide evidence that would point more firmly towards one or more of the several hypotheses discussed here.

References

Adeyokunnu, A. A. and Familusi, J. B. (1982). Prune belly syndrome in two siblings and a first cousin. *Am. J. Dis. Child.* **136**, 23–5.

Afifi, A. K., Rebeiz, J., Mire, J., Andonian, S. J. and Der Kaloustian, V. M. (1972). The myopathology of the prune belly syndrome. *J. Neurol. Sci.* **15**, 153–65.

Baird, P. A. and MacDonald, E. C. (1981). An epidemiologic study of congenital malformations of the anterior abdominal wall in more than half a million consecutive live births. *Am. J. Hum. Genet.* **33**, 470–8.

Bovicelli, L., Rizzo, N., Orsini, L. F. and Michelacci, L. (1980). Prenatal diagnosis of the Prune Belly Syndrome. *Clin. Genetics* **18**, 79–82.

Bronzini, E. and Moscatelli, P. (1973). L'aplasia della muscolatura della parete abdominale associata a malformazioni genito-urinarie in due fratellini. *Pathologica* **65**, 127–36.

Burke, E. C., Shin, M. H. and Kelalis, P. P. (1969). Prune belly syndrome. Clinical findings and survival. *Am. J. Dis. Child.* **117**, 668–71.

Burton, B. K. and Dillard, R. G. (1984). Brief clinical report: prune belly syndrome: observations supporting the hypothesis of abdominal over-distension. *Am. J. Med. Genet.* **17**, 669–72.

Fletcher, W. M. A. (1928). Congenital absence of the abdominal wall. *Med. J. Aust.* **1**, 435.

Frohlich, F. (1839). Der Mangol der Muskeln, insbesondere der Seitenbauch-muskeln. Dissertation, Würzberg.

Garlinger, P. and Ott, J. (1974). Prune belly syndrome: possible genetic implications. *Birth Defects Orig. Art. Series.* **10** (8), 173–80.

Garrett, W. J., Kassof, G. and Osborn, R. A. (1975). The diagnosis of fetal hydronephrosis, megaureter and urethral obstruction by ultrasonic echography. *Br. J. Obstet. Gynaecol.* **82**, 115–20.

Grenet, P., LeCalve, G., Badonal, J., Gallet, J. P. and Babinet, J. M. (1972). Aplasie congenitale de la paroi abdominale. *Ann. Pédiatr.* **19**, 523.

Geary, D. F., MacLuskey, I. B., Churchill, B. M. and McLorie, G. (1986). A broader spectrum of abnormalities in the prune belly syndrome. *J. Urol.* **135**, 324–6.

Harley, L. M., Chen, Y. and Rattner, W. H. (1972). Prune belly syndrome. *J. Urol.* **108**, 174–6.

Ives, E. J. (1974). The abdominal muscle deficiency triad syndrome: experience with ten cases. *Birth Defects Orig. Art. Series.* **10**, 127–35.

King, C. R. and Prescott, G. (1978). Pathogenesis of the prune-belly syndrome. *J. Pediatr.* **93**, 273–4.

Kohn, G. (1935). Agenesie des muscles de la paroi abdominale chez un nouveau-né. *Prog. Med.* **32**, 1328–32.

Moerman, P., Fryns, J.-P., Goddeeris, P. and Lauweryns, J. M. (1984). Pathogenesis of the prune belly syndrome: a functional urethral obstruction caused by prostatic hypoplasia. *Pediatrics* **73**, 420–75.

Nakayama, D. K., Harrison, M. R., Chinn, D. H. and De Lorimer, A. A. (1984). The pathogenesis of prune belly. *Am. J. Dis. Child.* **138**, 834–6.

Nunn, I. M. and Stephens, F. D. (1961). The triad syndrome: a composite anomaly of the abdominal wall, urinary system and testes. *J. Urol.* **86**, 782–94.

Okulski, T. A. (1977). The prenatal diagnosis of lower urinary tract obstruction using B-scan ultrasound: a case report. *J. Clin. Ultrasound* **5**, 268–70.

Osler, W. (1901). Congenital absence of the abdominal muscles with distended and hypertrophied urinary bladder. *Bull. Johns Hopkins Hosp.* **12**, 331–3.

Pagon, R. A., Smith, D. W. and Shepard, T. H. (1979). Urethral obstruction malformation complex: a cause of abdominal muscle deficiency and the 'prune belly'. *J. Pediatr.* **94**, 900–6.

Parker, R. W. (1895). Absence of abdominal muscles in an infant. *Lancet* **1**, 1252.

Petersen, D. S., Fish, L. and Cass, A. S. (1972). Twins with congenital deficiency of abdominal musculature. *J. Urol.* **107**, 670–2.

Qazi, Q. H., Kauffman, S., Sher, J. and Mapa, H. C. (1973). Chromosomal abnormality in prune belly syndrome. *Humangenetik* **20**, 265–7.

Riccardi, V. M. and Grum, C. M. (1977). The prune belly anomaly. Heterogeneity and superficial X-linkage mimicry. *J. Med. Genet.* **14**, 266–70.

Roberts, P. (1956). Congenital absence of the abdominal muscles with associated abnormalities of the genito-urinary tract. *Arch. Dis. Child.* **31**, 236–9.

Rogers, L. W. and Ostrow, P. T. (1973). The prune belly syndrome: report of 20 cases and description of a lethal variant. *J. Pediatr.* **83**, 786–93.

Sladezyk, Von E. (1967). Das gehaufte familiare Auftreten des angeborenen Bauchmuskelevanddefektes. *Zentbl. f. Chirurg.* **92**, 426–9.
Stephens, F. D. (1983). *Congenital malformations of the urinary tract.* pp. 483–511. Praeger, New York.
Texter, J. H. and Murphy, G. P. (1968). The right-sided syndrome: congenital absence of the right testis, kidney and rectus. Urologic diagnosis and treatment. *Johns Hopkins Med. J.* **122**, 224–8.
Weber, M. L., Rivard, G. and Perreault, G. (1978). Prune belly syndrome associated with congenital cystic adenomatoid malformation of the lung. *Am. J. Dis. Child.* **132**, 316–17.
Welling, P., Pfeiffer, R. A., Kosenow, W., Bleisener, J. A., Vernon Jones, K. and Haarmeyer, A. (1975). Beobachtungen zum Bauchmuskelaplasie-syndrome. *Z. Kinderheilk.* **118**, 315–35.
Willert, C., Cohen, H., Yu, Y.-M. T. and Madden, J. D. (1978). Association of prune belly syndrome and gastroschisis. *Am. J. Dis. Child.* **132**, 526–7.
Williams, D. I. and Burkholder, G. V. (1967). The prune belly syndrome. *J. Urol.* **98**, 244–51.
Woodhouse, C. R. J., Ransley, P. G. and Williams, D. I. (1982). Prune belly syndrome—report of 47 cases. *Arch. Dis. Child.* **57**, 856–9.

10.2.4. Vesico-ureteral reflux

Vesico-ureteral reflux as demonstrated by cystography is associated with congenital malformation affecting the insertion of the ureters into the bladder. The commonest associated malformations are ectopic insertion (Monticelli 1931), especially lateral ectopia (Ambrose 1969), a short intravesical ureteral segment or uretero-vesical junction (Burger 1972a), or ureteric duplication (Amar 1968; Frye *et al.* 1974). The milder cases tend to show some improvement with age.

There has been continuing controversy regarding the relationships of reflux, urinary tract infection, and nephropathy. It has been widely considered that urinary tract infection in patients with reflux results in pyelonephritis and renal scarring. Indeed a review claimed that in over 80 families with vesico-ureteral reflux the presence of renal scarring was always associated with recurrent urinary tract infection (British Medical Journal 1975). More recently Kerr and Pillai (1983) have argued, from their observation of identical twins concordant for vesico-ureteral reflux but discordant for pyelonephritis, that an environmental factor, presumably infection, is necessary for the development of pyelonephritis. This view may well be correct. Certainly up to a half of all cases of reflux are asymptomatic without evidence of either infection or renal damage, and there is a correlation between infection and the develoment of chronic pyelonephritis. However, it has been suggested that urinary reflux without infection may cause renal damage in some cases. There is evidence that renal scars result from reflux in infancy (Frye *et al.* 1974) and it is not always evident that there has been an associated infection. Furthermore reflux, although frequently present without infection, may nevertheless in at least some cases predispose to infection. This is suggested by the observation that the excess of patients of blood group P_1, which favours bacterial adhesion to urinary tract epithelial cells and which is seen in children with recurrent urinary tract infection without reflux (see Chapter 11), is not seen in similar children with reflux (Lomberg *et al.* 1983). Bailey (1973) has even argued that intrarenal reflux may damage the kidneys *in utero*. Lewy and Belman (1975) reported a family in which there was renal scarring apparently associated with non-obstructive, non-infectious vesico-ureteral reflux. Because of the difficulty of excluding past infection the only way this question could be resolved would be by a long term prospective follow-up, with frequent urine cultures, of a large number of infants with reflux.

Controversy also surrounds the role of genetic factors in the aetiology of vesico-ureteral reflux or its more serious complications. Mogg (1977) quotes an incidence of 26 per cent in children with recurrent urinary tract infection and of 5.6 per cent of the adult population. An estimate of 1 per cent is quoted for the population prevalance in infants and young children (De Vargas *et al.* 1978). The large majority of cases are sporadic but nevertheless there have been many reports of familial occurrence. Estimates of the frequency of a positive family history vary between about a tenth to a third of families seen (Geist and Antolak 1972; Mounger and Scott 1972; Bois *et al.* 1975; Dwoskin 1976; Jerkins and Noe 1982), with a higher frequency of affected relatives when the index case has required surgical correction (Mulcahy *et al.* 1970), or has renal scarring (Jerkins and Noe 1982). Jerkins and Noe (1982) found an overall incidence of reflux of 32 per cent among the sibs of index patients, but a 50 per cent incidence when the index patients had renal scarring compared with only 25 per cent of sibs of index patients without renal damage. The reported families with more than one affected relative divide into those with affected sibs only and those with affected individuals in more than one generation or in collateral branches. The more recent families with only sibs affected include two of the three families of Mulcahy and co-authors (1970), four of the seven families described by Burger's group (Burger and Smith 1971; Burger 1972a and b), six out of nine families studied by Schmidt and associates (1972), seven out of 10 families of Miller and Caspari (1972), six out of eight families of Amar (1972), all four families of Bredin and colleagues (1975), five families of Bois and co-authors (1975), one of Fried and co-authors' (1975) families, Mogg's (1977) family, and one of Chapman and co-workers' (1985) illustrative pedigrees. In some of these families parents have not been investigated and in others it will not have been possible to exclude reflux in infancy in a parent. It is notable that in none of these families is parental consanguinity recorded, and in most it is specifically excluded. Although there have been a few families with affected cousins (Geist and Antolak 1972; Mounger and Scott 1972; Schmidt *et al.* 1972; Lewy and Belman 1975) it would seem most unlikely that there is a form of vesico-ureteral reflux due to recessive inheritance sufficiently common to be shown up in this way. Hence, despite the number of families with affected members confined to one sibship, recessive inheritance for a significant proportion seems improbable. Families with affected members in more than one generation, mostly parent and children, include three of Burger's seven families, two of Miller and Caspari's families, four families of Bois and colleagues, two families reported by Ambrose (1969), two of Amar's eight families, five out of Chapman and colleagues' seven illustrative families, and single families of several other workers, (Tobenkin 1964; Mulcahy *et al.* 1970; Schmidt *et al.* 1972; Frye *et al.* 1974; Fried *et al.* 1975; Lewy and Belman 1975). The family reported by Lewy and Belman was particularly striking, involving a father, his daughter, and three sons, his first cousin once removed, his great uncle, and the latter's two children. This family demonstrates affected individuals over four generations and father-to-son transmission. Whereas most of the two or more generation families quoted above are as readily explained on a multifactorial basis as on a single gene basis with dominant expression, Lewy and Belman's family is more suggestive of autosomal dominance with incomplete penetrance. Family 1 of Chapman and coworkers 1985) contains six affected individuals in three generations with apparent complete penetrance. The only comparable family (Fig. 10.1) known to the author is one involving 14 individuals over three generations (Himsworth 1984). Whilst these three families may represent a rare single autosomal gene determination this is certainly not proved. Another interesting family is that of Middleton and others (1975) who reported a family with three affected brothers, three unaffected sisters, normal parents, but an affected maternal grandfather for which they suggest X-linked inheritance. Here again the case must be regarded as unproved.

Chapman and colleagues (1985) carried out a segregation analysis of 88 families containing at least one affected member. Their analysis indicated that a single major locus was the most important causal factor in reflux, with the mutant allele being dominant with a gene frequency of 0.16 per cent and 45 per cent penetrance.

The case for a multifactorial genetic basis for reflux, both sporadic and familial, acting at the vesico-ureteral junction (Atwell and Allen 1980), and subject to environmental influences such as age, infection and

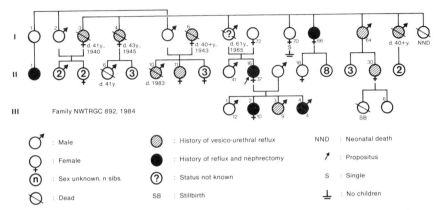

Fig. 10.1. Pedigree of a family with vesico-ureteral reflux in three generations. Reproduced with the permission of Prof. R. Himsworth (Himsworth 1984).

back pressure, has been argued by Burger (Burger and Smith 1971; Burger 1972b). He points out that the incidence of vesico-ureteral reflux of 1–2 per 1000 live births, and the increased incidence of first-degree relatives which is about 10- to 50-fold, are comparable to those in several other common malformations such as cleft-lip and palate, talipes, and neural tube defect.

The multifactorial case was supported by an extensive family study of 186 index patients with proved primary reflux carried out by C. O. Carter's group at the Institute of Child Health (De Vargas *et al.* 1978). Among these 186 patients there were two monozygotic twin pairs, (one pair concordant and the other discordant) and four dizygotic twin pairs (one pair concordant, one discordant, and two not investigated). Of the fully investigated young sibs three out of 20 (15 per cent) had reflux, and 10 out of 35 symptomatic parents had renal scarring.

Atwell and Allen (1980) in a study of 22 patients with a paraureteric diverticulum found an increased incidence of vesico-ureteral reflux and of duplication defects in the patients and their close relatives. They suggest that these three urinary tract anomalies comprise a syndrome complex with a multifactorial genetic basis which determines the length of the intravesical ureter. Atwell (1985) has produced further evidence in support of this hypothesis in another family study of 19 cases of pelvic-ureteric junction hydronephrosis in which he found nine further cases among the 71 first-degree relatives, along with three with pelvicalyceal duplication but only one with vesico-ureteral reflux. The genetic case is strengthened by reports of 10 monozygotic twin pairs, all but one pair concordant, at least for reflux (Stephens *et al.* 1955; Mebust and Foret 1972; Pochaczevsky *et al.* 1974; Hampel *et al.* 1975; Redman 1976; De Vargas *et al.* 1978; Kerr and Pillai 1983; Winearls and Hind 1983; Hayden and Koff 1984). Hayden and Koff reported triplets, a mono-zygotic pair with a dizygotic third triplet, concordant for reflux with infection. The fact that half of these twin pairs were discordant for urinary tract infection or pyelonephritic changes (Pochaczevsky *et al.* 1974; Redman 1976; Kerr and Pillai 1983; Winerals and Hind 1983) confirms that these complications, unlike the primary reflux, are not largely genetically determined. However, Bailey and Wallace (1978) found a barely significant excess of the major histocompatibility antigen HLA-B12 in patients with vesico-ureteral reflux and renal failure. Even if this were a true association, it is not clear from the nature of the study whether the HLA association is with reflux or its complicating nephropathy. Evidence that HLA antigens are associated with urinary tract infection rather than reflux comes from studies by MacDonald and colleagues (1976) who found an excess of HLA-A3 among reflux patients, and by Sengar and associates (1978, 1979) who studied 36 patients with urinary tract infection and found a significant increase in the frequency of HLA-BW16. When the patients were divided into those with or without vesico-ureteral reflux there were no significant differences between the two groups in HLA frequencies.

In conclusion it appears on present evidence that the occurrence of vesico-ureteral reflux, due to abnormalities of the vesico-ureteral junction, is strongly genetically determined on a multifactorial basis, and that subsequent urinary tract infection and nephropathy are largely environmentally determined but may be influenced by HLA antigen genes or genes closely linked to them. Nevertheless a strong case has been made for a single major gene, with irregular autosomal dominant inheritance, playing a major role in the aetiology of reflux. Even if this case is not accepted the possibility of it applying to a minority of families cannot be excluded.

For genetic counselling purposes Bois and colleagues (1975) estimate a 4 per cent risk of reflux for first-degree relatives of index patients with vesico-ureteral reflux. A higher risk would presumably be appropriate where there is strong family history.

Vesico-ureteral reflux may also occur as part of a syndrome, as for example in the imperforate anus, hand, foot and ear (Townes) syndrome. This was described by Townes and Brocks (1972) in a father and five out of seven of his children. They had imperforate anus, triphalangeal thumbs and other anomalies of hands and feet, with lop ears and sensori-neural deafness. Similar cases were described by Reid and Turner (1976), and Kurnit and colleagues (1978) who added renal hypoplasia and vesico-ureteral reflux or urethal valves. Inheritance is autosomal dominant.

References

Amar, A. D. (1968). Reflux in duplicated ureters. *Br. J. Urol.* **40**, 385–401.
—— (1972). Familial vesicoureteral reflux. *J. Urol.* **108**, 969–71.
Ambrose, S. S. (1969). Reflux pyelonephritis in adults secondary to congenital lesions of the ureteral orifice. *J. Urol.* **102**, 302–4.
Atwell, J. D. (1985). Familial pelviureteric junction hydronephrosis and its association with a duplex pelvicalyceal system and vesicoureteric reflux. A family study. *Br. J. Urol.* **57**, 365–9.
—— and Allen, N. H. (1980). The interrelationship between paraureteric diverticula, vesicoureteral reflux and duplication of the pelvicalicial collecting system: a family study. *Br. J. Urol.* **52**, 269–73.
Bailey, R. R. (1973). The relationship of vesico-ureteric reflux to urinary tract infection and chronic pyelonephritis—reflux nephropathy. *Clin. Nephrol.* **1**, 132–41.
—— and Wallace, M. (1978). HLA-B12 as a genetic marker for vesicoureteric reflux. *Br. Med. J.* **1**, 48–9.
Bois, E., Feingold, J., Benmaiz, H. and Briard, M. L. (1975). Congenital urinary tract malformations: epidemiologic and genetic aspects. *Clin. Genet.* **8**, 37–47.
Bredin, H. C., Winchester, P., McGovern, J. H. and Degnan, M. (1975). Family study of vesicoureteral reflux. *J. Urol.* **113**, 623–5.
British Medical Journal (anonymous) (1975). Vesicoureteral reflux and its familial distribution. *Br. Med. J.* **4**, 726.
Burger, R. H. (1972a). Congenitally short ureterovesical junction causing primary reflux—a common familial and hereditary trait. *Pediatr. Res.* **6**, 418.
—— (1972b). A theory on the nature of transmission of congenital vesicoureteral reflux. *J. Urol.* **108**, 249–54.
—— and Smith, C. (1971). Hereditary and familial vesicoureteral reflux. *J. Urol.* **106**, 845–51.
Chapman, C. J., Bailey, R. R., Janus, G. D., Abbott, G. D. and Lynn, K. L. (1985). Vesicoureteric reflux: segregation analysis. *Am. J. Med. Genet.* **20**, 577–84.
De Vargas, A., Evans, K., Ransley, P., Rosenberg, A. R., Rothwell, D., Sherwood, T., Williams, D. I., Barratt, T. M. and Carter, C. O. (1978). A family study of vesico-ureteric reflux. *J. Med. Genet.* **15**, 85–96.
Dwoskin, J. Y. (1976). Sibling uropathology. *J. Urol.* **115**, 726–7.
Fried, K., Yuval, E., Eidelman, A. and Beer, S. (1975). Familial primary vesicoureteral reflux. *Clin. Genet.* **7**, 144–7.
Frye, R. N., Patel, H. R. and Parsons, V. (1974). Familial renal tract abnormalities and cortical scarring. *Nephron* **12**, 188–96.
Geist, R. W. and Antolak, S. J. Jr. (1972). The clinical problems of children with sterile ureteral reflux. *J. Urol.* **108**, 343–6.
Hampel, N., Levin, D. R. and Gersh, I. (1975). Bilateral vesicoureteral reflux with pyelonephritis in identical twins. *Br. J. Urol.* **47**, 535–7.
Hayden, L. J. and Koff, S. A. (1984). Vesicoureteral reflux in triplets. *J. Urol.* **132**, 516–17.

Himsworth, R. (1984). Personal communication.

Jerkins, G. R. and Noe, H. N. (1982). Familial vesicoureteral reflux: a prospective study. *J. Urol.* **128**, 774–8.

Kerr, D. N. S. and Pillai, P. M. (1983). Identical twins with identical vesicoureteric reflux: chronic pyelonephritis in one. *Br. Med. J.* **286**, 1245–6.

Kurnit, D. M., Steel, M. W., Pinsky, L. and Dibbins, A. (1978). Autosomal dominant transmission of a syndrome of anal, ear, renal, and radial congenital malformations. *J. Pediatr.* **81**, 321–6.

Lewy, P. R. and Belman, A. B. (1975). Familial occurrence of nonobstructive noninfectious vesicoureteral reflux with renal scarring. *J. Pediatr.* **86**, 851–6.

Lomberg, H., Hanson, L. A., Jacobsen, B., Jodal, U., Leffler, H. and Svanborg Eden, C. (1983). Correlation of P blood group, vesicoureteral reflux, and bacterial attachment in patients with recurrent pyelonephritis. *New Engl. J. Med.* **308**, 1189–92.

MacDonald, I. M., Dumble, L. J. and Kincaid-Smith, P. (1976). HLA-A3, vesico-ureteric reflux and analgesic abuse. In *HLA and disease*, p. 255. INSERM, Paris.

Mebust, W. K. and Foret, J. D. (1972). Vesicoureteral reflux in identical twins. *J. Urol.* **108**, 635–6.

Middleton, G. W., Howards, S. S. and Gillenwater, J. Y. (1975). Sex-linked familial reflux. *J. Urol.* **114**, 36–9.

Miller, H. C. and Caspari, E. W. (1972). Ureteral reflux as genetic trait. *JAMA* **220**, 842–3.

Mogg, R. A. (1977). Familial and adult reflux. *Birth Defects Orig. Art. Series.* **13** (5), 365–6.

Monticelli, M. (1931). Enuresi uretorale congenita. *Pediatria* **39**, 401–26.

Mounger, E. J. and Scott, E. V. Z. (1972). Surgical correction of vesicoureteral reflux. *J. Urol.* **108**, 347–50.

Mulcahy, J. J., Kelalis, P. P., Stickler, G. B. and Burke, E. C. (1970). Familial vesicoureteral reflux. *J. Urol.* **104**, 762–4.

Pochaczevsky, R., Naysan, P. and Ratner, H. (1974). Congenital nonobstructive hydronephrosis and bilateral vesicoureteral reflux in identical twins. *Am. J. Roentgenol.* **120**, 398–401.

Redman, J. F. (1976). Vesicoureteral reflux in identical twins. *J. Urol.* **116**, 792–3.

Reid, I. S. and Turner, G. (1976). Familial anal abnormality. *J. Pediatr.* **88**, 992–4.

Schmidt, J. D., Hawtrey, C. E., Flocks, R. N. and Culp, D. A. (1972). Vesico-ureteral reflux, an inherited lesion. *JAMA* **220**, 821–6.

Sengar, D. P. S., Rashid, A. and Wolfish, N. M. (1978). Histocompatibility antigens and urinary tract abnormalities. *Br. Med. J.* **2**, 1146.

——, Rashid, A. and Wolfish, N. M. (1979). Familial urinary tract anomalies: association with the major histocompatibility complex in man. *J. Urol.* **121**, 194–7.

Stephens, F. D., Joske, R. A. and Simmons, R. T. (1955). Megaureter with vesicoureteric reflux in twins. *Aust. NZ J. Surg.* **24**, 192–4.

Tobenkin, M. I. (1964). Hereditary vesicoureteral reflux. *S. Med. J.* **57**, 139–47.

Townes, P. L. and Brocks, E. (1972). Hereditary syndrome of imperforate anus with hand, foot and ear anomalies. *J. Pediatr.* **81**, 321–6.

Winnearls, C. G. and Hind, C. R. K. (1983). Identical twins with identical vesicoureteric reflux. *Br. Med. J.* **286**, 1978.

10.3. URETHRAL

10.3.1. Hypospadias

Hypospadias may be secondary to chromosome abnormalities (see Chapter 3), to single gene defects, or to environmental induction as in progesterone administration to the mother in early pregnancy; or it may be primary. Whether primary or secondary hypospadias may be associated with chordee, meatal stenosis, cryptorchidism, or inguinal hernia. The defect varies in severity, the majority being of the relatively mild glandular or coronal forms, ranging through varying degrees of penile hypospadias to the rare severe peno-scrotal or perineo-scrotal forms.

It is difficult to assess the true incidence of the different aetiological groups of this common malformation since aetiology is often uncertain. Moreover, recent studies suggest that the incidence, in contrast to other malformations, is rising with an increased proportion of cases due to maternal hormone therapy (Czeizel 1985). Overall incidence has been previously estimated at between 0.8 and 8.2 per 1000. The trend has been for the higher incidence figures to be reported more recently. Early estimates were between 1 and 2 per 1000, as for example Campbell's (1951) figure of 1.6, in contrast to values of 4 to 8 per 1000 in more recent studies, such as the 4.0 of Lowry and Kliman (1976), the 4.4 of Leung and coworkers (1985), and the 8.2 found by Sweet and colleagues (1974). The last group reviewed eight earlier studies with incidence ranging from 0.8 to 7.6 per 1000. More recent studies (Avellan 1975; Czeizel *et al.* 1979; Kallen and Winberg 1982; Czeizel 1985; Matlai and Beral 1985) have observed a relatively high and increasing incidence. Matlai and Beral noted an approximate doubling of the incidence of hypospodias in England and Wales between 1964 and 1984, from 1.5 to 3.6 per 1000. Czeizel working in Hungary attributes the increase to the wide use of maternal hormone therapy and possibly to more effective treatment of subfertility. However, Baird (1985) and Leung and coworkers (1985) found no evidence for any increase in incidence in British Columbia between 1966 and 1981, but stated that hormonal therapy would be used much less than in Hungary. It has been postulated that the abrupt increase in incidence in Sweden between 1969 and 1971, with a subsequent steady rate (Kallen and Winberg 1982) suggests an artefactual basis, probably improved notification. This may be a factor in at least some of the other reported increases. However, a very similar abrupt increase in the same period has been recorded by the Liverpool Congenital Malformations Registry (Simpkin *et al.* 1985). The authors argue that this indicates a new, unidentified, environmental teratogen that has persisted. Aarskog (1970) in a series of 80 patients found five associated with a chromosomal anomaly and five with maternal progestin administration, that is, 6 per cent of the total each. Chen and Wooley (1971) found a similar proportion with chromosomal anomalies (two out of 26). Hence something like 15 per cent or more of cases of simple hypospadias are secondary and up to 85 per cent are primary, which would suggest a likely contemporary incidence of primary hypospadias of around 3 to 7 per 1000 live births, probably with some geographical variation. Sweet and colleagues (1974) in a study of 113 cases from Minnesota found coronal or glandular hypospadias in 7 per cent, penile in 10 per cent, and peno-scrotal in 3 per cent. They quote earlier studies that confirm the great preponderance of cases with the minimal form, 61 per cent in New York (Kennedy 1961) and 75 per cent in Denmark (Sorensen 1953). These latter studies also found a similar proportion of penile hypospadias to the Minnesota study, but had a higher proportion of patients with the severe form, possibly due to selective referral.

The most commonly observed type of chromosomal anomaly in hypospadias involves the sex chromosomes. Aarskog's (1970) five patients with chromosomal anomaly all involved the sex chromosomes with either XX/XY or XO/XY mosaicism, and all had severe peno-scrotal or perineo-scrotal hypospadias. Autosomal anomalies have also been reported in hypospadias as discussed in Chapter 3. Specific mention can be made here of a case separately reported by Aarskog (1969) with a duplication–deficiency syndrome due to inheritance of an unbalanced product of a familial reciprocal translocation between chromosomes 3 and 18.

Hypospadias is one feature of a number of inherited syndromes, of which autosomal recessive virilizing adrenal hyperplasia in the female has just been mentioned above. It is a near-constant feature, but of variable severity, in males with another autosomal recessive disorder, Smith–Lemli–Opitz syndrome, when it is usually associated with cryptorchidism (Smith *et al.* 1964; Blair and Martin 1966). Occasionally more serious urinary tract malformations occur in this syndrome, such as duplex renal systems, pelvi-ureteric or lower ureteric obstruction and ureteric reflux with bladder neck obstruction (Dallaire and Fraser 1966; Dallaire 1969). Halal and Farsky (1981) reported a possibly new irregular autosomal dominant syndrome in which the index patient was a boy with hypertelorism, bilateral ocular coloboma, and mental retardation and also had hypospadias. His father had only hypospadias but a brother had unilateral iris coloboma. The karytoype was normal. The authors consider the possibility that their family had the BBB syndrome with independent segregation of coloboma. However, the father–son involvement makes the probably X-linked BBB, or Opitz, syndrome unlikely. Both the BBB syndrome itself (Christian *et al.* 1969, Opitz *et al.*

1969) and the G syndrome (Opitz *et al.* 1969) are characterized by hypertelorism or telecanthus, hypospadias and cleft-lip, and palate. Further urinary malformations have been described in the BBB syndrome. Both syndromes show familial patterns strongly suggestive of X linkage although some authors have postulated autosomal dominance with father-to-son transmission (Funderburk and Stewart 1978; Farndon and Donnai 1983). The distinction between them rests on the addition of swallowing or respiratory difficulties associated with laryngo-tracheo-oesophageal anomalies in the G syndrome, and subtle differences in facial appearance, with a high broad nasal bridge with anteverted nostrils in the G syndrome. It has been suggested that this distinction merely represents variable expression of a single disorder (Cordero and Holmes 1978; Funderburk and Stewart 1978), and indeed it has been claimed that members of a single family show one or other syndrome (Parisian and Toomey 1978).

Another X-linked syndrome in which hypospadias is a feature, along with hypogonadism and gynaecomastia, is the form of male pseudohermaphroditism known as Reifenstein syndrome, or type I (Bowen *et al.* 1965). Despite the resemblance to Klinefelter syndrome the karyotype is 46,XY. Later research workers have produced evidence for partial androgen insensitivity in at least some patients with Reifenstein syndrome (Wilson *et al.* 1974; Amrhein *et al.* 1977; Keenan *et al.* 1977).

In the form of male pseudohermaphroditism known as type II there is pseudovaginal perineo-scrotal hypospadias (De Vaal 1955; Simpson *et al.* 1971; Wilson *et al.* 1974; Peterson *et al.* 1977). Affected males are usually brought up as girls but following masculinization at puberty tend to adopt a male gender role (Imperato-McGinley *et al.* 1979). There are normal levels of testosterone but low levels of dihydrotestosterone due to 5α-reductase deficiency (Imperato-McGinley *et al.* 1987; Peterson *et al.* 1985; Johnson *et al.* 1986). The autosomal recessive inheritance of this disorder has been established in a large Dominican family with much consanguinity (Imperato-McGinley *et al.* 1974, 1980, 1985; Akgun *et al.* 1986). Enzyme kinetic differences between families suggest genetic heterogeneity (Moore *et al.* 1975; Wilson 1975; Leshin *et al.* 1978).

In yet another form of male pseudohermaphroditism with gynaecomastia the external genitalia of males are female at birth but masculinize at puberty (Saez *et al.* 1971, 1972; Kohn *et al.* 1981). The primary defect is a deficiency of 17-ketoreductase activity (Saez *et al.* 1971, 1972). Autosomal recessive inheritance is confirmed by the inbred Arab family described by Kohn and colleagues (1981). Two affected sibs with perineal hypospadias were reported by Caufriez (1986).

Hypospadias has been reported as a feature of males with the crytophthalmos syndrome (Gupta and Saxena 1962), whereas females have fused labia and an enlarged clitoris (Fraser 1962), and patients of either sex may have renal malformations or agenesis, as discussed earlier (Fraser 1962, 1966). Hypospadias has also been reported as a feature of the Rapp–Hodgkin type of ectodermal dysplasia, which is a rare autosomal dominant anhidrotic form in which cleft-lip and palate may also occur (Rapp and Hodgkin 1968; Summitt and Hiatt 1971; Wannarachue *et al.* 1972), and in at least some families with Rieger syndrome, another autosomal dominant disorder with hypodontia, microcornea and iris hypoplasia with anterior synechiae, anal stenosis, and variable mild mental subnormality (Sadeghi-Nejad and Senior 1974; Jorgenson *et al.* 1978). In one family with Rieger syndrome there was also renal hypoplasia (Delmarcelle *et al.* 1958). Hess and colleagues (1974) described visual impairment, deafness, anomalous upper eyelids, large corneae, abnormal auricles, cryptorchidism, hypospadias, and spasticity in two brothers. They called this disorder the N syndrome after the initial letter of the boys' surname. Schmitt and others (1982) reported a three-generation family in which five females and three males were affected with a syndrome of bilateral radial hypoplasia with non-opposable triphalangeal thumbs and anterior maxillary diastema. All the affected males also had first-degree hypospadias. There was no male-to-male transmission but the fact that only two out of four daughters of an affected father were themselves affected make autosomal dominant inheritance probable. Autosomal recessive inheritance is almost certainly the case in the brachio-skeletal-genital syndrome. This was reported in three brothers in the family of first cousin parents (Elsahy and Waters 1971). The brothers had an identical syndrome of mental subnormality, maxillary hypoplasia and mandibular prognathism, dental cysts, a broad nasal bridge with hypertelorism, bifid uvular or partial cleft-palate, pectus excavatum, fused cervical spinous processes, Schmorl nodes, and peno-scrotal hypospadias. Another probable autosomal recessive syndrome is the Bowen syndrome. This consists of failure to thrive in an infant with feeble sucking and swallowing, finger flexion deformity, buphthalmos, malformed ears, small mandible, congenital heart defect, agenesis of the corpus callosum, enlarged clitoris in the female and hypospadias in the male, and early death. These abnormalities were found in a brother and sister in the second of the two families described by Bowen and coworkers (1964).

Hypospadias has been reported as an occasional feature in several further dysmorphic syndromes. These include the Shprintzen syndrome with autosomal, or possibly X-linked, dominant inheritance, characterized by cardiac defect, cleft-palate, and a prominent square nose (Shprintzen *et al.* 1981); the Leopard or multiple lentigenes syndrome, also with autosomal dominant inheritance (Moynahan 1962), in which unilateral renal agenesis has also been reported (Swanson *et al.* 1971);

the Dubowitz syndrome (Wilroy *et al.* 1978); and the Biemond II syndrome, as for example in the family of three brothers of Blumel and Kniker (1959) regarded by them as having Lawrence–Moon–Bardet–Biedl syndrome. Biemond II syndrome, like Dubowitz syndrome, is autosomal recessive. In addition hypospadias is occasionally seen in the fetal rubella syndrome and in the fetal syndromes associated with maternal hydantoin and trimethadione administration. Hypogonadism and hypospadias have been said to be common in Russell–Silver syndrome (Marks and Bergeson 1977) but Saal and colleagues (1985) found neither among 14 patients.

Hypospadias may also occur as one feature of a cluster of malformations not constituting a recognizable syndrome. In one such case a boy had hypospadias with chordee, unilateral duplex ureter, ureterocoele, and sacral agenesis. His identical twin brother was quite normal (Woodhouse and Crawfurd 1987), suggesting an intra-uterine environmental insult as the cause.

Other abnormalities of the male genitalia that are seen in specific syndromes include epispadias as an occasional finding in the autosomal recessive Ellis–van Creveld syndrome (Da Silva *et al.* 1980); the shawl or saddle scrotum of the Aarskog syndrome, which is either X linked or autosomal dominant with sex influence (Berry *et al.* 1980); the relatively large phallus seen in the autosomal recessive Robert's or pseudothalidomide (or SC) syndrome (Freeman *et al.* 1974); and the extraordinary autosomal dominant Ruvalcaba–Myhre syndrome in which from adolescence pigmented macular spots develop on the glans and shaft of the penis (Ruvalcaba *et al.* 1981). Apart from the relatively large phallus of Robert's syndrome there have also been occasional reports of polycystic kidney or horseshoe kidney in that disorder, as discussed in the section on fused kidneys.

Turning to simple hypospadias, a severe pseudovaginal perineo-scrotal form has been reported as being due to a single gene with autosomal recessive inheritance in some families (Opitz *et al.* 1972; Keenan 1980), also with androgen insensitivity. More remarkably recent evidence suggests that androgen insensitivity may even be involved in the aetiology of the common less severe non-inherited simple hypospadias. Svensson and Snochowski (1979) demonstrated decreased saturable methyltrienolone binding by preputial skin homogenates from boys with hypospadias. Their finding is supported by Keenan and colleagues (1984) who found reduced binding of 5α-dihydrotestosterone of genital skin fibroblasts of 26 affected boys compared with those from 18 controls. However, there was no correlation of the anatomic severity of the hypospadias and the degree of reduced androgen binding, suggesting that other factors are also involved. Hypospadias is thus the only common malformation for which there is evidence for a biochemically definable defect. As such it forms part of a spectrum of genetically distinct syndromes with androgen insensitivity. Complete insensitivity is seen in phenotypic females with testicular feminization, a 46,XY karyotype, and probably X linkage. Such individuals may have normal, deficient, or almost undetectable androgen receptor activity, indicating genetic heterogeneity of this extreme group. There are several syndromes of partial insensitivity with ambiguous genitalia or simple hypospadias. These include the Reifenstein and pseudovaginal perineo-scrotal hypospadias syndromes discussed above, and an apparently autosomal dominant syndrome of variable male pseudohermaphroditism with a qualitatively abnormal androgen receptor showing reduced affinity for 5α-dihydrotestosterone but not methyltrienolone (Pinksy *et al.* 1985).

Apart from the rare monogenic forms of hypospadias already described there have been a number of family studies of idiopathic simple hypospadias. One of the earliest such studies (Sorensen 1953) found an incidence of about 1 in 10 among brothers of affected boys, and suggested autosomal recessive inheritance of familial cases, but excluded this for the majority of cases on the basis of discordance in four monozygotic twin pairs. Reule and Ansell (1967) also reported discordance for hypospadias in an identical twin pair, but Lattimer (1944) observed a concordant identical pair. Chen and Wooley (1971) found six out of 62 brothers of their index cases to be affected, an incidence very close to that of Sorensen. They suggested polygenic inheritance and estimated heritability at 74 per cent. Sweet and colleagues (1974) also observed familial aggregation in that among 107 families of index cases there were seven in which two brothers were affected, two in which a father and son were affected, and two in which a father and two sons were affected. They also supported a multifactorial model of genetic predisposition, as did Czeizel and colleagues (1979) and Bauer and associates (1981). Lowry and Kliman (1976), on the other hand, postulated autosomal dominant inheritance in two families reported by them. These consisted of a father and two sons in one family, and five or six males with penile hypospadias in three or four generations with consistent male-to-male transmission in the other family. Taking all these reports together multifactorial genetic predisposition would seem the most likely explanation in most families with mild to moderate hypospadias, but single gene effects cannot be excluded in a minority of such families. This view might have to be revised if androgen insensitivity associated with hypospadias could be shown to segregate in a mendelian manner.

References

Aarskog, D. (1969). A familial 3/18 reciprocal translocation resulting in chromosome duplication-deficiency (3?+ −18q−). *Acta Paediatr. Scand.* **58**, 397–406.

—— (1970). Clinical and cytogenetic studies in hypospadias. *Acta Paediatr. Scand.* Suppl. **203**, 1–62.

Akgun, S., Ertel, N. H., Imperato-McGinley, J., Sayli, B. S. and Shackleton, C. (1986). Familial male pseudohermaphroditism due to 5-alpha-reductase deficiency in a Turkish village. *Am. J. Med.* **81**, 267–74.

Amrhein, J. A., Klingensmith, G. J., Walsh, P. C., McKusick, V. A. and Migeon, C. J. (1977). Partial androgen insensitivity: the Reifenstein syndrome revisited. *New Engl. J. Med.* **297**, 350–6.

Avellan, L. (1975). The incidence of hypospadias in Sweden. *Scand. J. Plast. Reconstr. Surg.* **9**, 129–39.

Baird, P. A. (1985). Incidence of hypospadias. *Lancet* **1**, 1162.

Bauer, S. B., Retik, A. B. and Colodny, A. H. (1981). Genetic aspects of hypospadias. *Urol. Clin. N. Am.* **8**, 559–64.

Berry, C., Cree, J. and Mann, T. (1980). Aarskog's syndrome. *Arch. Dis. Child.* **55**, 706–10.

Blair, H. R. and Martin, J. K. (1966). A syndrome characterised by mental retardation, short stature, cranio-facial dysplasia, and genital anomalies occurring in siblings. *J. Pediatr.* **69**, 457–9.

Blumel, J. and Kniker, W. T. (1959). Lawrence–Moon–Bardet–Biedl syndrome: review of the literature and a report of five cases including a family group with three affected males. *Texas Rep. Biol. Med.* **17**, 391–410.

Bowen, P., Lee, C. N. S., Zellweger, H. and Lindenburg, R. (1964). A familial syndrome of multiple congenital defects. *Bull. Johns Hopkins Hosp.* **114**, 402–14.

——, ——, Migeon, C. J., Kaplan, N. M., Whalley, P. J., McKusick, V. A. and Reifenstein, E. C. (1965). Hereditary male pseudohermaphroditism with hypogonadism, hypospadias, and gynecomastia (Reifenstein's syndrome). *Ann. Intern. Med.* **62**, 252–70.

Campbell, M. F. (1951). *Clinical pediatric urology.* W.B. Saunders, Philadelphia.

Caufriez, Z. (1986). Male pseudohermaphroditism due to 17-ketoreductase deficiency: report of a case without gynecomastia and without vaginal pouch. *Am. J. Obstet. Gynecol.* **154**, 148–9.

Chen, Y. C. and Wooley, P. V. (1971). Genetic studies on hypospadias in males. *J. Med. Genet.* **8**, 153–9.

Christian, J. C., Bixler, D., Blythe, S. C. and Merritt, A. D. (1969). Familial telecanthus with associated congenital anomalies. *Birth Defects Orig. Art. Series* **5** (2), 82–5.

Cordero, J. F. and Holmes, L. B. (1978). Phenotypic overlap of the BBB and G syndromes. *Am. J. Med. Genet.* **2**, 145–52.

Cote, G. B., Petmezaki, S. and Bastakis, N. (1979). A gene for hypospadias in a child with presumed tetrasomy 18p. *Am. J. Med. Genet.* **4**, 141–6.

Czeizel, A. (1985). Increasing trends in congenital malformations of male external genitalia. *Lancet* **1**, 462–3.

——, Toth, J. and Erodi, E. (1979). Aetiological studies of hypospadias in Hungary. *Hum. Hered.* **29**, 166–71.

Dallaire, L. (1969). Syndrome of retardation with urogenital and skeletal anomalies (Smith–Lemli–Opitz syndrome): clinical features and mode of inheritance. *J. Med. Genet.* **6**, 113–20.

—— and Fraser, F. C. (1966). The syndrome of retardation with urogenital and skeletal anomalies in siblings. *J. Pediatr.* **69**, 459–60.

Da Silva, E. O., Janovitz, D. and De Albuquerque, S. C. (1980). Ellis–van Creveld syndrome: report of 15 cases in an inbred kindred. *J. Med. Genet.* **17**, 349–56.

Delmarcelle, Y., de Clerck, P. and Pivont, A. (1958). Glaucome congénital associé à des malformations oculaires et somatiques dans deux générations successives. *Bull. Soc. Belge d'Ophthal.* **120**, 638–55.

De Vaal, O. M. (1955). Genital intersexuality in three brothers, connected with consanguineous marriages in the three previous generations. *Acta Paediatr.* **44**, 35–9.

Elsahy, N. I. and Waters, W. R. (1971). The brachio-skeletal-genital syndrome: a new hereditary syndrome. *Plast. Reconstr. Surg.* **48**, 542–50.

Farkas, L. G. (1970). Minor defects of the penis. Microforms or stigmata of hypospadias and epispadias. *Plast. Reconstr. Surg.* **45**, 480–6.

Farndon, P. A. and Donnai, D. (1983). Male to male transmission of the G syndrome. *Clin. Genet.* **24**, 446–8.

Fraser, G. R. (1962). Our genetical 'load'. A review of some aspects of genetical variation. *Ann. Hum. Genet.* **25**, 387–415.

—— (1966). XX chromosomes and renal agenesis. *Lancet* **1**, 1427.

Freeman, M. V. R., Williams, D. W., Schimke, R. N., Temtamy, S. A., Vachier, E. and German, J. (1974). The Roberts syndrome. *Clin. Genet.* **5**, 1–16.

Funderburk, S. J. and Stewart, R. (1978). The G and BBB syndromes: case presentations, genetics, and nosology. *Am. J. Med. Genet.* **2**, 131–44.

Gupta, S. P. and Saxena, R. C. (1962). Cryptophthalmos. *Br. J. Ophthalmol.* **46**, 629–32.

Halal, F. and Farsky, K. (1981). Brief clinical report: coloboma-hypospadias. *Am. J. Med. Genet.* **8**, 53–7.

Hess, R. O., Kaveggia, E. G. and Opitz, J. M. (1974). The N syndrome, a 'new' multiple congenital anomaly-mental retardation syndrome. *Clin. Genet.* **6**, 237–46.

Imperato-McGinley, J., Guerrero, L., Gautier, T. and Peterson, R. E. (1974). Steroid 5α-reductase deficiency in man: an inherited form of male pseudo-hermaphroditism. *Science* **186**, 1213–15.

——, Peterson, R. E., Gautier, T. and Sturla, E. (1979). Androgens and the evolution of male-gender-identity among male pseudohermaphrodites with 5α-reductase deficiency. *New Engl. J. Med.* **300**, 1233–7.

——, ——, Leshin, M., Griffin, J. E., Cooper, G., Draghi, S., Berenyi, M. and Wilson, J. D. (1980). Steroid 5α-reductase deficiency in a 65 year old male pseudohermaphrodite: the natural history, ultrastructure of the testes, and evidence for inherited enzyme heterogeneity. *J. Clin. Endocr. Metab.* **50**, 15–22.

——, ——, Gautier, T., Cooper, G., Danner, R., Arthur, A., Morris, P. L., Sweeney, W. J. and Shackleton, C. (1982). Hormonal evaluation of a large kindred with complete androgen insensitivity: evidence for secondary 5α reductase deficiency. *J. Clin. Endocr. Metab.* **54**, 931–41.

——, ——, ——, Arthur, A. and Shackleton, C. (1985). Decreased urinary C_{19} and C_{21} steroid 5α-metabolites in parents of male pseudohermaphrodites with 5α-reductase deficiency: detection of carriers. *J. Clin. Endocr. Metab.* **60**, 553–8.

Johnson, L., George, F. W., Neaves, W. B., Rosenthal, I. M., Christensen, R. A.,

Decristoforo, A., Schweikert, H.-U., Sauer, M. V., Leshin, M., Griffin, J. E. and Wilson, J. E. (1986). Characterization of the testicular abnormality in 5α-reductase deficiency. *J. Clin. Endocr. Metab.* **63**,1091–9.

Jorgenson, R. J., Levin, L. S., Cross, H. E., Yoder, F. and Kelly, T. E. (1978). The Rieger syndrome. *Am. J. Med. Genet.* **2**, 307–18.

Kallen, B. and Winberg, J. (1982). An aetiological study of hypospadias in Sweden. *Acta Paediatr. Scand.* Suppl. **293**, 1–21.

Keenan, B. S. (1980). Pseudovaginal perineoscrotal hypospadias: genetic heterogeneity. *Urol. Clin. N. Am.* **7**, 393–407.

——, Kirkland, J. L., Kirkland, R. T. and Clayton, G. W. (1977). Male pseudohermaphroditism with partial androgen insensitivity. *Pediatrics* **59**, 224–31.

——, McNeel, R. L. and Gonzales, E. T. (1984). Abnormality of intracellular 5α-dihydrotestosterone binding in simple hypospadias: studies on equilibrium steroid binding in sonicates of genital skin fibroblasts. *Pediatr. Res.* **18**, 216–20.

Kennedy, P. A. (1961). Hypospadias: a twenty year review of 489 cases. *J. Urol.* **85**, 814–17.

Kohn, G., Lasch, E. E. and Kosler, A. (1981). Male pseudohermaphroditism with post-pubertal gender role reversal in a large Arab kindred (abs.). *Sixth Int. Congr. Hum. Genet.*, Jerusalem, p. 259.

Lattimer, J. K. (1944). Similar urogenital anomalies in identical twins. *Am. J. Dis. Child.* **67**, 199–200.

Leshin, M., Griffin, J. E. and Wilson, J. D. (1978). Hereditary male pseudohermaphroditism associated with an unstable form of 5α-reductase. *J. Clin. Invest.* **62**, 685–91.

Leung, T. J., Baird, P. A. and McGillivray, B. (1985). Hypospadias in British Columbia. *Am. J. Med. Genet.* **21**, 39–48.

Lingard, A. (1884). The hereditary transmission of hypospadias and its transmission by indirect atavism. *Lancet* **1**, 703.

Lowry, R. B. and Kliman, M. R. (1976). Hypospadias in successive generations—possible dominant gene inheritance. *Clin. Genet.* **9**, 285–8.

Marks, L. J. and Bergeson, P. S. (1977). The Silver–Russell syndrome. *Am. J. Dis. Child.* **131**, 447–51.

Matlai, P. and Beral, V. (1985). Trends in congenital malformations of external genitalia. *Lancet* **1**, 108.

Moore, R. J., Griffin, J. E. and Wilson, J. D. (1975). Diminished 5α-reductase activity in extracts of fibroblasts cultured from patients with familial incomplete male pseudohermaphroditism, type 2. *J. Biol. Chem.* **250**, 7168–72.

Moynahan, E. J. (1962). Multiple symmetrical moles with psychic and somatic infantilism and genital hypoplasia. *Proc. R. Soc. Med.* **55**, 959–60.

Opitz, J. M., Frias, J. L., Gutenberg, J. E. and Pellett, J. R. (1969). The G syndrome of multiple congenital anomalies. *Birth Defects Orig. Art. Series* **5** (2), 95–101.

——, Summit, R. L. and Smith, D. W. (1969). The BBB syndrome: familial telecanthus with associated congenital malformations. *Birth Defects Orig. Art. Series* **5** (2), 86–94.

——, Simpson, J. L., Sarto, G. E., New, M. and German, J. (1972). Pseudovaginal perineoscrotal hypospadias. *Clin. Genet.* **3**, 1–26.

Parisian, S. and Toomey, K. E. (1978). Features of the G (Opitz–Frias) and BBB (hypospadias hypertelorism) syndrome in one family—are they a single disorder? *Am. J. Hum. Genet.* **30**, 62A.

Peterson, R. E., Imperato-McGinley, J., Gautier, T. and Sturla, E. (1977). Male pseudohermaphroditism due to steroid 5α-reductase deficiency. *Am. J. Med.* **62**, 170–90.

——, ——, —— and Shackleton, C. (1985). Urinary steroid metabolites in subjects with male pseudohermaphroditism due to 5α-reductase deficiency. *Clin. Endocrinol.* **23**, 43–53.

Pinsky, L., Kaufman, M. and Chudley, A. E. (1985). Reduced affinity of the androgen receptor for 5α-dihydrotestosterone but not methyltrienolone in a form of partial androgen resistance: studies on cultured genital skin fibroblasts. *J. Clin. Invest.* **75**, 1291–6.

Rapp, R. S. and Hodgkin, W. E. (1968). Anhidrotic ectodermal dysplasia: autosomal dominant inheritance with palate and lip anomalies. *J. Med. Genet.* **5**, 269–72.

Reule, G. R. and Ansell, J. S. (1967). Discordant occurrence of genitourinary defects in monozygotic twins. *J. Urol.* **97**, 1078–81.

Ruvalcaba, R. H. A., Myhre, S. and Smith, D. W. (1981). Sotos syndrome with intestinal polyposis and pigmentary changes of the genitalia. *Clin. Genet.* **18**, 413–16.

Saal, H. M., Pagon, R. A. and Pepin, M. G. (1985). Reevaluation of Russell–Silver syndrome. *J. Pediatr.* **107**, 733–7.

Sadeghi-Nejad, A. and Senior, B. (1974). Autosomal dominant transmission of isolated growth hormone deficiency in iris–dental dysplasia (Rieger's syndrome). *J. Pediatr.* **85**, 644–8.

Saez, J. M., De Peretti, E., Morera, A. M., David, M. and Bertrand, J. (1971). Familial male pseudohermaphroditism with gynecomastia due to a testicular 17-ketosteroid reductase defect. I. Study *in vivo*. *J. Clin. Endocrinol.* **32**, 604–10.

——, Morera, A. M., De Peretti, E. and Bertrand, J. (1972). Further *in vivo* studies in male pseudohermaphroditism with gynecomastia due to testicular 17-ketosteroid reductase defect (compared to a case of testicular feminization). *J. Clin. Endocrinol.* **34**, 598–600.

Schmitt, E., Gillenwater, J. Y. and Kelly, T. E. (1982). An autosomal dominant syndrome of radial hypoplasia, triphalangeal thumbs, hypospadias and maxillary diastema. *Am. J. Med. Genet.* **13**, 63–9.

Sedgwick, W. (1896). Notes on the influence of heredity in disease. *Br. Med. J.* 458–62.

Shprintzen, R. J., Goldberg, R. B., Young, D. and Wolford, L. (1981). The velo-cardio-facial syndrome: a clinical and genetic analysis. *Pediatrics* **67**, 167–72.

Simpkin, J. M., Owens, J. R. and Harris, F. (1985). Incidence of hypospadias. *Lancet* **1**, 384.

Simpson, J. L., New, M., Peterson, R. E. and German, J. (1971). Pseudovaginal perineoscrotal hypospadias (ppSH) in sibs. *Birth Defects Orig. Art. Series* **7** (6), 140–4.

Smith, D. W., Lemli, L. and Opitz, J. M. (1964). A newly recognized syndrome of multiple congenital anomalies. *J. Pediatr.* **64**, 210–17.

Sorensen, H. R. (1953). *Hypospadias with special reference to aetiology.* Munksgaard, Copenhagen.

Summitt, R. L. and Hiatt, R. L. (1971). Hypohidrotic ectodermal dysplasia with multiple associated anomalies. *Birth Defects Orig. Art. Series* **7** (8), 121–4.

Svensson, J. and Snochowski, M. (1979). Androgen receptor levels in preputial skin from boys with hypospadias. *J. Clin. Endocrinol. Metab.* **49**, 340–5.

Swanson, S. L., Santen, R. J. and Smith, D. W. (1971). Multiple lentigenes syndrome: new findings of hypogonadotrophism, hyposmia and unilateral renal agenesis. *J. Pediatr.* **78**, 1037–9.

Sweet, R. A., Schrott, H. G., Kurland, R. and Culp, O. S. (1974). Study of the incidence of hypospadias in Rochester, Minnesota, 1940–1970, and a case-control comparison of possible etiologic factors. *Mayo Clin. Proc.* **49**, 52–8.

Sykes, P. J. and Ho, L. C. Y. (1972). Hypospadias: a report on 193 treated cases. *Plastic Reconstr. Surg.* **50**, 452–7.

Wannarchue, N., Hall, B. D. and Smith, A. W. (1972). Ectodermal dysplasia and multiple defects (Rapp–Hodgkins type). *J. Pediatr.* **81**, 1217–18.

Wilroy, R. S. Jr., Tipton, R. E. and Summitt, R. L. (1978). The Dubowitz syndrome. *Am. J. Med. Genet.* **2**, 275–84.

Wilson, J. D. (1975). Dihydrotestosterone formation in cultured human fibroblasts: comparison of cells from normal subjects and patients with familial incomplete male pseudohermaphroditism, type 2. *J. Biol. Chem.* **250**, 3498–504.

——, Harrod, M. J., Goldstein, J. L., Hemsell, D. L. and MacDonald, P. C. (1974). Familial incomplete male pseudohermaphroditism, type I: evidence for androgen resistance and variable clinical manifestations in a family with Reifenstein syndrome. *New Engl. J. Med.* **290**, 1097–103.

Woodhouse, C. R. J. and Crawfurd, M. d'A. (1985). Monozygotic male twins discordant for hypospadias, duplex ureter and sacral agenesis (in preparation).

10.3.2. Hypoplasia or agenesis of the penis (micropenis)

Isolated micropenis is a very rare sporadic defect. However, genital hypoplasia in the male is a feature of several dysmorphic syndromes including the Cornelia de Lange syndrome in which Smith (1982) reports that four out of 17 male patients had a small penis. Male patients with Seckel syndrome (bird-headed dwarfism) may also show genital hypoplasia (Harper *et al.* 1967) and even hypoplastic or ectopic kidneys, or cloacal dystrophy (McKusick *et al.* 1967). Another disorder in which micropenis is common is the CHARGE association—a group of disorders in which varying combinations of coloboma, heart defect, choanal atresia, retarded growth, and genital and ear anomalies occur. Hall (1979) observed hypogenitalism in seven out of nine male cases; Pagon and colleagues (1981) in 11 out of 15 male cases; and Siebert and coworkers in one male and one female case. Pagon's group stated that two of their patients had renal anomalies without specifying the type. Davenport and associates (1986) found cryptorchidism and/or hypospadias in seven out of eight males with the CHARGE association. There are several other disorders in which hypogonadism with micropenis is a feature. These include atelencephaly (Siebert *et al.* 1986), the

Borjeson syndrome of severe mental subnormality, epilepsy, and hypogonadism, which is inherited in an X-linked recessive manner (Weber *et al.* 1978), and the Hallermann Strieff syndrome of microphthalmia, midfacial hypoplasia, hypotrichosis, and short stature, which is probably autosomal dominant with most cases being due to a fresh mutation (Fraser and Friedmann 1967). Micropenis and cryptorchidism are a regular feature of the Noonan syndrome of mental subnormality, neck webbing, pectus excavatum, and pulmonary stenosis most cases of which are sporadic but with occasional instances of parent–child transmission (Baird and DeJong 1972). Renal failure secondary to non-immune hydrops fetalis with severe hypoproteinaemia has also been reported in Noonan syndrome (Bawle and Black 1986). Micropenis and cryptorchidism also feature in the Robinow syndrome of short forearms, flat face, and genital hypoplasia, which is probably genetically heterogeneous (Wadia *et al.* 1978), and the Rothmund–Thomson syndrome of poikiloderma, cataract, small stature with small hands and feet, and other variable features of ectodermal dysplasia which is autosomal recessive (Hall *et al.* 1980). Another disorder with micropenis and cryptorchidism in males is the Prader–Willi syndrome of mental subnormality, small stature, small hands and feet, and infantile hypotonia. In a majority of cases with the complete clinical picture a small deletion within the long arm of chromosome 15 can be detected by high resolution banding techniques (Mattei *et al.* 1983; Niikawa and Ishikiriyama 1985). A small penis and testes with or without cryptorchidism are found in slightly less than half of all male patients with the autosomal recessive Fanconi's pancytopenia. Hypospadias is occasionally also present (Schroeder *et al.* 1976).

Finally, micropenis has been reported in one of two affected males, and vaginal septum or duplication in three females, with a new syndrome (Halal 1986). In addition to these genital anomalies the affected family members had upper limb abnormalities varying from postaxial polydactyly, through ectrodactyly, to upper limb hypoplasia with split hand. The syndrome showed an autosomal dominant pattern of inheritance.

References

Baird, P. A. and DeJong, B. P. (1972). Noonan's syndrome (XX and XY Turner phenotype) in three generations of a family. *J. Pediatr.* **80**, 110–14.

Bawle, E. V. and Black, V. (1986). Non-immune hydrops fetalis in Noonan's syndrome. *Am. J. Dis. Child.* **140**, 758–60.

Davenport, S. L. H., Hefner, M. A. and Mitchell, J. A. (1986). The spectrum of clinical features in CHARGE syndrome. *Clin. Genet.* **29**, 298–310.

Fraser, G. R. and Friedmann, A. I. (1967). *The causes of blindness in childhood.*

A study of 776 children with severe visual handicaps. p. 89. Johns Hopkins University Press, Baltimore.

Halal, F. (1986). A new syndrome of severe upper limb hypoplasia and Müllerian duct anomalies. *Am. J. Med. Genet.* **24**, 119–26.

Hall, B. D. (1979). Choanal atresia and associated multiple anomalies. *J. Pediatr.* **95**, 395–8.

Hall, J. C., Pagon, R. A. and Wilson, K. M. (1980). Rothmund–Thomson syndrome with severe dwarfism. *Am. J. Dis. Child.* **134**, 165–9.

Harper, R. G., Orti, E. and Baker, R. K. (1967). Bird-headed dwarfs (Seckel's syndrome). *J. Pediatr.* **70**, 799–804.

McKusick, V. A., Mahloudji, M., Abbott, M. H., Lindenberg, R. and Kepas, D. (1967). Seckel's bird-headed dwarfism. *New Engl. J. Med.* **277**, 279–86.

Mattei, J. F., Mattei, M. G. and Giraud, F. (1983). Prader–Willi syndrome and chromosome 15. *Hum. Genet.* **64**, 356–62.

Niikawa, N. and Ishikiriyama, S. (1985). Clinical and cytogenetic studies of the Prader–Willi syndrome: evidence of phenotype–karyotype correlation. *Hum. Genet.* **69**, 22–7.

Pagon, R. A., Graham, J. M., Zowana, J. and Yong, S.-I. (1981). Coloboma, congenital heart disease, and choanal atresia with multiple anomalies: CHARGE association. *J. Pediatr.* **99**, 223–7.

Schroeder, T. M., Tilgen, D., Kruger, J. and Vogel, F. (1976). Formal genetics of Fanconi's anemia. *Hum. Genet.* **32**, 257–88.

Siebert, J. R., Graham, J. M. Jr. and MacDonald, C. (1985). Pathologic features of the CHARGE association: support for involvement of the neural crest. *Teratology* **31**, 331–6.

——, Warkany, J. and Lemire, R. J. (1986). Atelencephalic microcephaly in a 21-week human fetus. *Teratology* **34**, 9–19.

Smith, D. W. (1982). *Recognizable patterns of human malformation,* 3rd edn. pp. 76–7. W.B. Saunders, Philadelphia.

Wadia, R. S., Shirole, D. B. and Dikshit, M. S. (1978). Recessively inherited costovertebral segmentation defect with mesomelia and peculiar facies (Covesdem syndrome)—a new genetic entity? *J. Med. Genet.* **16**, 162.

Weber, F. T., Frias, J. L., Julius, R. L. and Felman, A. H. (1978). Primary hypogonadism in the Borjeson–Forssman–Lehmann syndrome. *J. Med. Genet.* **15**, 63–6.

10.4. SECONDARY TO MISCELLANEOUS DYSMORPHIC SYNDROMES

10.4.1. Rubinstein–Taybi syndrome

This is a well-known syndrome of mental subnormality associated with short stature, microcephaly, downward slanting palpebral fissures, broad thumbs and great toes, and renal malformations (Rubinstein and Taybi 1963; Theile *et al.* 1978). The latter include renal agenesis, ureteral duplication and hydronephrosis (Rubinstein 1979). Smith (1982) states that malformations of the kidney are present in 50 per cent of cases, and

Beraud (1970) demonstrated 'rein multicaliciel', which from his description is probably an obstructive lesion.

Most cases are of sporadic occurrence. Simpson and Brissenden (1973) noted two out of 243 sibs of 112 patients to be affected, compared with a population incidence of 0.0003 per cent. Hence their estimate of a 1 per cent sib recurrence risk is a substantially increased risk. Gillies and Roussounis (1985) reported two familial cases which they considered support a polygenic aetiology. In one family the proband and an uncle had the complete syndrome, and three cousins showed reduced expression. In their second family a brother and sister were affected.

References

Beraud, C. (1970). Rein multicaliciel et syndrome de Rubinstein-Taybi. *J. Radiol. d'Electro. Med. Nucleaire* **51**, 197.

Gillies, D. R. N. and Roussounis, S. H. (1985). Rubinstein–Taybi syndrome: further evidence of a genetic aetiology. *Develop. Med. Child. Neurol.* **27**, 751–5.

Rubinstein, J. H. (1979). Broad thumb–hallux syndrome. In *Birth defects compendium*, 2nd edn., ed. Bergsma, D. p. 157. Alan R. Liss, New York.

—— and Taybi, H. (1963). Broad thumbs and toes and facial abnormalities. A possible mental retardation syndrome. *Am. J. Dis. Child.* **105**, 588–608.

Simpson, N. E. and Brissenden, J. E. (1973). The Rubinstein–Taybi syndrome: familial and dermatoglyphic data. *Am. J. Hum. Genet.* **25**, 225–9.

Smith, D. W. (1982). *Recognizable patterns of human malformation*, 3rd edn. p. 78. W. B. Saunders, Philadelphia.

Theile, U., Draf, U. and Heldt, J. P. (1978). Das Rubinstein–Taybi Syndrom. *Dtsch Med. Wschr.* **103**, 1505–10.

10.4.2. Apert and Saethre–Chotzen syndromes

These two syndromes are variants of acrocephalo-syndactyly. There is craniosynostosis, often with facial asymetry, and syndactyly of hands and feet in both disorders. They are distinguished by a flattened midface, often with a prominent supraorbital ridge, proptosis, downward-slanting palpebral fissures and frequent cleft patale or bifid uvula in Apert syndrome but ptosis, often unilateral, telecanthus, prominent crus of ear, and low frontal hairline in Saethre–Chotzen. Syndactyly is severe in Apert syndrome involving all the digits, or at least the ulnar four digits, in the hands, whereas it is mild in Saethre–Chotzen. When not involved in the syndactyly the thumbs are broad in both disorders. Both are probably autosomal dominant but expression is variable in Saethre–Chotzen and most cases of Apert syndrome are sporadic, presumably occurring as a result of fresh mutation. Patients with Apert syndrome may have polycystic kidneys or hydronephrosis, and similar renal abnormalities have been reported in Saethre–Chotzen (Bartsocas *et al.* 1970; Cohen 1977).

References

Bartsocas, C. S., Weber, A. L. and Crawford, J. D. (1970). Acrocephalosyndactyly type III: Chotzen's syndrome. *J. Pediatr.* **77**, 267–72.

Cohen, M. M. Jr. (1977). Genetic perspectives on craniosynostosis and syndromes with craniosynostosis. *J. Neurosurg.* **47**, 886–98.

10.4.3. Poland anomaly

This is one of two curiously unilateral disorders in this section. It comprises a unilateral deficiency of the pectoralis minor and usually of the sternal head of pectoralis major, often with absence of the nipple in the overlying skin. This defect is associated with limb and chest defects on the same side, most often a syndactyly of the hand but in the more severe cases including ipsilateral rib anomalies and even hypoplasia of the hand or even arm. Renal anomaly is an occasional further association (Ireland *et al.* 1976). Occurrence is sporadic.

Reference

Ireland, D. C. R., Takayama, N. and Flatt, A. E. (1976). Poland's syndrome: a review of forty-three cases. *J. Bone Jt. Surg.* **58A**, 52–8.

10.4.4. Thrombycytopenia–radial aplasia (TAR) syndrome

This autosomal recessive disorder combines skeletal and haematological defects. The skeletal defect consists of bilateral radial aplasia with ulnar hypoplasia but persistence of the thumbs. Haematologically there is thrombocytopenia with absent or defective megakaryocytes, and anaemia. There may be associated malformations of internal organs including the heart and the kidneys (Hall *et al.* 1969).

Reference

Hall, J. G., Levin, J., Kuhn, J. P., Ottenheimer, E. J., van Berkum, K. A. P. and McKusick, V. A. (1969). Thrombocytopenia with absent radius (TAR). *Medicine* **48**, 411–39.

10.4.5. CHILD syndrome

The acronym CHILD stands for Congenital Hemidysplasia with Ichthyosiform erythroderma and Limb Defects. The syndrome constitutes the second unilateral anomaly to be described in this section and is even more curious than the Poland anomaly, being both more severe and probably genetically determined. The skin lesion affects half of the body, usually the right half, with a sharp midline line of demarcation. In addition to erythroderma there is hyperkeratosis of nails on the same side. Ipsilateral skeletal defects vary from phalangeal hypoplasia to absence of a whole limb. The scapulae, pelvis, and vertebrae may also be involved. There may be ipsilateral visceral anomalies including renal defects, such as ipsilateral renal agenesis (Happle *et al.* 1980) and heart defects. Nineteen out of 20 reported patients have been girls, including two sisters (Falek *et al.* 1968), and a girl and her maternal and great maternal aunts (Kontras *et al.* 1975a and b). The suggestion that inheritance is X linked dominant, usually lethal in the male, is supported by the observation of 11 unaffected sisters to only three unaffected brothers of probands.

References

Falek, A., Heath, C. W., Ebbin, A. J. and McLean, W. R. (1968). Unilateral limb and skin deformities with congenital heart disease in two siblings: a lethal syndrome. *J. Pediatr.* **73**, 910–13.

Happle, R., Koch, H. and Lenz, W. (1980). The CHILD syndrome: congenital hemidysplasia with ichthyosiform erythroderma and limb defects. *Eur. J. Pediatr.* **134**, 27–33.

Kontras, S. B., Kataria, S., Eaton, A. P. and Flowers, F. P. (1975a). Congenital unilateral ichthyosiform erythroderma with ipsilateral hypoplasia of upper and lower limbs. *Birth Defects Orig. Art. Series* **11**(5), 333–4.

——, ——, —— and —— (1975b). Case report 27. *Syndrome Identification* **3**, 3–6.

10.4.6. EEC syndrome

EEC is another acronym, standing in this disorder for Ectrodactyly-Epidermal dysplasia–Clefting syndrome. Inheritance is autosomal dominant with very variable expression and even incomplete penetrance. The hair is fair, thin, and sparse, and the skin also pale and hyperkeratotic. The irides are blue and there is photophobia, often associated with lacrimal duct defects. There is cleft-lip with or without cleft-palate, and the lip may be cleft bilaterally. The limb defects vary from syndactyly to ectrodactyly. Renal anomalies, usually obstructive, are an occasional finding (Preus and Fraser 1973; Gorlin *et al.* 1976; London *et al.* 1985).

References

Gorlin, R. J., Pinborg, J. J. and Cohen, M. M. (1976). *Syndromes of the head and neck*, 2nd edn. McGraw-Hill, New York.
London, R., Heredia, R. M. and Israel, J. (1985). Urinary tract involvement in EEC syndrome. *Am. J. Dis. Child.* **139**, 1191–3.
Preus, M. and Fraser, F. C. (1973). The lobster claw defect, cleft lip/palate, tear duct anomaly and renal anomalies. *Clin. Genet.* **4**, 369–75.

10.4.7. Oculo-auriculo-vertebral (Goldenhar) syndrome

This syndrome, which involves the first and second branchial arches, is also known as the facio-auriculo-vertebral syndrome. As with many dysmorphic syndromes expression is variable, to the extent that many of the features in a particular patient may be unilateral.

The principle features that may be present are facial hypoplasia involving the malar region, maxilla, and mandible especially the ramus and condyle and the temporomandibular joint; severe malformation of the ear with microtia and preauricular tags and pits similar to the malformations seen in Treacher–Collins syndrome; hemivertebrae or hypoplastic vertebrae in cervical, or less often thoracic or lumbar region; and epibulbar dermoids of the conjunctiva or coloboma of the eyelids. Cardiac defects and renal anomalies, such as renal aplasia, duplication defects, and ectopia (Sugiura 1971), are occasional findings. This disorder is almost certainly genetically heterogeneous (Setzer *et al.* 1981).

References

Setzer, E. S., Ruiz-Castaneda, N., Severn, C., Ryden, S. and Frias, J. L. (1981). Etiologic heterogeneity in the oculo-auriculo-vertebral syndrome. *J. Pediatr.* **98**, 88–90.
Sugiura, Y. (1971). Congenital absence of the radius with hemifacial microsomia, ventricular septal defect and crossed renal ectopia. *Birth Defects Orig. Art. Series* **7**(7), 109–16.

10.4.8. VATER association

This is the last of the acronyms in this section, standing for Vertebral defects, Anal atresia, Tracheo-Esophageal fistula with esophageal atresia and Radial or Renal dysplasia (Quan and Smith 1973). Cardiac defects and a single umbilical artery are also commonly seen and the acryonym VACTERL has been used for the extended association, where C stands for cardiac, R for renal, and L for limb defects. Temtamy and Miller (1974) estimate that renal anomalies are present in 53 per cent of cases, and Barry and Auldist (1974) describe unilateral agenesis or hypoplasia and dysplasia as the renal anomalies to be found. The occurrence is sporadic.

References

Barry, J. E. and Auldist, A. W. (1974). The VATER association. *Am. J. Dis. Child.* **128**, 769–71.

Quan, L. and Smith, D. W. (1973). The VATER association, Vertebral defects, Anal atresia, T-E fistula with esophageal atresia, Radial and Renal dysplasia: a spectrum of associated defects. *J. Pediatr.* **82**, 104–7.

Temtamy, S. A. and Miller, J. D. (1974). Extending the scope of the VATER association: definition of a VATER syndrome. *J. Pediatr.* **85**, 345–9.

10.4.9. Familial extrahepatic biliary atresia

Krauss (1964) noted reports of five families in which two or more sibs had extrahepatic biliary atresia, and cardiac and renal malformations. There have been other reports of familial biliary atresia, including one pair of sibs with consanguineous parents, but not necessarily with renal malformation.

Reference

Krauss, A. N. (1964). Familial extrahepatic biliary atresia. *J. Pediatr.* **65**, 933–7.

10.4.10. Camptomelic dysplasia

This skeletal dysplasia with dwarfism was first described by Bound and coworkers (1952) as a disorder with congenital bowing of the tibiae. Further cases were reported by others (Bain and Barrett 1959; Spranger *et al.* 1970; Hoefnagel *et al.* 1972; Schmickel *et al.* 1973) to give a picture of infants of low birth weight who fail to thrive, with central nervous system disorder including apnoeic attacks, skeletal defects including anterior bowing of tibiae and femora with a dimple at the point of maximum convexity, scapula hypoplasia and flat facies, and neonatal death from respiratory failure.

Khajavi and colleagues (1976) delineated three distinct varieties of camptomelic dysplasia: a relatively common long-limbed form with bowing of otherwise normal femora and tibiae, and two rare short-limbed forms. The short-limbed forms are associated with short, wide, bowed long bones in both upper and lower limbs, and are distinguished by the fact that in one variety there is also craniosynostosis with a clover-leaf skull deformity.

There have been occasional reports of genito-urinary anomalies in this disorder. Mellows and coworkers (1980) described hydronephrosis in one of two affected sisters with the long-limbed variety. Pauli and Pagon (1980) reported a boy with the long-limbed variety who had hypospadias and bifid scrotum, and mentioned similar previously published cases. Gorlin and Langer (1978) commented that hydronephrosis and hydroureter was present in the autopsied cases reviewed by them.

Inheritance has usually been regarded as autosomal recessive on the basis of several reports of affected sibs (Stuve and Wiedemann 1971; Mellows *et al.* 1980; Fryns *et al.* 1981). Gorlin and Langer (1978) reviewed 11 cases and note parental consanguinity as well as sib occurrence. Cremin and colleagues (1973) have also described parental consanguinity. A high proportion of female cases of the long-limbed type have a male karyotype: 46,XY, indicating that in these cases there is a failure of the normal mechanism of sex determination (Schmickel *et al.* 1973; Hoefnagel *et al.* 1978). Fryns and associates (1981) reported prenatal diagnosis.

References

Bain, A. D. and Barrett, H. S. (1959). Congenital bowing of the long bones: report of a case. *Arch. Dis. Child.* **34**, 516–24.

Bound, J. P., Finlay, H. V. L. and Rose, F. C. (1952). Congenital anterior angulation of the tibia. *Arch. Dis. Child.* **27**, 179–84.

Cremin, B. J., Orsmond, G. and Beighton, P. (1973). Autosomal recessive inheritance in camptomelic dwarfism. *Lancet* **1**, 488–9.

Fryns, J. P., van den Berghe, K., van Assche, A. and van den Berghe, H. (1981). Prenatal diagnosis of campomelic dwarfism. *Clin. Genet.* **19**, 199–201.

Gorlin, R. J. and Langer, L. O. (1978). Dyssegmental dwarfism (?s): lethal anisospondylic camptomicromelic dwarfism. *Birth Defects Orig. Art. Series* **14**(6B), 193–7.

Hoefnagel, D., Wurster, D., Carey, D., Harris, G. J. and Pilliod, J. (1972). Camptomelic dwarfism. *Lancet* **1**, 1068.

——, Wurster-Hill, D. H., Dupree, W. B., Benirschke, K. and Fuld, G. L. (1978). Camptomelic dwarfism associated with XY-gonadal dysgenesis and chromosome anomaly. *Clin. Genet.* **13**, 489–99.

Khajavi, A., Lachman, R., Rimoin, D., Schimke, R. N., Dorst, J., Handmaker, S., Ebbin, A. and Perreault, G. (1976). Heterogeneity in the camptomelic syndromes. *Radiology* **120**, 641–7.

Mellows, H. J., Pryse-Davies, J., Bennett, M. J. and Carter, C. O. (1980). The camptomelic syndrome in two female siblings. *Clin. Genet.* **18**, 137–41.

Pauli, R. M. and Pagon, R. A. (1980). Abnormalities of sexual differentiation in camptomelic dwarfs. *Clin. Genet.* **18**, 223–5.

Schmickel, R. D., Heidelberger, K. P. and Poznanski, A. K. (1973). The campomelique syndrome. *J. Pediatr.* **82**, 299–302.

Spranger, J., Langer, L. O. and Maroteaux, P. (1970). Increasing frequency of a syndrome of multiple osseous defects? *Lancet* **2**, 716.
Stuve, A. and Wiedemann, H.-R. (1971). Congenital bowing of the long bones in two sisters. *Lancet* **2**, 495.

10.4.11. Weyers syndrome

Weyers reported two unrelated patients with preaxial digital deficiency due to absence or hypoplasia of ulnar and fibular rays, antecubital pterygia, reduced sternal segments, and congenital malformations of the spleen and kidneys (1957). One of his patients also had cleft-lip and -palate, and the other had maxillary hypoplasia, dental deformities, and hypoplasia of the lateral end of the clavicle. Further cases have been reported by others (De la Chapelle *et al.* 1972; Elejalde *et al.* 1985). The renal malformations are mainly hydronephrosis but are not invariable. In the second of Elejalde and colleagues' cases hydronephrosis was bilateral but was gross on the left side, filling most of the abdominal cavity. Inheritance is probably autosomal recessive, sibs having been reported by De la Chapelle and colleagues (1972) and by Elejalde and colleagues (1985). The latter group report a prenatal diagnosis by ultrasound at 19 weeks on their second infant.

References

De la Chapelle, A., Maroteaux, P., Havu, N. and Granroth, G. (1972). Une rare dysplasie osseuse lethale de transmission recessive autosomique. *Arch. Fr. Pédiatr.* **29**, 759–70.
Elejalde, B. R., de Elejalde, M. M., Booth, C., Kaye, C. and Hollison, L. (1985). Prenatal diagnosis of Weyers syndrome (deficient ulnar and fibular rays with bilateral hydronephrosis). *Am. J. Med. Genet.* **21**, 439–44.
Weyers, H. (1957). Das Oligdactylie Syndrom des Menschen und seine Parellel-mutation bei der Hausmaus. *Ann. Paediatr.* **189**, 351–70.

10.4.12. Digito-reno-cerebral syndrome

Eronen and others (1985) have recently reported a family in which the propositus, a boy, and two sisters who were first cousins and also double second cousins of the propositus, had a previously unreported acro-renal syndrome. The mother of the propositus had also had seven miscarriages at 9–17 weeks, including four macerated fetuses. The parents were un-related but came from the same area of Finland. All three affected members of the family had complete absence of terminal phalanges and nails of all fingers and toes. The propositus had unilateral renal agenesis, whereas one of his two cousins had bilateral cystic renal dysplasia and the other had recurrent urinary tract infection but died without this being fully elucidated. All three had convulsions starting within the neonatal period associated in one with microcephaly, and in the other two with lateral ventricle dilatation. The propositus at 10 months was severely mentally retarded and had bilateral optic atrophy.

In view of the family history the disorder is likely to be autosomal recessive.

References

Eronen, M., Somer, G., Gustafsson, B. and Holmberg, C. (1985). New syndrome: a digito-reno-cerebral syndrome. *Am. J. Med. Genet.* **22**, 281–5.

11. Renal tract infection

There has long been an interest in the role of genetic factors in human infection, in terms both of the virulence of the infecting organism and of the resistance of the patient. As far as the renal tract is concerned this interest has been stimulated by the work of several groups, mainly Swedish and Finnish, who have shown that bacterial adhesion to urinary tract epithelial cells is necessary for the establishment of pyelonephritic infection (Svanborg Eden *et al.* 1976, 1978; Fowler and Stamey 1977; Kallenius and Winberg 1978) and that this adhesion is determined by bacterial surface adhesins and by host epithelial cell receptors (Kallenius *et al.* 1980a and b, 1981b). Most urinary tract infections are due to *Escherichia coli.* To ascend against the urine flow the bacteria need to adhere to the epithelial surface, and strains unable to do so merely produce an asymptomatic bacteriuria or at most cystitis. The severity of infection correlates with the ability of the infecting strain to adhere to human uroepithelial cells *in vitro* (Svanborg Eden *et al.* 1976). Greater adhesion to such cells has been reported in patients with frequent urinary tract infections compared with healthy controls (Fowler and Stamey 1977; Kallenius and Winberg 1978; Svanborg Eden and Jodal 1979), possibly due to a higher receptor incidence (Svanborg Eden and Jodal 1979). *E. coli* adherence and urinary tract infection have recently been reviewed by Svanborg Eden (1986).

The adherence of pyelonephritogenic *E. coli* is determined by P-blood-group-specific adhesins (Korhonen *et al.* 1980, 1981) on the filamentous protein pili or fimbriae of the bacteria, termed P fimbriae (Brinton 1965). The degree of adherence correlates with the ability of the bacteria to cause a D-mannose-resistant specific haemagglutination of human erythrocytes (Kallenius and Molby 1979; Kallenius *et al.* 1980c; Hagberg *et al.* 1981; Korhonen *et al.* 1981) or synthetic particle agglutination (Svenson *et al.* 1982), a phenomenon which is more readily quantifiable than epithelial cell adhesion and which has therefore been widely used in the study of bacterial virulence for the urinary tract. Kallenius and colleagues (1981a), using inhibition of haemagglutination in the presence of mannose by P antigen, found that 33 out of 35 (91 per cent) of the *E. coli* strains causing acute pyelonephritis in children carried P fimbriae, whereas only 19 per cent and 14 per cent respectively of the strains causing cystitis or asymptomatic bacteriuria did so. Only 7 per cent of *E. coli* isolated from faeces of healthy controls carried P fimbriae. Similar findings were later reported by the same group (Vaisanen *et al.* 1981) who found that 29 out of 32 (91 per cent) of *E. coli* strains isolated from children with pyelonephritis showed mannose-resistant haemagglutination. P specificity associated with specific *E. coli* O and K antigens was found in 81 per cent of these mannose-resistant haemagglutinating strains and another separate X specificity in a further 19 per cent. In contrast Harber and associates (1982a) found that all but one of the urinary pathogens isolated from 20 female patients with urinary tract infection were non-fimbriate and non-adherent when freshly isolated, although after repeated subcultures 14 out of 20 strains developed fimbriae and became adherent. They argued from this evidence that adherence is not after all a virulence factor for bacteria once they have entered the urinary tract. However, as subsequently pointed out by Makela and Korhonen (1982) and by Svanborg Eden and colleagues (1982) only three of their patients had acute pyelonephritis, the remainder having cystitis (seven patients), or were symptomless (10 patients). However, the experimental conditions differed from those of the Scandinavian workers. Sussman and others (1982) produced evidence that a filtration step in Harber and associates' procedure was likely to remove fimbriated in preference to non-fimbriated organisms.

More recently Kallenius and Svenson's group, in collaboration with American workers, have confirmed the pathogenicity of P-fimbriated *E. coli* (Dominigue *et al.* 1985). They used a P-receptor-specific particle agglutination test to identify P-fimbriated bacteria among over 2000 isolates from patients with bacteriuria. The patients were male and female and ranged in age from infancy to 91 years. Ten per cent of all isolates, all *E. coli*, were P fimbriated. These comprised 21.5 per cent of all *E. coli* isolates. In cases of non-obstructive acute pyelonephritis all of the infecting bacteria were P fimbriated, whereas in the presence of urinary tract obstruction infection was associated with a variety of bacterial strains, with or without P fimbriae. In non-obstructive pyelonephritis biological characteristics of the infecting bacteria, other than P fimbriation, were unrelated to virulence. Kallenius and Svenson's group have provided further confirmation of the pathogenicity of P-fimbriated *E. coli* in children with urinary tract infection (Elo *et al.* 1985). They isolated P-fimbriated *E. coli* from 77 per cent of cases of pyelonephritis compared with 22–23 per cent in cystitis or asymptomatic bacteriuria. The frequency of P fimbriae in organisms isolated was related to clinical severity, but not to the presence or absence of reflux or obstruction.

Another recent study found that the DNA of all of 12 pyelonephritic strains of *E. coli* hybridized to a gene probe for the P-fimbrial adhesin, compared with only 29 per cent of control strains (O'Hanley *et al.* 1985). The authors defined this adhesin as one binding to the GAL—GAL epithelial cell surface receptor described below. They also found hybridization of a probe for a haemolysin gene to nine out of the 12 pyelonephritic strains, but only 14 per cent of control strains. Despite Harber and associates' (1982b) defence of their position, and support for that position from one other group (Schwatz *et al.* 1982), the balance of evidence must now be regarded as being in favour of specific fimbrial antigens acting as virulence factors through adherence to urinary tract epithelial cells. These bacterial antigens are of course themselves genetically determined, and appear to be plasmid encoded (Morris *et al.* 1982; Normark *et al.* 1983). Although P fimbriae are the predominant specific type of adhesin found in association with upper urinary tract infection they are not the only one. The X-specific factor that recognizes an unidentified receptor on the host cell surface, discovered by Vaisanen and colleagues (1981), has already been mentioned. The same group have reported the isolation of a strain with a blood-group-M-specific haemagglutinin (Vaisenen *et al.* 1982).

The P fimbriae of a majority of pyelonephritogenic *E. coli* isolated from children bind to a receptor on the surface of erythrocytes, and uroepithelial cells, which is a carbohydrate-forming part of the glycosphingolipid of the P-blood-group system (Kallenius *et al.* 1980a and b; Leffler and Svanborg Eden 1980). The receptor on red blood cells has been shown to be a disaccharide of the constitution α-D-galactopyranosyl-β-D-galactopyranoside (α-D-Gal$p$-(1→4)-β-D-Gal$p$) (Kallenius *et al.* 1980a and b). Kallenius and Winberg (1978) noted that uroepithelial cells from girls prone to upper urinary tract infections have a greater capacity for binding pyelonephritogenic *E. coli* than similar cells from healthy controls. Red cells of the very rare p̄ blood group do not bind virulent *E. coli* as they lack the receptor for P fimbriae (Kallenius *et al.* 1980b). A group of 30 individuals with the p̄ phenotype has been identified in one Swedish county and represent about half of all known p̄ subjects (Cedergren 1973). None of these individuals has had urinary tract infection. Kallenius and colleagues (1981b) studied the binding of pyelonephritogenic *E. coli* by uroepithelial cells from patients of P_1, P_2, and p̄ phenotypes. The cells from p̄ subjects bound the bacteria to a significantly less extent than those from P_1 or P_2 subjects. Furthermore the binding by uroepithelial cells from P_1 subjects was blocked by α-D-Gal$p$-(1→4)-β-D-Gal$p$ thus demonstrating that this dissacharide is absent from uroepithelial, as well as red blood, cells of p̄ subjects, and that it is the receptor for P-fimbriated *E. coli*. There is also evidence that the P_1 phenotype is more common than P_2 among children with recurrent urinary tract infection (Lomberg *et al.* 1981). Lomberg and associates (1983) have also demonstrated that the high frequencies of P_1 blood group and of bacterial attachment in girls with recurrent pyelonephritis do not hold when there is an associated vesico-ureteral reflux.

Most of the above studies relate to children, mainly girls. The only comparable study to have been undertaken in adult women is that of Domingue and colleagues (1985) discussed above. Further adult studies are obviously needed. There have, however, been a few studies of ABO and secretor phenotypes among adult patients. Cruz-Coke and colleagues (1965) found that Chilean patients of blood group B had a 50 per cent greater probability of contracting *E. coli* urinary tract infections than those of other blood groups. A Scottish study of 319 girls and women, aged 10–80 years, with recurrent urinary tract infection confirmed this finding (Kinane *et al.* 1982). Women of blood groups B and AB who were non-secretors had a relative risk of urinary tract infection of 3.12 compared with women of other types. Further confirmation comes from a study in Texas (Ratner *et al.* 1986). The mechanism of this susceptibility has not been investigated .

Finally plasmid encoded haemolysins also influence the virulence of nephropathogenic *E. coli* (Hughes *et al.* 1982; Waalwijk *et al.* 1982; Hacker *et al.* 1983). Hacker and colleagues in an experimental study in mice found that cloned haemolysin genes from pyelonephritogenic *E. coli* determined different levels of toxicity.

References

Brinton, C. C. Jr. (196). The structure, function, synthesis and genetic control of bacterial pili and a molecular model for DNA and RNA transport in gram-negative bacteria. *Trans. NY Acad. Sci.* **27**, 1003–54.

Cedergren, B. (1973). Population studies in northern Sweden. IV. Frequency of the blood type p̄. *Hereditas* **73**, 27–30.

Cruz-Coke, R., Parades, L. and Monengro, A. (1965). Blood groups and urinary microorganisms. *J. Med. Genet.* **2**, 185–8.

Domingue, G. J., Roberts, J. A., Laucirica, R., Ratner, M. H., Bell, D. P., Suarez, G. M., Kallenius, G. and Svenson, S. (1985). Pathogenic significance of P-fimbrited *Escherichia coli* in urinary tract infections. *J. Urol.* **133**, 983–9.

Elo, J., Tallgren, L. G., Väisänen, V., Korhonen, T. K., Svenson, S. B., and Makela, P. H. (1985). Association of P and other fimbriae with clinical pyelonephritis in children. *Scand. J. Urol. Nephrol.* **19**, 281–4.

Fowler, J. E. Jr. and Stamey, T. A. (1977). Studies of introital colonization in women with recurrent urinary infections. VII. The role of bacterial adherence. *J. Urol.* **117**, 442–76.

Hacker, J., Hughes, C., Hof, H. and Goebel, W. (1983). Cloned hemolysin genes from *Escherichia coli* that cause urinary tract infection determine different levels of toxicity in mice. *Infect. Immunol.* **42**, 57–63.

Hagberg, L., Jodal, U., Korhonen, T. K., Lidin-Janson, G., Lindberg, U. and Svanborg-Eden, C. (1981). Adhesion, hemagglutination, and virulence of *Escherichia coli* causing urinary tract infections. *Infect. Immunol.* **31**, 564–70.

Harber, M. J., Chick, S., MacKenzie, R. and Asscher, A. W. (1982a). Lack of adherence to epithelial cells by freshly isolated urinary antigens. *Lancet* **1**, 586–8.

——, MacKenzie, R. K. and Asscher, A. W. (1982b). Bacterial adherence and the urinary tract (letter). *Lancet* **1**, 1352–3.

Hughes, C., Philips, R. and Roberts, A. P. (1982). Serum resistance among *Escherichia coli* strains causing urinary tract infection in relation to O type and the carriage of hemolysin, colicin and antibiotic resistance determinants. *Infect. Immunol.* **35**, 270–5.

Kallenius, G. and Mollby, R. (1979). Adhesion of *Escherichia coli* to human periurethral cells correlated to mannose-resistant agglutination of human erythrocytes. *FEMS Microbiol. Lett.* **5**, 295–9.

—— and Winberg, J. (1978). Bacterial adherence to periurethral epithelial cells in girls prone to urinary-tract infections. *Lancet* **2**, 540–3.

——, Mollby, R., Svenson, S. B., Winberg, J. and Hultberg, H. (1980a). Identification of a carbohydrate receptor recognized by uropathogenic *Escherichia coli*. *Infection*, suppl. 3, S288–S293.

——, ——, ——, ——, Lundblad, L., Svenson, S. and Cedergren, B. (1980b). The P^k antigen as receptor for the haemagglutinin of pyelonephritic *Escherichia coli*. *FEMS Microbiol. Lett.* **7**, 297–302.

——, ——, ——, Helin, I., Hultberg, H., Cedergren, B. and Winberg, J. (1981a). Occurrence of P-fimbriated *Escherichia coli* in urinary tract infections. *Lancet* **2**, 1369–72.

——, Svenson, S. B., Mollby, R., Cedergren, B., Hultberg, H. and Winberg, J. (1981b). Structure of carbohydrate part of receptor on human uroepithelial cells for pyelonephritogenic *Escherichia coli*. *Lancet* **2**, 604–6.

——, Mollby, R. and Winberg, J. (1980c). *In vitro* adhesion or uropathogenic *Escherichia coli* to human periurethral cells. *Infect. Immunol.* **28**, 972–80.

Kinane, D. F., Blackwell, C. C., Brettle, R. P., Weir, D. M., Winstanley, F. P. and Elton, R. A. (1982). ABO blood group, secretor state, and susceptibility to recurrent urinary tract infection in women. *Br. Med. J.* **285**, 7–9.

Korhonen, T. K., Eden, S. and Svanborg-Eden, C. (1980). Binding of purified *Escherichia coli* pili to human urinary tract epithelial cells. *FEMS Microbiol. Lett.* **7**, 237–40.

——, Leffler, H. and Svanborg-Eden, C. (1981). Binding specificity of pilated strains of *Escherichia coli* and *Salmonella typhimurium* to epithelial cells, *Saccharomyces cerevisiae* cells, and erythrocytes. *Infect. Immunol.* **32**, 796–804.

Leffler, H. and Svanborg, Eden, C. (1980). Chemical identification of a glycosphingolipid receptor for *Escherichia coli* attaching to human urinary tract epithelial cells and agglutinating human erythrocytes. *FEMS Microbiol. Lett.* **8**, 127–34.

Lomberg, H., Jodal, U., Svanborg Eden, C., Leffler, H. and Samuelsson, B. (1981). P_1 blood group and urinary tract infection. *Lancet* **1**, 551–2.

——, Hanson, L. A., Jacobsson, B., Jodal, U., Leffler, H. and Svanborg Eden, C. (1983). Correlation of P blood group, vesicoureteral reflux, and bacterial attachment in patients with recurrent pyelonephritis. *New Engl. J. Med.* **308**, 1189–92.

Makela, P. H. and Korhonen, T. K. (1982). Bacterial adherence and urinary tract infection (letter). *Lancet* **1**, 961.

Morris, J. A., Thorns, C. J., Scott, A. C. and Sojka, W. J. (1982). Adhesive properties associated with the Vir plasmid: a transmissible pathogenic characteristic associated with strains of invasive *Escherichia coli*. *J. Gen. Microbiol.* **128**, 2097–103.

Normark, S., Lark, D., Hull, R., Norgren, M., Baga, M., O'Hanley, P., Schoolnik, G. and Falkow, S. (1983). Genetics of digalactoside-binding adhesin from a uropathogenic *Escherichia coli* strain. *Infect. Immunol.* **41**, 942–9.

O'Hanley, P., Low, D., Romero, I., Lark, D., Vosti, K., Falkow, S. and Schoolnik, G. (1985). Gal–Gal binding and hemolysin phenotypes and genotypes associated with uropathogenic *Escherichia coli*. *New Engl. J. Med.* **313**, 414–20.

Ratner, J. J., Thomas, V. L. and Forland, (1986). Relationships between human blood groups, bacterial pathogens, and urinary tract infections. *Am. J. Med. Sci.* **292**, 87–91.

Schwatz, J., Menoret, P., Begue, P. and Lasfargues, G. (1982). Bacterial adherence and urinary tract infection (letter). *Lancet* **2**, 108.

Sussman, M., Parry, S. H., Rooke, D. M. and Lee, M. J. S. (1982). Bacterial adherence and the urinary tract (letter). *Lancet* **1**, 1352.

Svanborg, Eden, C. (1986). Review: bacterial adherence in urinary tract infections caused by *Eschericia coli*. *Scand. J. Urol. Nephrol.* **20**, 81–8.

—— and Jodal, U. (1979). Attachment of *Escherichia coli* to sediment epithelial cells from UTI prone and healthy children. *Infect. Immunol.* **26**, 837–40.

——, Hanson, L. A., Jodal, U., Lindberg, U. and Sohl Akerlund, A. (1976). Variable adhesion to normal human urinary tract epithelial cells of *Escherichia coli* strains associated with various forms of urinary tract infection. *Lancet* **2**, 490–2.

——, Hagberg, L., Hanson, L. A., Lomberg, H., Orskov, I. and Orkov, F. (1982). Bacterial adherence and urinary tract infection (letter). *Lancet* **1**, 961–2.

——, Eriksson, B., Hansson, L. A., Jodal, U., Kaijser, B., Lidin Janson, G., Lindberg, U. and Olling, S. (1978). Adhesion to normal human uroepithelial cells of *Escherichia coli* from children with various forms of urinary tract infection. *J. Pediatr.* **93**, 398–403.

Svenson, S. B., Kallenius, G., Mollby, R., Hultberg, H. and Winberg, J. (1982). Rapid identification of P-fimbriated *Escherichia coli* by a receptor-specific particle agglutination test. *Infection* **10**, 209–14.

Vaisanen, V., Elo, J., Tallgren, L. G., Siitonen, A., Makela, P. H., Svanborg-Eden, C., Kallenius, G., Svenson, S. B., Hultberg, H. and Korhonen, T. (1981). Mannose-resistant haemagglutination and P antigen recognition are characteristic of *Escherichia coli* causing primary pyelonephritis. *Lancet* **2**, 1366–9.

——, Korhonen, T. K., Jokinen, M., Gahmberg, C. G. and Ehnholm, C. (1982). Blood group M specific haemagglutinin in pyelonephritogenic *Escherichia coli* (letter). *Lancet* **1**, 1192.

Waalwijk, C., Van den Bosch, J. F., Mallaren, D. M. and De Graaff, J. (1982). Hemolysin plasmid encoding for the virulence of a nephropathogenic *Escherichia coli* strain. *Infect. Immunol.* **35**, 32–7.

12. Urinary tract neoplasia

12.1. RENAL

12.1.1. Wilms' tumour (nephroblastoma, embryonal carcinoma)

Wilms' tumour is one of the well-recognized tumours occurring in young children. About three-quarters of patients are under 4 years of age at the time of diagnosis. Patients with bilateral tumours tend to present earlier than those with a unilateral tumour, exceptionally even at birth. At the opposite extreme Wilms' tumour rarely presents in adult life (Roth *et al.* 1984). The onset is usually insidious, with gradual abdominal enlargement, so that the tumour may have metastasized before the development of symptoms. A rare presentation of nephroblastoma, in association with nephrotic syndrome, has been observed in sibs (Zunin and Soave 1964). Klapproth (1959) reported 45 new cases and analysed 1351 reported cases in one of the earlier reviews. It is the second most common malignant tumour of childhood, accounting for about 20 per cent of tumours in this age group (Robbins 1967).

As there are several other renal tumours, mostly less malignant than Wilms', that are congenital or infantile in onset diagnosis can only be made histologically. Wilms' tumours usually remain encapsulated until fairly large but eventually extend into the surrounding renal parenchyma and into omentum and adjacent viscera. Microscopically there are sheets of embryonic connective tissue cells with dark nuclei that here and there form tubular or rosette-like glandular structures (Fig. 12.1). Epithelial cells may be present, forming solid cords and strands of cells, and even abortive glomerular-like structures may be seen. Tumour cells bind antibodies to cytokeratin and epithelial membrane antigens similarly to normal renal tissue (Wick *et al.* 1986). Occasionally muscle (fetal rhabdomyomatosis), cartilage or myxomatous tissue may be present. A papillary Wilms' tumour with renal carcinoma like foci has recently been described (Kodet and Marsden 1985).

Bolande (1974) has reviewed the differential diagnosis of congenital and infantile primary renal tumours. Apart from true Wilms' tumour, which is in fact rare within the first few months of life, there are three main types of renal tumour seen: congenital mesoblastic nephroma of infancy, well-differentiated epithelial nephroblastoma, and nephroblastomatosis or nodular renal blastema. The most common of these

606

(A)

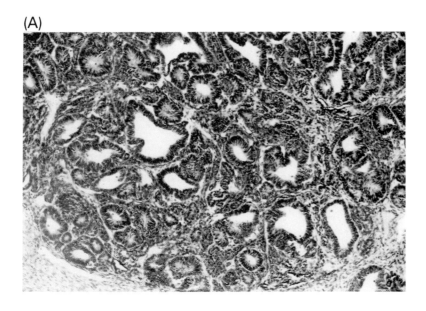

(B)

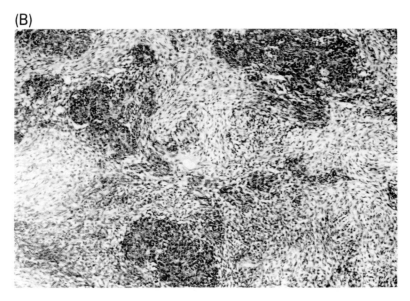

Fig. 12.1. Histological appearance of Wilms' tumour, kindly provided by Dr A. Price, (A) well differentiated, (B) undifferentiated (both ×100) and photographed by the Medical Illustration Department, Clinical Research Centre.

early renal tumours is congenital mesoblastic nephroma of infancy (fetal renal hamartoma or leiomyomatous hamartoma). It is a large, usually congenital, tumour with a fibrous stroma containing dysplastic tubules and glomeruli, angioid, and cartilagenous elements (Fig. 12.2) (Bolande 1973; Marsden and Newton 1986). Thus its histological appearance is very akin to that of non-tumerous renal dysplasia, suggesting a possibly similar origin. As might be expected it is nearly always benign and amenable to simple nephrectomy. In only a few instances have such tumours proved to be malignant.

Another comparatively rare benign tumour is the well-differentiated epithelial nephroblastoma. It is a single well-circumscribed tumour with distinct tubules or cysts of renal epithelium. Connective tissue stroma is

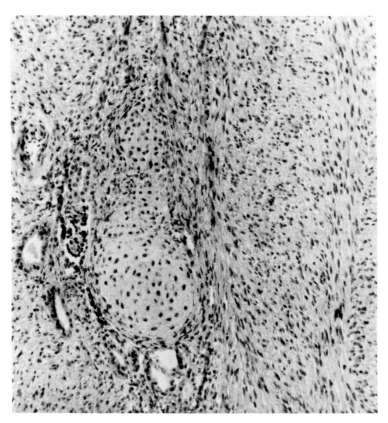

Fig. 12.2. Congenital mesoblastic nephroma of infancy (×120). Reproduced with permission from Bolande (1973) Congenital mesoblastic nephroma in infancy. In *Perspectives in pediatric pathology*, Vol. 1, eds. H. S. Rosenberg and R. P. Bolande, Copyright 1973 by Year Book Medical Publishers, Inc., Chicago.

inconspicuous. Several distinct patterns may be seen including benign multilocular cystic nephroma or polycystic nephroma consisting of large cysts lined by low cuboidal epithelium (Bolande 1971; Egerdie *et al.* 1986), tubular Wilms' tumour consisting of cysts and tubules similar in appearance to mature renal tubules, and papillary adenoma with infolded tubular lining.

Diffuse nephroblastomatosis or nodular renal blastema is a less well-defined congenital renal defect. It consists of small, often microscopic, discrete subcapsular nodules of primitive metanephric epithelium. The nodules are usually bilateral but can be unilateral. They are usually only incidental autopsy findings, being found in 1 in 200–400 autopsies on infants under the age of 4 months (Hou and Holman 1961; Potter 1961; Bove *et al.* 1969; Shanklin and Sotelo-Avila 1969). Since they are rarely observed over this age it is presumed that most of these lesions regress. Exceptionally the nodules may be massive, becoming confluent, and result in renal enlargement. Some such cases have been diagnosed as multicentric Wilms' tumour, or alternatively give rise to true tumours, as for example in the sporadic cases of Neuhauser (1960), Gyepes and Bucko (1964), Bishop and Hope (1966), and Anderson and colleagues (1968). The dysgenetic changes in the kidneys of Cochran and Froggatt's (1967) sibs may be of similar origin. Nodular renal blastema shows an association with malformation, not only of the kidney itself as in trisomy 18 (Bove *et al.* 1969), but of other tissues such as splenic agenesis and liver malformation (Vlachos and Tsakraklides 1968) and Klippel-Trenaunay syndrome (Mankad *et al.* 1974). A familial form of diffuse nephroblastomatosis has been described in an Israeli Yemenite kindred with second-cousin parents, consisting of six affected infants out of a family of seven, with fetal gigantism and visceromegaly, hypoglycaemia with hyperplasia of the Islets of Langerhans, odd facies, and renal hamartomas (Liban and Kozenitzky 1970; Perlman *et al.* 1973, 1975). One of the affected children in this family developed Wilms' tumour. Neri and colleagues (1984), who reported a further family with two affected sibs, proposed the term 'Perlman syndrome' for this apparently autosomal recessive disorder. A further possible case with associated Wilms' tumour was reported by Greenberg and associates (1986).

It has been suggested by Knudson and Strong (1972) and others that these nodular lesions constitute a nephroblastoma-in-situ that may give rise to subsequent true Wilms' tumour. Indeed Bove and coworkers (1969) found nodular renal blastema in eight out of 46 kidneys removed for Wilms' tumour, which in five of these was bilateral. More recent studies suggest that nephroblastomatosis is a precursor lesion in up to 50 per cent of Wilms' tumours and in almost all bilateral cases (Machin and McCaughey 1984). Bove and coworkers (1969) and Vlachos and

Tsakraklides (1968) found cystic and dysplastic changes in kidneys with nephroblastomatosis, once again hinting at a common origin, as with congenital mesoblastic nephroma. Recently Machin and McCaughey (1984) have described a new type of nephroblastomatosis, a deep cortical or intralobular multifocal form, rather than the usual superficial type, in four children with Wilms' tumour. These children had tumours with a distinct histological picture, the fetal rhabdomyomatous type. The eventual elucidation of the relationship between these various types of renal developmental lesion will have to await future studies.

Returning to the consideration of true Wilms' tumour, estimates of incidence vary surprisingly little. Leck (1977) basing his figures on the University of Manchester Children's Tumour Registry, and using cases presenting under the age of 15 years from 1954 to 1973, gives an annual incidence per million of 5.5 and a cumulative incidence per thousand live-born children of 0.08. This compares closely with Cochran and Froggat's (1967) earlier estimate of 1 per 10 000 live-births and with American (Young and Miller 1975), Japanese (Hanawa 1978), and other British (Mott 1975) estimates of annual incidence per million of 8, 5, and 5 respectively. However, Glen and Rhame (1961) estimated an annual incidence of only 2 per million. Despite the insidious onset survival has greatly improved, since the introduction of radiotherapy and cytotoxic drug therapy, to over 70 per cent at 5 years (Leck 1977). In the American study the annual incidence of 8 per million was the same in Blacks and Whites (Young and Miller 1975). Cochran and Froggatt (1967), on the basis of a review of published cases from 13 different countries, found that both kidneys were involved in 4.1 per cent of cases. In what proportion these bilateral cases represent independent development of nephroblastoma in each kidney, whether against a background of diffuse nephroblastomatosis or not, or metastasis from one kidney to the other is not known. Cochran and Froggatt argue that the true incidence of bilateral involvement is probably higher as not all cases come to autopsy and furthermore that some unilateral cases would have become bilateral if the patient had lived longer. On the other hand, they ignore the likelihood that bilateral cases will have been more fully reported. Other estimates of the proportion of bilateral cases have varied from 0.5 per cent in the United States (Abeshouse 1957) and 1.4 per cent in Britain (Riches *et al.* 1951) to Wilms' own early estimate of 7.2 per cent (Wilms' 1899). Knudson and Strong (1972) give a figure of 5–10 per cent of all Wilms' tumours being bilateral, compared to 21 per cent of hereditary Wilms' tumours. In an analysis of 103 reported bilateral cases they found, as with familial cases, an earlier age of onset and an exponential decrease with age in the proportion of cases not yet diagnosed. This pattern is not seen with unselected unilateral cases.

Like diffuse nephroblastomatosis Wilms' tumour itself shows a remarkable association with certain malformations suggesting a teratogenic origin. The earliest reported such association was with hemihypertrophy. Lenstrup recorded this association in a description of eight cases of hemihypertrophy over 50 years ago (Lenstrum 1927). Although numerous subsequent reports of this association have appeared (Riedel 1952; Bjorklund 1955; Sulas 1955; Scarabicchi *et al.* 1960; Schaeffer 1960; Benson *et al.* 1963; Barber and Spiers 1964; Hart and Naunton 1964; Miller *et al.* 1964; Miller 1966; Fraumeni *et al.* 1967; Boxer and Smith 1970) the incidence of this combined abnormality must be very low. Fraumeni and colleagues (1967) record seven instances of hemihypertrophy among 225 patients with Wilms' tumour. The association has in every case involved unilateral Wilms' tumour, which is usually associated with superficial multifocal nephroblastomatosis (Machin 1980); but the hemihypertrophy has varied, being total or partial, ipsilateral, contralateral, or even crossed (Bjorklund 1955). Miller and others (1964), in a study of congenital malformations among 440 cases of childhood Wilms' tumour, found three with hemihypertrophy and 13 other instances described by the authors listed above prior to 1964. Wilms' tumour developing in a kidney with nephroblastomatosis has recently been reported in association with hemihypertrophy (Mottu *et al.* 1981). In view of the extreme rarity of hemihypertrophy it is most improbable that this association is a chance one.

There have also been several reports of the association of Wilms' tumour with other urinary tract abnormalities, especially horseshoe kidney and duplication defects (Lathem and Smith 1962; Snyder *et al.* 1962; Miller *et al.* 1964; Bond 1975). Bond (1975) studied 87 cases of Wilms' tumours of which 11 were bilateral. She found a 10-fold increase in associated urinary tract abnormalities in the bilateral compared with the unilateral cases. Furthermore the urinary tract malformations were confined to those patients with bilateral tumours arising simultaneously, with none among the patients showing sequential bilateral tumours. Unfortunately Miller and colleagues (1964) in their earlier and larger study did not separate out their bilateral from their unilateral cases. However, among their total of 440 cases there were 18 with horseshoe or fused kidney, duplication defects, or other urinary tract anomalies. Among the 23 boys in their series five had hypospadias and 11 had undescended testes. As in Bond's series this clearly represents an excess.

Miller and colleagues (1964) also found an excess of multiple pigmented naevi and haemangiomata, four of each, among their 440 cases of Wilms' tumour. Miller (1969) also observed one patient with multiple neurofibromatosis, an association subsequently reported on two further occasions (Kung and Nyman 1973; Walden *et al.* 1977).

Wilms' tumour has been reported in pseudohermaphrodite patients (Stump and Garrett 1954; Angstrom 1965; Denys *et al.* 1967; Drash *et al.* 1970), and particularly in male pseudohermaphrodites with nephritis (Barakat *et al.* 1974), in which combination it is known as the Drash syndrome. The associated chronic glomerulopathy may present as nephrotic syndrome or as proteinuria with renal failure and usually leads to death in infancy. Some 55 per cent of patients with pseudohermaphroditism and nephritis develop Wilms' tumours (Eddy and Mauer 1985).

Other rare disorders in which Wilms' tumour occurs with increased frequency are Wiedemann–Beckwith syndrome, in which 1 in 20 patients develop this tumour, (Reddy *et al.* 1972; Sotelo-Avila *et al.* 1980), hyperprolinaemia in one family only (Perry *et al.* 1968), and in another family a syndrome of unusual facies, short stature, chromosome aberration, and aminoaciduria (Lynch *et al.* 1974).

The most remarkable association with Wilms' tumour is that of bilateral aniridia, first reported by Brusa and Torricelli (1953) in a single case. Subsequently Miller and colleagues (1964) observed this rare anomaly in six of their 440 Wilms' tumour patients, a frequency of 1 in 73, and Shannon and associates (1983) found it in 1 in 43 Wilms' tumour patients in the United Kingdom. This compares with a birth frequency of aniridia estimated at 1 in 50 000 by Shaw and colleagues (1960) for Michigan. Two-thirds of their patients with aniridia had an affected parent and they considered the remainder to be new mutants. In contrast none of Miller and colleagues' (1964) six patients with aniridia and Wilms' tumours had an affected parent. Indeed only one instance of autosomal dominant aniridia in a patient with Wilms' tumours has been recorded (Fraumeni and Glass 1968). About a third of all patients with sporadic aniridia have Wilms' tumour (Fraumeni 1969), and, allowing for fresh mutations among other sporadic aniridia cases, it would seem probable that most, if not all, sporadic cases are either due to the gene mutation associated with inherited aniridia or occur as part of the aniridia–Wilms' tumour syndrome. Since Miller and colleagues' (1964) report many further instances of the association have been described (Fontana *et al.* 1965; Schroeder and Cardle 1965; DiGeorge and Harley 1966; Zimmerman and Font 1966; Schweisguth 1967; Mackintosh *et al.* 1968; Flanagan and DiGeorge 1969; Miller 1969; Woodard and Levine 1969; Gandhi *et al.* 1970; Ledlie *et al.* 1970; Haicken and Miller 1971; Bond 1975; Pilling 1975; Pendergrass 1976). Four out of the 26 cases (15 per cent) in which this is reported (Zimmerman and Font 1966; Fraumeni and Glass 1968; Mackintosh *et al.* 1968) have bilateral tumours, similar to the 21 per cent of bilateral cases among hereditary tumours. Several of the reported patients, including one of Miller and colleagues' (1964) original six cases, have had additional urinary tract malformations (Miller 1966); a number, including three of the cases of Miller and colleagues (1964), have been mentally retarded, with or without microcephaly. These further anomalies, which may be seen in association with sporadic aniridia without Wilms' tumour, have led to the definition of a broader syndrome: the AGR triad of anirida, genito-urinary abnormalities and mental retardation, associated in almost half of the cases with Wilms' tumour (then sometimes abbreviated to the WAGR tetrad). The genito-urinary abnormalities observed include a further type of tumour, gonadoblastoma (Anderson *et al.* 1978; Junien *et al.* 1980; Turleau *et al.* 1981).

In describing this triad or tetrad Riccardi and his colleagues (Franke *et al.* 1978, 1979; Riccardi *et al.* 1978) made the remarkable discovery, by using chromosome analysis in early metaphase, that it was associated with a minute constitutional deletion within the short arm of chromosome 11. They observed this deletion, which varied in length but in all cases included band 11p13, in lymphocytes and cultured skin fibroblasts of six patients, two of whom had Wilms' tumour. Park Gerald (1979) confirmed the presence of this deletion in a further nine patients with aniridia and Wilms' tumour, and suggested that the relevant region of the chromosome 11 short arm carries a series of linked loci for aniridia, Wilms' tumour, genito-urinary abnormality, and mental retardation, probably in that order. The development of Wilms' tumour would require a further step to account for the fact that only half of the patients with the complete AGR triad develop Wilms' tumour. It is notable that several of the previously reported patients with aniridia and Wilms' tumour have had chromosomal analysis by conventional culture and banding techniques without any abnormality being detected.

It is becoming apparent that the 11p13 deletion is present in most, if not all, patients with the AGR triad or aniridia and Wilms' tumour, as in Shannon and colleagues' (1983) study in which all of eight children investigated had the deletion, and that of Nakagome and coworkers (1984) in which all of six had it. Junien and associates (1980) assigned the catalase locus to the 11p13 band and suggested that this linkage could be used to identify cases of aniridia needing follow-up for Wilms' tumour or gonadoblastoma. Recently a study of one patient with aniridia and Wilms' tumour, and another with the AGR triad, both included in Nakagome and coworkers study, has permitted the more precise regional localization of both the catalase locus and the WAGR cluster to 11p1305–1306 (Narahara *et al.* 1984). They suggested that the catalase locus is distal to the WAGR locus. An apparently exceptional case was that of a child with aniridia and Wilms' tumour reported as having a translocation, t(8p+; 11q−) (Ladda *et al.* 1974). The authors interpreted this child as having a small interstitial deletion of the short arm of chromosome 8. However, this patient has been reinvestigated by Franke and colleagues (1979) and shown to have a complex translocation with deletion of the 11p13 band. This patient subsequently developed hypertension and focal glomerular sclerosis in his remaining kidney, possibly due to hyperfiltration (Case Records of the Massachusetts General Hospital 1985). Familial occurrence of aniridia–Wilms' tumour with 11p13 deletion has been reported (Yunis and Ramsay 1980), as has familial aniridia alone in association with a translocation t(4;11)– (q22;p13) (Simola *et al.* 1983). In this latter case the authors suggest there is either a submicroscopic deletion at 11p13 or a position effect. The patient of Fraumeni and Glass (1968) with familial aniridia and Wilms' tumour has not been studied by the prometaphase technique and may have a different genetic basis from the deletion cases. The 11p13 deletion is not usually seen in either normal or tumour tissue from sporadic Wilms' tumour cases without any features of the AGR triad (Nakagome *et al.* 1984), but has been reported in tumour, but not normal, tissue from one case (Kaneko *et al.* 1981); and in blood from another case with Wilms' tumour, chordee, and cryptorchidism, but no aniridia and no evidence of mental retardation (Turleau *et al.* 1984b). They suggest a gene order of centromere, catalase, Wilms' tumour, aniridia. This places catalase at the opposite side of the Wilms' gene to that proposed by Narahara and others (1984). The 11p13 deletion has also been reported in a 46,XY true hermaphrodite with Wilms' tumour but normal irides and normal intelligence, and in a boy who died at 1 hour with multiple congenital abnormalities but without Wilms' tumour or aniridia (Gustavson *et al.* 1984). An analysis of five patients with the anirida syndrome and 11p13 deletion revealed deletion of the catalase gene in four of them, and of two cell surface marker genes on 11p in two of them. None had lost the β-globin or calcitonin gene (van Heyningen *et al.* 1985). The authors conclude that the catalase gene is proximal to the Wilms'-aniridia cluster, in agreement with Turleau and colleagues (1984b). Deletion of one of the cell surface marker genes, E7, was also observed by one other group (Scoggin *et al.* 1985).

It has recently been demonstrated that postzygotic events resulting in chromosome 13 rearrangements bring about mutations that, acting together in a recessive manner with a presumed pre-existing inherited mutation on the homologous chromosome 13, induce childhood retinoblastoma (Benedict *et al.* 1983; Cavanee *et al.* 1983). This observation has stimulated several groups to apply independently recombinant DNA techniques to the analysis of Wilms' tumour in a search for analogous chromosomal alterations. The starting point for their studies, which have been published together in a single issue of *Nature* (10 May 1984) (Fearon *et al.* 1984; Koufos *et al.* 1984; Orkin *et al.* 1984; Reeve *et al.*

1984), has been the 11p13 deletion observed in cells from many Wilms' tumour patients, discussed above. In the retinoblastoma studies available DNA probes made it possible to distinguish certain rearrangements, such as mitotic non-disjunction with loss of the wild type chromosome and mitotic recombination, from one another. In the case of Wilms' tumour the available probes all hybridize to the tip of chromosome 11 short arm, distal to the WAGR cluster at 11p13, and such distinctions were more difficult to make. However, by comparing DNA polymorphisms, detected by the probes, in normal and tumour tissue of the same patients it is possible to demonstrate that a site on chromosome 11 which is heterozygous in the normal tissue has become apparently homozygous, or hemizygous, in the tumour. From this it can be concluded that there has been a loss, or defective alteration, of the site recognized by the probe on one homologue, and along with it loss of the wild type Wilms' tumour locus, rendering this locus functionally defective in both members of the chromosome 11 pair within the tumour. The probes utilized have been ones that recognize sequences flanking the insulin gene, the β-globin gene cluster, the parathormone gene, the c-Ha-*ras*-1 oncogene, and a random restriction fragment length polymorphism (RFLP).

Koufos' group from Cincinnati (Koufos *et al.* 1984), using the insulin gene 5′ flanking, β-globin, c-Ha-*ras*-1, and RFLP probes, found loss of heterozygosity in tumour tissue with two or more probes in five out of seven patients studied. Furthermore in several instances the intensity of the hybridization bands obtained for the allele remaining in the tumour tissue was greater than in the corresponding normal tissue. This suggests that a recombinational event had occurred with loss of the wild type allele and reduplication of the chromosome segment carrying the tumour-predisposing mutation, rather than a simple loss of the wild type chromosome through mitotic non-disjunction.

Orkin and coworkers (1984) from Harvard studying seven patients detected heterozygosity for at least one DNA polymorphism in the normal tissues of all seven, with probes for β-globin and the c-Ha-*ras*-1 oncongene. Probes for the insulin gene 5′ flanking and for the parathormone genes were uninformative. In only one case was the heterozygosity observed in normal tissue lost in the tumour, but in that case heterozygosity detected with three separate β-globin gene probes and the c-Ha-*ras*-1 probe were all lost, and the tumour was shown to be homozygous for the paternal chromosome 11. As with the Cincinnati group the intensity of the bands on the autoradiographs from the Southern blot hybridization experiments appears to exclude a simple chromosomal loss, and to imply some mechanism of chromosomal reduplication.

Reeve and colleagues (1984) from Dunedin, New Zealand, working with a probe for c-Ha-*ras*-1, studied four Wilms' tumour cases and in two of these found that one of two alleles detected in the normal tissue was absent in the tumour in Southern blots, and in the first case also on *in situ* hybridization. In the first case the tumour was shown on karyotype analysis to carry a balanced translocation involving the 11p13 band; 46,XX, t(11;12)(p13;q13). The authors postulated that in this case there had been a submicroscopic deletion at the 11p13 breakpoint but recognized the difficulty in this interpretation, arising from earlier evidence that the Wilms' tumour–aniridia locus and the c-Ha-*ras*-1 locus are two bands apart on the short arm of chromosome 11. An alternative interpretation is a position effect from the translocation leading to inactivation of the Wilms' locus, but even this does not account for the apparent loss of one c-Ha-*ras* allele. A third hypothesis, which would take account of the genetic distance between the 11p13 gene cluster and the terminal 11p15 band, is that there may be some instability of the DNA of the chromosome 11 short arm with transposition of loci within the 11p13→pter region. Thus if the c-Ha-*ras*-1 locus were transposed to 11p13 and either deleted or involved in a recombinational transfer, along with the Wilms' tumour locus, to the homologous chromosome 11 at the time of the break giving rise to the 11;12 translocation this would account for the development of the Wilms' tumour and the loss of a c-Ha-*ras*-1 allele.

A similar mechanism could account, in other cases, for the association of Wiedemann–Beckwith syndrome, which is possibly due to duplication in the 11p15 region (Waziri *et al.* 1983; Turleau *et al.* 1984a), and Wilms' tumour, and even for the discrepancy between different groups of workers' claims for the WAGR–catalase gene order. 11p15 duplication has not been detected in all patients with Wiedemann–Beckwith syndrome who have had high resolution banding (Nakagome *et al.* 1984). However, the difficulties of high resolution banding analysis are illustrated by one case of aniridia–Wilms' tumour reported by Nakagome and colleagues. This boy had an 11p deletion, which was also present in his clinically normal mother. In a follow-up letter (Nakagome and Nagahara 1985) they reported further studies which showed that the mother, and a sister, were balanced carriers of an insertion from chromosome 11 to chromosome 12. Recently Koufos and colleagues (1985) have carried out similar studies on tumours from patients with hepatoblastomas or rhabdomyosarcomas. They have demonstrated loss of heterozygosity for loci on the short arm of chromosome 11 in tumours from constitutionally heterozygous patients, similar to that observed in Wilms' tumours. They also showed that there is no such loss of heterozygosity for loci on other chromosomes in the same tumours, nor for several DNA polymorphisms on chromosome 11 in Ewings' or osteogenic sarcomas from other patients. They proposed that their evidence for the operation of similar mechanisms involving chromosome 11 in at least three embryonal tumour types, taken together with the known predisposition of Wiedemann–Beckwith patients to develop any of these types of embryonal tumour, suggests a common pathogenetic mechanism for all embryonal tumours. These issues will only be finally resolved when a probe for the Wilms' locus itself becomes available.

Finally Fearon and associates (1984) at Johns Hopkins studied six cases and found evidence for somatic deletions in the tumours of four of these. They worked with probes for γ-globin, insulin, c-Ha-*ras*-1, and parathormone. In all six of their patients they detected heterozygosity for γ-globin gene polymorphisms, in five out of six with the insulin probe, in four with the c-Ha-*ras*-1 probe, and in three with the parathormone probe. This group also observed increased intensity of the band for the remaining allele in tumour tissue from patients showing deletion of one allele, again implying a duplication event. Thus in exactly half of the patients studied (12/24) in these four reports functional loss of a marker allele due to a chromosomal mechanism was detected. In most of these 12 there is evidence for a duplication of the remaining allele, and in one a possible position effect, or gene transposition, associated with a translocation.

More recently Michalopoulos and colleagues (1985) produced hybrid clones from human fibroblasts from a patient with the aniridia–Wilms' tumour association and Chinese hamster cells. The parental human line contained two alleles for the Ha-*ras*-1 gene by restriction fragment length polymorphism. One hybrid clone contained a single human chromosome 11 with a visible 11p13 deletion. DNA from this clone contained only one Ha-*ras*-1 allele and also insulin, Aγ and Gγ globin, and calcitonin genes, but no sequences homologous to human catalase cDNA. The clone also expressed human lactate dehydrogenase A activity. The authors concluded that the 11p deletion was distal to LDH A but proximal to the other genes dected. Raizis and others (1985) have demonstrated mitotic recombination in Wilms' tumour between the 11p13 deletion and the parathyroid hormone locus. This locus has been localized to 11p15 by *in situ* hybridization, along with the β-globin and insulin genes, and the HRAS 1 oncogene (Zabel *et al.* 1985). Kittur and colleagues (1985), using classical linkage of RFLPs adjacent to known genes on 11p have established a gene order on 11p of: centromere-catalase-Wilms'-aniridia cluster-calcitonin-parathormone-β-globin-c-Ha-ras/insulin-like growth factor II/insulin. Insulin-like growth factor II (IGF II), localized to 11p15, shows markedly increased expression in sporadic Wilms' tumours compared to normal tissues, possibly reflecting the embryonic origin of the tumour (Reeve *et al.* 1985; Scott *et al.* 1985). These studies are a remarkable confirmation of Knudson's and Strong's (1974) hypothesis, based on epidemiological evidence and discussed more fully below, of a two-step mutational origin of Wilms' and other embryonic tumours of childhood, and of the fact that it is too simplistic to discount genetic factors in the causation of disorders that are mostly non-familial.

Other chromosomal abnormalities have been described in patients with Wilms' tumour without aniridia, but are probably chance associations. These include 18 trisomy (Geiser and Schindler 1969), trisomy 8 mosaicism confined to cultured fibroblasts (Niss and Passarge 1976; Nakamura *et al.* 1985), a translocation between a B and C group chromosome (Giangiacoma *et al.* 1975), and XX/YY mosaicism (Denys *et al.* 1967). Soulie and colleagues (1985) have reported the finding of a 3;17 translocation in fibroblasts cultured from tumour tissue of a child with bilateral Wilms' tumour. The parents had normal karyotypes.

It is notable that Wilms' tumour with aniridia, in contrast to that seen in association with hemihypertrophy, pseudohermaphroditism or Wiedemann–Beckwith syndrome and even some familial cases, is not associated with superficial multifocal nephroblastomatosis (Machin 1980).

The great majority of cases of Wilms' tumour are sporadic. Knudson and Strong (1972) found no familial cases among 93 unilateral and four bilateral cases from one hospital and Miller and colleagues (1964) found only two instances of familial Wilms' tumour among 440 cases from six hospitals. In a later study Miller (1968) found only one concordant sib pair and no twin pairs among 1205 cases. Draper and coworkers (1977) carried out a study based on interviews with families of children with neoplasia indentified in the Marie Curie/Oxford survey of Childhood Cancers through death certification of deaths of children with neoplasia since 1953, and cancer registration since 1962, throughout Great Britain. They were able to identify only one pair of male twins both with Wilm's tumours, and no other affected sibs. Nevertheless there have been many reports of familial occurrence including some in the United Kingdom during the period of Draper and coworkers' survey. Some early reports lacked either precise histological diagnosis or adequate family data but were probably familial Wilms' tumour (Walker 1897; Deuticke 1931; Fischer-Wasels 1933; Bobio 1935). Maslow (1940) reported histologically confirmed Wilms' tumour in three sibs, with a fourth possibly affected sib. Further reports of families with affected sibs followed (Mackay 1945; Silver 1947; Chapian 1948; Collins 1955; Snyder *et al.* 1962; Miller *et al.* 1964; Zunin and Soave 1964; Bishop and Hope 1966; Cochran and Froggatt 1967; Miller 1968, 1971; Tsunoda *et al.* 1969; Wilbur 1971; Meadows *et al.* 1974). Cochran and Froggatt (1967) described two affected sisters, the first reported sibs with bilateral Wilms' tumours. There has been a single report of parental consanguinity (British Empire Cancer Campaign: 29th Annual Report 1951).

There have been eight reports of concordant monozygotic or presumed monozygotic, twins (Gaulin 1951; Miller *et al.* 1964; Franklin 1965; Hewitt *et al.* 1966; Murphy 1968; Ledlie *et al.* 1970; Leen and Williams 1971; Draper *et al.* 1977). Juberg and associates (1975) described a family in which monozygotic twin brothers were discordant for Wilms' tumour but another male sib was affected. They argued that this discordance was evidence for environmental causation, a view challenged by Knudson and Strong (1975) who pointed out twin discordance was entirely compatible with their two-mutation hypothesis. Francke and collegues (1978) included in their study a pair of monozygotic twin sisters concordant for aniridia, mental subnormality, and a deletion of the 11 short arm but discordant for Wilms' tumour.

There have also been several reports of affected individuals in more than one generation of the same family. Fitzgerald and Hardin (1955) reported Wilms' tumour in a father and two of this three daughters, histologically confirmed in the two daughters. Brown and coworkers (1972) subsequently reported Wilms' tumour in the only child of the surviving affected daughter of Fitzgerald and Hardin's family. Strom (1957) described the family of a healthy man in which two out of his five children were affected. A further child by another marriage, together with the father's sister and aunt were also affected. Unfortunately only one of these cases was histologically proved. Owings and Radokovich (1959) described Wilms' tumour in a mother and her child. Kaufman and others (1973) reported Wilms' tumour in a father and son, as did Jolles (1973). Knudson and Strong (1972) in a review of data on 58 familial cases, including all of those mentioned above, pointed out that the familial cases have an earlier onset, of about 2 years of age, compared with 3–4 years for all Wilms' tumour cases, and have bilateral tumours in 21 per cent of cases compared with only 5–10 per cent for all Wilms' tumour cases. Wilms' tumour has also been reported as occurring in five cousins in a single family (Cordero *et al.* 1980). The report of Wilms' tumour in a child, and of hypernephroma in her grandmother, is presumably a purely chance association (Banham and Jolles 1946). Several explanations for these rare familial cases are feasible. Some might be due to an undetected environmental factor persisting within a family. They could be due to one or more single genes determining a phenocopy of the usual sporadic Wilms' tumour. The sporadic tumours themselves may be due to fresh mutations of a gene which with survival of affected individuals would show dominant inheritance. If this were so then the few instances of two generation affected families on record might be due to the same gene. Knudson and Strong (1972) have argued that this is so for bilateral Wilms' tumour, as has been shown for bilateral retinoblastoma (Schappert-Kimmijser *et al.* 1966). They further postulated that the development of Wilms' tumour in a genetically predisposed individual requires an additional somatic mutation. On this model 37 per cent of heterozygotes for the germinal mutation do not develop tumours, and 15 per cent with more than one somatic mutation develop bilateral tumours. Sporadic unilateral cases would require two sequential somatic mutations. This model is analogous to that proposed earlier by Knudson (1971) for retinoblastoma, but, as the authors recognized, survival rates for Wilms' tumour have up to the present time been too low to provide the direct confirmation that exists for retinoblastoma. Knudson and Strong (1972) also pointed out that the aniridic cases showed a similar early age of onset to the familial and bilateral non-aniridic cases. In view of the subsequent demonstration of the 11p13 deletion in the WAGR syndrome this strongly supports the hypothesis that the deletion involves separate genes whose loss leads to aniridia and other features of the AGR triad on the one hand and Wilms' tumour on the other. This possibility was foreseen by Knudson and Strong. They also observed that the hemihypertrophy with Wilms' tumour cases, and those with associated genito-urinary anomaly but no aniridia, followed the age of onset pattern of sporadic unilateral cases, suggesting that these cases likewise depend on postzygotic events. The role of somatic mutation in sporadic cases is further supported by the findings on normal and tumour tissues investigated with chromosome 11 DNA probes discussed above. Knudson and Strong recognized that their two-mutational model did not account for the frequency of Wilms' tumour in sibs with normal parents. They accepted that this was too high to be accounted for by low penetrance. A similar phenomenon was observed in retinoblastoma and Knudson and Strong suggested that it may be due to 'delayed mutation' (Auerbach 1956; Neel 1962), possibly induced by a vertically transmitted tumour virus that becomes integrated into the host genome, analogous to the variant of avian myeloblatsosis virus that induces renal tumours but not leukaemia (Lacour *et al.* 1970). An alternative hypothesis that meets the objections regarding affected sibs with normal parents has been proposed by Matsunaga (1981). He concluded that inheritance in familial cases of Wilms' tumour, less than 1 per cent of all cases, was autosomal dominant with variable penetrance and expressivity. He noted that 20 per cent of familial cases were bilateral, compared with only 3 per cent of sporadic cases, and speculated as to whether all bilateral cases were hereditary. Matsunaga proposed what he termed a 'host resistance model' in familial Wilms' tumour to account for the variable penetrance and expression. This is essentially a modifier gene model in which possession of the tissue specific suppressor genes results in a failure of tumour induction in carriers of the Wilms' major gene. He argued that there was no evidence for a vertically transmitted tumour virus and quoted in support of his hypothesis a significant correlation between first-degree relatives with Wilms' tumour in the proportion with bilateral tumours and in the age at diagnosis, especially for parent:child correlations. For genetic counselling purposes he gave an average risk of developing Wilms' tumour for children of unaffected carrier parents of 0.30, and for children of survivors with familial unilateral or bilateral Wilms' tumour of 0.40 and 0.50 respectively. The risk for children of survivors with sporadic unilateral tumour he gave as only 2–4 per cent.

Another possible explanation of the relatively high incidence of affected sibs among familial cases is that a proportion of both familial and sporadic cases are inherited in mendelian recessive manner. This was suggested by the observation of Imray and colleagues (1984) of increased sensitivity to mitomycin C of lymphoblastoid cell lines from five patients with Wilms' tumour and six of their parents. Their data indicated increased sensitivity to mitomycin C in both parents in the two families where both were studied. Two of their five cases were of sporadic occurrence, two were sibs, and one had an affected cousin. They suggested, however, in response to a comment on the implications of their observations for the genetics of Wilms' tumour (Crawfurd 1984), that this sensitivity to mitomycin C is not necessarily linked to the Wilms' tumour gene but may merely reflect a defect in DNA repair or recombination that may generate the homozygosity or hemizygosity of the Wilms' tumour gene necessary for its expression (Smith and Imray 1984). However, patients with Wilms' tumour show none of the features common to other disorders in which there is a known or suspected defect in DNA repair.

In formulating their genetic hypotheses, neither Knudson and Strong, nor Matsunaga, take account of the different histological types of Wilms' tumour. Delemarre and colleagues (1982) have classified Wilms' tumour according to the degree of differentiation, and whether differentiation is epithelial, blastemal, or mixed. The more undifferentiated, anaplastic or sarcomatous, tumours carry the worst prognoses, and multicystic nephroblastomas, and also mesoblastic nephroma, carry the most favourable prognoses. Recently the same group have described another histological type, also with relatively favourable prognosis, the fibroadenomatous type seen in about 2.5 per cent of all cases (Delemarre *et al.* 1984). A further type is the fetal rhabdomyomatous type seen in association with intralobular multifocal nephroblastomatosis (Machin and McCaugley 1984), which is itself liable to be misdiagnosed as nephroblastoma.

The gene probe studies discussed above essentially confirm the main thesis of Knudson and Strong's theory, of a two-step mutational model of

Wilms' tumour induction, rather than Matsunaga's main gene plus modifier gene hypothesis. However, Knudson and Strong argued that familial cases were due to an inherited germ line gene mutation acting together with a second somatic mutation, and that sporadic cases were due to two somatic mutations. The recent studies were carried out on sporadic cases and revealed that a surprisingly high proportion, about half, of the 'second', somatic, mutations are chromosomal events. The presumed initial event must on this basis be a constitutional, or germ-line, mutation at the gene or at least at submicroscopic level, rather than a somatic one as postulated by Knudson and Strong for sporadic cases. This being so one could postulate that the initial constitutional mutation is a fresh mutation in some sporadic cases and inherited in other sporadic and all familial cases. Several questions still remain unanswered. The incidence of affected sibs with normal parents is unexplained, as is the much higher proportion of familial cases in retinoblastoma compared with Wilms' tumour. The analysis of the molecular basis will be greatly simplified when DNA probes for the 11p13 region itself become available. When that happens studies of both sporadic and familial cases, of unilateral and bilateral cases, and of uncomplicated Wilms' tumour and of tumours associated with the AGR triad or hemihypertrophy will be necessary. DNA studies of the different histological types of tumour will also be essential. One interesting hypothesis is that the constitutional mutation in Wilms' tumour may be an oncogene (Green and Wyke 1985).

Data for genetic counselling are also as yet inadequate. There have been too few offspring of affected individuals to provide empirical estimates of the risk for children. Leck (1972), on the basis of a 10-fold increase in the observed number of concordantly affected sib pairs compared with expected, estimated a relative risk for sibs of affected children of 10. Assuming a live-born incidence of 1 in 10 000 this gives a sib risk of 1 in 1000 for Wilms' tumour overall. Knudson and Strong (1972) estimated the penetrance for hereditary Wilms' tumour at 0.63 and the proportion of all Wilms' tumours that are hereditary as 0.38. On the assumption that 8 per cent of cases are bilateral, then all bilateral and 30 per cent of unilateral survivors would be at a 1 in 2 risk of hetro-zygosity for offspring with a 63 per cent risk of tumour development, that is, a risk of 32 per cent for tumours in the offspring of gene carriers. This compares well, perhaps fortuitously, with Matsunaga's estimate of 30 per cent. It would be reasonable to use this 1 in 3 risk provis-ionally for the offspring of all bilateral survivors, unilateral but familial survivors, and for further sibs when more than one sib has already been affected. If 30 per cent of unilateral survivors are in fact hereditary then the risk for offspring of sporadic unilateral survivors can be estimated as approximately 1 in 10 (0.32×0.3) on Knudson and Strong's hereditary hypothesis, but only 2–4 per cent on Matsunaga's hypothesis. Such cases will, of course, at present form only a small minority of all cases seen for genetic counselling in relation to Wilms' tumour, the majority of which will be sporadic cases whose parents wish to know the sib risk. Estimates of risks for sibs of such sporadically affected children with normal parents are difficult to make as the proportion of either bilateral cases, or the purported 30 per cent of unilateral hereditary cases that do not have a fresh mutation of the germinal gene, is unknown. Draper and colleagues (1977), considering the sib recurrence risks for all childhood malignant neoplasms excluding leukaemia and lymphoma, estimated this at about 1 in 400 with recurrence being usually concordant for type of tumour. However, since none of their concordant sib pairs both had Wilms' tumour this 1 in 400 may be an overestimate for Wilms' tumour. It would, therefore, be reasonable to use the 1 in 1000 risk derived for Leck's data, which is partially based on Draper and colleagues' data, for unilateral, non-familial, Wilms' tumour not associated with aniridia. This relatively low sporadic case sib risk is in line with the negligible risk under Matsunaga's hypothesis.

In summary, Wilms' tumour is a mainly sporadic and unilateral tumour of early childhood, occurring in a minority of cases in association with hemihypertrophy as a unilateral, presumably unifocal tumour; in association with renal malformations and/or nodular renal blastema, especially when the tumour is bilateral, and in the case of association with nodular blastema multifocal; and in about half of all patients with the aniridia, genito-urinary, mental retardation syndrome. This last syndrome, with or without Wilms' tumour is associated with a deletion in the chromosome segment designated 11p13. Duplication within a neighbouring chromosomal segment, 11p15, has been reported in Wiedemann–Beckwith syndrome, about 5 per cent of cases of which have Wilms' tumour. There are well-documented instances of exceptional familial occurence of Wilms' tumour involving sibs, or parent and child, for which there is no evidence for any environmental cause. Recent studies using DNA probes for the distal short arm of chromosome 11 have provided strong support for the theory of a two-step mutational hypothesis for the origin of this tumour, involving either a germ-line mutation followed by a somatic mutation or two sequential somatic mutations. Recurrence risks for sibs of sporadic, unilateral cases are low, probably about 1 in 1000; but are higher for children of surviving sporadic, unilaterally affected patients, probably of the order of 2 to 10 per cent; and higher still, at about 1 in 3, for children of patients with bilateral or familial tumours, or for children with two or more affected sibs.

References

Abeshouse, B. S. (1957). The management of Wilms' tumor as determined by national survey and review of the literature. *J. Urol.* **77**, 792–813.

Anderson, E. E., Herlong, J. H., Harper, J. M., Small, M. P. and Atwill, W. H. (1968). Bilateral Wilms' tumor. Diagnosis and management. *Clin. Pediatr. (Phila)* **7**, 596–9.

Anderson, S. R., Geertinger, P., Larsen, H.-W., Mikkelsen, M., Parving, A., Vestermark, S. and Warburg, M. (1978). Aniridia, cataract and gonadoblastoma in a mentally retarded girl with deletion of chromosome 11: a clinicopathological case report. *Ophthalmologia* **176**, 171–7.

Angstrom, T. (1965). Nephroblastoma in a case of agonadism. *Cancer* **18**, 857–62.

Auerbach, C. (1956). A possible case of delayed mutation in man. *Ann. Hum. Genet.* **20**, 266–9.

Banham, A. R. and Jolles, B. (1946). Kidney tumours in a child and her grandmother. *Br. Med. J.* **2**, 774.

Barakat, A. Y., Papadopoulov, Z. L., Chandra, R. S., Hollerman, C. E. and Calcagno, P. L. (1974). Pseudohermaphroditism, nephron disorder and Wilms' tumour: a unifying concept. *Pediatrics* **54**, 366–9.

Barber, R. and Spiers, P. S. (1964). Oxford survey of Childhood Cancers, Progress Report II: Relatives of cases and controls. *Monthly Bulletin of the Ministry of Health and the Public Health Laboratory Service*, **23**, 46–52.

Benedict, W. F., Murphee, A. L., Banerjee, A., Spina, C. A., Sparkes, M. C. and Sparks, R. S. (1983). Patient with a chromosome 13 deletion: evidence that the retinoblastoma gene is a recessive cancer gene. *Science* **219**, 973–5.

Benson, P. F., Vulliamy, D. G. and Taubman, J. O. (1963). Congenital hemihypertrophy and malignancy. *Lancet* **1**, 468–9.

Bishop, H. C. and Hope, J. W. (1966). Bilateral Wilms' tumors. *J. Pediatr. Surg.* **1**, 476–87.

Bjorklund, S.-I. (1955). Hemihypertrophy and Wilms' tumor. *Acta Paediatr.* **44**, 287–92.

Bobbio, L. (1935). Tumeurs renales congenitales (dysembryomes renaux) familiales chez des heredo-syphilitiques. *Arch. Mal. Reins.* **9**, 571–4.

Bolande, R. P. (1971). Benignity of neonatal tumours and concept of cancer regression in early life. *Am. J. Dis. Child.* **122**, 12–14.

—— (1973). Congenital mesoblastic nephroma of infancy. *Perspect. Pediatr. Pathol.* **1**, 227–50.

—— (1974). Congenital and infantile neoplasia of the kidney. *Lancet* **2**, 1497–9.

Bond, J. V. (1975). Bilateral Wilms' tumour. Age at diagnosis, associated congenital anomalies, and possible pattern of inheritance. *Lancet* **2**, 482–4.

Bove, K. E., Koffler, H. and McAdams, A. J. (1969). Nodular renal blastema. Definition and possible significance. *Cancer* **24**, 323–32.

Boxer, L. A. and Smith, D. L. (1970). Wilms' tumor prior to onset of hemihypertrophy. *Am. J. Dis. Child.* **120**, 564–5.

British Empire Cancer Campaign (1951). *Twenty-ninth Annual Report.* pp. 133–42.

Brown, W. T., Puranik, S. R., Altman, D. H. and Hardin, H. C. Jr. (1972). Wilms' tumor in three successive generations. *Surgery* **72**, 756–61.

Brusa, P. and Torricelli, C. (1953). Nephroblastoma di Wilms ed affezioni Renali Congenite Nella Casistica dell' I.P.P.A.I. di Milano. *Minerva Pediatr.* **5**, 457–63.

Case Records of the Massachusetts General Hospital (1985). Case 17—1985. *New Engl. J. Med.* **312**, 111–19.

Cavanee, W. K., Dryja, T. P., Phillps, R. A., Benedict, W. F., Godbout, R., Gallie, B. L., Murphree, A. L., Strong, L. C. and White, R. L. (1983). Expression of recessive alleles by chromosomal mechanisms in retinoblastoma. *Nature* **305**, 779–84.

Chapian, M. A. (1948). Wilms' tumor: Report of 2 cases in the same family. *Rhode Island Med. J.* **31**, 105–9.

Cochran, W. and Froggatt, P. (1967). Bilateral nephroblastoma in two sisters. *J. Urol.* **97**, 216–20.

Collins, V. P. (1955). Wilms' tumor: Its behaviour and prognosis. *J. Louisiana Med. Soc.* **107**, 474–80.

Cordero, J. F., Li, F. P., Holmes, L. B. and Gerald, P. S. (1980). Wilms' tumor in five cousins. *Pediatrics.* **66**, 716–9.

Crawfurd, M. d'A. (1984). Mutant genes in Wilms' tumour (letter). *Lancet* **2**, 97.

Delemarre, J. F. M., Sandstedt, B., Gerard Marchant, R. and Tournade, M. F. (1982). S.I.O.P. nephroblastoma trials and studies. Morphological aspects. In *Pediatric oncology: Proc. of the Internat. Soc. of Paediatric Oncology Marseille, 15–19 September 1981*, eds. Rayhaud, A., Clement, R., Lebreuil, G. and Bernard, J. L. pp. 261–72. Excerpta Medica, Amsterdam.

——, —— and Tournade, M. F. (1984). Nephroblastoma with fibroadenomatous-like structures. *Histopathology* **8**, 55–62.

Denys, P., Malvaux, P., Van Den Berge, H., Tanghe, W. L. and Proesmans, W. (1967). Association d'un syndrome anatomopathologique de pseudohermaphrodisme masculin, d'une tumeur de Wilms', d'une nephropathie parenchymateuse et d'un mosaicisme XX/YY. *Arch. Fr. Pediatr.* **24**, 729–39.

Deuticke, P. (1931). Nierentumoren. *D. Z. Chir.* **231**, 767–97.

DiGeorge, A. M. and Harley, R. D. (1966). The association of aniridia, Wilms' tumor and genital abnormalities. *Arch. Ophthalmol.* **75**, 796–8.

Draper, G. J., Heaf, M. M. and Kinnear Wilson, L. M. (1977). Occurrence of childhood cancers among sibs and estimation of familial risks. *J. Med. Genet.* **14**, 81–90.

Drash, A., Sherman, F., Hartmann, W. H. and Blizzard, R. M. (1970). A syndrome of pseudohermaphroditism, Wilms' tumour, hypertension, and degenerative renal disease. *J. Pediatr.* **76**, 585–93.

Eddy, A. A. and Mauer, S. M. (1985). Pseudohermaphroditism, glomerulopathy, and Wilms' tumor (Drash syndrome): frequency in end-stage renal failure. *J. Pediatr.* **106**, 584–7.

Egerdie, R. B., Buckspan, M. B., Klotz, P. G., Steinhardt, M. I. and Pritzker, K. P. H. (1986). Bilateral multilocular renal cysts. *J. Urol.* **135**, 346–8.

Fearon, E. R., Vogelstein, B. and Feinberg, A. P. (1984). Somatic deletion and duplication of genes on chromosome 11 in Wilms' tumours. *Nature* **309**, 176–8.

Fischer-Wasels, B. (1933). Zur Erforschung und Bekompfung bosartiger Geschevulste. *Dtsch. Med. Wschr.* **59**, 1489–94.

Fitzgerald, W. L. and Hardin, H. C. Jr. (1955). Bilateral Wilms' tumor in a Wilms' tumor family: case report. *J. Urol.* **73**, 468–74.

Flanagan, J. C. and DiGeorge, A. M. (1969). Sporadic aniridia and Wilms' tumor. *Am. J. Ophthalmol.* **67**, 558–81.

Fontana, V. J., Ferrara, A. and Perciaccante, R. (1965). Wilms' tumor and associated anomalies. *Am. J. Dis. Child.* **109**, 459–61.

Francke, U., Riccardi, V. M., Hittner, H. M. and Borges, W. (1978). Interstitial del(11p) as a cause of the aniridia-Wilms' tumor association: band localization and a heritable basis. *Am. J. Hum. Genet.* **30**, 81A.

——, Holmes, L. B., Atkins, L. and Riccardi, V. M. (1979). Aniridia–Wilms' tumor association: evidence for specific deletion of 11p13. *Cytogenet. Cell Genet.* **24**, 185–92.

Franklin, A. W. (1965). Personal communication quoted by Cochran, W. and Froggatt, P. (1967). *J. Urol.* **97**, 216–20.

Fraumeni, J. F., Jr. (1969). The aniridia–Wilms' tumor syndrome. *The clinical delineation of birth defects.* II. Malformation syndromes. pp. 198–201. National Foundation, New York.

—— and Glass, A. G. (1968). Wilms' tumor and congenital aniridia. *JAMA* **206**, 825–8.

——, Geiser, C. F. and Manning, M. D. (1967). Wilms' tumour and congenital hemihypertrophy: report of five new cases and review of literature. *Pediatrics* **40**, 886–99.

Gandhi, R. K., Deshmukh, S. S. and Waingankar, V. S. (1970). Wilms' tumor with aniridia. *J. Pediatr. Surg.* **5**, 571.

Gaulin, E. (1951). Simultaneous Wilms' tumors in identical twins. *J. Urol.* **66**, 547–50.

Geiser, C. F. and Schindler, A. M. (1969). Long survival in a male with 18 trisomy syndrome and Wilms' tumor. *Pediatrics* **44**, 111–16.

Gerald, P. S. (1979). Cited by Culliton, B. J. and Waterfall, W. K. (1979). Symposium on genetics. *Br. Med. J.* **4**, 1059–60.

Giangiacomo, J., Penchansky, I., Monteleone, P. L. and Thompson, J. (1975). Bilateral neonatal Wilms' tumor with B-C chromosomal translocation. *J. Pediatr.* **86**, 98–102.

Glenn, J. F. and Rhame, R. C. (1961). Wilms' tumor: epidemiological experience. *J. Urol.* **85**, 911–18.

Green, A. R. and Wyke, J. A. (1985). Anti-oncogenes: a subset of regulatory genes involved in carcinogenesis. *Lancet* **2**, 475–7.

Greenberg, F., Stein, F., Gresik, M. V., Finegold, M. J., Carpenter, R. J., Riccardi, V. M. and Beaudet, A. L. (1986). The Perlman familial nephroblastomatosis syndrome. *Am. J. Med. Genet.* **24**, 101–10.

Gustavson, K.-H., Anneren, G. and Wranne, L. (1984). Two cases of 11p13 interstitial deletion and unusual clinical features. Papers presented at the Third Nordic Conference of Medical Genetics; *Clin. Genet.* **26**, 247–9.

Gyepes, M. T. and Burko, H. (1964). Diffuse bilateral Wilms' tumor simulating multicystic renal disease. *Radiology* **82**, 1029–31.

Haicken, B. N. and Miller, D. R. (1971). Simultaneous occurrence of congenital aniridia, hamartoma and Wilms' tumor. *J. Pediatr.* **78**, 497–502.

Hanawa, Y. (1978). In *All Japan Children's Cancer Registration 1969–1973*, pp. 31–72. Children's Cancer Association of Japan, Tokyo.

Hart, C. W. and Naunton, R. F. (1964). The ototoxicty of chloroquine phosphate. *Arch. Otolaryng.* **80**, 407–12.

Hewitt, D., Lashof, J. C. and Stewart, A. M. (1966). Childhood cancer in twins. *Cancer* **19**, 157–61.

Hou, L. T. and Holman, R. L. (1961). Bilateral nephroblastomatosis in a premature infant. *J. Pathol. Bact.* **82**, 249–55.

Imray, F. P., Smith, P. J., Relf, W. and Kidson, C. (1984). Wilms' tumour: association with cellular sensitivity to mitomycin C in patients and first degree relatives. *Lancet* **1**, 1148–51.

Jolles, B. (1973). Wilms' tumour in a father and son. *Lancet* **1**, 207.

Juberg, R. C., St Martin, E. C. and Hundley, J. R. (1975). Familial occurrence of Wilms' tumor: nephroblastoma in one of monozygous twins and in another sibling. *Am. J. Hum. Genet.* **27**, 155–64.

Junien, C., Turleau, C., De Grouchy, J., Said, R., Rethore, M.-O., Tenconi, R. and Dufier, J. L. (1980). Regional assignment of catalase (CAT) gene to band 11p13: associated with the aniridia–Wilms' tumor–gonadoblastoma (WAGR) complex. *Ann. Genet.* **23**, 165–8.

Kaneko, Y., Egves, M. C. and Rowley, J. D. (1981). Interstitial deletion of short arm of chromosome 11 limited to Wilms' tumor cells in a patient without aniridia. *Cancer Res.* **41**, 4577–8.

Kaufman, R. L., Vietti, T. J. and Wabner, C. I. (1973). Wilms' tumour in father and son. *Lancet* **1**, 43.

Kittur, S. D., Hoppener, J. W. M., Antonarakis, S. E., Davies, J. D. J., Meyer, D. A., Maestri, N. E., Jansen, M., Korneluk, R. G., Nelkin, B. D. and Kazazian, H. H. Jr. (1985). Linkage map of the short arm of human chromosome 11: location of the genes for catalase, calcitonin, and insulin-like growth factor II. *Proc. Nat. Acad. Sci.* **82**, 5064–7.

Klapproth, H. J. (1959). Wilms' tumor: a report of 45 cases with an analysis of 1,351 cases reported in the world literature from 1940–1958. *J. Urol.* **81**, 633–48.

Knudson, A. G. Jr. (1971). Mutation and cancer: statistical study of retinoblastoma. *Proc. Nat. Acad. Sci.* **68**, 820–3.

—— and Strong, L. C. (1972). Mutation and cancer: a model for Wilms' tumor of the kidney. *J. Nat. Cancer. Inst.* **48**, 313–24.

—— and —— (1975). Familial Wilms' tumour (letter). *Am. J. Hum. Genet.* **27**, 809–10.

Kodet, R. and Marsden, H. B. (1985). Papillary Wilms' tumour with carcinoma-like foci and renal cell carcinomas in childhood. *Histopathol.* **9**, 1091–1102.

Koufos, A., Hansen, M. F., Lampkin, B. C., Workman, M. L., Copeland, N. G., Jenkins, N. A. and Cavanee, W. K. (1984). Loss of alleles at loci on chromosome 11 during genesis of Wilms' tumour. *Nature* **309**, 170–2.

Kung, F. H. and Nyman, W. L. (1973). In *Cancer medicine.* eds. Holland, J. and Frei, E. III. p. 198. Lee & Febiger, Philadelphia.

Lacour, F., Delain, E., Gerard-Marchant, R. *et al.* (1970). Dysembryome nephroblastique 'lignee DNV' du poulet. Observations de 10 generations de transmission experimentale. *C.R. Acad. Sci. (Paris)* **271**, 141–4.

Ladda, R., Atkins, L., Littlefield, J., Neurath, P. and Marimuthu, K. M. (1974). Computer assisted analysis of chromosomal abnormalities: detection of a deletion in aniridia Wilms' tumor syndrome. *Science* **185**, 784–7.

Lathem, J. E. and Smith, K. H. (1962). Wilms' tumor in horseshoe kidney: surviving case. *J. Urol.* **88**, 25–8.

Leck, I. (1977). Congenital malformations and childhood neoplasms. *J. Med. Genet.* **14**, 321–6.

Ledlie, E. M., Mynors, L. S., Draper, G. J. and Gorbach, P. D. (1970). Natural history and treatment of Wilms' tumour: an analysis of 335 cases occurring in England and Wales 1962–1966. *Br. Med. J.* **4**, 195–200.

Leen, L. S. and Williams, I. G. (1971). Bilateral Wilms' tumor. Seven personal cases with observations. *Cancer* **28**, 802–6.

Lenstrup, E. (1927). Eight cases of hemihypertrophy. *Acta. Paediatr.* **6**, 205–13.

Liban, E. and Kozenitzky, I. L. (1970). Metanephric hamartomas and nephroblastomatosis in siblings. *Cancer* **25**, 885–8.

Lynch, H. T., Reed, W. and Mulcahy, G. M., Krush, A. J., Sweet, R. A., Kaplan, A. and Villacorte, G. (1974). A familial syndrome characterised by peculiar facies, small stature, chromosomal aberrations and aminoaciduria. *Birth Defects Orig. Art. Series.* **10**(8), 35–51.

Machin, G. A. (1980). Persistent renal blastema (nephroblastomatosis) as a frequent precursor of Wilms' tumor: a pathological and clinical review. Part I. Nephroblastomatosis in context of embryology and genetics. *Am. J. Ped. Hematology/Oncology* **2**, 165–72. Part II. Significance of nephroblastomatosis in the genesis of Wilms' tumor. *ibid.*, pp. 253–61.

—— and McCaughey, W. T. E. (1984). A new precursor lesion of Wilms' tumour (nephroblastoma): introlobar multifocal nephroblastomatosis. *Histopathology* **8**, 35–53.

Mackay, H. (1945). Congenital bilateral megalo-ureters with hydronephrosis: a remarkable family history. *Proc. R. Soc. Med.* **38**, 567–8.

Mackinstosh, T. F., Girdwood, T. G., Parker, D. J. and Strachan, I. M. (1968). Aniridia and Wilms' tumour (nephroblastoma). *Br. J. Ophthalmol.* **52**, 846–8.

Mankad, V. N., Gray, G. F. and Miller D. R. (1974). Bilateral nephroblastomatosis and Klippel Trenaunay syndrome. *Cancer* **33**, 1462–7.

Marsden, H. B. and Newton, W. A. (1986). New look at mesoblastic nephroma. *J. Clin. Path.* **39**, 508–13.

Maslow, L. A. (1940). Wilms' tumor: Report of three cases and a possible fourth one in the same family. *J. Urol.* **66**, 547–50.

Matsunaga, E. (1981). Genetics of Wilms' tumor. *Hum. Genet.* **57**, 231–46.

Meadows, A. T., Lichtenfeld, J. L. and Koop, C. E. (1974). Wilms' tumor in three children of a woman with congenital hypertrophy. *New Engl. J. Med.* **291**, 23–4.

Michalopoulos, E. E., Bevilacqua, P. J., Stokoe, N., Powers, V. E., Willard, H. F. and Lewis, W. H. (1985). Molecular analysis of gene deletion in aniridia–Wilms' tumor association. *Hum Genet.* **70**, 157–62.

Miller, R. W. (1966). Relation between cancer and congenital defects in man. *New Engl. J. Med.* **275**, 87–93.

—— (1968). Deaths from childhood cancer in sibs. *New Engl. J. Med.* **279**, 122–8.

—— (1969). Childhood cancer and congenital defects. A study of U.S. death certificates during the period 1960–1966. *Pediatr. Res.* **3**, 389–97.

——, Fraumeni, J. F. and Manning, M. D. (1964). Association of Wilms' tumor with aniridia, hemihypertrophy and other congenital malformations. *New Engl. J. Med.* **270**, 922–7.

Mott, M. G. (1975). Nephroblastoma (Wilms' tumour). *Br. J. Hosp. Med.* **13**, 161–80.

Mottu, D., Wyss, M., Cox, J. and Paunier, L. (1981). Nephroblastomatose et tumeur de Wilms' associees a une hemihypertrophie. *Helv. Paeidatr. Acta.* **46**, 87–95.

Murphy, M. L. (1968). Curability of cancer in childhood. *Cancer* **22**, 779–84.

Nakagome, Y. and Nagahara, N. (1985). High resolution studies in patients with aniridia-Wilms' tumour association. *Hum. Genet.* **70**, 289.

——, Ise, T., Sakurai, M., Nakajo, T., Okamoto, E., Takano, T., Nakahuri, Y., Tsuchida, Y., Nagahara, N., Takada, Y., Ohsawa, Y., Sawaguchi, S., Toyosaka, A., Kobayashi, N., Matsunaga, E. and Saito, S. (1984). High-resolution studies in patients with aniridia-Wilms' tumor association, Wilms' tumor or related congenital abnormalities. *Hum. Genet.* **67**, 245–8.

Nakamura, Y., Nakashima, H., Fukuda, S., Hashimoto, T. and Maruyama, M. (1985). Bilateral cystic nephroblastomas and multiple malformations with trisomy 8 mosaicism. *Hum. Pathol.* **16**, 754–6.

Narahara, K., Kikkawa, K., Kimira, S., Kimoto, H., Ogata, M., Kasai, R., Hamawaki, M. and Matsvoka, K. (1984). Regional mapping of catalase and Wilms' tumor-aniridia, genito-urinary abnormalities, and mental retardation triad loci to the chromosome segment 11p1305–p1306. *Hum. Genet.* **66**, 181–5.

Neel, J. V. (1962). Mutations in the human population. In *Methodology in human genetics.* ed. Burdette, W. J. pp. 203–24. Holden-Day, San Francisco.

Neri, G., Martini-Neri, M. E., Katz, B. E. and Opitz, J. M. (1984). The Perlman syndrome: familial renal dysplasia with Wilms' tumor, fetal gigantism and multiple congenital anomalies. *Am. J. Med. Genet.* **19**, 195–207.

Neuhauser, E. B. D. (1960). Case records of the Massachusetts General Hospital, Case 46372. Presentation of case. *New Engl. J. Med.* **263**, 557–60.

Niss, R. and Passarge, E. (1976). Trisomy 8 restricted to cultured fibroblasts. *J. Med. Genet.* **13**, 229–34.

Orkin, S. H., Goldman, D. S. and Sallan, S. E. (1984). Development of homozygosity for chromosome 11p markers in Wilms' tumour. *Nature* **309**, 172–4.

Owings, R. S. and Radakovich, M. (1959). Wilms' tumour: an evaluation of prognosis and treatment. *Surgery* **46**, 864–9.

Pendergrass, T. W. (1976). Congenital anomalies in children with Wilms' tumor. *Cancer* **37**, 403–8.

Perlman, M., Goldberg, G. M., Barziv, J. and Danovitch, G. (1973). Renal hamartomas and nephroblastomatosis with fetal gigantism: a familial syndrome. *J. Pediatr.* **83**, 414–18.

——, Levin, M. and Wittels, B. (1975). Syndrome of fetal gigantism, renal hamartomas, and nephroblastomatosis with Wilms' tumor. *Cancer* **35**, 1212–17.

Perry, T. L., Hardwick, D. F., Lowry, R. B. and Hansen, S. (1968). Hyperprolinaemia in two successive generations of a North American Indian family. *Ann. Hum. Genet.* **31**, 401–8.

Pilling, G. P. (1975). Wilms' tumor in seven children with congenital aniridia. *J. Pediatr. Surg.* **10**, 87–96.

Potter, E. L. (1961). *Pathology of the fetus and infant,* 2nd edn, p. 199. Year Book Medical Publishers, Chicago.

Raizis, A. M., Becroft, D. M., Shaw, R. L. and Reeve, A. E. (1985). A mitotic recombination in Wilms' tumor occurs between the parathyroid hormone locus and 11p13. *Hum. Genet.* **70**, 344–6.

Reddy, J. K., Schimke, R. N., Chang, C. H. J., Svoboda, D. J., Slaven, J. and Therou, L. (1972). Beckwith–Wiedemann syndrome. Wilms' tumor, cardiac hamartoma, persistent visceromegaly, and glomerulonephritis in a 2-year-old boy. *Arch. Pathol.* **94**, 523–2.

Reeve, A. E., Eccles, M. R., Wilkins, R. J., Bell, G. I. and Millow, L. J. (1985). Expression of insulin-like growth factor—II transcripts in Wilms' tumour. *Nature* **317**, 258–60.

——, Housiaux, P. J., Gardner, R. J. M., Chewings, W. E., Grindley, R. M. and Millow, L. J. (1984). Loss of a Harvey *ras* allele in sporadic Wilms' tumour. *Nature* **309**, 174–6.

Riccardi, V. M., Sujansky, E., Smith, A. C. and Francke, U. (1978). Chromosomal imbalance in the aniridia–Wilms' tumor association: 11p interstitial deletion. *Pediatrics* **61**, 604–10.

Riches, E. W., Griffiths, I. H. and Thackray, A. C. (1951). New growths of the kidney and ureter. *Br. J. Urol.* **23**, 297–356.

Riedel, H. A. (1952). Adrenogenital syndrome in male child due to adreno-cortical tumor: report of a case with hemihypertrophy and subsequent development of embryoma (Wilms' tumor). *Pediatrics* **10**, 19–27.

Robbins, S. L. (1967). *Pathology,* 3rd end. W.B. Saunders, Philadelphia.

Roth, D. R., Wright, J., Cawood, C. D. and Pranke, D. W. (1984). Nephro-blastoma in adults. *J. Urol.* **132**, 108–10.

Scarabicchi, S., Massimo, L. and Tortorolo, G. (1960). L'emiipertrofia e il tumore de Wilms. *Minerva Pediatr.* **12**, 1368–71.

Schaeffer, E. (1960). Halbseitenriesenwuchs und Wilms' tumor. *Monatschr. f. Kinderh.* **108**, 504–6.

Schappert-Kimmijser, J., Hemmes, G. D. and Nijland, R. (1966). The heredity of retinoblastoma. *Ophthalmologica (Basel)* **151**, 197–213.

Schroeder, A. J. and Cardle (1965). Cited by Miller, R. W. (1966). Relation between cancer and congenital defects in man. *New. Engl. J. Med.* **272**, 89–93. and by DiGeorge and Hanley (1966) q.v.

Schweisguth, O. (1967). Personal communication cited by Fraumeni and Glass (1968), q.v.

Scoggin, C. H., Fisher, J. H., Shoemaker, S. A., Morse, H., Leigh, T. and Riccardi, V. M. (1985). The E7-associated cell-surface antigen: a marker for the 11p13 chromosomal deletion associated with aniridia-Wilms' tumor. *Am. J. Hum. Genet.* **37**, 883–9.

Scott, J., Cowell, J., Robertson, M. E., Priestley, L. M., Wadley, R., Hopkins, B., Pritchard, J., Bell, G. I., Rall, L. B., Graham, C. F. and Knott, T. J. (1985). Insulin-like growth factor-II gene expression in Wilms' tumour and embryonic tissues. *Nature* **317**, 260–2.

Shanklin, D. R. and Sotelo-Avila, C. (1969). *In situ* tumours in fetuses, newborns and young infants. *Biol. Neonat.* **14**, 286–316.

Shannon, R. S., Mann, J. R., Harper, E., Harnden, D. G., Morten, J. E. N. and Herbert, A. (1983). Wilms' tumour and aniridia: clinical and cytogenetic features. *Arch. Dis. Child.* **57**, 685–90.

Shaw, M. W., Falls, H. F. and Neel, J. V. (1960). Congenital aniridia. *Am. J. Hum. Genet.* **12**, 389–415.

Silver, H. K. (1947). Wilms' tumor (embryoma of the kidney). *J. Pediatr.* **31**, 643–50.

Simola, K. O. J., Knuvtila, S., Kaitila, I., Pirkola, A. and Pohja, P. (1983). Familial aniridia and translocation t(4;11)–(q22;p13) without Wilms' tumor. *Hum. Genet.* **63**, 158–61.

Smith, P. J. and Imray, F. P. (1984). Mutant genes in Wilms' tumor. (reply to letter). *Lancet* **2**, 97.

Snyder, W. H. Jr., Hastings, T. N. and Pollock, W. (1962). Retroperitoneal tumors. In *Pediatric surgery,* Vol. 2. eds. Benson, C. D., Mustard, W. T., Ravitch, M..M., Snyder, W. H. and Welch, K. J. Chapter 527, pp. 1020–55.Year Book Medical Publishers, Chicago.

Soulie, J., Rousseau-Merck, M.-F., Mouly, H. and Nezelof, C. (1985). Bilateral nephroblastoma associated with a 3;17 translocation. *Cytogenet. Cell Genet.* **39**, 64–6.

Sotelo-Avila, C., Gonzalez-Crussi, F. and Fowler, J. W. (1980). Complete and incomplete forms of Beckwith–Wiedemann syndrome: their oncogenic potential. *J. Pediatr.* **96**, 47–50.

Strom, T. (1957). A Wilms' tumour family. *Acta. Paediatr.* **46**, 601–4.

Stump, T. A. and Garrett, R. A. (1954). Bilateral Wilms' tumor in a male pseudo-hermaphrodite. *J. Urol.* **72**, 1146–52.

Sulas, V. (1955). Du di un caso di emipertrofia e tumore di Wilms. *Neoplasia* **8**, 299–303.

Tsunoda, A., Ishida, M. and Omi, K. (1969). Bilateral Wilms' tumor: A case report and a survey of nineteen cases in Japanese literature. *Acta. Pediatr. Jap.* **11**, 1–7.

Turleau, C., De Grouchy, J., Dufier, J. L., Phuc, L. H., Schmelck, P. H., Rappaport, R., Nihoul-Fekete, C. and Diebold, N. (1981). Aniridia, male pseudohermaphroditism, gonadoblastoma, mental retardation and del 11p13. *Hum. Genet.* **57**, 300–6.

——, ——, Chavin-Colin, F., Martelli, H., Voyer, M. and Charlas, R. (1984a). Trisomy 11p15 and Beckwith Wiedemann syndrome. A report of two cases. *Hum. Genet.* **67**, 219–21.

——, ——, Nihoul-Fekete, C., Dufier, J. L., Chavin-Colin, F. and Junien, C. (1984b). Del 11p13/nephroblastoma without aniridia. *Hum. Genet.* **67**, 455–6.

Vlachos, J. and Tsakraklides, V. (1968). A case of renal dysplasia and its relation to 'bilateral nephroblastomatosis'. *J. Pathol. Bact.* **95**, 560–2.

Walden, P. A. M., Johnson, A. G. and Bagshawe, K. D. (1977). Wilms' tumour and neurofibromatosis. *Br. Med. J.,* **1**, 813.

Walker, G. (1897). Sarcoma of the kidney in children: A critical review of the pathology, symptomatology, prognosis and operative treatment as seen in one hundred and forty five cases. *Ann. Surg.* **26**, 529–602.

Waziri, M., Patil, S. R., Hanson, J. W. and Bartley, J. A. (1983). Abnormality of chromosome 11 in patients with features of Beckwith–Wiedemann syndrome. *J. Pediatr.* **102**, 873–6.

Wick, M. R., Manivel, C., O'Leary, T. P. and Cherwitz, D. L. (1986). Nephroblastoma: a comparative immunocytochemical and lectin-histochemical study. *Arch. Pathol. Lab. Med.* **110**, 630–5.

Wilbur, J. (1971). Personal communication to Knudson and Strong (1972). *J. Nat. Cancer Inst.* **48**, 313–24.

Wilms, M. (1899). Die Mischgeschwulste. Vol. I: Die Mischgeschwulste der Niere. Verlag Arthur Georgi, Leipzig.

Woodward, J. R. and Levine, M. K. (1969). Nephroblastoma (Wilms' tumor) and congenital aniridia. *J. Urol.* **101**, 140–3.

Van Heyningen, V., Boyd, P. A., Seawright, A., Fletcher, J. M., Fantes, J. A., Buckton, K. A., Spowart, G., Porteous, D. J., Hill, R. E., Newton, M. S. and Hastie, N. D. (1985). Molecular analysis of chromosome 11 deletions in aniridia-Wilms tumor syndrome. *Proc. Nat. Acad. Sci.*, **82**, 8592–6.

Young, J. L. Jr. and Miller, R. W. (1975). Incidence of malignant tumors in U.S. children. *J. Pediatr.* **86**, 254–8.

Yunis, J. J. and Ramsay, N. K. C. (1980). Familial occurrence of the aniridia-Wilms' tumor syndrome with deletion 11p13-14.1 *J. Pediatr.* **96**, 1027–30.

Zabel, B. U., Kronenberg, H. M., Bell, G. I. and Shows, T. B. (1985). Chromosome mapping of genes on the short arm of human chromosome 11: parathyroid hormone gene is at 11p15 together with the genes for insulin, C-Harvey-*ras* 1, and β-hemoglobin. *Cytogen. Cell. Genet.* **39**, 200–5.

Zimmerman, L. E. and Font, R. L. (1966). Congenital malformations of the eye. Some recent advances in knowledge of the pathogenesis and histopathological characteristics. *JAMA* **196**, 684–92.

Zunin, C. and Soave, F. (1964). Association of nephrotic syndrome and nephroblastoma in siblings. *Ann. Pediatr. (Basel),* **203**, 29–38.

12.1.2. Hypernephroma (renal carcinoma or adenocarcinoma, Gravitz tumour)

This is a relatively common tumour for which there are only a few reports of familial occurrence. Clemmesen (1942) reported a unique family in which two out of 15 sibs had hypernephromas and six had polycystic kidneys. Valleteau de Mouillac and coworkers (1974) described an even more remarkable family in which four out of seven sibs developed eosinophilic carcinomas of the left kidney. At least two of these, as well as other members of the family, had von Recklinghuasen's neurofibromatosis. This family may represent an example of malignant change in neurofibromata which may occur in the kidney, as in any other organ of the body. However, malignant neurofibromata usually become sarcomatous rather than carcinomatous (Sands *et al.* 1975). Renovascular hypertension due to renal artery stenosis is another renal complication of neurofibromatosis (Feinman and Yakovac 1970; Muller-Wiefel 1978). Further reports of affected sibs include those of Rusche (1953), Franksson and colleagues (1972), who reported four sibs with multiple bilateral tumours and a fifth with a solitary tumour, and Lyons and associates (1977). Brinton (1960) described three sibs with hypernephroma whose father had been treated for renal tumour. Steinberg and others (1972) also reported occurrence in a parent and child. Mathieson (1986) reported a family in which four out of six sibs, and the daughter of one of them, had renal carcinoma. Cytogenetic studies were not undertaken.

Renal carcinoma has been reported as developing within the cystic kidneys of Von Hippel Lindau disease (Kaplan *et al.* 1961; Melmon and Rosen 1964; Case Records of the Massachusetts General Hospital 1966; Nagendron and Dimond 1984), and in one family as occurring in over 80 per cent of those members affected with Von Hippel Lindau disease (Lee *et al.* 1977). Renal cell carcinoma has also been reported in association with phaeochromocytoma (Hadorn 1963; Fairchild *et al.* 1979). In Hadorn's family three sibs had phaeochromocytoma.

Braun and colleagues (1975) in a study of three families found an association with the major histocompatibility type HLA-W17. However, Kuntz and coworkers (1978) found no significant excess of B8 or B17, but did find an excess of AW30/31. Germenis and associates (1984) found an association of renal carcinoma with the 3F allele of the third component of complement, and with the Gc2 gene, but not with haptoglobin or transferrin phenotypes.

Cohen and colleagues (1979) have described a remarkable family in which there had been 10 members, over three generations, with bilateral renal cell carcinoma of multifocal origin. An apparently balanced translocation, involving the short arm of chromosome 3 and the long arm of chromosome 8 (e.g. t(3;8)(p21;q24)), was present in all of the affected individuals available for study. Knudson (1979) commenting on this paper estimates that in this family any member carrying the translocation has an 87 per cent risk of developing renal carcinoma by the age of 59 years. The breakpoint on chromsome 3 was subsequently revised to 3p14.2 (Wang and Perkins 1984). In another family renal carcinomas, present over three generations, are associated with a 3;11 translocation limited to tumour tissue. The breakpoint on chromosome 3 was again at 3p13 or 14, which is a fragile site (Pathak *et al.* 1982). The chromosome 8 breakpoint in Cohen and colleagues' family is at the site of the C-*myc* oncogene, and Drabkin and coworkers (1985) have shown that in the chromosome rearrangement in this family c-*myc* is translocated from chromosome 8 to the derivative chromosome 3.

In typical non-familial renal carcinoma the tumour and urine consistently bind a monoclonal antibody to a retrovirus p30-related antigen (Wahlström *et al.* 1985).

References

Braun, W. E., Strimlan, C. V., Negron, A. G., Straffon, R. A., Zachary, A. A., Bartee, S. L. and Grecek, D. R. (1975). The association of W17 with familial renal cell carcinoma. *Tissue antigens* **6**, 101–4.

Brinton, L. F. (1960). Hypernephroma—a familial occurrence in one family. *JAMA* **173**, 888–90.

Case Records of the Massachussets General Hospital. *New Engl. J. Med.* **275**, 950–9.

Clemmesen, J. (1942). Familiaert malignt Hypernephrome i en Slaegt med herditaer cystenyre. *Nordish Medicine* **14**, 1472–6.

Cohen, A. J., Li, F. P., Berg, S., Marchetto, D. J., Tsai, S., Jacobs, S. C. and Brown, R. S. (1979). Hereditary renal-cell carcinoma associated with a chromosomal translocation. *New Engl. J. Med.* **301**, 592–5.

Drabkin, H. A., Bradley, C., Hart, I., Bleskan, J., Li, F. P. and Patterson, D. (1985). Translocation of c-*myc* in the hereditary renal cell carcinoma associated with a t(3;8) (p14.2;q24.13) chromosomal translocation. *Proc. Nat. Acad. Sci.* **82**, 6980–4.

Fairchild, R. S., Kyner, J. L., Hermreck, A. and Schimke, R. N. (1979). Neuroblastoma, pheochromocytoma and renal cell carcinoma: occurrence in a single patient. *JAMA* **242**, 2210–11.

Feinman, N. L. and Yakovac, W. C. (1970). Neurofibromatosis in childhood. *J. Pediatr.* **76**, 339–46.

Franksson, C., Bergstrand, A., Ljungdahl, G. M. and Nordenstam, H. Renal carcinoma (hypernephroma) occurring in 5 siblings. *J. Urol.* **108**, 58–61.

Germenis, A., Dimopoulos, M.-A., Fertakis, A. and Dimopoulos, C. (1984). Genetic markers in renal adenocarcinoma. *J. Urol.* **132**, 173–4.

Hadorn, W. (1963). Hypernephroide und paraganglionaere Mischgeschwuelste der Nebenniere bei drei Geschwistern. *Helv. Med. Acta.* **30**, 291–6.

Kaplan, C., Sayre, G. P. and Greene, L. F. (1961). Bilateral nephrogenic carcinomas in Lindau–von Hippel disease. *J. Urol.* **86**, 36–42.

Knudson, A. G. Jr. (1979). Persons at high risk of cancer. *New Engl. J. Med.* **301**, 606–7.

Kuntz, B. M. E., Schmidt, G. D., Scholz, S. and Albert, E. D. (1978). HLA-antigens and hypernephroma. *Tissue Antigens* **12**, 407–8.

Lee, K. R., Wulfsberg, E. and Kepes, J. J. (1977). Some important radiological aspects of the kidney in Hippel–Lindau syndrome: the value of prospective study in an affected family. *Radiology* **122**, 649–53.

Lyons, A. R., Logan, H. and Johnston, G. W. (1977). Hypernephroma in two brothers. *Br. Med. J.* **3**, 816–17.

Mathieson, P. W. (1986). Renal carcinoma with a strong family history. *Br. J. Urol.* **58**, 458–9.

Melmon, K. L. and Rosen, S. W. (1964). Lindau's disease. Review of the literature and study of a large kindred. *Am. J. Med.* **36**, 595–617.

Muller-Wiefel, D. E.. (1978). Renovaskulare Hypertension bei Neurofibromatose von Recklinghausen. *Monatschr. Kinderheilk.* **126**, 113–18.

Nagendran, V. and Dimond, A. H. (1984). Renal carcinoma in Lindau's disease. *Postgrad. Med. J.* **60**, 624–5.

Pathak, S., Strong, L. C., Ferrell, R. E. and Trindade, A. (1982). Familial renal carcinoma with a 3;11 chromosome translocation limited to tumour cells. *Science* **217**, 939–41.

Rusche, C. (1953). Silent adenocarcinoma of the kidneys with solitary metastases occurring in brothers. *J. Urol.* **70**, 146–51.

Sands, M. J., McDonough, M. T., Cohen, A. M., Rutenberg, H. L. and Eisner, J. W. (1975). Fatal malignant degeneration in multiple neurofibromatosis. *JAMA* **233**, 1381–2.

Steinberg, S. M., Brodovsky, H. S. and Goepp,C. E. (1972). Renal carcinoma in mother and daughter. *Cancer* **29**, 222–5.

Valleteau de Moulliac, M., Ganansia, R., Hors, J., Letexier, A. and Morin, M. (1974). Cancer du rein familial et system H.L.A. Quatre cancers du rein gauche dans une fratrie. *La Nouvelle Presse Medicale* **3**(24), 1539–42.

Wahlström, T., Suni, J., Nieminen, P., Närvänen, A., Lehtonen, T. and Vaheri, A. (1985). Renal cell adenocarcinoma and retrovirus p30-related antigen excreted to urine. *Lab. Invest.* **53**, 464–9.

Wang, N. and Perkins, K. L. (1984). Involvement of renal 3p14 in t(3;8) hereditary renal carcinoma. *Cancer Genet. Cytogenet.* **11**, 479–81.

12.1.3. Klippel–Trenaunay–Weber syndrome

The typical haemangiomas of this disorder may involve the kidneys. There is little evidence to support a genetic basis for the syndrome although Lindenauer (1965) did report an affected brother and sister.

Reference

Lindenauer, S. M. (1965). The Klippel–Trenaunay–Weber syndrome: varicosity, hypertrophy and hemangioma with no arteriovenous fistula. *Ann. Surg.* **162**, 303–14.

12.1.4. Linear sebaceous naevus (Jadassohn syndrome)

Jadassohn (1895) first described this midfacial naevus, and Feurerstein and Mims (1962) added the clinical features of convulsions and mental retardation. Other abnormalities have subsequently been recognized, especially ocular abnormalities including colobomata (Marden and Venters 1966; Bianchine 1970). Bianchine suggested that the hamartomatous naevus was potentially premalignant.

Lansky and colleagues (1972) reported three cases including one girl who died at 9 months of age. At autopsy she was found to have bilateral multiple renal nodules and cysts, which histologically proved to be nodular nephroblastomatosis.

True familial occurrence has not been reported but minor features were present in relatives of Bianchine's case. The father had convulsions, mild mental subnormality, and a haemangioma of the forehead. A paternal aunt had convulsions. Twin sisters had ocular abnormalities and were retarded, another sister had ocular abnormalities and convulsions while the eldest sister was normal.

References

Bianchine, J. W. (1970). The nevus sebaceus of Jadassohn: a neurocutaneous syndrome and a potentially premalignant lesion. *Am. J. Dis. Child.* **120**, 223–8.

Feurerstein, R. C. and Mims, L. C. (1962). Linear nevus sebaceus with convulsions and mental retardation. *Am. J. Dis. Child.* **104**, 675–9.

Jadassohn, J. (1895). Bemerkungen zur Histologie der systematisierten Naevi und über 'Talgdrusen-Naevi' (Part II). *Arch. Dermatol. Syph.* **33**, 355–408.

Lansky, L. L., Funerburk, S., Cuppage, F. E., Schimke, R. N. and Diehl, A. M. (1972). Linear sebaceous nevus syndrome. *Am. J. Dis. Child.* **123**, 587–90.

Marden, P. M. and Venters, H. D. (1966). A new neurocutaneous syndrome. *Am. J. Dis. Child.* **112**, 79–81.

12.2. LOWER URINARY TRACT

12.2.1. Cancer of the ureter

There has been a single familial report of this tumour, occurring in a mother and son (Burkland and Juzek 1966). Fujita and colleagues (1984) have demonstrated somatic activation of a Ha-*ras*-proto-oncogene in a papillary transitional cell carcinoma of the renal pelvis.

12.2.2. Bladder tumours

Transitional cell carcinoma of the bladder (bladder cancer) is the most common tumour of the urinary tract. Familial carcinoma of the bladder appears to be uncommon, the significant association being with environmental factors. The few reports of familial occurrence include those of Fraumeni and Thomas (1967), McCullough and colleagues (1975), Sharma and coworkers (1976) and Cartwright (1979). Cartwright in a study of 1261 patients found that 7.6 per cent of them knew of an affected first or second-degree relative. In a comparison with controls this incidence was not significantly increased. Cartwright postulated that there may nevertheless be common genes conferring susceptibility.

Herring and others (1979) observed an excess of the blood group A gene among patients compared with controls, confirming earlier studies pointing in the same direction. However, in another study blood group A patients had lower grade tumours and lower mortality rates compared to group O patients (Srinivias *et al.* 1986). Several groups have reported on HLA gene frequencies in transitional cell carcinoma but the results have been somewhat inconsistent. Terasaki and coworkers (1977) found a weak association with HLA BW35, whilst Herring and others (1979) observed significant associations with HLA-B5 and -CW4. A probably important genetic association is that with acetylator status based on an enzyme polymorphism of hepatic *N*-acetyltransferase. A Scandinavian study first provided evidence of a relative excess of the slow acetylator phenotype among patients with carcinoma of the bladder (Lower *et al.* 1979; Wolf *et al.* 1980), in that among the patients 65 per cent were of the slow phenotype compared with 50 per cent of controls. Similar results were obtained more recently by workers in this country (Cartwright *et al.* 1982; Woodhouse *et al.* 1982; Evans *et al.* 1983) but without reaching statistical significance in the individual studies. Evans and colleagues in a combined analysis of their own findings with those of the groups of Lower, Cartwright and Woodhouse found a significant association of slow acetylator phenotype with bladder cancer ($P<0.01$). Cartwright's group also found a significant excess of slow acetylators among patients with more severe carcinoma or carcinoma-in-situ, and among those patients previously exposed occupationally to dyestuff chemical intermediates. Exposed patients had a 96 per cent frequency of slow phenotype compared with 59 per cent among non-exposed patients. Mommsen and Wolf (1985) found the excess of slow acetylators in patients with carcinoma *in situ* to be less than in patients without. However, Miller and Cosgriff (1983) in an American study on only 26 patients found no excess of slow acetylators among bladder cancer patients, even among those with occupational exposure to carcinogens ($P=0.00056$). In view of these conflicting findings further research into acetylator phenotype is needed in order to determine whether or not screening of prospective workers in the dye and rubber industries, using the comparatively simple dapsone method of Cartwright and colleagues (1982), would be justified.

Another exciting recent development in relation to this tumour has been the discovery that in certain cell lines (T24 and EJ) derived from patients with bladder carcinoma an oncogene, c-*ras*H or c-Ha-*ras*-1, homologous with the v-*ras* gene of the Harvey rat sarcoma virus (Der *et al.* 1982) and assigned to human chromosome 11, band 11p15 (de Martinville *et al.* 1983), has undergone a point mutation. This oncogene has now been fully sequenced (Capon *et al.* 1983) and the mutation identified as a guanine to cytosine transversion, resulting in a glycine to valine amino acid substitution in the gene product protein p21 (Reddy 1982; Tabin *et al.* 1982; Taparowsky *et al.* 1982) within the first of four exons (Capon *et al.* 1983). The precise role of the mutant form of protein p21 in carcinogenesis is unclear. A claim that the mutant oncogene was present in normal as well as tumour tissue of a patient (Muschel *et al.*

1983) has been withdrawn. It has been shown that the NIH3T3 cells used in experimental studies of transformation by transfected oncogenes are already partially transformed, and that c-Ha-*ras*-1 oncogene from the EJ bladder carcinoma cell line will not transform normal fibroblasts unless they have already been immortalized by carcinogenesis (Newbold and Overell 1983). However, if a second oncogene, such as *myc*, is introduced with the *ras* gene then normal fibroblasts may be transformed (Land *et al.* 1983). Thus bladder carcinogenesis is at least a two-step process, reminiscent of the similar hypothesis for Wilms' tumour already discussed. The frequency of the *ras* oncogene in bladder tumours, and the relative roles of oncogenes, carcinogens, and associated genotypes such as ABO, HLA, and acetylator genotype remain to be elucidated. An indication of oncogene frequency comes from the work of Fujita and colleagues (1984) who demonstrated the presence of the activated allele of the Ha-*ras* oncogene in tumour cells from two out of 23 randomly selected urinary tract (mainly bladder) tumours. Thus this evidence suggests that around 10 per cent of such tumours contain the active Ha-*ras* oncogene. Whether or not oncogenes, other than c-Ha-*ras*, are involved in naturally occurring bladder carcinoma is not yet known. Nor is their mode of action understood. Recently Gay and Walker (1983) have described homology of the *ras* oncogene product with other proteins such as mitochondrial ATP synthetase. This approach may eventually yield clues to the mode of action of bladder carcinoma oncogenes, and it is of course known that other oncogenes are homologous to, or even are, growth factors.

Another intriguing observation is the assignment of the c-Ha-*ras* 1 oncogene to a region of chromosome 11 near to that for the deletion in the Wilms' tumour–aniridia syndrome. Nevertheless, the oncogene is not involved in the WAGR tetrad deletion (de Martinville and Francke 1983; Huerre *et al.* 1983), and maps along with the β-globin gene cluster, the insulin gene, the parathormone gene, and the calcitonin gene, distal to 11p13. Huerre and colleagues locate the c-Ha-*ras* 1 locus to 11p15.1→11p15.5. The possibility that this is not just a chance synteny has been discussed earlier in this chapter under Wilms' tumour. As with Wilms' tumour an appreciable proportion of bladder carcinoma patients show a loss of genes on the short arm of chromosome 11, at least when probed with the c-Ha-*ras*-1 or insulin gebe probes (Fearon *et al.* 1985).

Neal and coworkers (1985) have shown that invasiveness and the degree of dedifferentiation of bladder carcinoma is positively correlated with the density of epidermal growth factor receptors on the cell surface. Control samples failed to stain for the receptor.

The involvement of the bladder, and lower urinary tract in general, in multiple neurofibromatosis has been reviewed earlier (p. 446).

References

Burkland, C. E. and Juzek, R. H. (1966). Familial occurrence of carcinoma of the ureter. *J., Urol.* **96**, 697–701.

Capon, D. J., Ellson, Y. C., Levinson, A. D., Seeburg, P. H. and Goeddel, D. V. (1983). Complete nucleotide sequences of the T24 human bladder carcinoma oncogene and its normal homologue. *Nature* **302**, 33–7.

Cartwright, R. A. (1979). Genetic association with bladder cancer. *Br. Med. J.* **3**, 798.

Cartwright, R. A., Glashan, R. W., Rogers, H. J., Ahmad, R. A., Barham-Hall, D., Higgins, E. and Kahn, M. A. (1982). Role of acetyltransferase phenotypes in bladder carcinogenesis: a pharmocogenetic epidemiological approach to bladder cancer. *Lancet* **2**, 842–5.

Clark, S. S., Marlett, M., Prudencio, R. and Dasgupta, T. K. (1977). Neurofibromatosis of the bladder in children: case report and literature review. *J. Urol.* **118**, 654–6.

De Martinville, B. and Francke, U. (1983). The c-Ha-*ras* 1, insulin and beta-globin loci map outside the deletion associated with aniridia–Wilms' tumour. *Nature* **305**, 641–3.

——, Giacalone, J., Shih, C., Weinberg, R. A. and Francke, U. (1983). Oncogene from human EJ bladder carcinoma is located on the short arm of chromosome 11. *Science* **219**, 498–501.

Der, C. J., Krontiris, T. G. and Cooper, G. M. (1982). Transforming genes of human bladder and lung carcinoma cell lines are homologous to the *ras* genes of Harvey and Kirsten sarcoma viruses. *Proc. Nat. Acad. Sci.* **79**, 3637–40.

Evans, D. A. P., Eze, L. C. and Whibley, E. J. (1983). The association of the slow-acetylator phenotype with bladder cancer. *J. Med. Genet.* **20**, 330–3.

Fearon, E. R., Feinberg, A. P., Hamilton, S. H. and Vogelstein, B. (1985). Loss of genes on the short arm of chromosome 11 in bladder cancer. *Nature* **318**, 377–80.

Fraumeni, J. F. and Thomas, L. B. (1967). Malignant bladder tumors in a man and his three sons. *JAMA* **201**, 507–9.

Fujita, J., Yoshida, O., Yuasa, Y., Rhim, J. S., Hatanaka, M. and Aaronson, S. A. (1984). Ha-*ras* oncogenes are activated by somatic alterations in human urinary tract tumours. *Nature* **309**, 464–6.

Gay, N. J. and Walker, J. E. (1983). Homology between human bladder carcinoma oncogene product and mitochondrial ATP-synthetase. *Nature* **301**, 262–4.

Herring, D. W., Cartwright, R. A. and Williams, D. O. R. (1979). Genetic associations of transitional cell carcinoma. *Br. J. Urol.* **51**, 73–7.

Huerre, C., Despoisse, S., Gilgenkrantz, S., Lenoir, G. M. and Junien, C. (1983). c-Ha-*ras* 1 is not deleted in aniridia–Wilms' tumour association. *Nature* **305**, 638–41.

Land, H., Parada, L. F. and Weinberg, R. A. (1983). Tumorigenic conversion of primary embryo fibroblasts requires at least two cooperating oncogenes. *Nature* **304**, 596–602.

Lower, G. M., Nillson, T., Nelson, C. E., Wolf, H., Gamsky, T. E. and Bryan, G. T. (1979). *N*-acetyltransferase phenotype and the risk of urinary bladder cancer: approaches in molecular epidemiology. Preliminary results in Sweden and

Denmark, *Envir. Hlth Perspect.* **29**, 71–9.

McCullough, D. L., Lamm, D. L., McLaughlin, A. P. and Gittes, R. F. (1975). Familial transitional cell carcinoma of the bladder. *J. Urol.* **113**, 629–35.

Miller, M. E. and Cosgriff, J. M. (1983). Acetylator phenotype in human bladder cancer. *J. Urol.* **130**, 65–6.

Mommasen, S. and Wolf, H. (1985). N-acetyltransferase phenotypes in bladder tumour patients with and without carcinomas *in situ* in selected biopsy sites. *Scand. J. Urol. Nephrol.* **19**, 203–4.

Muschel, R. J., Khoury, G., Lebowitz, P., Koller, R. and Dhar, R. (1983). The human c-*ras* H oncogene: a mutation in normal and neoplastic tissue from the same patient. *Science* **219**, 853–6.

Neal, D. E., Bennett, M. K., Hall, R. R., Marsh, C., Abel, P. D., Sainsbury, J. R. C. and Harris, A. L. (1985). Epidermal-growth factor receptors in human bladder cancer: comparison of invasive and superficial tumours. *Lancet* **1**, 366–8.

Newbold, R. F. and Overell, R. W. (1983). Fibroblast immortality is a prerequisite for transformation by E J c-Ha-*ras* oncogene. *Nature* **304**, 648–51.

Reddy, E. P., Reynolds, R. K., Santos, E. and Barbacid, M. (1982). A point mutation is responsible for the acquisition of transforming properties by the T24 human bladder carcinoma oncogene. *Nature* **300**, 149–52.

Sharma, S. K., Bapna, B. C. and Singh, S. M. (1976). Familial profile of transitional cell carcinoma. *Br. J. Urol.* **48**, 442.

Srinivas, V., Alikhan, S., Hoisington, S., Varma, A. and Gonder, M. J. (1986). Relationships of blood groups and bladder cancer. *J. Urol.* **135**, 50–2.

Tabin, C. J., Bradley, S. M., Bargmann, C. I., Weinberg, R. A., Papageorge, A. G., Scolnick, E. M., Dhar, R., Lowy, D. R. and Chang, E. H. (1982). Mechanism of activation of a human oncogene. *Nature* **300**, 143–9.

Taparowsky, E., Suard, Y., Fasano, O., Shimizu, K., Goldfarb, M. and Wigler, M. (1982). Activation of the T24 bladder carcinoma transforming gene is linked to a single amino acid change. *Nature* **300**, 762–5.

Terasaki, P. I., Perdue, S. T. and Mickey, M. R. (1979). HLA frequencies in cancer. A second study. In *The genetics of human cancer.* ed. Milvihill, J. J. pp. 321–7. Raven Press, New York.

Wolf, H., Lower, G. M. and Bryan, G. T. (1980). Role of *N*-acetyltransferase phenotype in human susceptibility to bladder carcinogenic arylamines. *Scand. J. Urol. Nephrol.* **14**, 161–5.

Woodhouse, K. W., Adams, P. C., Clothier, A., Mucklow, J. C. and Rawlins, M. D. (1982). *N*-acetylation phenotype in bladder cancer. *Hum. Toxicol.* **1**, 443–5.

General references

Black, Sir Douglas and Jones, F. F. (eds.) (1979). *Renal disease,* 4th edn. Blackwell Scientific Publications, Oxford, London, Edinburgh and Melbourne.

de Wardener, H. E. (1985). *The kidney: an outline of normal and abnormal function.* 5th edn. Churchill Livingstone, Edinburgh.

Earley, L. W. and Gottschalk, C. W. (eds.) (1979). *Straus and Welt's diseases of the kidney,* 3rd edn. Little Brown, Boston.

Emery, A. E. H. (1975). *Elements of medical genetics,* 4th edn. Churchill Livingstone, Edinburgh and London.

—— (1976). *Methodology in medical genetics.* Churchill Livingstone, Edinburgh, London, and New York.

—— and Rimoin, D. L. (eds.) (1983). *Principles and practice of medical genetics,* 2 vols. Churchill Livingstone, Edinburgh.

Fraser Roberts, J. A. and Pembrey, M. E. (1978). *An introduction to medical genetics,* 7th edn. Oxford University Press.

Gates, R. R. (1946). *Human Genetics,* 2 vols. Chapters XIII (Vol. 1) and XXXI (Vol. 2). pp. 519–80, 1414–28. Macmillan, New York.

Harris, H. (1972). Chapter 27. Genetic Aspects of Renal Disease. In *Renal Disease,* 3rd edn. Ed. Sir Douglas Black. pp. 781–804. Blackwell Scientific, Oxford, London, Edinburgh, and Melbourne.

Kemp, T. (1951). Genetics and disease, Chapter 28. *Disease of internal organs.* pp. 249–50. Oliver & Boyd, Edinburgh and London.

Lynch, H. T. and Egan, J. P. (1973). Chapter 18. The kidney and urogenital tract. In *Clinical genetics,* 2nd edn. ed. Sorsby, A. Butterworth, London.

Murphy, E. A. and Chase, G. A. (1975). *Principles of genetic counselling.* Year Book Medical Publishers, Chicago.

Osman, A. A. (1934). Hereditary renal diseases. In *The chances of morbid inheritance,* ed. Blacker, C. P. pp. 280–8. H. K. Lewis, London.

Rubin, M. I. and Barratt, T. M. (eds.) (1975). *Pediatric nephrology.* Williams & Wilkins, Baltimore.

Seldin, D. W. and Giebisch, G. (eds.) (1985). *The kidney: physiology and pathophysiology,* (2 vols.). Raven Press, New York.

Sorsby, A. (1953). *Clinical genetics,* 1st edn. Butterworth, London.

Stanbury, J. B., Wyngaarden, J. B. and Frederickson, D. S. (1978). *The metabolic basis of inherited disease,* 4th edn. McGraw-Hill, New York.

——, ——, ——, Goldstein, J. L. and Brown, M. S. (1983). *The metabolic basis of inherited disease.* 5th edn. McGraw-Hill, New York.

Stevenson, A. C. and Davidson, B. C. C. (1976). *Genetic counselling,* 2nd edn. Heinemann, London.

Suki, W. N. and Eknoyan, G. (eds.) (1981). *The kidney in systemic disease.* 2nd edn. John Wiley, Chichester, New York.

Thompson, J. S. and Thompson, M. W. (1980). *Genetics in medicine* 3rd edn. W.B. Saunders, Philadelphia, London, and Toronto.

Touraine, A. (1955). *L'Heredite en Medicine.* pp. 215–18 and 784–98. Masson, Paris.

Wilcox, C. S. (1984). The Kidney. Chapter 4 in *Clinical physiology*, 5th edn. Eds. Campbell, E. J. M., Dickinson, C. J., Slater, J. D. H., Edwards, C. R. W. and Sikora, K. pp. 154–217. Blackwell Scientific Publications, Oxford, and Edinburgh.

Winter, R. M. (1984). Genetics. Chapter 18 in *Clinical physiology*, 5th edn. Eds. Campbell, E. J. M., Dickinson, C. J., Slater, J. D. H., Edwards, C. R. W. and Sikora, K. pp. 611–50. Blackwell Scientific Publications, Oxford and Edinburgh.

Index

(Page numbers in italic show the major entries for each topic)

643

hemizygote or hemizygous 4, 7, 84, 196, 615
heparan sulphate-rich anionic sites, *see* proteoglycan
hepatic and central nervous system malformation syndrome 544
hepatic cysts 460, 467, 493–4
hepatic fibrosis 490, 495–6
   congenital 456, 460, *463–4*, 485, 494
hepatic N-acetyltransferase 637
hepatoblastoma 522, 616
hepatolenticular degeneration, *see* Wilson's disease
hereditary degnerate nephropathy, *see* nephronophthisis
heritability 390
hermaphroditism
   female 539, 558
   male 461, 495, 581
   true 614
heterochromatic 13
heterozygote or heterozygous 4–7, 10, 15–16, 70, 110, 189, 195–6, 201, 203, 207, 209, 211, 242–5, 250, 254, 258, 267, 275, 318, 334, 432, 434, 542, 620
   detection or diagnosis 14–16, 77, 81, 84, 95, 98, 101–2, 109, 111–12, 137, 140–1, 143, 150–4, 165, 180, 195–6, 203, 207, 238, 275, 373, 376, 422, 441, 472
   loss of heterozygosity 522, 615–17, 638
hexacosanoic and hexacosenoic acids 176
hexosaminidase 93
   A 93, 97
   B 93, 97
hiatus hernia 370
highly variable region 473
hip dysplasia 568
hippuric acid or hippurate 35
   P-amino-hippuric acid 35
histidinuria 253
HLA antigens 15, 101, 263, 290, 298–300, 361, 399–400, 405, 428, 438, 576, 633, 636–8
Holt–Oram syndrome 56
homogentisic acid 69
   oxidase 69
homozygote or homozygous 4–7, 10, 16, 70, 77, 95, 150, 238, 242–4, 254, 261, 267, 351, 551, 615
'Hopewell' 275
horseshoe kidney 40, 42–3, 45, 47–8, 55–6, 527, 532, 544, 550, *553–5*, 557, 562, 583, 611
host resistance model 620
Huntington's chorea 4, 14, 16, 77
Hurler syndrome 72, 134
   Hurler/Scheie syndrome 72
hutterite cerebro-osteo-nephrodysplasia 370
hybridization
   nucleic acid 11–12, 138, 615
   in situ 13, 616

somatic cell 13, 71–2, 85–6, 98, 152, 196, 617
hydrocephalus 57, 370, 519
hydrogen ions 32, 35, 226
hydronephrosis 40, 42–3, 45–51, 53, 55, 56–7, 188, 273, 432, 439, 446, 501, 504–5, 532, 544, 554, 561–2, 568, 575, 591, 593, 597–8
   congenital 556–9
hydroureter 40, 42–3, 47–8, 50, 55, 273, 446, 505, 544, 556, 558–9, 562, 568–9, 597
hydroxycholcalciferol, 25- or 1, 25-, *see* vitamin D
1 α-hydroxylase 232, 266
hydroxylysine 344
p-hydroxyphenlactic acid 160
p-hydroxyphenylpyruvic acid 160
   oxidase 160
hydroxyproline 29, 250, 344, 371
hydroxypyruvate 191
hyp, mouse 227–8
hyperammonaemia 181
hypercalcaemia 167, 382
hypercalciuria (or hypercalcinuria) *211–17*, 220–1, 279, 281–2, 288
hyperchloraemic acidosis 256, 281, 376, 389, 444
hypercholesterolaemia, familial 15
hypercystinuria 224, 240
hyperdibasicaminoaciduria 240–1
hyperglycollic aciduria 191
hyperhydroxyprolinaemia 250
hyperimmunoglobulinaemia D with periodic fever 127
hyperkalaemia 280, 293–4
hyperlipidaemia, type III 15
hypermagnesaemia 260
hypernephroma, *see* renal cell carcinoma
hyperoxaluria 77, *188–91*, 213–14
   type I: glycolic aciduria 76, 168, *188–91*
   type II: L-glyceric aciduria 76, 168, 188, *191*
   atypical primary 191
hyperparathyroidism, familial 185–6
   neonatal primary 186, 261
   primary 211, 264
   secondary 212
hyperphosphataemia 264
hyperprolinaemia 250, 319, 335, *371–3*, 612
   type I 372–3
   type II 372–3
hyperprostaglandin E syndrome 290
hypertelorism 384, 464, 543, 580, 582
hypertelorism, coloboma, mental retardation, hypospadias syndrome 580
hypertension 134, 290, 295, 311, 382, 416, 444, 447–9, 481, 502, 553–4, 614
   essential 390–4
   in rats 391
   and low sodium, high potassium diet 392